The Philadelphia Guide: Inpatient Pediatrics

Third Edition

NOTICE

Medicine is an ever-changing science. As new research and clinical experience broaden our knowledge, changes in treatment and drug therapy are required. The authors and the publisher of this work have checked with sources believed to be reliable in their efforts to provide information that is complete and generally in accord with the standards accepted at the time of publication. However, in view of the possibility of human error or changes in medical sciences, neither the authors nor the publisher nor any other party who has been involved in the preparation or publication of this work warrants that the information contained herein is in every respect accurate or complete, and they disclaim all responsibility for any errors or omissions or for the results obtained from use of the information contained in this work. Readers are encouraged to confirm the information contained herein with other sources. For example and in particular, readers are advised to check the product information sheet included in the package of each drug they plan to administer to be certain that the information contained in this work is accurate and that changes have not been made in the recommended dose or in the contraindications for administration. This recommendation is of particular importance in connection with new or infrequently used drugs.

The Philadelphia Guide: Inpatient Pediatrics

Third Edition

Edited by

Samir S. Shah, MD, MSCE
Director, Division of Hospital Medicine
James M. Ewell Endowed Chair
Attending Physician in Hospital Medicine and Infectious Diseases
Cincinnati Children's Hospital Medical Center
Professor, Department of Pediatrics
University of Cincinnati College of Medicine
Cincinnati, Ohio

Jeanine C. Ronan, MD, MS, MSEd
Program Director, Pediatrics Residency Program
Children's Hospital of Philadelphia
Associate Professor of Clinical Pediatrics
Perelman School of Medicine at the University of Pennsylvania
Philadelphia, Pennsylvania

Marina Catallozzi, MD, MSCE
Associate Professor of Pediatrics and Population and Family Health at
Columbia University Irving Medical Center
Vice Chair for Education, Department of Pediatrics
Director, Pediatric Medical Student Education
Director, Medical Education Scholarly Project Track
Columbia University, Vagelos College of Physicians & Surgeons
Morgan Stanley Children's Hospital at NewYork Presbyterian Hospital
Director, General Public Health Program
Faculty Co-Leader, Sexuality Sexual and Reproductive Health Certificate
Mailman School of Public Health
New York

Gary Frank, MD
Chief Quality and Patient Safety Officer
Children's Healthcare of Atlanta
Adjunct Associate Professor of Pediatrics, Department of Pediatrics
Emory University School of Medicine
Atlanta, Georgia

New York   Chicago   San Francisco   Athens   London   Madrid   Mexico City
Milan   New Delhi   Singapore   Sydney   Toronto

The Philadelphia Guide: Inpatient Pediatrics, Third Edition.

Copyright © 2022, 2016 by McGraw Hill. All rights reserved. Printed in the United States of America. Except as permitted under the United States Copyright Act of 1976, no part of this publication may be reproduced or distributed in any form or by any means, or stored in a data base or retrieval system, without the prior written permission of the publisher.

1 2 3 4 5 6 7 8 9 LCR 26 25 24 23 22 21

ISBN: 978-1-260-11788-2
MHID: 1-260-11788-X

This book was set in Minion Pro Regular by MPS Limited.

The editors were Leah Carton and Christie Naglieri.
The production supervisor was Richard Ruzycka.
Project Management was provided by Poonam Bisht, MPS Limited.
The cover designer is W2 Design.

This book is printed on acid-free paper.

Library of Congress Cataloging-in-Publication Data
Names: Shah, Samir S., editor. | Ronan, Jeanine C., editor. | Catallozzi,
    Marina, editor. | Frank, Gary, 1971- editor.
Title: The Philadelphia guide : inpatient pediatrics / edited by Samir S.
    Shah, Jeanine C. Ronan, Marina Catallozzi, Gary Frank.
Description: Third edition. | New York : McGraw-Hill Education, [2021] |
    Includes bibliographical references and index. | Summary: "Focusing
    specifically on caring for pediatric patients in the hospital setting,
    this unique handbook addresses more than 350 of the most commonly
    encountered inpatient pediatric medical conditions. Unlike similar
    handbooks on the subject, The Philadelphia Guide goes beyond diagnostic
    strategies to include complete treatment and management guidelines"—
    Provided by publisher.
Identifiers: LCCN 2020053596 | ISBN 9781260117882 (paperback ; alk. paper)
    | ISBN 9781260117899 (ebook)
Subjects: MESH: Pediatrics | Handbook
Classification: LCC RJ61 | NLM WS 39 | DDC 618.92—dc23
LC record available at https://lccn.loc.gov/2020053596

McGraw Hill books are available at special quantity discounts to use as premiums and sales promotions or for use in corporate training programs. To contact a representative, please visit the Contact Us pages at www.mhprofessional.com

To our mentors for sharing their wisdom and knowledge
To our families for providing love and support for all of our endeavors
To our patients for teaching us and to their families for trusting us

We are very grateful for Dr. Lisa B. Zaoutis. Through her mentorship and guidance, we developed our wisdom in pediatrics, our love of teaching, and our commitment to providing compassionate care.

Contents

Contents

Contributors

Paul L. Aronson, MD, MHS, Associate Professor of Pediatrics and of Emergency Medicine, Deputy Director, Pediatric Residency Program, Yale School of Medicine, New Haven, Connecticut

Amanda Barone Pritchard, MD, Assistant Professor of Pediatrics, Division of Pediatric Genetics, Metabolism, and Genomic Medicine, C.S. Mott Children's Hospital, Michigan Medicine, Ann Arbor, Michigan

Rosara Bass, MD, MS, Fellow Physician, Gastroenterology, Hepatology and Nutrition, Children's Hospital of Philadelphia, Philadelphia, Pennsylvania

Esther Berko, MD, PhD, Fellow, Divisions of Hematology and Oncology, Children's Hospital of Philadelphia, Philadelphia, Pennsylvania

Elizabeth J. Bhoj, MD, PhD, Attending Physician, Division of Human Genetics, Children's Hospital of Philadelphia, Philadelphia, Pennsylvania; and Assistant Professor of Pediatrics, Perelman School of Medicine at the University of Pennsylvania, Philadelphia, Pennsylvania

Gil Binenbaum, MD, MSCE, Attending Surgeon, Division of Pediatric Ophthalmology, Children's Hospital of Philadelphia, Philadelphia, Pennsylvania

Mercedes M. Blackstone, MD, Attending Physician, Pediatric Emergency Medicine, Children's Hospital of Philadelphia, Philadelphia, Pennsylvania; and Associate Professor of Clinical Pediatrics, Perelman School of Medicine at the University of Pennsylvania, Philadelphia, Pennsylvania

Erin Blevins, MD, MSCEd, Attending Pediatric Surgeon Department of Pediatric General, Thoracic, and Fetal Surgery, University of California Davis Medical Center, Sacramento, California

Donald L. Boyer, MD, MSEd, FAAP, Attending Physician, Division of Critical Care Medicine, Children's Hospital of Philadelphia, Philadelphia, Pennsylvania; and Assistant Professor of Anesthesiology and Critical Care Medicine, Perelman School of Medicine at the University of Pennsylvania, Philadelphia, Pennsylvania

Jennifer M. Brady, MD, Attending Physician, Perinatal Institute, Cincinnati Children's Hospital Medical Center, Cincinnati, Ohio; and Associate Professor, Department of Pediatrics, University of Cincinnati, College of Medicine, Cincinnati, Ohio

Terri Brown-Whitehorn, MD, Attending Physician, Division of Allergy and Immunology, Children's Hospital of Philadelphia, Philadelphia, Pennsylvania; and Professor of Clinical Pediatrics, Perelman School of Medicine the University of Pennsylvania, Philadelphia, Pennsylvania

Diane P. Calello, MD, Associate Professor of Emergency Medicine, Medical Director, New Jersey Poison Control Center, Rutgers–New Jersey Medical School, Newark, New Jersey

Peter Capucilli, MD, Fellow, Division of Allergy and Immunology, Children's Hospital of Philadelphia, Philadelphia, Pennsylvania

Joann Spinale Carlson, MD, Assistant Professor of Pediatrics, Division of Pediatric Nephrology and Hypertension, Rutgers/Robert Wood Johnson Medical School, New Brunswick, New Jersey

Pi Chun Cheng, MD, MS, Attending Physician, Division of Pulmonary and Sleep Medicine, Children's Hospital of Philadelphia, Philadelphia, Pennsylvania; and Assistant Professor,

Department of Pediatrics, Perelman School of Medicine at the University of Pennsylvania, Philadelphia, Pennsylvania

Kathleen Chiotos, MD, MSCE, Assistant Professor of Anesthesia, Critical Care, and Pediatrics, Perelman School of Medicine at the University of Pennsylvania, Philadelphia, Pennsylvania; and Attending Physician, Division of Critical Care Medicine and Division of Infectious Diseases, Children's Hospital of Philadelphia, Philadelphia, Pennsylvania

Stephanie L. Clark, MD, MPH, Assistant Professor, Division of Nephrology, The Children's Hospital of Philadelphia, Philadelphia, Pennsylvania

Máire Conrad, MD, MS, Assistant Professor of Pediatrics, Perelman School of Medicine at the University of Pennsylvania, Philadelphia, Pennsylvania; and Attending Physician, Division of Gastroenterology, Hepatology, and Nutrition, Children's Hospital of Philadelphia, Philadelphia, Pennsylvania.

Stefanie L. Davidson, MD, Attending Surgeon, Division of Pediatric Ophthalmology, Children's Hospital of Philadelphia, Philadelphia, Pennsylvania

Jeannine Del Pizzo, MD, Attending Physician, Division of Emergency Medicine, Children's Hospital of Philadelphia, Philadelphia, Pennsylvania; and Assistant Professor of Clinical Pediatrics, Perelman School of Medicine at the University of Pennsylvania, Philadelphia, Pennsylvania

Conor Devine, MD, Attending Surgeon, Division of Otolaryngology, Children's Hospital of Philadelphia; and Assistant Professor, Department of Pediatrics, Perelman School of Medicine at the University of Pennsylvania, Philadelphia, Pennsylvania

Marissa Di Giovine, MD, Assistant Professor of Neurology, Perelman School of Medicine at the University of Pennsylvania, Philadelphia, Pennsylvania; and Attending Physician, Division of Neurology, Children's Hospital of Philadelphia, Philadelphia, Pennsylvania

James Dodington, MD, Assistant Professor of Pediatrics and of Emergency Medicine, Yale School of Medicine, New Haven, Connecticut

Fabian Engelbertz, MD, Clinical Director, MVZ Kinder- und Jugendmedizin, Kölner Norden Cologne, Germany

Sarah Fesnak, MD, Attending Physician, Division of Emergency Medicine, Children's Hospital of Philadelphia, Philadelphia, Pennsylvania; and Assistant Professor of Clinical Pediatrics, Perelman School of Medicine at the University of Pennsylvania, Philadelphia, Pennsylvania

Julie Fierro, MD, MPH, Assistant Professor of Pediatrics, Perelman School of Medicine at the University of Pennsylvania, Division of Pulmonary and Sleep Medicine, Children's Hospital of Philadelphia, Philadelphia, Pennsylvania

Erin G. Brown, MD, Pediatric Surgeon, Shriners Hospitals for Children – Northern California, University of California Davis Health System, Sacramento, California

Rebecca D. Ganetzky, MD, Attending Physician, Division of Human Genetics, Children's Hospital of Philadelphia, Philadelphia, Pennsylvania; and Assistant Professor of Pediatrics, Perelman School of Medicine at the University of Pennsylvania, Philadelphia, Pennsylvania

Theodore Ganley, MD, Director of Sports Medicine, Children's Hospital of Philadelphia, Philadelphia, Pennsylvania; and Professor of Orthopedic Surgeon, Perelman School of Medicine at the University of Pennsylvania, Philadelphia, Pennsylvania

Jeffrey S. Gerber, MD, PhD, Associate Professor of Pediatrics, Perelman School of Medicine at the University of Pennsylvania, Philadelphia, Pennsylvania; and Attending Physician, Division of Infectious Diseases, Children's Hospital of Philadelphia, Philadelphia, Pennsylvania

John Germiller, MD, PhD, Attending Surgeon, Division of Pediatric Otolaryngology, Children's Hospital of Philadelphia, Philadelphia, Pennsylvania; and Associate Professor of Clinical Otorhinolaryngology/Head and Neck Surgery, Perelman School of Medicine at the University of Pennsylvania, Philadelphia, Pennsylvania

Vi L. Goh, MD MS, Assistant Professor of Pediatrics, University of Pennsylvania School of Medicine, Philadelphia, Pennsylvania; Attending Physician, Division of Gastroenterology, Hepatology and Nutrition, Children's Hospital of Philadelphia, Philadelphia, Pennsylvania

Selasie Q. Goka, MD, Attending Physician, Division of Nephrology, Children's Hospital of Philadelphia, Philadelphia, Pennsylvania

Kandace Gollomp, MD, Attending Physician, Division of Hematology, Children's Hospital of Philadelphia; Assistant Professor, Department of Pediatrics, Perelman School of Medicine at the University of Pennsylvania, Philadelphia, Pennsylvania

Matthew Grady, MD, Director, Primary Care Sports Medicine Fellowship and Attending Physician, Division of Orthopaedic Surgery, Children's Hospital of Philadelphia, Philadelphia, Pennsylvania; and Associate Professor of Clinical Pediatrics, Perelman School of Medicine at the University of Pennsylvania, Philadelphia, Pennsylvania

Lori Handy, MD, MSCE, Assistant Professor of Pediatrics, Perelman School of Medicine at the University of Pennsylvania, Philadelphia, Pennsylvania; and Attending Physician, Division of Infectious Diseases, Children's Hospital of Philadelphia, Philadelphia, Pennsylvania

Soma Jyonouchi, MD, Attending Physician, Division of Allergy and Immunology, Children's Hospital of Philadelphia, Philadelphia, Pennsylvania; Assistant Professor of Pediatrics, Perelman School of Medicine at the University of Pennsylvania, Philadelphia, Pennsylvania

Robert P. Kavanagh, MD, Assistant Professor, Department of Pediatrics, Division of Pediatric Critical Care, Penn State Hershey Children's Hospital, Penn State College of Medicine, Philadelphia, Pennsylvania

Katie Kennedy, MD, Attending Physician, Division of Allergy and Immunology, Children's Hospital of Philadelphia, Philadelphia, Pennsylvania

Marissa Kilberg, MD, MSEd, Attending Physician, Division of Endocrinology and Diabetes, Children's Hospital of Philadelphia, Philadelphia, Pennsylvania; and Assistant Professor of Clinical Pediatrics, Perelman School of Medicine at the University of Pennsylvania, Philadelphia, Pennsylvania

Amy Kim, MD, Attending Physician, Department of Child and Adolescent Psychiatry and Behavioral Sciences, Children's Hospital of Philadelphia, Philadelphia, Pennsylvania; and Associate Professor of Clinical Psychiatry, Perelman School of Medicine at the University of Pennsylvania, Philadelphia, Pennsylvania

Eimear Kitt, MD, Attending Physician, Division of Infectious Diseases, Associate Medical Director, Department of Infection Prevention and Control, Children's Hospital of Philadelphia, Philadelphia, Pennsylvania

Kelley Kovatis, MD, Attending Neonatologist, Christiana Care Health System, Newark, Delaware, Maryland

F. Wickham Kraemer III, MD, Associate Professor of Clinical Anesthesiology and Critical Care, Section Chief, Acute and Chronic Pain Management, Children's Hospital of Philadelphia, Philadelphia, Pennsylvania; and Associate Professor, Perelman School of Medicine at the University of Pennsylvania, Department of Anesthesiology and Critical Care, Philadelphia, Pennsylvania

Juhee Lee, MD, Attending Physician, Division of Allergy and Immunology, Children's Hospital of Philadelphia, Philadelphia, Pennsylvania

Emily Liebling, MD, Assistant Professor of Pediatrics, Perelman School of Medicine, University of Pennsylvania; and Division of Rheumatology, Children's Hospital of Philadelphia, Philadelphia, Pennsylvania

Arul M. Lingappan, MD, Attending Anesthesiologist, Department of Anesthesiology and Critical Care, Children's Hospital of Philadelphia, Philadelphia, Pennsylvania; and Clinical Instructor, Perelman School of Medicine at the University of Pennsylvania, Department of Anesthesiology and Critical Care, Philadelphia, Pennsylvania

Katherine Lord, MD, Attending Physician, Division of Endocrinology and Diabetes, Children's Hospital of Philadelphia, Philadelphia, Pennsylvania; and Assistant Professor of Clinical Pediatrics, Perelman School of Medicine at the University of Pennsylvania, Philadelphia, Pennsylvania

Jennifer Louis-Jacques, MD, MPH, Attending Physician, Division of General Pediatrics, UVA Children's Hospital; and Associate Professor, Department of Pediatrics, University of Virginia School of Medicine, Charlottesville, North Carolina

Maria R. Mascarenhas, MBBS, Professor of Pediatrics, Perelman School of Medicine, University of Pennsylvania, Philadelphia, Pennsylvania; and Section Chief, Nutrition Division of Gastroenterology, Hepatology and Nutrition, Children's Hospital of Philadelphia, Philadelphia, Pennsylvania

Peter Mattei, MD, Associate Professor, Department of Surgery, Perelman School of Medicine of the University of Pennsylvania, Philadelphia, Pennsylvania; and Attending Surgeon, Division of General, Thoracic and Fetal Surgery, Children's Hospital of Philadelphia, Philadelphia, Pennsylvania

Zachary B. R. McClain, MD, Attending Physician, Craig-Dalsimer Division of Adolescent Medicine, Children's Hospital of Philadelphia, Philadelphia, Pennsylvania; and Assistant Professor, Department of Pediatrics, Perelman School of Medicine at the University of Pennsylvania, Philadelphia, Pennsylvania

Jennifer McGuire, MD, MSCE, Assistant Professor of Neurology and Pediatrics, Perelman School of Medicine at the University of Pennsylvania, Philadelphia, Pennsylvania; and Attending Physician, Division of Neurology, Children's Hospital of Philadelphia, Philadelphia, Pennsylvania

Jay Mehta, MD, Associate Professor of Clinical Pediatrics, Perelman School of Medicine, University of Pennsylvania, Philadelphia, Pennsylvania; and Attending Physician, Pediatric Rheumatology, Children's Hospital of Philadelphia, Philadelphia, Pennsylvania

Amanda Muir, MD, Attending Physician, Division of Gastroenterology, Hepatology, and Nutrition, Children's Hospital of Philadelphia, Philadelphia, Pennsylvania; Assistant Professor of Pediatrics, Perelman School of Medicine at the University of Pennsylvania, Philadelphia, Pennsylvania

Regina Myers, MD, Instructor of Pediatrics, Perelman School of Medicine at the University of Pennsylvania Philadelphia, Pennsylvania; and Attending Physician, Division of Oncology, Children's Hospital of Philadelphia, Philadelphia, Pennsylvania

Haley Newman, MD, Pediatric Resident, Children's Hospital of Philadelphia, Philadelphia, Pennsylvania

Matthew J. O'Connor, MD, Attending Physician, Division of Cardiology, Children's Hospital of Philadelphia, Philadelphia, Pennsylvania; Associate Professor of Pediatrics, Perelman School of Medicine at the University of Pennsylvania, Philadelphia, Pennsylvania

Howard B. Panitch, MD, Professor of Pediatrics, Perelman School of Medicine at the University of Pennsylvania, Philadelphia, Pennsylvania; and Director of Clinical Programs, Division of Pulmonary Medicine, Children's Hospital of Philadelphia, Philadelphia, Pennsylvania

Melissa Desai Patel, MD, MPH, Section Chief of Pediatric Hospital Medicine, Children's Hospital of Philadelphia, Philadelphia, Pennsylvania; and Associate Clinical Assistant Professor of Pediatrics, Perelman School of Medicine at the University of Pennsylvania, Philadelphia, Pennsylvania; and Medical Director of Sedation Services, Attending Physician, Division of General Pediatrics, Children's Hospital of Philadelphia, Philadelphia, Pennsylvania

Rosemary Peterson, MD, Attending Physician, Pediatric Rheumatology, Dell Children's Medical Center, Austin, Texas

Joseph Picoraro, MD, Assistant Professor, Department of Pediatrics, Columbia University Medical Center, New York, New York; and Attending Physician, Division of Gastroenterology, Hepatology, and Nutrition, Morgan Stanley Children's Hospital, New York, New York

Leila Posch, MD, Clinical Assistant Professor of Pediatrics, Keck School of Medicine, University of Southern California, Los Angeles, California; and Attending Physician, Division of Infectious Diseases, Children's Hospital of Los Angeles, Los Angeles, California

Nicole Pouppirt, MD, Attending Physician, Division of Neonatology, Ann and Robert H. Lurie Children's Hospital of Chicago, Chicago, Illinois; and Assistant Professor, Department of Pediatrics, Northwestern University, Feinberg School of Medicine, Chicago, Illinois

Chitra Ravishankar, MD, Professor of Pediatrics, Division of Cardiology, Children's Hospital of Philadelphia, Philadelphia, Pennsylvania; Attending Physician, Division of Cardiology, Children's Hospital of Philadelphia, Philadelphia, Pennsylvania; and Professor, Department of Pediatrics, Perelman School of Medicine at the University of Pennsylvania, Philadelphia, Pennsylvania

Anne Reilly, MD, Attending Physician, Division of Oncology, Children's Hospital of Philadelphia, Philadelphia, Pennsylvania; and Professor of Clinical Pediatrics, Perelman School of Medicine, University of Pennsylvania, Philadelphia, Pennsylvania

Christopher B. Renjilian, MD, MBE, Fellow, The Craig-Dalsimer Division of Adolescent Medicine, Children's Hospital of Philadelphia, Philadelphia, Pennsylvania; and Resident, Pediatrics, Children's Hospital of Philadelphia, Philadelphia, Pennsylvania

Madeline H. Renny, MD, Postdoctoral fellow, Department of Population Health Clinical Instructor, Departments of Emergency Medicine and Pediatrics, New York University Grossman School of Medicine, New York, New York

Jeanine C. Ronan, MD, MS, MSEd, Program Director, Pediatrics Residency Program, Children's Hospital of Philadelphia, Philadelphia, Pennsylvania; and Associate Professor of Clinical Pediatrics, Perelman School of Medicine at the University of Pennsylvania, Philadelphia, Pennsylvania

Joseph W. Rossano, MD, MS, Professor of Pediatrics at Children's Hospital of Philadelphia, Division of Cardiology, University of Pennsylvania Perelman School of Medicine, Philadelphia, Pennsylvania

Samuel A. Rosenblatt, MD, MSEd, Assistant Professor, Department of Anesthesiology and Critical Care Medicine, Children's Hospital of Philadelphia and the Perelman School of Medicine at the University of Pennsylvania, Philadelphia, Pennsylvania

Rebecca L. Ruebner, MD, MSCE, Assistant Professor of Pediatrics, Division of Pediatric Nephrology, Johns Hopkins University School of Medicine, Baltimore, Maryland

Richard Rutstein, MD, Attending Physician, Division of General Pediatrics, Children's Hospital of Philadelphia, Philadelphia, Pennsylvania; and Professor, Department of Pediatrics, Perelman School of Medicine at the University of Pennsylvania, Philadelphia, Pennsylvania

Jill J. Savla, MD, MSCE, Attending Physician, Division of Cardiology, Children's Hospital of Philadelphia, Philadelphia, Pennsylvania; and Assistant Professor, Department of Pediatrics, Perelman School of Medicine at the University of Pennsylvania, Philadelphia, Pennsylvania

Andrew P. Steenhoff, MBBCh, DCH, Medical Director, Global Health Center; Attending Physician, Division of Infectious Diseases, Children's Hospital of Philadelphia, Philadelphia, Pennsylvania; and Associate Professor, Department of Pediatrics, Perelman School of Medicine at the University of Pennsylvania, Philadelphia, Pennsylvania

Kara N. Shah, MD, PhD, Attending Dermatologist, Optima Dermatology in Cincinnati, Cincinnati, Ohio

Salwa Sulieman, DO, Attending Physician, Division of Infectious Diseases, Nemours/Alfred I. duPont Hospital for Children, Wilmington, Delaware

Dava Szalda, MD, MSHP, Division of Oncology, Children's Hospital of Philadelphia, Philadelphia, Pennsylvania; and Assistant Professor of Pediatrics, Perelman School of Medicine, University of Pennsylvania, Philadelphia, Pennsylvania

Rebecca Tenney-Soeiro, MD, MSEd, Associate Professor of Pediatrics, Division of General Pediatrics, Children's Hospital of Philadelphia, Philadelphia, Pennsylvania

Catharyn A. Turner II, MEd, MD, Attending Physician, Department of Child and Adolescent Psychiatry and Behavioral Sciences, Children's Hospital of Philadelphia, Philadelphia, Pennsylvania

Brian Vernau, MD, Attending Physician, Division of Orthopedic Surgery, Children's Hospital of Philadelphia, Philadelphia, Pennsylvania

Tara L. Wenger, MD, PhD, Division of Genetic Medicine, University of Washington, Seattle, Washington

Char Witmer, MD, MSCE, Attending Physician, Division of Hematology, Children's Hospital of Philadelphia, Philadelphia, Pennsylvania; and Assistant Professor of Pediatrics, Perelman School of Medicine at the University of Pennsylvania, Philadelphia, Pennsylvania

Preface

The care of a hospitalized child has evolved dramatically since the publication of earlier editions of *The Philadelphia Guide: Inpatient Pediatrics*. As the first two editions were published, a common question was "What is a Hospitalist?" Hospital system pressures fueled by increasing patient complexity, changes in reimbursement models, and emphasis on value of care contributed to expansion of the hospitalist model. Hospital medicine is now the fastest growing specialty in modern history and the hospitalist model of care—a phrase coined a quarter century ago—is ensconced in virtually all hospitals. Furthermore, Pediatric Hospital Medicine is an official sub-specialty certified by the American Board of Pediatrics. Hospital Medicine has assumed even greater importance during the coronavirus disease 2019 (COVID-19) pandemic. Hospitalists have been on the frontlines caring for patients suffering from this new and mysterious disease while simultaneously redesigning systems of care. For example, they led the development of new care algorithms to manage a rare but serious COVID-19 complication termed multisystem inflammatory syndrome in children (MIS-C) and managed patient flow to accommodate the atypical seasonality of common viruses. (Who could have imagined hospital capacity issues in summer as a result of respiratory syncytial virus?) Hospitalists have also been at the forefront of public health, advocating for the wellbeing of children with efforts to resume safe schooling, increase rates of immunization against COVID-19, enforce masking policies to mitigate SARS-CoV transmission, expand mental health services, and reduce gun violence. The role of the hospitalist has fundamentally changed as these one-time generalists who became specialists have once again demonstrated their range. The question "What is a Hospitalist?" is being asked yet again but with different intent. Hospitalists provide clinical care, conduct practice-changing research, lead quality and safety efforts of hospital and its health system as well as community child advocacy efforts, improve health information systems, and so much more. They are a model speciality for innovation, collaboration, and patient-centered care.

As we prepared the third edition, Hospital Medicine remained our core focus. We believe that *Inpatient Pediatrics* should provide clinicians with the vital information necessary to make management decisions in the care of hospitalized children. Once again, we are fortunate that over 80 leading experts in pediatric hospital medicine and pediatric subspecialty care, many with roots at The Children's Hospital of Philadelphia, share their collective wisdom by contributing to this book.

Designed to be an invaluable resource on the hospital wards, *Inpatient Pediatrics* features:

• Practical diagnostic strategies
• Extensive differential diagnosis suggestions
• Up-to-date treatment and management guidelines
• Alphabetical organization within chapters for rapid access
• Structured format with consistent headings throughout
• Bulleted format for efficient and effective presentation of relevant information
• Print and electronic versions to maximize portability and ensure access to information whenever and wherever necessary

Appendices cover normal vital signs, as well as rapid access to pediatric dosages for emergency, airway, and rapid sequence intubation medications, and cardioversion.

As many clinicians are involved in the care of children, this book is ideal for practitioners of all levels, from residents to attending physicians, physician assistants, advanced practice

nurses, pediatric nurses, and health practitioners from all disciplines involved in the care of a hospitalized child.

The goal of this book is to provide a single reference with sufficient detail to guide diagnostic and therapeutic decisions for a wide range of conditions. We believe that the consistent format, detailed focus on diagnosis and management, and comprehensive coverage of topics have accomplished that goal, enabling you to give the best possible care to your patients.

Samir S. Shah, MD, MSCE
Jeanine C. Ronan, MD, MS, MSEd
Marina Catallozzi, MD, MSCE
Gary Frank, MD

List of Abbreviations

3TC	Lamivudine
AAP	American Academy of Pediatrics
ABC	Airway, breathing, circulation
ABG	Arterial blood gas
ABR	Auditory brainstem response
ACC	American College of Cardiology
ACE	Angiotensin converting enzyme
ACh	Acetylcholine
ACLS	Advanced cardiac life support
ACOG	American College of Obstetrics and Gynecology
ACPA	Anti-citrullinated peptide antibodies
ACTH	Adrenocorticotropic hormone
ADEM	Acute disseminated encephalomyelitis
ADH	Anti-diuretic hormone
ADHD	Attention deficit hyperactivity disorder
AFP	Alpha-fetoprotein
AG	Anion gap
AGA	Appropriate for gestational age
AHA	American Heart Association
AIDP	Acute inflammatory demyelinating polyradiculoneuropathy
AIDS	Acquired immune deficiency syndrome
AIH	Autoimmune hepatitis
AIHA	Autoimmune hemolytic anemia
AIN	Autoimmune neutropenia
AKI	Acute kidney injury
ALCL	Anaplastic large cell lymphoma
ALL	Acute lymphoblastic leukemia
ALP	Alkaline phosphatase
ALT	Alanine aminotransferase
ALTE	Apparent life-threatening event
AML	Acute myeloid leukemia
ANA	Anti-nuclear antibody
ANC	Absolute neutrophil count
ANCA	Anti-neutrophil cytoplasmic antibody
AOM	Acute otitis media
AP	Anterior-posterior

APAP	Acetaminophen
APRV	Airway pressure release ventilation
aPTT	Activated partial thromboplastin time
ARB	Angiotensin Receptor Blockers
ARDS	Acute respiratory distress syndrome
ARFID	Avoidant or restrictive food intake disorder
ARR	Absolute risk reduction
ART	Anti-retroviral treatment
ASA	Aspirin
ASAL	Argininosuccinic acid lyase
ASAS	Argininosuccinic acid synthetase
ASCA	Anti-Saccharomyces cerevisiae antibody
ASD	Atrial Septal Defect
ASO	Anti-streptolysin O
AST	Aspartate aminotransferase
ATN	Acute tubular necrosis
ATP	Adenosine triphosphate
ATV	Atazanavir
AUB	Abnormal uterine bleeding
AV	Atrioventricular
BCG	Bacille-Calmette Guerin
BLL	Blood lead level
BLPAP	Bi-level positive airway pressure
BMI	Body mass index
BMP	Basic metabolic panel
BMT	Bone marrow transplantation
BP	Blood pressure
BPD	Bronchopulmonary dysplasia
BRUE	Brief resolved unexplained event
BSA	Body surface area
BUN	Blood urea nitrogen
BV	Bacterial vaginosis
CA-MRSA	Community-acquired methicillin-resistant *Staphylococcus aureus*
CAH	Congenital adrenal hyperplasia
CAKUT	Congenital abnormalities of the kidney and urinary tract
CAP	Community-acquired pneumonia
CAR	Chimeric antigen receptor
cART	Combination anti-retroviral treatment
CAVC	Common atrioventricular canal

CBC	Complete blood count
CBD	Common bile duct
CCAM	Congenital Cystic Airway Malformation
CCK	Cholecystokinin
CD	Crohn's disease
CDC	Centers for Disease Control and Prevention
CDH	Congenital diaphragmatic hernia
CF	Cystic fibrosis
CFU	Colony forming units
CGD	Chronic granulomatous disease
CHD	Congenital heart disease
CHED	Congenital hereditary endothelial dystrophy
CHF	Congestive heart failure
CHSD	Congenital hereditary stromal dystrophy
CIPO	Chronic intestinal pseudo-obstruction
CKD	Chronic kidney disease
CLABSI	Central line-associated bloodstream infection
CML	chronic myeloid leukemia
CMP	Comprehensive metabolic panel
CMV	Cytomegalovirus
CN	Cranial nerve
CNS	Central nervous system
CO	Carbon monoxide
CO2	Carbon dioxide
CoNs	Coagulase-negative Staphylococcus
COVID-19	Coronavirus disease 2019
CPAP	Continuous positive airway pressure
CPDA	Citrate-phosphate-dextrose-adenine
CPK	Creatine phosphokinase
CPP	Cerebral perfusion pressure
CPR	Cardiopulmonary resuscitation
CPS	Carbamoyl phosphate synthetase
Cr	Creatinine
CR	Cardiorespiratory
CrCl	Creatinine clearance
CRH	Cortisol-releasing hormone
CRP	C-reactive protein
CRRT	Continuous renal replacement therapy
CSF	Cerebrospinal fluid

CSV	Continuous spontaneous ventilation
CT	Computed tomography
CTA	Computed tomography angiography
CV	Cardiovascular
CVC	Central venous catheter
CVID	Common variable immune deficiency
CVP	Central venous pressure
CVR	CCAM Volume Ratio
CVVH	Continuous veno-venous hemofiltration
CXR	Chest radiograph
DASH	Dietary Approaches to Stop Hypertension
DBP	Diastolic blood pressure
DCM	Dilated Cardiomyopathy
DHEA	Dihydroepiandrostenedione
DHT	Dihydrotestosterone
DI	Diabetes insipidus
DIC	Disseminated intravascular coagulation
DIHS	Drug-induced hypersensitivity syndrome
DKA	Diabetic ketoacidosis
DLBCL	diffuse large B-cell lymphoma;
DM	Diabetes mellitus
dMAI	Disseminated Mycobacterium avium intercellulare
DNA	Deoxyribonucleic acid
DOAC	Direct oral anticoagulant
DOC	Deoxycorticosterone
DORV	Double outlet right ventricle
DRESS	Drug rash with eosinophilia and systemic symptoms
DRI	Dietary reference intakes
DRV	Daruavir
DTG	Dolutegravir
DTR	Deep tendon reflex
DVT	Deep vein thrombosis
EAR	Estimated average requirement
EBNA	Epstein-Barr Nuclear Antibody
EBV	Epstein-Barr virus
ECF	Extracellular fluid
ECG	Electrocardiogram
ECMO	Extracorporeal membranous oxygenation
ED	Emergency department

EEG	Electroencephalogram
EIA	Enzyme immmnosorbent assay
EMG	Electromyography
EMLA	Eutectic mixture of local anesthetics
EN	Enteral nutrition
EOS	Early onset sepsis
EPAP	Expiratory positive airway pressure
EPS	Extra-pyramidal symptoms
ERCP	Endoscopic retrograde cholangiopancreatography
ERV	Expiratory reserve volume
ESR	Erythrocyte sedimentation rate
ETT	Endotracheal tube
FAA	Fumarylacetoacetate
FAO	Fatty acid oxidation
FAOD	Fatty acid oxidation disorders
FDA	Food and Drug Administration
FENa	Fractional excretion of sodium
FEV-1	Forced expiratory volume -1
FFA	Free fatty acids
FFP	Fresh frozen plasma
FHR	Familial hypophosphatemic rickets
FiO2	Fraction of inspired oxygen
FISH	Fluorescent in situ hybridization
FN	False negative
FP	False positive
FRC	Functional residual capacity
FTA-ABS	Fluorescent treponemal antibody absorption
FTC	Emtricitabine
FVC	Forced vital capacity
FWD	Free water deficit
G-tube	Gastrostomy tube
G6PD	Glucose-6-phosphate dehydrogenase
GA	Gestational age
GABHS	Group A beta-hemolytic *Streptococcus*
GALT	galactose-1-phosphate uridyltransferase
GAS	Group A *Streptococcus*
GBS	Group B *Streptococcus*
GC	*Gonococcus*
GCS	Glasgow coma score

GCSF	Granulocyte-colony stimulating factor
GER	Gastroesophageal reflux
GERD	Gastroesophageal reflux disease
GFR	Glomerular filtration rate
GGT	Gamma glutamyl transferase
GH	Growth hormone
GI	Gastrointestinal
GIR	Glucose infusion rate
GJ	Gastrojejunostomy
GK	Galactokinase
GM-CSF	granulocyte-macrophage colony-stimulating factor;
GN	Glomerulonephritis
GSD	Glycogen storage disease
GU	Genitourinary
GVHD	Graft-versus-host disease
Gy	Gray unit
H2RA	H2 receptor antagonist
HAV	Hepatitis A virus
Hb	Hemoglobin
HbA	Hemoglobin A
HbF	Fetal hemoglobin
HBIG	Hepatitis B immune globulin
HbS	Hemoglobin S
HBsAb	Hepatitis B surface antibody
HBsAg	Hepatitis B surface antigen
HBV	Hepatitis B virus
HCT	Hematocrit
HCV	Hepatitis C virus
HDL	High density lipoprotein
HEENT	Head, eyes, ears, nose, throat
HELLP	Hemolysis, elevated liver enzymes, and low platelet count
HFOV	High frequency oscillatory ventilation
HGA	Human granulocytic anaplasmosis
HHH	Hyperorinthinemia-Hyperammonemia-Homocitrullinuria
HHV-6	Human herpes virus-6
HHV-7	Human herpes virus-7
HIT	Heparin-induced thrombocytopenia
HIV	Human immunodeficiency virus
HLA	Human leukocyte antigen

HLA-B27	Human leukocyte antigen B27
HLH	Hemophagocytic lymphohistiocytosis
HLHS	Hypoplastic left heart syndrome
HME	Human monocytic ehrlichiosis
HPO	Hypothalamic-Pituitary-Ovarian
HPV	Human papilloma virus
HR	Heart rate
HSCT	Hematopoietic stem cell transplantation
HSP	Henöch-Schonlein purpura
HSV	Herpes simplex virus
HUS	Hemolytic-uremic syndrome
IAP	Intrapartum antibiotics
IBD	Inflammatory bowel disease
IBD-U	Inflammatory bowel disease -unspecified
IBS	Irritable bowel syndrome
IC	Inspiratory capacity
ICP	Intracranial pressure
ICU	Intensive care unit
IDM	Infant of a diabetic mother
IDU	Injection drug use
IEM	Inborn errors of metabolism
IFN	Interferon
Ig	Immunoglobulin
IGF	Insulin-like growth factor
IGF-BP1	Insulin-like growth factor binding protein-1
IGRA	Interferon-gamma release assay
IL-1	Interleukin-1
ILCOR	International Liaison Committee on Resuscitation
IM	Intramuscular
IMRT	intensity-modulated radiation therapy;
IMV	Intermittent mandatory ventilation
INH	Isoniazid
INR	International normalized ratio
INSTI	Integrase strand transfer inhibitors
IO	Intraosseus
IOP	Intraocular pressure
IP	Interphalangeal
IPAP	Inspiratory positive airway pressure
IRIS	Immune reconstitution inflammatory syndrome

ITP	Immune thrombocytopenia purpura
IUD	Intrauterine device
IUGR	Intrauterine growth restriction
IV	Intravenous
IVF	Intravenous fluids
IVH	Intraventricular hemorrhage
IVIG	Intravenous immunoglobulin
JDM	Juvenile dermatomyositis
JIA	Juvenile idiopathic arthritis
JMML	juvenile myelomonocytic leukemia;
LCHAD	long-chain 3-hydroxyacyl-CoA dehydrogenase
LDH	Lactate dehydrogenase
LES	Lower esophageal sphincter
LET	Lidocaine, epinephrine, and tetracaine
LFT	Liver function test
LGA	Large for gestational age
LGTQ+	Lesbian, gay, bisexual, transgender, and questioning
LH	Lutenizing hormone
LHR	Lung-Head ratio
LILT	Longitudinal lengthening and tailoring procedure
LLQ	Left lower quadrant
LLSB	Left Lower Sternal Border
LMA	Laryngeal mask airway
LMP	Last menstrual period
LMWH	Low molecular weight heparin
LOC	Loss of consciousness
LOS	Late onset sepsis
LP	Lumbar puncture
LR	Likelihood ratio
LSD	Lysosomal storage disease
LTBI	Latent tuberculosis infection
LVH	Left ventricular hypertrophy
LVNC	Left Ventricular Noncompaction
MAC	Mycobacterium avium complex
MADD	Multiple acyl-CoA dehydrogenase deficiency
MAI	Mycobacterium avium intercellulare
MAO	Monamine oxidase
MAOI	Monamine oxidase inhibitor
MAP	Mean arterial pressure

MAS	Macrophage activation syndrome
MCAD	Medium-chain acyl CoA dehydrogenase
MCH	Mean corpuscular hemoglobin
MCHC	Mean corpuscular hemoglobin concentration
MCV	Mean corpuscular volume
MDAC	Multiple-dose activated charcoal
MDI	Metered dose inhaler
MDMA	3,4-Methylenedioxymethamphetamine (ecstasy)
MDS	myelodysplastic syndrome;
MEN	Multiple endocrine neoplasia
MG	Myasthenia gravis
MHA-TP	Microhemagglutination-assay Treponema pallidum
MLB	Microlaryngoscopy and bronchoscopy
MMA	Methylmalonic acid
MMR	Measles, mumps, rubella
MODY	Mature onset diabetes of the young
MPGN	Membranoproliferative glomerulonephritis
MPS	Mucopolysacharidoses
MRA	Magnetic resonance arteriography
MRI	Magnetic resonance imaging
MRSA	Methicillin-resistant *Staphylococcus aureus*
MRV	Magnetic resonance venography
MSAF	Meconium-stained amniotic fluid
MSH	Melanocyte-stimulating hormone
MSM	Men who have sx with men
MSSA	Methicillin-sensitive *Staphylococcus aureus*
MSUD	Maple syrup urine disease
MTCT	Maternal-to-child transmission
MuSK	Muscle-specific kinase
MVC	Motor vehicle crash
NAAT	Nucleic acid amplification test
NAC	N-acetylcysteine
NAIT	Neonatal alloimmune thrombocytpenia
NAPQI	N-acetyl-p-benzoquinone-imine
NARP	Neuropathy, ataxia, retinitis pigmentosa
NAS	Neonatal abstinence syndrome
NAT	Non-accidental trauma
NBL	Neuroblastoma
NBS	Newborn screening

ND	Nasoduodenal
NEC	Nectotizing enterocolitis
NEMO	Nuclear factor-kappa B essential modulator deficiency syndrome
NG	Nasogastric
NHL	Non-Hodgkin lymphoma
NICU	Neonatal intensive care unit
NIF	Negative inspiratory force
NIPS	Non-invasive prenatal screening
NJ	Nasojejunal
NMDA	anti-N-methyl-D-aspartate
NMO	Neuromyelitis optica
NNRTI	Non-nucloside reverse transcriptase inhibitor
NP	Nasopharyngeal
nPEP	Non-occupational post-exposure prophylaxis
NPL	Nasopharyngolaryngoscopy
NPO	Nil per os
NPV	Negative predictive value
NRP	Neonatal resuscitation program
NRTI	Nucleoside reverse transcriptase inhibitors
NS	Normal saline
NSAID	Non-steroidal anti-inflammatory drug
NSSI	Non-suicidal self injury
NTBC	2-(2-nitro-4-trifluoromethyl-benzoyl)-1,3-cyclohexanedione
O2	Oxygen
OAE	Otoacoustic emissions
OCP	Oral contraceptive pill
OI	Opportunistic infection
OME	Otitis media with effusion
ORIF	Open reduction, internal fixation
OSA	Obstructive sleep apnea
OTC	Ornithine transcarbamylase
OTC	Over-the-counter
PA	Pulmonary atresia
PA	Posterior-Anterior
$PaCO_2$	Arterial partial pressure of carbon dioxide
PAH	Phe hydroxylase
PALS	Pediatric advanced life support
PAO_2	Alveolar partial pressure of oxygen
PaO_2	Arterial partial pressure of oxygen

P_{atm}	Atmospheric pressure
PBD	Peroxisomal biogenesis disorders
PCA	Patient controlled analgesia
PCOS	Polycystic ovary syndrome
PCP	Phencyclidine
PCr	Plasma creatinine
PCR	Polymerase chain reaction
PCV	Pneumococcal conjugate vaccine
PDA	Patent ductus arteriosus
PE	Pulmonary embolus
PEA	Pulseless electrical activity
PEEP	Positive end expiratory pressure
PEG	Polyethylene glycol
PEP	Post-exposure prophylaxis
PES	Pediatric Endocrine Society
PET	Partial exchange transfusion
PFT	Pulmonary function test
PGE1	Prostaglandin E_1
PH2O	Partial pressure of water vapor
PI	Protease inhibitors
PICU	Pediatric intensive care unit
PID	Pelvic inflammatory disease
PIP	Positive inspiratory pressure
PKU	Phenylketonuria
PMA	Post-menstrual age
PN	Parenteral nutrition
PNET	peripheral neuroectodermal tumor;
PO	Per os
PPD	Purified protein derivative
PPHN	Persistent pulmonary hypertension
PPI	Proton pump inhibitor
PPMS	Primary progressive multiple sclerosis
PPSV	Pneumococcal polysaccharide vaccine
PPV	Positive predictive value
pRBC	Packed red blood cell
PRES	Posterior reversible encephalopathy syndrome
PRG	Percutaneous radiologic gastrostomy
PRVC	Pressure-regulated volume control
PS	Pressure support

PSV	Pressure support ventilation
PT	Prothrombin time
PTH	Parathyroid hormone
PTSD	Post-traumatic stress disorder
PTT	Partial thromboplastin time
PTU	Propylthiouracil
PUCAI	Pediatric ulcerative colitis activity index
PUD	Peptic ulcer disease
PVC	Premature ventricular contraction
PVL	Periventricular leukomalacia
PVNS	Pigmented villonodular synoitis
PVR	Pulmonary Vascular Resistance
RAL	Raltegravir
RBC	Red blood cell
RDA	Recommended daily allowance
RDS	Respiratory distress syndrome
RDW	Red cell distribution width
REE	Resting energy expenditure
RF	Rheumatoid factor
RFS	Refeeding syndrome
RI	Reticulocyte index
RIG	Rabies immune globulin
RLQ	Right lower quadrant
RMSF	Rocky Mountain spotted fever
RNA	Ribonucleic acid
RNP	Anti-ribonuclear protein
ROM	Range of motion
ROP	Retinopathy of prematurity
RPR	Rapid plasma reagin
RR	Respiratory rate
RRMS	Relapsing remitting multiple sclerosis
RRR	Relative risk reduction
RSBI	Rapid shallow breathing index
RSV	Respiratory syncytial virus
RT	Radiation therapy
RTA	Renal tubular acidosis
RUQ	Right upper quadrant
RV	Residual volume
SABA	Short-acting beta-agonist

SARI	Serotonin antagonist/reuptake inhibitor
SARS-CoV-2	Severe acute respiratory syndrome coronavirus-2
SBE	Subacute bacterial endocarditis
SBI	Serious bacterial infection
SBP	Systolic blood pressure
SC	Subcutaneous
SCAR	Severe cutaneous adverse reactions
SCD	Sickle cell disease
SCFE	Slipped femoral capital epiphysis
SCID	Severe combined immune deficiency
SCN	Severe congenital neutropenia
SCT	Stem cell transplant
SD	Standard deviation
SEM	Skin, eye, mucosa
SGA	Small for gestational age
SIADH	Syndrome of inappropriate antidiuretic hormone secretion
SIDS	Sudden infant death syndrome
SIMV	Synchronized intermittent mandatory ventilation
SIRS	Systemic inflammatory response syndrome
SJS	Stevens–Johnson Syndrome
SLE	Systemic lupus erythematosus
SMS	Superior mediastinal syndrome
SSKI	Saturated solution of potassium iodide
SSRI	Selective serotonin release inhibitor
SSSS	Staphylococcal scalded skin syndrome
STEC	Shiga toxin producing Escherichia coli
STEP	Serial transverse enteroplasty
STI	Sexually transmitted infection
SUID	Sudden unexplained infant death
SV	Stroke volume
SVC	Superior vena cava
SVCS	superior vena cava syndrome
SVR	Systemic Vascular Resistance
T4	Thyroxine
TA-TMA	Transplant-associated thrombotic microangiopathy
TAC	Truncus arteriosus communis
TAF	Tenofovir alafenamide
TAPVC	Total anomalous pulmonary venous connection
TAPVR	Total anomalous pulmonary venous return

TAR	Thrombocytopenia absent radii
TB	Tuberculosis
TBI	Traumatic brain injury
TBII	Thyroid binding inhibitory immunoglobulin
TBW	Total body water
TCA	Tricarboxylic acid
TcB	Transcutaneous bilirubin
Td	Tetanus-diphtheria
TDD	Total daily dose
TDF	Tenofovir disoproxil fumarate
TEC	Transient erythroblastopenia of childhood
TEF	Tracheoesophageal fistula
TEN	Toxic epidermal necrolysis
TFP	Trifunctional protein
TGA	Transposition of the great arteries
THC	Tetrahydrocannabinol
TIA	Transient ischemic attack
TIBC	Total iron binding capacity
TINU	Tubular intersitital nephritis
TIPS	Trans-jugular intrahepatic portal shunt
TLC	Total lung capacity
TLS	tumor lysis syndrome;
TMP-SMX	Trimethoprim-sulfamethoxazole
TN	True negative
TNF	Tumor necrosis factor
TOA	Tubo-ovarian abscess
TOF	Tetraology of Fallot
TP	True positive
tPA	tissue plasminogen activator
TPN	Total parenteral nutrition
TRALI	Transfusion-related acute lung injury
TSB	Total serum bilirubin
TSH	Thyroid stimulating hormone
TSI	Thyroid stimulating immunoglobulin
TSS	Toxic shock syndrome
TSST-1	Toxic shock syndrome toxin-1
TST	Tuberculin skin test
TTN	Transient tachypnea of the newborn
TTP	Thrombotic thrombocytopenic purpura

UA	Urinalysis
UAC	Umbilical artery catheter
UC	Ulcerative colitis
UCD	Urea cycle disorders
UCr	Urine creatinine
UPD	Uniparental disomy
URI	Upper respiratory infection
USPSTF	United States Preventative Services Task Force
UTI	Urinary tract infection
UV	Ultraviolet
UVC	Umbilical venous catheter
V/Q	Ventilation/Perfusion
VC	Volume control
VCA	Viral capsid antigen
VCUG	Voiding cystourethrogram
VDDR	Vitamin D-dependent rickets
VDRL	Venereal Diseases Research Laboratory
VEGF	Vascular endothelial growth factor
VKDB	Vitamin K deficient bleeding
VL	Viral load
VLBW	Very low birth weight
VLCAD	Very long chain acyl CoA Dehydrogenase
VP	Ventriculo-peritoneal
VSD	Ventricular septal defect
VUR	Vesicoureteral reflux
vWD	von Willebrand disease
vWF	von Willebrand factor
VZV	Varicella zoster virus
WAS	Wiskott-Aldrich syndrome
WBC	White blood cell
WBI	Whole bowel irrigation
WHO	World Health Organization
XLA	X-linked agammaglobulinemia

The Philadelphia Guide: Inpatient Pediatrics

Third Edition

1

Adolescent Medicine

Christopher B. Renjilian, MD, MBE
Jennifer Louis-Jacques, MD, MPH
Zachary B. R. McClain, MD

SETTING THE STAGE FOR COMMUNICATION WITH ADOLESCENTS AND PARENTS

Effective communication with adolescents and parents in the health care setting can be essential to the advancement of the adolescent's health.

Potential challenges include:
- Lack of adolescent experience in carrying out health-related conversations.
- Lack of established trust, on the part of the adolescent and/or the parent, in the health care provider.
- Tension between adolescent and parental interests.
- Tension between the adolescent's emerging autonomy and authority of the parents/guardians.
- Tension between the adolescent's desire to maintain privacy/autonomy and the adolescent's simultaneous reliance on adults (and adult-controlled resources) to carry out life tasks, including those related to health care.
- The possibility of discovering information (e.g., suicidal ideation reported trauma, abuse, neglect) that obligates the health care provider to act in a way that may disrupt the adolescent's life or family unit, in pursuit of overriding goals such as adolescent safety.

Effective communication can be facilitated by "setting the stage" at the beginning of the encounter. This refers to establishing ground rules for the conversation and sets the expectation that you will speak with the parent and adolescent together, as well as the adolescent independently.

Setting the stage can help adolescents and parents to
- Know what to expect from the encounter.
- Develop trust in the health care team.
- Be more at ease.
- Avoid conflict.
- Focus their interests on the adolescent's health.
- Avoid entering legal/ethical dilemmas unknowingly.

A conversation to set the stage should meet four key objectives. The adolescent needs to know
- Why a health care provider will ask personal questions.
- What the health care provider will do with the information.
- What might be gained by sharing personal information with the health care provider.
- Their rights to privacy/confidentiality and the limitations of privacy/confidentiality.

A step-by-step guide to setting the stage appears next.

STEP-BY-STEP GUIDE TO SETTING THE STAGE

With the adolescent and the parent together
- **Begin the conversation with the adolescent and parent.**
  ✓ Make introductions and establish the purpose of the visit.
  ✓ Explain that you will "set the stage."

- **Establish roles.**
  - ✓ Emphasize the adolescent's participation in providing history.
  - ✓ Underscore the parent's role as a resource and support.
- **Set the expectation for one-on-one communication with the adolescent**
  - ✓ Frame this as routine practice.
  - ✓ This promotes adolescent development and creates opportunity for privacy.
  - ✓ It also creates an opportunity for a separate discussion with the parent(s).

With the adolescent and parent together or the adolescent alone

- **Explain why you will ask personal questions.**
  - ✓ Frame this as routine practice.
  - ✓ Link this to your ability to fully address the adolescent's issues(s) and give them opportunity for independence.
- **Privacy and the limitations of privacy**
  - ✓ State that the adolescent's information will be kept private within the medical team.
  - ✓ Tell the adolescent that information will be shared outside of the medical team only with permission.
  - ✓ State that concerns for immediate safety (suicide, homicide, abuse) override privacy.
- **Disclosure is a choice**
  - ✓ The adolescent is in control of the information they choose to share.
  - ✓ The adolescent is free to defer or decline to answer a question.
- **Your commitment to nonjudgmental and honest communication**
  - ✓ Affirm that providers do not judge adolescents on their behaviors.
  - ✓ Affirm that your goal is to listen carefully and to make connections between personal information and health.
  - ✓ Affirm a commitment to honesty and transparency with the adolescent.
- **Confirm understanding and solicit questions**

In a first-time encounter or one with adolescents who have no experience with provider private time, all of the points should be covered to facilitate future communication. In a repeat encounter or one with adolescents who have experience with provider private time, the conversation can be abbreviated.

DETAILED STEP-BY-STEP GUIDE TO SETTING THE STAGE

Sample phrases for this conversation appear in italics.

- **Begin the conversation with the adolescent and parent.**
  - ✓ Introductions:
    Introduce yourself. Give your name, pronouns, discipline, level of training, and relationship to the team.
    Ask the adolescent to say their first and last name and to tell you what name they like to be called and their pronouns (e.g., he/him, she/her, they/them).
    Ask the adolescent to introduce who is in the room with them. If needed, clarify what these people like to be called (e.g., do they have different last names; try not to call an adolescent's parent "mom").
  - ✓ State your general purpose in plain language.
    I'm here learn to more about what brought you into the hospital.
    I'd like to review some of the information that you've already provided, and to clarify a few details.
  - ✓ Explain that you are about to set the stage for your conversation:
    Before we begin, I'd like for you to know what you can expect from this conversation.

- **Establish roles.**

Prioritize the adolescent's participation in providing the history and set expectations for the order of adolescent and parent communication. This can facilitate the flow of information, while limiting interruptions, conflict, and competition.

✓ State why and how this should happen.

✓ To the adolescent:

> *Part of my job is to help prepare you to speak with health care providers on your own when you are an adult. When you were younger, doctors probably asked your parents all the questions. Today, you will notice that I address most of my questions to you. We are here to talk about your health, and you are the expert on your life, including how your body feels. When I ask a question, I'd like to hear from you first.*

> *If you need help answering a question, or if we need more information, that's when we'll turn to your parent/guardian. When that happens, I'd like for you to listen carefully to their answers, so that you can learn how you might answer a similar question in the future.*

✓ To the parent:

> *Hearing from your adolescent first may help us both to learn valuable information. At a minimum, it helps us learn what they already know and do not know about their health history.*

> *I'd like for you to listen carefully to what they say.*

> *We will still need your help today. You are an expert on what their health was like when they were younger, and you are an expert on what it has been like to see their health from the outside looking in.*

- **Set the expectation for one-on-one communication with the adolescent.**

✓ State that your goals include speaking with the adolescent one on one.

✓ Frame this objective as a routine practice.

✓ Be sure to set this expectation at the beginning of the encounter. Doing so can reduce any fears that private communication is a reaction to some element of the history or a sign of distrust of the parent. This also clears the path for individual conversations in the future. When presented this way, significant parental resistance to private communication with the adolescent is unusual. If it occurs, it is a clue about the nature of the parent–adolescent relationship.

✓ To both:

> *We'll begin the conversation by speaking all together.*

✓ To adolescent:

> *Later in the conversation, I'd like to take some time to speak with you one on one. Have you ever spoken with a doctor one on one before?*

> [Wait for response. If answer is a confident "Yes," then you can set the stage more quickly as a "review" of information that was most likely delivered in the past, based on your best judgment. Typically, this includes a brief review of privacy and its limitations. It is always prudent to review the limitations of confidentiality.]

> *Great. There are two reasons for us two speak one on one:*

> *First, remember that part of my job is to help prepare you to speak with health care providers on your own someday. Taking some time to speak one on one is practice.*

> *Second, we've learned that many adolescents are more comfortable asking and answering some questions about their health when they have some privacy. We've learned that it's important to create opportunities for all adolescents to do this as a matter of our routine practice.*

3

✓ To parent (optional, but encouraged):

I've also learned that parents often appreciate the opportunity to speak one on one with the health care team. I'd be happy to speak with you independently as well. [Watch to see how parent responds. Their response can indicate underlying concerns or the expectation that more information will need to be covered after the adolescent speaks independently. Remember to have as many conversations at the bedside with the adolescent to avoid loss of trust.]

- **Explain why you will ask personal questions.**
  ✓ This must be discussed.
  ✓ It can be successfully reviewed with the parent and adolescent together or with the adolescent alone, depending on your personal approach.

Key Points

- It is routine for health care providers to ask questions that may feel personal or private to the adolescent.
- It is often essential to cover personal topics to fully address the adolescent's primary problem. In other cases, discussion of personal topics is incorporated into an understanding of their health more generally.
- Adolescents should begin to expect this as a routine part of care in any setting, even as they continue into adulthood.
  ✓ To the adolescent:

My job is to help young people, and I (along with my team) know how to do that. I want to make sure you stay safe and alive and that you have a positive future.

I'd like for you to know that I think about the health of all adolescents in a broad sense. This means that I think about the kinds of things that help adolescents to stay healthy, and the things that get in the way. It means that I think about the health of the body, as well as the health of the mind and spirit.

As I think about the problem(s) that brought you into the hospital, there may be some key pieces of information that I need to clarify to help make sure that I am considering all the causes of your problem(s) and that I'm treating you in the best possible way.

I may ask you some questions that may feel personal or private, and I want you to know that I am asking those questions with these goals in mind.

- **Privacy and the limitations of privacy**
  ✓ This must be discussed.
  ✓ It can be successfully reviewed with the parent and adolescent together or with the adolescent alone, depending on your personal approach.

Key Points

- Personal information is kept private and cannot be shared beyond the medical team directly responsible for the adolescent's care.
- Information shared during a one-on-one conversation with the adolescent will not be shared with family members, unless the adolescent gives permission for you to do so.
- Concerns for the immediate safety of the patient or others (e.g., suicidal or homicidal ideation, child abuse) overrides privacy.
  ✓ To the adolescent:

I keep your information private. This rule applies whenever you speak with a health care provider. It applies when I speak with you and your family together, as well as when I speak with you one on one.

I may need to share some of your information with other members of the medical team, but only those who are responsible for your care. I cannot share your personal information with anyone else without your permission. The same goes for other members of the medical team that work in the hospital.

But remember, my most important job is to save lives. In some cases, this takes priority above all else. For example, if your life was in immediate danger because you were going to kill yourself or someone else, or if there was an adult abusing you, you and I would have to work together to get other people involved to keep you safe.

I've also learned that young people cannot always take care of their health without the help of an adult. Let's imagine that you and I spoke privately about your health and we agreed that you needed the help of an adult to carry out a plan to keep yourself healthy. In most cases, who is it that we would turn to for help?

[Wait for adolescent's response, which can provide important clues.]

In most cases, it is your parent/guardian but that is not always true. If this were ever to happen, you and I would work together to figure out the best way to communicate with your parent/guardian or another adult who can be helpful in a way that respects your personal information and helps to keep you safe and healthy.

<u>Important Tips</u>

- Say "private" rather than "confidential." Many adolescents believe "confidential" means that you have confidence in them.
- Do not say "secret." Secrecy connotes shame or stigma.
- Say "kill" rather than "harm" or "hurt." "Kill" communicates the immediate risk of danger to self/others more accurately and explicitly. Adolescents know we believe that a wide range of behaviors—including smoking or recreational drug use—may harm or hurt them, but these harmful behaviors do not typically require reporting that violates an adolescent's privacy.
- Become familiar with adolescent healthcare privacy laws in your state/municipality and reflect these accurately in your discussion.
- **Disclosure is a choice.**
  ✓ Be clear that the adolescent is ultimately in control of what information is shared.
  ✓ Your respect for privacy includes respecting when the adolescent does not want to share personal information with you.
  ✓ When adolescents understand that they are in control and that you respect their privacy, they may be empowered to reveal their personal boundaries, and less inclined to feel coerced or that their only option to maintain privacy is to provide misleading or deceptive information.
  ✓ To the adolescent:
    Just because I ask a question does not mean you have to answer it. I want you to feel very free to say, "I don't want to talk about that today," or "I'd rather keep that private." I will always respect that.

    I would much rather you tell me that you would prefer to keep something private, than for you to feel you have to give me the "right" answer even if it is not completely true.

    Remember, I don't read minds. If you tell me something that is not truthful, I won't know.

    As a doctor, I do my best work when I have complete information. I can also do a great job when I can see clearly what I do know and what I do not know. I won't be able to do my job as well, if I can't tell the difference between truths and nontruths or if I am not working with good information.

- **Your commitment to nonjudgmental and honest communication**
  - ✓ Many adolescents have learned to see adults as sources of discipline or criticism.
  - ✓ Reframe your role as an honest broker of health information, whose role is not to judge behaviors, but to see them in the context of health.
  - ✓ To the adolescent:

    I can guarantee you my honesty. You can ask me anything about your health, and I'll be honest. When you ask, I'll share what I know. When I don't know the answer, I'll share that with you, too.

    I can't punish you and don't want to. I take care of lots of adolescents and really respect all—all kinds of adolescents and adolescents who do all sorts of things. I don't judge you on your behavior. Instead, I listen and respect your honesty. When possible, I share information with you so that you can protect your own health.

- **Confirm understanding and solicit questions**

BRIEF PSYCHOSOCIAL ASSESSMENT

Periodic psychosocial assessment is recommended as an essential component of routine adolescent care. In the acute hospital setting, a brief psychosocial assessment can generate information that finetunes the differential diagnosis, directs the treatment plan, and detects "red flags" in the health and behavioral history that merit further attention. Two classic cases highlight the potential value of a brief psychosocial screen.

Case 1: A young man presents with abdominal pain, poor appetite, and weight loss. The brief psychosocial assessment can help clinicians evaluate the likelihood of primary diagnoses including major depression, an eating disorder, or stimulant use. Further, the assessment may uncover relevant and more pressing concerns, such as comorbid suicidal ideation.

Case 2: A young woman presents with abnormal uterine bleeding. The brief psychosocial assessment (which includes a sexual history) can inform clinicians about the relative likelihood of pelvic inflammatory disease, pregnancy, contraceptive use/misuse, or anovulatory cycles.

Beyond this, clinical conversations that occur around the brief psychosocial assessment, and follow from it, can foster youth development and youth participation in their health care and build connections between the youth and the health care team.

The SSHADESS Screen
The American Academy of Pediatrics recommends the "SSHADESS" Screen (**Box 1-1**) as an initial tool for the brief psychosocial assessment of youth. SSHADESS is an acronym to denote topic domains that should be covered during the assessment.

General Approach
The psychosocial screen is typically completed during a private one-on-one interview with the youth. Topics should generally be covered in the following order.

- Begin with an assessment of the young person's strengths and then move progressively from topics that are often perceived by youth as less personal/sensitive to those that are more so.
- Progression helps the clinician to identify areas of strength and risk. This can help with strength-based counseling efforts later in the interaction.
- Progression can provide early opportunities for the youth to become more comfortable with the interaction (by first addressing topics that are easier to discuss) and for the clinician to earn the youth's trust.

BOX 1-1   THE SSHADESS SCREEN

Strengths
School
Home
Activities
Drugs/Substance Use
Emotions/Eating/Depression
Sexuality
Safety

Worrisome responses require a deeper level of questioning than what is included here. Sample questions that might be included in a SSHADESS screen are included below.

Sample Introduction: *I'd like to take some time to get to know you a little better*

- **Strengths**
  - ✓ *How would you describe yourself?*
  - ✓ *How would your closest friends describe you?*
  - ✓ *Tell me about your strengths.*
  - ✓ *What do you like doing?*
  - ✓ *Tell me what you're most proud of.*

- **School**
  - ✓ *Where do you go to school? What grade are you in this year?* [note whether the grade differs from that expected based on the adolescent's age]
  - ✓ *What do you enjoy most/least about school?*
  - ✓ *Do you feel like you are doing your best at school? If not, why not—what's getting in the way?*
  - ✓ *Are there supports in place to help you do your best in school?* [Examples: Individualized education plan, accommodations like extra time on tests, other resources]
  - ✓ *What are your grades like this year? Are they any different from last year?*
  - ✓ *What would you like to do when you get older?*

- **Home**
  - ✓ *Who do you live with?*
  - ✓ *Have there been any changes in your family or home life?*
  - ✓ *Could you talk to your family if you were upset or stressed?*
  - ✓ *Who would you go to first?*

- **Activities**
  - ✓ *What kinds of things do you do outside of school or just for fun?*
  - ✓ *Tell me about your friends. What are they like? What kinds of people are they?*
  - ✓ *Are your friends treating you well?*
  - ✓ *Are you spending as much time with your friends as you used to?*
  - ✓ *Do you have a close friend or an adult you can trust outside of your family?*

Sample transition: *"As a doctor, I always think about how medications fit into a young person's life. We've already reviewed your medications. In the same way, I also have to think about what other substances might be part of a young person's life."*

- **Drugs/Substance Use**
  - ✓ *Do any of your friends talk about smoking cigarettes, taking drugs, or drinking alcohol?*
  - ✓ *How does this make you feel?*
  - ✓ *How have substances fit into your life?*

✓ *Do you smoke cigarettes, use e-cigarettes or vape? Do you drink alcohol? Have you tried sniffing glue, smoking weed, or using pills or other drugs?*

✓ *When/if you use a substance, how does it make you feel, or what does it do for you?*

✓ *Have you considered changing how substances fit into your life?*

Sample transition: *"I'd like to take some time to understand how you see your mental health."*

- **Emotions/Eating/Depression**

✓ *Would you say that you've been feeling mentally strong and ready for life's challenges, or have you been feeling stressed and overwhelmed?*

✓ *How does who you appear to be on the outside fit who you are on the inside?*

✓ *Would you describe yourself as a healthy eater? Have you been trying to gain or lose weight? Tell me why.*

✓ *Have you been feeling … stressed, bored, irritated, down, sad, depressed, nervous?*

✓ *Have you been having more trouble sleeping lately? If so, what kind of trouble?*

✓ *Have you thought of killing yourself or someone else?*

✓ *Have you ever tried to kill yourself?*

Sample Transition: *"As I think about your health, I also want to take a moment to talk about sexuality and relationships."*

- **Sexuality**

✓ *Tell me about your friends. Are people dating, in relationships, or hooking up?*

✓ *Have you had crushes or felt attraction to other people?*

✓ *How have relationships and sexuality been a part of your life?*

✓ *Is there anyone special in your life right now?*

✓ *Tell me about that person. What are they like?*

✓ *Are you comfortable with your sexual feelings?*

✓ *Do you find that you are attracted to guys, girls, or both?*

✓ *What kinds of things have you done sexually?*

✓ *What parts of your body have you used to be sexual with another person?*

✓ *What kind of steps do you take to protect yourself?*

✓ *Have you ever been worried that you (or your partner) could be pregnant?*

✓ *Have you ever been tested for a sexually transmitted infection?*

✓ *Have you ever been worried about or had a sexually transmitted infection?*

✓ *Do you have goals for your sexual health that we can help you to accomplish during this visit?*

Sample Transition: *"Finally, I want to check in with you about safety."*

- **Safety**

✓ *Do you feel safe on your way to school and in school?*

✓ *Are there a lot of fights at your school or in your neighborhood?*

✓ *Is there bullying? Have you been bullied? How much do you have to worry about bullying?*

✓ *What kinds of things would make you mad enough to fight?*

✓ *Do people you know feel like they need to carry weapons to protect themselves?*

✓ *How about you? Do you carry weapons?*

✓ *When is the last time that you saw a gun?*

✓ *If you decided to carry a gun, would you know where to find one?*

✓ *Has anyone ever touched you physically or sexually when you didn't want them to?*

✓ *How safe do you feel in your relationship?*

✓ *Does your partner get jealous?*

✓ *Do you ever get into fights with your partner? Physical fights?*

✓ *Have you ever seen people in your family or home hurt each other? Say mean things? Throw things or hit each other?*

Key Points

Avoid temptation to provide feedback (negative or positive) during the assessment.

When given too early, negative feedback can create shame and positive feedback can create an expectation that the youth should continue to deliver only praiseworthy answers. Both perceptions can impact a young person's willingness to disclose personal information when it counts most.

Instead, reserve feedback about behaviors for the end of the interview or interaction, when it can be put in context and connections can be drawn to a bigger picture understanding of their health.

Remember:

Youth deserve our praise for engaging in the *process* of good communication, perhaps even more than they require feedback on specific behaviors.

Recognize and praise youth when they participate in communication that required them to trust in your abilities, overcome personal fears about disclosure, or apply extra effort to articulate something difficult to express.

In this way, we can earn their trust—and the privilege of hearing their personal information when it matters most.

SUPPORTING AND DISCUSSING YOUTH ACROSS THE GENDER IDENTITY SPECTRUM

Health care providers should consistently demonstrate an openness to patients who identify with a gender that is different or more expansive than the sex they were assigned at birth.

The demonstration of openness may be more important than asking a directed question, or obtaining a definitive answer, during any particular health care encounter.

Youth who identify with a gender that is different or more expansive than the sex they were assigned at birth will notice cues about how open or closed you are to their identity—perhaps more so than any direct questions you ask about the topic.

These youths are at high risk for depression, anxiety, and suicidal ideation. Consistent support from health care providers and family members can be lifesaving. Even more broadly, demonstrations of openness and support by health care providers conveys a basic respect for persons—to which all youth are entitled.

Often, there are several opportunities during an encounter when health care providers can create an opening for adolescents to reveal more about their identities and "test the waters" before committing to full disclosure. Clinicians can introduce themselves with their pronouns and invite the adolescent and parent to share their pronouns. Gender identity can be approached again tat the beginning of the psychosocial assessment or when discussing emotions or sexuality.

Key Points

• Ask adolescents whether they have a name that they use other than the name that appears on their chart. Make a point to ask when the parent is present in the room and also when the youth is alone. Let them know that their pronouns and name can be changed in the chart or electronic medical record and ask if it is ok to share with the larger team and if their parent is aware.

• As with all adolescents, avoid language that assumes the gender identity of romantic and sexual partners based on the adolescent's gender identity. Choose nongendered language:

✓ *Is there anyone special in your life?*

✓ *Tell me about your significant other/partner/special person. What are they like?*

9

- Consider asking questions that create an opening for all adolescents to reveal themselves, without assuming that gender identity is (or is not) at stake:
  ✓ *Tell me about how the person you appear to be on the outside fits who you are on the inside?*
- Consider a more specific follow-up question:
  ✓ *How does being a boy or girl (sex assigned at birth), fit for you?* (Be prepared for any answer.)

  Individual expression of gender identity, and popular terminology around gender identity, can evolve. Avoid assumptions or premature closure of the conversation. If a young person discloses that their gender identity differs from their assigned sex at birth, follow with appreciation for their trust in you, and ask them to elaborate:
  Thank you for sharing that with me. Tell me more about what that means for you.

- Helpful follow-up questions include:
  ✓ *Have they shared this information with anyone else. If so, who?*
  ✓ *Are there concerns about privacy?*
  ✓ *Are there ways they believe you can help to support them?*
  ✓ *Does they have preferred pronouns (e.g., he/him/his, she/her/hers, they/them/theirs, ze/zim/zirs)?*
  ✓ *How should the medical team address or refer to the adolescent privately or when family is present (with regards to pronouns (e.g., he/him/his, she/her/hers, they/them/theirs, ze/zim/zirs) and name)?*

ABNORMAL UTERINE BLEEDING

AUB is bleeding from the uterine endometrium unrelated to an anatomic lesion. AUB can be identified as menstrual cycles that occur less than 21 or more than 45 days apart, bleeding lasting more than 7 days, or blood loss greater than 40 mL per cycle.

ETIOLOGY

- Anovulatory cycles (over 75% of cases)
  ✓ Commonly occurs in first 2–5 years after menarche
  ✓ Immaturity of the hypothalamic-pituitary-ovarian (HPO) axis leads to ovarian estrogen production that doesn't consistently reach level needed to trigger an LH surge, which in turns leads to failure to ovulate each month.
  ✓ No ovulation results in: of no corpus luteum, no progesterone secretion, unopposed estrogen secretion, continuously stimulated endometrium without stromal support, lining outgrowing blood supply, leading to the endometrium breaking down with variable shedding, necrosis, and irregular bleeding.

DIFFERENTIAL DIAGNOSIS

- Anovulatory cycles: Immaturity of HPO axis
- Pregnancy: Ectopic, threatened or incomplete abortion, placenta previa, hydatidiform mole
- Sexually transmitted infection (STI): Vaginitis (e.g., *Trichomonas*), cervicitis (e.g., gonorrhea, *Chlamydia*), pelvic inflammatory disease (i.e., endometritis)
- Endocrinopathy causing anovulation: Thyroid disease (hypothyroidism, hyperthyroidism), hyperprolactinemia (e.g., prolactinoma, dopamine antagonists), adrenal disorders (e.g., Addison disease, Cushing disease), PCOS, or other disorder of androgen excess
- Systemic disease causing anovulation: Chronic renal failure, systemic lupus erythematosus
- Hematologic disorder: Thrombocytopenia (e.g., idiopathic thrombocytopenic purpura, leukemia), defects in platelet function (e.g., von Willebrand disease), coagulation disorders

- Medications: Direct effect on hemostasis (e.g., warfarin, chemotherapeutic agents), indirect effect by altering hormone levels (e.g., breakthrough bleeding with hormonal contraception)
- Trauma: Laceration to vaginal mucosa or cervix
- Foreign body: Retained tampon or condom, for example
- Endometriosis
- Structural abnormalities (rare): Uterine polyps, myoma, cervical hemangioma, arteriovenous malformation, neoplasm

CLINICAL MANIFESTATIONS

- Bleeding pattern can help guide evaluation
  - ✓ Consider hematologic disorder if normal cyclic intervals with increased bleeding during each cycle, especially if has been occuring since menarche
  - ✓ Normal intervals with bleeding between cycles may suggest infection (particularly chlamydia), pregnancy, or foreign body
  - ✓ Endocrinopathy, anovulatory cycles, and medication effects are suggested by lack of cycle regularity
- The physical exam may be unremarkable, especially if the bleeding is due to anovulatory cycles.
- There may be evidence of anemia (e.g., pallor, lethargy) or hypovolemia, depending on the amount of blood loss.
- Signs and symptoms will reflect underlying the etiology. For example:
  - ✓ Prolactinoma: Headaches, visual changes, nipple discharge
  - ✓ Thyroid disease: Diarrhea or constipation, palpitations, skin changes, heat or cold intolerance
  - ✓ Bleeding disorder: Epistaxis and gingival bleeding, easy bruising
  - ✓ Sexually transmitted infection: Fever, abdominal pain, vaginal discharge, dysuria
  - ✓ Retained foreign body: Foul smelling odor and discharge
  - ✓ PCOS: Acne, hirsutism, acanthosis nigricans, weight gain

DIAGNOSTICS

Clinical Assessment

- Obtain menstrual history: Last menstrual period, age at menarche, cycle length (counting from day 1 of menses to day 1 of subsequent menses), frequency of tampon/pad changes, presence of premenstrual symptoms (cramping is often is a marker for ovulatory cycles due to prostaglandin secretion, bloating, moodiness)
- Obtain sexual history in confidential manner.
- Ask about symptoms of anemia (e.g., dizziness or lightheadedness).
- Assess hemodynamic stability (pulse, blood pressure, orthostatic vital signs).
- Pay special attention to: nutritional status, visual fields (i.e., pituitary lesions), thyroid size, breast exam (for galactorrhea), evidence of androgen excess (hirsutism, acne), ecchymoses or petechiae, sexual maturity rating
- Perform pelvic exam (including bimanual exam) if patient has ever been sexually active or to visualize source of bleeding. External exam may be sufficient, especially in patients who have never been sexually active.

Studies

- Pregnancy test: On every adolescent female presenting with vaginal bleeding, regardless of report of sexual activity
- Complete blood count with differential

- STI testing: Nucleic acid amplification testing for *Neisseria gonorrhoeae*, *Chlamydia trachomatis*, and *Trichomonas vaginalis* via urine or cervical swabs.
- Prothrombin time and partial thromboplastin time
- Depending on the history, consider testing for von Willebrand disease, thyroid-stimulating hormone, prolactin level, LH, follicle-stimulating hormone, serum androgens (e.g., free testosterone, dehydroepiandrosterone-S, androstenedione)
- Pelvic ultrasound if mass palpated on bimanual exam, unable to perform bimanual exam, or if concern about structural abnormalities exists.

MANAGEMENT

- Depends on severity of bleeding and degree of anemia
- Hormonal therapy is the mainstay of treatment: Use a monophasic OCP to provide hemostasis (estrogen) and stabilize the endometrium (progesterone). Ideally, the OCP should contain 30 μg of estrogen with second-generation progestin (levonorgestrel, norgestrel). Rarely, OCPs containing 50 μg of estrogen can be used in cases of severe AUB. *Note*: Must ask about contraindications to estrogen use specified in the CDC Medical Eligibility Criteria for Contraceptive Use. Category 3 or 4 conditions warrant use of progesterone-only options. In adolescents, it is particularly important to ask about migraine with aura and family history of clots (https://www.cdc.gov/reproductivehealth/contraception/mmwr/mec/summary.html).
- Treat underlying pathology (e.g., infection, endocrinopathy)
- Adjunct management: Menstrual diaries, iron supplementation, NSAIDs

AUB MANAGEMENT

Bleeding without anemia: Bleeding of prolonged duration or frequent due to shortened cycles with no anemia defined as Hgb greater than 12 g/dL

- Reassurance and observation with menstrual calendar
- Use of NSAIDs (antiprostaglandin effects useful for bleeding)
- Can consider use of OCP especially if contraception needed

Bleeding with mild anemia: Bleeding that is of prolonged duration or more frequent due to shortened cycles with mild anemia as defined by Hgb 10–11 g/dL

- Iron supplementation and NSAIDs
- OCP daily until anemia improves
- If estrogen is contraindicated:
  ✓ Norethindrone acetate (Aygestin) 5 mg daily to suppress menses.

Bleeding with moderate anemia: Bleeding that is of prolonged duration or more frequent due to shortened cycles with moderate anemia as defined by Hgb 7–10 g/dL

- Iron supplementation and NSAIDs
- OCP BID until bleeding stops then taper to daily until follow up
- If estrogen is contraindicated:
  ✓ Norethindrone acetate (Aygestin) 5–10 mg daily to suppress menses.

Bleeding with severe anemia: Bleeding that is of prolonged duration or more frequent due to shortened cycles with severe anemia as defined by Hgb <7 g/dL

- Inpatient admission indicated for treatment including potential blood transfusions (rarely necessary)
- Iron supplementation
- OCP (containing 30–35 μg of estrogen) every 8 hours until bleeding slows or stops then every 12 hours until hematocrit >30. Can increase to every 6 hours if bleeding does not slow down or add antifibrinolytic therapy (tranexamic acid or aminocaproic acid)
- Give antiemetics as needed prior to each OCP dose
- If not tolerating oral medications or if hemodynamically unstable, can use high-dose conjugated estrogen (Premarin). Give 25 mg intravenously every 4 hours for two to three doses to control bleeding. An OCP should be started within 24–48 hours after the initiation of IV estrogen to provide progestin for endometrial stabilization; this will prevent estrogen withdrawal bleeding.
- If estrogen is contraindicated:
  ✓ Norethindrone acetate (Aygestin) 5–10 mg every 6 hours until bleeding stops then tapered to every 8 hours a day for 3 days, and then twice a day for at least 2 weeks or until follow up.
  ✓ Medroxyprogesterone 10–20 mg every 6–12 hours until bleeding stops then tapering as tolerated to maintain control of bleeding.

Use of transfusion should be made on case by case basis taking into consideration hemodynamic stability, clinical status and response to therapy.

PELVIC INFLAMMATORY DISEASE (PID)

PID is a clinical condition referring to infection and inflammation involving the female upper genital tract including endometritis, salpingitis, tubo-ovarian abscess, and pelvic peritonitis. PID is a common and morbid complication of some STIs, in particular *Chlamydia trachomatis* (most commonly) and *Neisseria gonorrhoeae*.

EPIDEMIOLOGY

- 4.4% self-reported lifetime prevalence in sexually experienced women (18–44 years of age)
- Approximately 1 million U.S. women are diagnosed with PID each year. The true incidence of PID and its complications have been difficult to ascertain because no national surveillance or reporting requirements exist, national estimates are limited by insensitive clinical diagnostic criteria, and definitive diagnosis can be challenging.
- Major cause of other reproductive health problems, including infertility, ectopic pregnancy, abscess formation, and chronic pelvic pain
- Risk factors for PID include sexually active and age ≤25 years, history of PID, current or past infection with gonorrhea or chlamydia, male partner with gonorrhea or chlamydia, multiple partners or partner with multiple partners, douching, IUD insertion with previous 3 weeks, bacterial vaginosis (BV), and low socioeconomic status (may be surrogate marker for decreased access to care).
- Adolescent girls are at risk for PID because of
  ✓ Presence of cervical ectropion (columnar epithelium on exocervix rather than squamous epithelium) facilitates STI pathogen adherence.
  ✓ Disproportionate exposure to nongonococcal organisms (e.g., *C. trachomatis*).
  ✓ Low levels of local protective antibodies.

ETIOLOGY

- Microorganisms ascend from the lower genital tract (cervix) to infect the upper genital tract (uterus, fallopian tubes, etc.), resulting in an inflammatory response (prostaglandin release, edema, exudate and tissue destruction).
- Most cases of PID are considered to be polymicrobial.
- *C. trachomatis* and *N. gonorrhoeae* are the most commonly implicated organisms.
- Several microorganisms that comprise the vaginal flora (anaerobes, *Gardnerella vaginalis*, *Haemophilus influenzae*, *Streptococcus agalactiae*, enteric gram-negative organisms) and other pathogens (genital mycoplasmas, cytomegalovirus, and *Ureaplasma urealyticum*) have also been associated with PID.

CLINICAL MANIFESTATIONS

- Symptoms can range from none to severe.
- Lower abdominal pain is the most common presentation.
- Other symptoms may include fever, abnormal vaginal discharge, dyspareunia, dysuria, AUB, or right upper quadrant pain (consistent with perihepatitis or Fitz–Hugh–Curtis syndrome secondary to capsular inflammation).

DIAGNOSTICS

- The clinical diagnosis of acute PID is imprecise. The most common clinical presentations (e.g., lower abdominal pain) are nonspecific, but the use of diagnostic criteria to increase specificity has a significant impact on sensitivity. Because of the high risk of adverse outcomes with untreated PID and its later impact on fertility, it is recommended that health care providers maintain a low threshold for the diagnosis of PID and err on the side of overtreatment.
- Minimum criteria in women with lower abdominal pain: Uterine tenderness, adnexal tenderness, or cervical motion tenderness on bimanual examination
- Additional criteria to increase specificity: (WBCs on vaginal wet preparation, abnormal cervical or vaginal mucopurulent discharge, oral temperature greater than 38.3°C, elevated erythrocyte sedimentation rate or C-reactive protein, laboratory documentation of infection with *C. trachomatis* or *N. gonorrhoeae*
- PID is less likely if no WBCs are found on the wet preparation of the vaginal secretions.
- Most specific criteria for the diagnosis of PID include: Endometrial biopsy with evidence of endometritis, transvaginal ultrasound or MRI demonstrating thickened fallopian tubes or tubo-ovarian complex/abscess, and laparoscopic abnormalities consistent with PID
- Laparoscopy is the gold standard, but is usually not warranted for diagnosis.

MANAGEMENT

- Regardless of laboratory results, treatment for PID must include coverage of *C. trachomatis*, *N. gonorrhoeae*, anaerobes, gram-negative organisms, and streptococci.
- Because early treatment is an important part of the strategy to prevent adverse outcomes from PID, many clinical situations may warrant empiric therapy even while an evaluation for other causes of the presenting illness is still underway.
- Criteria for hospitalization: Pregnancy; poor clinical response to oral therapy; failure to follow or tolerate outpatient oral therapy; severe illness evidenced by nausea, vomiting,

or high fever; TOA; inability to rule out a surgical abdomen (e.g., appendicitis). Note that adolescence is no longer a criterion for hospitalization.
- Parenteral regimens (adapted from the CDC STI treatment guidelines):
  - ✓ Regimen A: Cefotetan 2 g intravenously (IV) every 12 hours OR cefoxitin 2 g IV every 6 hours PLUS doxycycline 100 mg orally (preferable because it has the same bioavailability and avoids the pain associated with infusion) or IV every 12 hours; discontinue IV therapy 24 hours after clinical improvement and complete total of 14 days of doxycycline; for TOA, can add clindamycin or metronidazole for increased anaerobic coverage.
  - ✓ Regimen B: Clindamycin 900 mg IV every 8 hours PLUS gentamycin loading dose IV or intramuscularly (IM) (2 mg/kg of body weight) followed by a maintenance dose (1.5 mg/kg) every 8 hours; discontinue IV therapy 24 hours after clinical improvement and complete total of 14 days of doxycycline 100 mg orally twice a day or clindamycin 450 mg orally four times a day (clindamycin has better anaerobic coverage for a TOA).
  - ✓ Alternative parenteral regimens exist but have not been as well studied.
- Outpatient regimens (adapted from the CDC STI treatment guidelines):
  - ✓ Ceftriaxone 250 mg IM in a single dose OR cefoxitin 2 g IM in a single dose (given with probenecid 1 g orally) OR other parenteral third-generation cephalosporin (ceftizoxime or cefotaxime) PLUS doxycycline 100 mg orally twice a day for 14 days
  - ✓ Additional anaerobic coverage may be provided by adding metronidazole 500 mg orally twice a day for 14 days to the above regimen.
  - ✓ Alternative oral regimens using fluoroquinolones are no longer recommended owing to changing resistance patterns for *N. gonorrhoeae*. However, if parenteral cephalosporin therapy is not feasible, use of fluoroquinolones (levofloxacin 500 mg orally once daily or ofloxacin 400 mg twice daily for 14 days) can be considered to be low community prevalence and individual risk for gonorrhea.
  - ✓ Expect clinical improvement within 3 days after initiating outpatient treatment; if no improvement appears, patient may require hospitalization, additional testing, or surgical intervention.
- Partners who have had sexual contact with the patient during the 60 days before symptoms occurred should be treated empirically for *C. trachomatis* and *N. gonorrhoeae*.
- Instruct patients to abstain from sexual intercourse until patient and current partner have both completed treatment regimen and are free from symptoms.
- All women diagnosed with PID should be offered HIV testing at the time of diagnosis.
- Repeat screening for re-infection of all women who have been diagnosed with chlamydia or gonorrhea is recommended 3–6 months after treatment
- PID risk can be reduced through regular STI screening for all women, especially those at high risk, treating any suspected PID, promoting safe sex practices (condom use), and enhancing vaginal health (avoiding douching, treating BV)

EMERGENCY CONTRACEPTION

Emergency contraception is a method of contraception in which a drug or IUD is used after unprotected intercourse.

INDICATIONS

- Pregnancy prevention following unprotected vaginal intercourse, contraceptive failure (e.g., broken condom, missed or late doses of hormonal contraceptives), sexual assault
- Most effective within 120 hours or less after event

OPTIONS

- Three general classes of hormonal emergency contraception are currently approved for use in the United States (see **Table 1-1**):
  - ✓ Progestin-only oral regimens including levonorgestrel (e.g., Plan B, Next Choice)
  - ✓ Novel progestin receptor agonist/antagonist oral regimens including ulipristal (Ella)
  - ✓ Combination estrogen and progestin oral regimens using alternative dosing of combination OCPs, also known as the Yuzpe regimen
- Nonhormonal methods of emergency contraception are currently limited to insertion of the copper IUD. This IUD is currently the most effective method of emergency contraception and affords continued long-acting reversible contraception.

TABLE 1-1	Emergency Contraception Regimens*		
Regimen Name	**Pills per Dose/Color (Repeat Once in 12 Hours)**	**Advantages of Regimen†**	**Disadvantages of Regimen**
Yuzpe Regimen (Combined Estrogen/Progestin)			
Preven	2 blue	• 75% efficacy	• 72-hour window
Ovral, Ogestrel	2 white		
Alesse, Levlite	5 pink	• Preven comes with patient info book and urine pregnancy test	• Side effects including nausea/vomiting common
Aviane	5 orange		
Nordette, Levlen	4 light-orange	• Patient may already have OCPs	• Cannot be used in individuals in which estrogen is contraindicated (refer to CDC Medical Eligibility Criteria for Contraceptive Use)‡
Levora, Lo/Ovral	4 white	• Established safety/efficacy	
Low-Ogestrel	4 yellow		
Triphasil, Tri-Levlen, Trivora	4 pink	• Can continue as contraception	
Progestin Only			
Plan B	1 white	• 89% efficacy	• 72-hour window
Ovrette	20 yellow	• Plan B comes with patient info kit	
		• More effective than combined	
		• Fewer side effects	
IUD	NA	• 99% efficacy	• Contraindicated for those with or at risk of STIs, other pelvic infections, anatomic anomalies, and in immunocompromised patients
		• Can be inserted up to 5 days after unprotected sex	
		• Can continue as contraception	

*Most effective when given in first 12 hours of unprotected sex.
†Applies to medications with a particular regimen unless specifically noted.
‡http://www.cdc.gov/reproductivehealth/UnintendedPregnancy/USMEC.htm
IUD = intrauterine device; NA = not applicable; OCPs = oral contraceptive pills; STIs, sexually transmitted infections.

CONTRAINDICATIONS

- All regimens: Pregnancy, hypersensitivity to drug components, undiagnosed vaginal bleeding
- Method-specific contraindications
  - ✓ Progestin-only oral regimens: No contraindications
  - ✓ Progestin receptor agonist/antagonist: Unclear if safe to use in pregnancy
  - ✓ Combination OCPs: Same as above, but also include contraindications to estrogen exposure (e.g., history of thrombophilia, thromboembolic disease, migraine with aura or neurologic changes; refer to CDC Medical Eligibility Criteria for Contraceptive Use)
  - ✓ Copper IUD: Abnormal genital tract anatomy, infection at the time of insertion

MECHANISM OF ACTION

- Inhibits or delays ovulation
- Disrupts follicular development
- Impairs corpus luteum
- Creates unfavorable environment for sperm function
- Alters endometrium, likely interfering with implantation; unclear if such alteration also occurs with hormonal emergency contraception

ADVERSE EFFECTS

- Occur mostly with combined emergency contraception (containing estrogen): Nausea/vomiting; dizziness; fatigue; breast tenderness, altered menstrual cycle
- Copper IUD may cause cramping or increased menstrual flow; also low risk of uterine perforation upon insertion

SAFETY

- Short course of therapy leads to few complications

ANTICIPATORY GUIDANCE

- Nausea/vomiting: Common in combined regimen; can be reduced by pretreatment with oral antiemetic (e.g., metoclopramide 10 mg or meclizine 25–50 mg) given 1 hour before emergency contraception
- Effect on menstrual cycle: Next menses may be early or late but should come within 21 days.
- Effect on pregnancy: Levonorgestrel and combined OCP regimens do not affect established pregnancy or lead to birth anomalies; data on progestin receptor agonist/antagonist and pregnancy still unclear.
- Progestin-only methods less effective with BMI >25
- Follow-up: Not required but recommended for contraceptive counseling and/or pregnancy testing if no menses in 21 days

ANOREXIA NERVOSA

DSM-V criteria* for AN are summarized below.
- Restriction of energy intake compared to requirements, which leads to significantly low weight
- Intense fear of gaining weight or behaviors that sabotage weight gain

*Note: DSM-V no longer sets a specific percent of ideal body weight but states that "significantly low weight" for developmental stage is less than is minimally normal or normally expected (for children and adolescents). DSM-V removes amenorrhea as a criterion for anorexia as it did not apply to males, females on contraceptives, or premenarchal females.

- Disturbance in the way in which one's body weight or shape is experienced
- *Restricting type:* During the prior 3 months with AN, the person has not achieved weight loss through being regularly engaged in binge eating or purging behavior (self-induced vomiting, use of laxatives/diuretics/enemas) but through dieting and excessive exercise.
- Binge eating/purging type: During the prior 3 months with AN, the person has regularly engaged in binge eating or purging behavior (self-induced vomiting, use of laxatives/ diuretics/enemas).

Note: ARFID (Avoidant Restrictive Food Intake Disorder) is now a diagnosis in the DSM-V. As with anorexia, there is a restriction in the amount of food eaten, but there is no associated distortion of body size or fear of weight gain.

EPIDEMIOLOGY

- Estimated to affect 1% of adolescents and young adults
- Age at presentation ranges from 10 to 25 years
- Increasing prevalence in adolescent males, non-White populations, and lower socioeconomic groups; more common among individuals involved in sports or activities where size and body shape impact success
- Bimodal age at onset at 14 and 18 years corresponding with life transitions (i.e., puberty, moving from high school to college or work)
- Mortality rates range from 1.8 to 5.9% (usually because of cardiac complications or suicide)

ETIOLOGY

- Exact etiology unknown; likely multifactorial in origin, including:
- Genetic: Increased risk with first-degree relatives with an eating disorder
- Neurotransmitters: Serotonin and its relationship to hunger and satiety
- Psychological: Theories range from sociocultural influences, perfectionism and rigidity, identity conflicts, and weight-related teasing.

CLINICAL MANIFESTATIONS

- Typically presents with a refusal to maintain a minimally normal weight
- Menstrual irregularities
- Frequently, patients do not report symptoms, but family members are concerned about significant weight loss, secondary amenorrhea, dizziness, lack of energy, gastrointestinal symptoms (e.g., constipation), and/or pale skin.
- Depending on amount of weight loss, clinical findings can range from normal to problems such as orthostasis, bradycardia, hypothermia, hypotension, dry skin, lanugo hair, thinning hair, brittle nails, peripheral edema, acrocyanosis, and findings suggestive of purging such as eroded tooth enamel, Russell sign (scars on knuckles), or parotid enlargement.
- External evidence of self-harm, such as scars from cutting on the extremities

DIAGNOSTICS

- Must consider the differential diagnosis for weight loss and exclude malabsorption and catabolic states
- Clinical information is vital. Questions should focus on disordered thinking and behavior. Screening questions (e.g., SCOFF questionnaire) can be helpful:
  ✓ Do you make yourself sick because you feel uncomfortably full?
  ✓ Do you worry you have lost control over how much you eat?
  ✓ Have you recently lost more than one stone (6.3 kg [14 lb]) in a 3-month period?
  ✓ Do you believe yourself to be fat when others say you are too thin?
  ✓ Would you say that food dominates your life?

Give 1 point for every yes; scores of 2 or more indicate anorexia nervosa or bulimia.

- Laboratory studies are not diagnostic of anorexia nervosa. **Table 1-2** suggests tests to obtain in the initial assessment of a patient in whom anorexia nervosa is suspected. Further tests should be ordered on the basis of clinical suspicion for other diseases.
- Electrocardiography: Indicated for bradycardia less than 50 bpm to rule out prolonged QTc or dysrhythmias. Low voltage, ST-segment depression, or conduction abnormalities may also be seen.

TABLE 1-2 Laboratory Studies in Anorexia Nervosa

Study	Rationale/Interpretation
Serum chemistries	Hyponatremia—water loading or inappropriate regulation of ADH
	Hypophosphatemia—severe malnutrition
	Hypokalemic, hypochloremic metabolic alkalosis—vomiting
	Acidosis—laxative abuse
	Hypoglycemia
	High blood urea nitrogen and creatinine—dehydration with or without purging
Complete blood-cell count	High hemoglobin—dehydration
	Anemia—chronic disease and/or iron deficiency
	Leukopenia and thrombocytopenia
Liver-function tests (including prealbumin)	Prealbumin and albumin—evaluate nutritional status
	Abnormal liver enzymes—fatty liver infiltration
Cholesterol, triglycerides	Elevated owing to abnormal lipoprotein metabolism
Erythrocyte sedimentation rate	Normal to low in anorexia
Urinalysis	Low specific gravity—water loading
Morning cortisol level	Rule out adrenal insufficiency
Thyroid-function tests	Euthyroid sick sinus syndrome—normal or low thyroid-stimulating hormone and normal thyroxine
	Rule out hyperthyroidism or hypothyroidism
β-human chorionic gonadotropin	Rule out pregnancy
Prolactin	Rule out prolactinoma
LH, FSH, estradiol (females), testosterone (males)	Evaluate hormonal suppression, rule out ovarian failure
Amylase, lipase	Evidence of purging, rule out pancreatitis
Celiac panel (IgA tissue transglutaminase, antiendomysial antibodies	Rule out celiac disease
Labs as indicated	HIV Ag/Ab testing, PPD, FOBT
Nutrition labs	Vitamins B_1, B_{12}, and D, zinc

Ab = antibody; ADH = antidiuretic hormone; Ag = antigen; FOBT = fecal occult blood test; FSH = follicle-stimulating hormone; LH = luteinizing hormone; PPD = purified protein derivative.

- Dual-energy x-ray absorptiometry: Evaluate bone density in patients who have been amenorrheic for longer than 6 months
- Imaging: Chest x-ray, brain magnetic resonance imaging, barium enema, and upper gastrointestinal series with small bowel follow-through should be considered on the basis of clinical concern for other conditions as an explanation for symptoms.

MANAGEMENT

- Indications for inpatient treatment are listed in **Table 1-3**.
- Interdisciplinary team: This team comprises a physician, dietician, mental health professional, and social worker and should generate a coordinated consistent plan of care and be available for team meetings with patient and family; family-based therapy is the gold standard treatment for AN.
- Fluids/electrolytes/nutrition:
  ✓ Correction of dehydration
  ✓ Blind weights with the patient wearing only a gown at same time and on the same scale each day are best. Expected rate of weight gain is 0.9–1.4 kg (2–3 lb) per week.
- Refeeding syndrome: Constellation of cardiac, neurologic, and hematologic complications as phosphate shifts from extracellular to intracellular compartments in patients with total-body phosphate depletion secondary to malnutrition
  ✓ Risk factors: Moderate to severe anorexia (10% or more below ideal body weight)
  ✓ Prevention: Slow refeeding with or without phosphorus supplementation (in patients with normal renal function)
  ✓ Monitoring: Telemetry, frequent vital signs, and electrolytes, especially phosphorus, potassium, and magnesium
  ✓ Clinical manifestations: Cardiac arrest, delirium, congestive heart failure
- Cardiovascular: Telemetry for patients with significant bradycardia, dysrhythmias, and electrolyte abnormalities until resolution of conditions
- Gastrointestinal: Control of constipation with stool softeners (avoid laxatives)
- Endocrinology:
  ✓ Osteopenia: Weight gain is the best therapy; a multivitamin with 400 IU of vitamin D and 1200–1500 mg/day of elemental calcium is recommended.

TABLE 1-3	Criteria for Hospital Admission for Children, Adolescents, and Young Adults with Anorexia Nervosa
Criteria for Hospital Admission	
<75% of ideal body weight or failure of outpatient management	
Refusal to eat	
Heart rate <50 beats per minute daytime or <45 beats per minute nighttime	
Hypotension (<90/50 mm Hg)	
Orthostatic changes in pulse (20 beats per minute or blood pressure <10 mm Hg)	
Temperature <96°F	
Arrhythmia (e.g., prolonged QTc interval)	

Adapted with permission from Rosen DS; American Academy of Pediatrics Committee on Adolescence: Identification and management of eating disorders in children and adolescents, *Pediatrics* 2010 Dec;126(6):1240–1253.

✓ Amenorrhea: Menses will resume with adequate weight gain and improved nutritional status; no hormonal therapy is required.
- Psychiatry:
  ✓ Safety and compliance: One-on-one observation by qualified staff with experience with eating disorders is required, especially at the beginning of treatment.
  ✓ Mental-status abnormalities improve with correction of malnourished state. Most interventions should begin after patient is medically stable.
  ✓ Psychotherapy: Cognitive behavioral therapy is the most effective treatment.
  ✓ Pharmacotherapy: Indicated only for treatment of comorbid disorders (i.e., depression, obsessive–compulsive disorder). There is no FDA-approved drug for the treatment of anorexia nervosa.

TANNER STAGING

- Used to define male and female pubertal development (see **Table 1-4**).
- It is critical to explain to the adolescent patient what you are doing when assessing Tanner stage. Say, "as part of your development through adolescence it is important that I check where you are in pubertal development."
- Tanner staging is helpful because it demonstrates normal progression through puberty or identifies delayed puberty; it also determines hallmarks of pubertal development such as growth spurts, menarche (females), and spermarche (males)

TABLE 1-4	Tanner Staging	
Males		
Stage	**Testes development**	**Penis development**
I	Prepubertal (<4 mL)	Prepubertal
II	Testes enlarge (≥4 mL), scrotum reddens and changes texture	Slight enlargement
III	Larger	Longer
IV	Scrotum darkens	Larger, wider with development of glans
V	Adult size	Adult size
Stage	**Female breast development**	
I	Prepubertal	
II	Breast and papilla elevated as small mound with palpable subareolar bud, areolar diameter increased	
III	Enlargement and elevation of whole breast	
IV	Areola and papilla form secondary areolar mound	
V	Mature breast contour, nipple projects	
Stage	**Male and female pubic hair development**	
I	None	
II	Sparse, short, straight, at base of penis or medial border of labia	
III	Darker, longer, coarser, and curlier, sparsely over pubic bones	
IV	Coarse, curly, resembles adult hair; but spares thighs	
V	Adult distribution with inverse triangle pattern and spread to medial thighs	

Allergy and Asthma

Peter Capucilli, MD
Terri Brown-Whitehorn, MD

ANAPHYLAXIS

Anaphylaxis is an acute, potentially life-threatening systemic allergic reaction. It is most commonly triggered by interaction of an allergen with specific IgE antibody bound to mast cells and basophils, leading to cell activation and mediator release. Non–IgE-mediated direct mast-cell degranulation can also result in mediator release.

EPIDEMIOLOGY

- Lifetime prevalence for all triggers is 0.05–2%.
- Incidence is thought to be increasing.
- Food is the most common cause of anaphylaxis, affecting up to 8% of young children and 3–4% of adults.
- Drugs are the second most common cause of anaphylaxis.
- Approximately 1% of all cases of anaphylaxis (all causes) have a fatal outcome in the United States (including ~200 from food).

ETIOLOGY

- Major causes are food (milk, egg, soy, wheat, peanut, tree nut, fish, and shellfish), medications (antibiotics, aspirin, NSAIDs, biologics, chemotherapeutics, muscle relaxants, blood products, radiocontrast media), latex, insect stings (especially bee venom), and allergy immunotherapy
- Rare causes include
  - ✓ Exercise-induced anaphylaxis—reaction triggered by exertion, cardiovascular exercise, or fast-paced walking. Reaction may be food-dependent (anaphylaxis occurs with exercise only after eating a specific food) or independent of food exposure.
  - ✓ Alpha-1,3-galactose (alpha-gal syndrome)—tick-related immune response following a bite by a Lone Star tick. Patients experience characteristic a delayed mild-to-severe systemic allergic reaction after ingestion of red meat.
  - ✓ Idiopathic anaphylaxis—may be related to hormone cycle, rare hidden food additives or underlying mast-cell instability.

DIFFERENTIAL DIAGNOSIS

- Other causes of shock: Hypovolemic, cardiogenic, and septic
- Cardiopulmonary instability: Myocardial infarction, pulmonary embolism, pneumothorax, vasovagal reaction
- Allergic/immunologic: Status asthmaticus, scombroid poisoning, hereditary angioedema, non–IgE-mediated reactions (serum sickness, DRESS, leukotriene-mediated reactions)
- Oncologic/hematologic: Carcinoid syndrome, pheochromocytoma, systemic mastocytosis (which increases risk of anaphylaxis)

PATHOPHYSIOLOGY

- Previous exposure to an allergen (antigen) leads to allergen-specific IgE antibody production.
  - ✓ IgE binds to the surface of mast cells and basophils.

✓ Upon subsequent exposure, the antigen binds cell-bound IgE, triggering cell activation and degranulation.

✓ Sometimes, there is no known prior allergen exposure and reaction occurs on the first known exposure.

• Mediators involved include histamine, arachidonic acid derivatives (prostaglandins and leukotrienes), tryptase, bradykinin, and platelet-activating factor.

✓ These mediators cause smooth-muscle spasm (bronchi, coronary arteries, and gastrointestinal tract), increased vascular permeability, vasodilation, and complement activation.

✓ Conditions that may develop include urticaria, angioedema, wheezing, emesis, diarrhea, hypotension, and occasionally altered mental status.

• Nonimmunologic (previously known as anaphylactoid) reactions result from non–IgE-mediated degranulation of mast cells and basophils. This can occur with radiocontrast media, NSAIDs, opiates, and other agents

CLINICAL MANIFESTATIONS

• Exposure to a known allergen and/or prior history of anaphylaxis is a helpful sign, but it is not always present.

• Onset is typically within 30 minutes after exposure to allergens. Symptoms typically progress very rapidly. At times, reactions may occur up to 2 hours after exposure

• When treated, symptoms usually resolve within a few hours. Outside of having a biphasic reaction, symptoms do not persist unless the patient is reexposed to the trigger.

• Biphasic responses can occur in up to 20% of adult cases (1.5–14.7% in pediatric studies) with recurrence of symptoms 8–10 hours later.

✓ Seen more frequently following severe initial reactions with biphasic response being less severe in nature

• Cutaneous (80–90% of patients): Urticaria, pruritus, flushing, and angioedema. Patients with severe manifestation of anaphylaxis do not always present with skin findings.

• Respiratory (60% of patients): Lower airway symptoms include wheezing, cough, stridor, chest tightness, and dyspnea. Upper airway symptoms include sneezing, congestion/rhinorrhea, dysphonia, laryngeal edema (drooling), and hoarseness.

• Gastrointestinal (45% of patients): Nausea, vomiting, abdominal pain, diarrhea

• Cardiovascular (45% of patients): Chest pain, palpitations, tachycardia or bradycardia, dysrhythmia, hypotension, shock, cardiac arrest

• Central nervous system (15% of patients): Feeling of "impending doom," anxiety, headache, confusion, mental status change, and/or behavior changes. In younger children, this may manifest as irritability, fatigue, or cessation of play.

• Anaphylaxis can progress within minutes to shock, arrhythmia, and cardiac arrest. Death is most often from upper and/or lower airway obstruction or cardiovascular collapse.

DIAGNOSTICS

• Diagnosis is clinical and early intervention is lifesaving.

• The plasma tryptase level is usually elevated if obtained <4 hours after the start of symptoms, though tryptase is often normal in food-induced anaphylaxis.

• Electrocardiography may show dysrhythmia, ischemic changes, or signs of myocardial infarction, and cardiac enzymes can be elevated.

MANAGEMENT

First Line

• ABCs [airways, breathing, circulation], airway management as needed, supplemental oxygen

- Epinephrine 1:1000 injection or epinephrine auto-injector; repeat every 3–5 minutes as needed.
- Auto-injectors are recommended to decrease risk of error. Administer epinephrine IM as soon as anaphylaxis is recognized.
  Dosing:
  > Neonates:
  > IM: <5 kg: 0.01 mg/kg of body weight (0.1 mL/kg of 0.1 mg/mL solution) every 3–5 minutes, as needed
  > Infants and children:
  > IM epinephrine auto-injector:
  > > 5–24 kg: 0.15 mg
  > > ≥25 kg: 0.3 mg
- Isotonic intravenous fluid resuscitation for hypotension, progressing to volume expanders and/or vasoactive infusions if inadequate response to IM epinephrine
- Supine position, feet elevated
- Racemic epinephrine should be given *only* if preparing for endotracheal intubation
- Extremis: IV epinephrine infusions (note dose)

Second Line

- Diphenhydramine (H_1-antihistamine) 1 mg/kg IV or orally (maximum, 50 mg per dose); every 6 hours (maximum, 300 mg/day) OR cetirizine (H_1-antihistamine) PO (less sedating)
- Nebulized albuterol (β-adrenergic agonist) 2.5–5 mg/3 mL (or inhaled albuterol via metered dose inhaler and spacer) for wheezing/chest tightness, used in conjunction with epinephrine if not resolved after epinephrine administration
- Famotidine (H_2 antihistamine) 0.25–0.5 mg/kg IV (maximum 20 mg/dose); or orally 0.5 mg/kg (maximum 40 mg/dose)
- Hydrocortisone 2 mg/kg IV (maximum, 60 mg) once, then 1 mg/kg IV every 6 hours. Alternatives: methylprednisolone 1–2 mg/kg IV, then 1 mg/kg/dose every 6 hours; or oral prednisone 2 mg/kg once then 1 mg/kg/dose (maximum, 60 mg). There is no evidence to support glucocorticoid treatment beyond the acute setting.
- If patient is taking a β-adrenergic blocking agent (i.e., beta-blocker) and symptoms of anaphylaxis are not responsive to epinephrine IM, consider giving glucagon.
- There is no evidence to indicate the optimal length of time for therapy.
  - ✓ Many children receive therapy with resolution of symptoms and do not need further treatment.
  - ✓ If a patient is being discharged from the hospital, some clinicians will prescribe 24 hours of antihistamines with or without oral steroids based on the assessment of symptoms.

Admission to Hospital

- Hospitalization should be considered for patients with one or more of the following:
  - ✓ Current severe reaction with hypotension or need for IV fluid bolus
  - ✓ Need for more than one dose of epinephrine
  - ✓ History of severe reaction or biphasic reaction
  - ✓ History of severe asthma or in a current asthma exacerbation
  - ✓ Progression or persistence of symptoms
  - ✓ Parent/caregiver or clinician concerned about ability to return to care and/or unsafe discharge plan

Follow-up Care

- Patients who do not require hospitalization should be observed for at least 4 hours.

- Upon discharge:
  - ✓ Prescribe an epinephrine auto-injector and train patient/caregivers in its proper use. (Families should have epinephrine in hand at time of discharge, if possible.)
  - ✓ Develop an anaphylaxis action plan and review with patient and caregivers.
  - ✓ Educate patient/family about allergen avoidance if an allergen has been identified.
  - ✓ List identified allergen in the medical record.
  - ✓ Refer for an allergy consultation.

Children's Hospital of Philadelphia (CHOP) Anaphylaxis Pathway—Emergency (https://www.chop.edu/clinical-pathway/anaphylaxis-emergent-care-clinical-pathway)

Authors: J. Lee, MD; T. Brown-Whitehorn, MD; N. Tsarouhas, MD; B. Rodio, RN; L. Zielinski, RN; J. Molnar, CRNP

CHOP Anaphylaxis Pathway—Inpatient (https://www.chop.edu/clinical-pathway/anaphylaxis-inpatient-clinical-pathway)

Authors: T. Brown-Whitehorn, MD; J. Spergel, MD, PhD; J. Lavelle, MD; S. O'Neill, PharmD; J. Lamaina, RN, MSN; R. Sutton, MD; D. Davis, MD

ANGIOEDEMA AND URTICARIA

Urticaria refers to transient, raised, pruritic, erythematous, blanching skin lesions. Angioedema is a transient, often asymmetric, swelling in the deep dermis and subcutaneous or submucosal tissues with little or no pruritus. Angioedema and urticaria often occur together. A hereditary form of isolated angioedema also exists.

EPIDEMIOLOGY

- Acute urticaria/angioedema, lasting <6 weeks, is seen in up to 20% of the population.
- Chronic urticaria/angioedema, lasting ≥6 weeks, is seen in 0.5% of the population.

ETIOLOGY

Acute Urticaria/Angioedema

- Causes of acute urticaria/angioedema include
  - ✓ Infections: most often viral, but has been associated with parasites and certain bacteria
  - ✓ Foods (Symptoms do not last >24 hours after exposure.)
  - ✓ Contact reaction
  - ✓ Environmental allergen exposure (e.g., licked by dog, rolling in grass)
  - ✓ Medications (NSAIDs, aspirin, Angiotensin converting enzyme (ACE) inhibitors)
  - ✓ Insect stings, activities that increase body temperature (cholinergic)
  - ✓ Physical triggers (cold, heat, water, vibration, sunlight)
  - ✓ Idiopathic (estimated 1–14% in children)

Chronic Urticaria and Angioedema

- A specific cause of chronic urticaria and angioedema is rarely found, especially in pediatric patients. Rare causes include underlying autoimmune urticaria, malignancy, thyroid disorders, and mast-cell disease, such as urticaria pigmentosa or systemic mastocytosis.

PATHOPHYSIOLOGY

- IgE-mediated: Previous allergen (antigen) exposure leads to production of allergen-specific IgE antibody. IgE binds to surface of mast cells and basophils. Upon subsequent exposure, the antigen binds cell-bound IgE, leading to cell activation and degranulation, resulting in urticaria and/or angioedema.

- Non–IgE-mediated: Nonspecific activation and degranulation of mast cells and/or basophils. Triggers are physical stimuli (e.g., cold, heat, pressure, vibration, water, sunlight), complement factors (e.g., C3a, C4a, and C5a), and some medications (e.g., NSAIDs, opiates).
- Autoimmune urticaria: Chronic idiopathic urticaria is a diagnosis of exclusion. In 30–40% of cases an autoantibody against the IgE receptor on mast cells and basophils is identified. Rarely, anti-IgE antibodies are demonstrated. Thyroid autoantibodies may be seen, but they have value only in the context of abnormal thyroid hormone levels.

DIFFERENTIAL DIAGNOSIS

- Viral exanthem, contact dermatitis, papular urticaria, erythema multiforme, urticarial vasculitis, and systemic lupus erythematosus

CLINICAL MANIFESTATIONS

- Individual urticarial lesions are transient, lasting <2–3 hours, resolve, and reappear in another area. An individual lesion does not last >24 hours.
- Dermatographism may be seen when stroking of the skin leads to linear wheals (occurs in 2–5% of population).

DIAGNOSTICS

- Diagnosis is clinical.
- Allergy testing for acute urticaria is useful if a specific food or environmental trigger is suspected on the basis of the history.
  - ✓ If hives last longer than 24 hours, then reaction is unlikely to be secondary to a food allergen exposure.
  - ✓ Broad-panel food testing, especially to foods tolerated in the diet, is not recommended.
- Extensive studies to determine viral infectious etiology are not routinely recommended, as identification of a specific infectious cause does not typically change management.
- Consider a skin biopsy and dermatology referral when individual urticarial lesions persist >24 hours or are atypical in appearance.
- Laboratory workup should be considered for chronic urticaria if there are additional worrisome symptoms (e.g., joint pain/swelling, bruising, fatigue, fever, weight loss) that may be suggestive of autoimmune, myeloproliferative, oncologic, endocrine, or vasculitis disorder or if there is a family history of angioedema.

MANAGEMENT

- If a trigger is identified, avoidance is advised.
- Acute cases usually self-resolve.
- Treatment is aimed at decreasing pruritus and providing comfort.
- First-generation (e.g., diphenhydramine) or second-generation (nonsedating) H_1-antihistamines (e.g., cetirizine, fexofenadine) are used for primary management.
  - ✓ Second-generation (nonsedating) antihistamines may be used initially to avoid sedation side effects associated with first-generation antihistamines. Second-generation antihistamines also require less frequent dosing than first-generation antihistamines.
  - ✓ If symptoms are not well controlled, high-dose H_1-antihistamines are used in combination with H_2-antihistamines (e.g., ranitidine).
  - ✓ In chronic urticaria, in addition to H_1- and H_2-antihistamines, scheduled dosing of H_1- and H_2-antihistamines as well as additional medications may be considered (**Figure 2-1**).
- Glucocorticoids can reduce symptoms; however, they are not recommended long term, as acute worsening of symptoms may occur when stopped.

STEP 4
Add an alternative agent
- Omalizumab or cyclosporine
- Other antiinflammatory agents, immunosuppressants, or biologics

STEP 3
Dose advancement of potent antihistamine (e.g., hydroxyzine or doxepin) as tolerated

STEP 2
One or more of the following:
- Dose advancement of second-generation antihistamine used in Step 1
- Add another second-generation antihistamine
- Add H_2-antagonist
- Add leukotriene receptor antagonist
- Add first-generation antihistamine to be taken at bedtime

STEP 1
- Monotherapy with second-generation antihistamine
- Avoidance of triggers (e.g., NSAIDs) and relevant physical factors if physical urticaria/angioedema syndrome is present

- Begin treatment at step appropriate for patient's level of severity and previous treatment history.
- At each level of the step approach, medication(s) should be assessed for patient tolerance and efficacy.
- **"Step-down" in treatment is appropriate at any step, once consistent control of urticaria/angioedema is achieved.**

FIGURE 2-1 Treatment Algorithm for Chronic Urticaria. Reproduced with permission from Bernstein JA, Lang DM, Khan DA, et al: The diagnosis and management of acute and chronic urticaria: 2014 update, J Allergy Clin Immunol 2014 May;133(5):1270-1277.

- Cyproheptadine is useful in cold-induced urticaria.
- Initial acute urticaria after ingestion of food or medication may progress to anaphylaxis, which warrants epinephrine use.
- NSAIDs should be avoided entirely with acute or chronic urticaria or angioedema as they may exacerbate symptoms via leukotriene pathway mechanism

ANGIOEDEMA—HEREDITARY FORMS

EPIDEMIOLOGY

- Hereditary angioedema (HAE) is a rare disease, accounting for about 2% of angioedema cases.
  - ✓ Its prevalence is about 1/10,000–1/50,000.
- Inheritances is autosomal dominant. However, family history can be negative because of variable penetrance and variation in age at disease onset.

ETIOLOGY

- Type I (85%): Low or absent protein C1 inhibitor (C1-INH) with concurrent poor protein function
- Type II (15%): Normal/high levels of C1-INH, but the protein is nonfunctioning
- Type III: Rare, more severe, and more common in women. Underlying mediator remains unidentified, but has been associated with estrogen and coagulation factor XII mutations. Level and function of C1-INH may be normal.

PATHOPHYSIOLOGY

- Without proper levels or function of C1-INH, there is unopposed activation of the first component of the classical complement pathway. Angioedema occurs because of the formation of bradykinin and complement factors.
- The acquired forms exist where a lymphoproliferative disorder leads to production of a monoclonal antibody that neutralizes existing C1-INH.

DIFFERENTIAL DIAGNOSIS

- Allergic reactions, malignancy, allergic urticaria/angioedema, rheumatologic disease, ACE-inhibitor–induced angioedema

CLINICAL MANIFESTATIONS

- Angioedema, without urticaria, lasting 1–4 days
- A prodromal reticular rash may present prior to onset.
- Affected areas include the skin and mucous membranes, larynx, and bowel wall.
- Episodes are often spontaneous, but known triggers include trauma, surgery (including dental work), emotional stress, infection, exogenous estrogen, and menstruation.

DIAGNOSTICS

- Serum C4 level is the best screening test. C4 level will be low secondary to complement consumption via complement pathway activation due to loss of C1-INH inhibition. (The sample should be placed on ice, otherwise complement levels can be falsely low.)
- C1-INH level and function can also be measured and can differentiate among the forms of HAE (see types above).

MANAGEMENT

Acute Treatment

- Plasma-derived C1-INH (Berinert)
  ✓ Approved for pediatric patients
- Recombinant kallikrein inhibitor (ecallantide)
  ✓ Approved for patients >16 years of age
- Recombinant bradykinin-2 receptor inhibitor (icatibant)
  ✓ Approved for patients >18 years of age
- If the above are not available, consider fresh frozen plasma, as it contains C1-INH.

  Dose: 2 units for adults; 10 mL/kg for children

- IV fluids and pain medications (avoid opiates if possible, as they can cause nonimmune-mediated mast-cell degranulation)
- Co-management and referral to a board-certified allergist/immunologist is highly recommended to discuss long-term management and prophylaxis.

Chronic/Prophylactic Treatment

- Plasma-derived C1-INH (Cinryze) IV infusions every 3–4 days
- Plasma-derived C1-INH (Haegarda) subcutaneous infusion for short-term prophylaxis
- Androgens (danazol or stanozolol) increase hepatic C1-INH synthesis—not recommended as first-line therapy because of significant side effects and availability of alternative medication options.

Short-Term Prophylaxis Prior to Surgery/Trauma

- Plasma-derived C1-INH on the day of surgery

DRUG ALLERGY

CLASSIFICATION

- Modified Gel–Coombs classification of hypersensitivity reactions (**Table 2-1**)
- Nonimmunologic-mediated (pseudoallergic) reactions: Due to nonimmune degranulation of mast cells and basophils (e.g., vancomycin, radiocontrast dye, opiates, NSAID-induced urticaria)

CLINICAL MANIFESTATIONS

- Hives, angioedema, and anaphylaxis-type symptoms occurring within minutes to hours after exposure suggest type I hypersensitivity.
- Cough within 10 days after the start of drug administration (e.g., nitrofurantoin) with peripheral eosinophilia and migratory infiltrates suggests pulmonary drug hypersensitivity.
- Maculopapular exanthem within days after the start of drug administration (e.g., amoxicillin) suggests a T-cell–mediated reaction.
- Skin reaction always occurring in the same area suggests a fixed drug eruption.

TABLE 2-1	Classification of Hypersensitivity Reactions	
Classification Type	**Immunoreactants**	**Clinical Presentation**
I	Mast cell-mediated, IgE-dependent	Anaphylaxis, urticaria, angioedema, asthma, allergic rhinitis
IIa	Antibody-mediated cytotoxic reaction	Immune cytopenia
IIb	Antibody-mediated cell-stimulating reactions	Graves disease, chronic idiopathic urticaria
III	Immune complex-mediated	Serums sickness, vasculitis
IVa	Th1 cell-mediated, macrophage activation	Type 1 diabetes Contact dermatitis (also IVc)
IVb	T helper cell type 2 (Th2)-mediated, eosinophilic inflammation	Persistent asthma and allergic rhinitis
IVc	Cytotoxic T-cell–mediated (perforin, granzyme B)	Stevens–Johnson syndrome, toxic epidermal necrolysis syndrome
IVd	T-cell-mediated, neutrophilic inflammation	Acute generalized exanthematous pustulosis, Behçet disease

- Lichenification/eczema occurring 1–3 days after the start of drug administration (e.g., hydrochlorothiazide) suggests photoallergic reaction.
- Fine pustules, fever, and neutrophilia occurring days after the start of drug administration suggest acute generalized exanthematous pustulosis.
- Rash and fever with lymphadenopathy, arthralgia, gastrointestinal symptoms, and proteinuria occurring after 1–3 weeks after the start of drug administration suggest serum sickness or serum sickness–like reaction.
- Rash and fever with eosinophilia, facial edema, and organ involvement (e.g., liver, kidney, lymph nodes) 2–8 weeks after drug administration suggest DRESS.
- Mucosal erosion, target lesions, epidermal necrosis, and multiorgan involvement occurring days to weeks after the start of drug administration suggest SJS/TEN.

RISK FACTORS FOR DRUG ALLERGY

- Host factors include patient's genetics, history of prior allergic reaction, underlying concomitant diseases (e.g., HIV, cystic fibrosis), and female sex.
- Drug factors include high dose, repetitive courses, high molecular weight of drug, and IV administration.

DIAGNOSTICS

- Serum tryptase
  - ✓ High positive predictive value, but low negative predictive value in perioperative anaphylaxis
- Skin-prick testing and specific IgE testing:
  - ✓ For patients who have reaction to penicillin, skin testing is available.
  - ✓ Skin testing for other drugs has not been validated but may be helpful.
  - ✓ Neither skin nor specific IgE tests are diagnostic for cytotoxic, immune complex, or cell-mediated drug-induced allergic reactions.

MANAGEMENT

- Stop the medication.
- If anaphylaxis occurs, follow treatment as outlined in Anaphylaxis section.
- Drug avoidance
- Drug desensitization is used when there is a history of immediate reaction, there are no alternative drugs, and the drug is medically necessary. This is best performed by an allergist in a critical care setting, as anaphylaxis may develop.

COMMONLY IMPLICATED DRUGS

- Antibiotics
  - ✓ Penicillin can cause all types of reactions, from type I to type IV
  - ✓ Sulfa antibiotics
  - ✓ Cephalosporin antibiotics
  - ✓ Carbapenem
  - ✓ Neomycin (topical)
- Chemotherapeutics
  - ✓ Type I reactions are reported for almost all commonly used agents and range from mild skin reactions to severe anaphylaxis.
  - ✓ Paclitaxel and docetaxel produce non-IgE–mediated (anaphylactoid) reactions in up to 42% of patients on first administration but rarely with subsequent cycles.
  - ✓ Platinum compounds (cisplatin, carboplatin) can produce type I reactions
- Asparaginase can produce type I and pseudoallergic reactions.

- Local anesthetics
  - ✓ Allergy testing is available.
- Muscle relaxants
  - ✓ Can cause an IgE or pseudoallergic reaction
- Antiepileptics
  - ✓ Carbamazepine, lamotrigine, phenytoin (associated with delayed drug reactions such as DRESS and SJS)
- Natural rubber latex (NRL)
  - ✓ High-risk groups include those with a history of multiple surgeries (especially genito-urinary and abdominal surgery) and those with occupations in which latex gloves are frequently used.
  - ✓ Positive skin-prick test to a reliable crude NRL extract is more sensitive than specific IgE to latex to confirm diagnosis.
- NSAIDs and aspirin
  - ✓ For patients with history of urticaria or angioedema in reaction to NSAID exposure, avoidance is recommended. If required, graded challenge protocol may be used.
  - ✓ Various reactions can be seen (**Table 2-2**).
  - ✓ Aspirin exacerbated respiratory disease is characterized by aspirin- or NSAID-induced respiratory reaction in patients with underlying asthma
- Radiocontrast media
  - ✓ Can cause a non-IgE–mediated reaction that is unpredictable. If there is a history of prior reaction, pretreatment protocols may prevent reaction: a corticosteroid (e.g., prednisone) given at 13 hours, 7 hours, and 1 hour prior to procedure and an antihistamine (e.g., diphenhydramine) given1 hour prior. Reaction is not related to underlying shellfish allergy.

TABLE 2-2	Classification of NSAID Reactions*		
Type of Reaction	**Description**	**Timing of Reaction**	**Cross Reactivity**
NSAID-exacerbated cutaneous disease	Urticaria or angioedema exacerbated by NSAID use	0.5–6 hours	All NSAIDs, including aspirin, usually excluding COX-2 inhibitors and acetaminophen
NSAID-induced urticaria/ angioedema	Urticaria or angioedema precipitated by NSAID use	Minutes to 24 hours	All NSAIDs, including aspirin, usually excluding COX-2 inhibitors and acetaminophen
Single NSAID-induced angioedema or anaphylaxis	IgE-mediated, immediate reaction following NSAID use	Minutes to 2 hours	Single-NSAID–specific, usually able to tolerate other NSAIDs, aspirin, and acetaminophen
NSAID-induced delayed hypersensitivity reaction	T-cell–mediated cutaneous eruption, SJS, TEN	>24 hours	Single-NSAID–specific is typical, usually able to tolerate other NSAIDs, aspirin, acetaminophen

*Excludes aspirin-exacerbated respiratory disease (AERD)
COX = cyclooxygenase; NSAID = nonsteroidal antiinflammatory drug; SJS = Stevens–Johnson syndrome; TEN = toxic epidermal necrolysis.

TABLE 2-3	Implications of Inaccurate Penicillin Allergy Labeling

- Penicillin (PCN) is the most commonly reported drug allergy.
- Estimates suggest that only 10–20% of those considered to have a PCN allergy are actually allergic.
- Most patients with previous PCN allergy outgrow their allergy after roughly 10 years, but most maintain allergy label for longer.
- Patients who carry a PCN allergy label are more likely to be prescribed antibiotics that are
  - ✓ Broad-spectrum
  - ✓ Associated with more side effects
  - ✓ More expensive
  - ✓ Less effective for certain conditions
- PCN allergy–labeled patients also have
  - ✓ Higher rates of *Clostridiodes difficile*, vancomycin-resistant *Enterococcus*, and methicillin-resistant *Staphylococcus aureus* infections
  - ✓ Higher health care costs
  - ✓ Longer hospital stays
  - ✓ More frequent hospital admissions

- Penicillin allergy
  - ✓ Most commonly reported drug allergy, although the vast majority of patients considered to be allergic may tolerate penicillin after evaluation (**Table 2-3**).
  - ✓ Reactions to penicillin (PCN) can be immediate (e.g., IgE-mediated anaphylaxis) or delayed (e.g., DRESS, SJS).
  - ✓ If a PCN allergy is suspected (immediate or delayed), consultation or referral to an allergist for further evaluation is warranted.
  - ✓ Factors that suggest likely IgE-mediated allergy are immediate onset of symptoms (minutes to a few hours) following initial doses of a course of antibiotics, classic IgE-mediated symptoms (hives, angioedema, vomiting, wheezing, anaphylaxis), and recurrent and reproducible symptoms with exposure to same drug or derivatives.
  - ✓ Factors that suggest unlikely IgE-mediated allergy are general or nonhives rash following completion of a course of antibiotics or toward end of a course of antibiotics (i.e., rash development after the last dose of a 10-day course), lack of other IgE-mediated symptoms, symptoms suggestive of delayed drug reaction (fever, malaise, elevated inflammatory markers, mucosal involvement, skin cracking or peeling, toxic appearance).
  - ✓ PCN allergy mimics: Viral exanthem, roseola, Reye syndrome, viral urticaria and/or angioedema, delayed drug reaction.
  - ✓ PCN-specific allergen skin-prick testing and possible oral challenge should be considered for suspected IgE-mediated reactions only. Patients with a distant history (>10 years) of IgE-mediated PCN allergy should be referred for skin-prick testing.
  - ✓ Skin-prick testing is not useful for delayed drug rashes or severe delayed allergic reactions such as DRESS, SJS, and serum sickness.
  - ✓ Patients who experience severe delayed reactions (DRESS, SJS, serum sickness) should avoid PCN derivatives indefinitely.
  - ✓ Guidelines for PCN allergy evaluation and treatment can be found at CHOP Penicillin Allergy Pathway (https://www.chop.edu/clinical-pathway/penicillin-drug-allergy-clinical-pathwayby Lee J, Swami S, Grundmeier R, et al.).

NON-IgE–MEDIATED FOOD ALLERGY

This section focuses on non-IgE–mediated reactions, some of which may be seen in the inpatient setting, including food protein–induced proctocolitis, food protein–induced enterocolitis (or food protein–induced enterocolitis syndrome), and eosinophilic esophagitis.

FOOD PROTEIN–INDUCED PROCTOCOLITIS

EPIDEMIOLOGY

• Food protein–induced proctocolitis occurs in 2–6% of infants in developed countries. Approximately 60% are breastfed. The most common foods triggers are milk and soy.

CLINICAL MANIFESTATIONS

• Healthy-appearing infants who present with streaks of blood or mucus in stools without fissure or identifiable cause
• Unlike those with food protein–induced enterocolitis, these babies are well and are often treated as outpatients.

DIAGNOSTICS

• Diagnosis is made by history.
• Resolution of symptoms following elimination of food from diet (maternal and/or infant) suggests the diagnosis.
• Some babies may have associated iron deficiency anemia.

MANAGEMENT

• Stop offending food(s)—most often milk and soy, because of high rate of cross reactivity in some babies.
• For breastfed babies, maternal dietary restrictions of milk and/or soy is successful.
• Seventy percent of formula-fed infants respond to partially hydrolyzed milk–based formulas, but others may require transition to amino acid–based formula.
• Reintroduction of food around 12 months of age should be attempted, as typical natural history is resolution by this time, but some babies outgrow at a later date, most by 15–18 months of age.

FOOD PROTEIN–INDUCED ENTEROCOLITIS (FPIES)

EPIDEMIOLOGY

• FPIES occurs in 0.16% of infants.
• Most infants have symptoms when ingesting food directly rather than through breast milk after the mother's ingestion.
• Most common triggers in the United States are milk, soy, rice, and oats.
• Other causes include chicken, fish, sweet potatoes, and legumes.

CLINICAL MANIFESTATIONS

• Acute FPIES: Ill-appearing infant who presents 2 hours after ingestion of a food with severe vomiting and lethargy, often followed by diarrhea; may also have hypotension (15–20% may present with hypovolemic shock) and hypothermia
• Chronic FPIES: Ill-appearing infant who presents with more chronic symptoms of abdominal pain, vomiting, failure to thrive, and abnormal stools (chronic diarrhea that may contain mucous or blood)

DIFFERENTIAL DIAGNOSIS

- Acute FPIES: Sepsis, surgical or acute abdomen, malrotation, other causes of shock
- Chronic FPIES: Structural abnormalities, gastroesophageal reflux disease, infection, cyclic vomiting, metabolic disorder, inflammatory bowel disease, behavioral issues

DIAGNOSTICS

- Based on history as there is no confirmatory test.
- Sometimes, an elevated white blood-cell count with neutrophilia is observed.
- If the diagnosis is unclear, a special food challenge is recommended.

MANAGEMENT

- **Acute Management**
  - ✓ Rehydration: Oral rehydration or normal saline fluid boluses
  - ✓ Supportive care
  - ✓ Epinephrine usually does not help.
  - ✓ Ondansetron (IV or IM) has been used with success in some patients.
  - ✓ Avoid trigger foods.
  - ✓ Slowly introduce new foods.
- **Chronic Management**
  - ✓ Avoid known triggers.
  - ✓ Elemental formula may be necessary.
  - ✓ Slowly introduce new foods.
- Most children will outgrow these issues by school age (sometimes by 3 years of age).
- Food challenge in a hospital setting may be appropriate.

EOSINOPHILIC ESOPHAGITIS

EPIDEMIOLOGY

- 1 in 2000 patients in developed countries
- 5–10% of pediatric patients with poorly controlled gastroesophageal reflux

CLINICAL MANIFESTATIONS

- Infants: Regurgitation, frequently spitting up or arching back, abdominal pain, food refusal, at times failure to thrive
- Children: Abdominal pain, regurgitation, vomiting, burning feeling similar to acid reflux, gagging or difficulty swallowing, food aversions, poor weight gain
- Adolescent/adults: Difficulty swallowing, food or pill impaction, regurgitation, abdominal pain

DIFFERENTIAL DIAGNOSIS

- Esophageal reflux, eosinophilic gastroenteritis, Crohn's disease, inflammatory bowel disease, celiac disease, medication, infection, hypereosinophilic syndrome, graft-versus-host disease

DIAGNOSTICS

- Diagnosis is made when patient has a clinical history compatible with this disorder and esophageal eosinophilia (minimum of 15 eosinophils per high-power field) without an alternative diagnosis.

- Classically, patients could be differentiated as proton-pump inhibitor–responsive or requiring food elimination and topical steroid treatment.

MANAGEMENT

- If food or medication impaction is present, removal is top priority.
- This disorder is often co-managed by gastroenterology, allergy, and nutrition specialists.
- Dietary therapy: Food elimination based on most common causes of eosinophilic esophagitis and patient's diet (milk, soy, egg, and/or wheat), allergy testing, or switch to elemental formula (for infants).
- Medical management: Systemic steroids for severe symptoms for short-term therapy. Alternative option for management includes swallowed steroids (viscous budesonide or inhaled steroids). When used, patients should not eat or drink for 30 minutes after dosing.
- May require esophageal dilatation if narrowing is severe (confirmed by barium swallow examination).
- Repeat endoscopy following either dietary or medical management to assess progress

ASTHMA

Asthma is the diffuse, chronic inflammatory disease of large and small airways punctuated by acute exacerbations of airflow obstruction that are at least partially reversible.

EPIDEMIOLOGY

- Affects approximately 1 in 11 children in the United States
- Nearly 1 in 5 children with asthma will present to the emergency department for asthma-related care.
- Higher prevalence in African Americans, Hispanics, and inner-city youth

PATHOPHYSIOLOGY

- Triggers: Allergic (e.g., pet dander, dust mites, pollen), nonspecific stimuli (e.g., smoke, exercise, chemical spray), and infections (e.g., viral, bacterial, fungal)
- Mast cells in airway mucosa release mediators (e.g., histamine, leukotrienes, platelet-activating factor) that cause biphasic immune response:
  ✓ Early (begins within minutes): Bronchoconstriction
  ✓ Late (begins 6–8 hours later): Hypersecretion of mucus, airway edema, epithelial desquamation, and infiltration of inflammatory cells
- Airway obstruction with nonuniform ventilation and atelectasis leads to ventilation/perfusion mismatch. Hyperinflation leads to decreased compliance and increased work of breathing. Increased intrathoracic pressure impairs venous return and reduces cardiac output.

CLINICAL MANIFESTATIONS

- Acute episodes of cough, wheeze, shortness of breath, increased work of breathing, chest pain
- Symptoms can occur outside of viral illness (triggers include exercise, emotional upset, weather change, allergen, irritants [e.g., smoke exposure])
- Family history of asthma and/or atopy is common.
- Relief from asthma medications used in the past may be helpful.
- Comorbid conditions can aggravate flares: Sinusitis, rhinitis, gastroesophageal reflux disease (GERD), obstructive sleep apnea (OSA), allergic bronchopulmonary aspergillosis (ABPA)

Physical Exam Findings

- General: Well-appearing versus ill- or toxic-looking, cough, audible wheeze
- Vital signs: Tachycardia, tachypnea, pulsus paradoxus (systolic blood pressure drop >10 mm Hg with inspiration); decreased pulse oximetry level
- Respiratory: Breathlessness, nasal flaring, accessory muscle use, prominence of ribs or clavicles with inspiration, increase in chest-wall diameter, wheezing (polyphonic), decreased breath sounds, prolonged expiratory phase
- Mental status: altered mental status (somnolent or anxious) is a concern for respiratory insufficiency

DIFFERENTIAL DIAGNOSIS

- Anatomic:
  - ✓ Extrinsic to airway (e.g., bronchial or tracheal stenosis, tracheomalacia, vascular ring, lymphadenopathy, tumor);
  - ✓ Intrinsic to airway (e.g., foreign body, laryngeal web, pulmonary sequestration, bronchial adenoma)
- Inflammatory/infectious: Allergic rhinitis and sinusitis, viral or obliterative bronchiolitis, pneumonia, atypical pneumonia, hypersensitivity pneumonitis, pulmonary hemosiderosis
- Genetic/metabolic: Cystic fibrosis, primary immunodeficiency, ciliary dysfunction, alpha$_1$-antitrypsin deficiency
- Other: Vocal-cord dysfunction, aspiration from swallowing dysfunction or gastroesophageal reflux, habit cough (psychogenic cough), heart disease

DIAGNOSTICS

- Spirometry (in children ≥5 years)
  - ✓ Values are compared to age-, height-, sex-, and race-matched references.
  - ✓ In obstructive conditions like asthma: Decrease in forced expiratory volume in 1 second (FEV_1) and FEV_1/forced vital capacity (FVC) (whereas normal or increased FEV_1/FVC with reduced FVC suggests a restrictive disorder)
  - ✓ In severe cases, FVC can also be reduced because of air trapping.
  - ✓ Reversibility: Increase in FEV_1 ≥12% and ≥10% of predicted after short-acting bronchodilator
  - ✓ Like FEV_1/FVC, decreased forced expiratory flow at 25–75% of FVC ($FEF_{25-75\%}$) correlates with poorer PC_{20} (methacholine concentration causing a 20% fall in FEV_1), peak expiratory flow variability, and bronchodilator response, but has more variability
- Peak expiratory flow (PEF): Spirometry is recommended over PEF for diagnosis, as there is wide variability in published PEF values. It may be useful in the acute setting to compare to patient's personal best value.
- Bronchoprovocation (methacholine, histamine, cold air, exercise): Useful if asthma suspected and spirometry equivocal
- Methacholine challenge: If negative, then helpful in excluding a diagnosis of asthma
  - ✓ A PC_{20} cutoff of 8–16 mg/mL is optimal in identifying patients with asthma.
  - ✓ A positive test is seen in asthma, but also in allergic rhinitis, cystic fibrosis, and chronic obstructive pulmonary disease (COPD).
- Skin testing or ImmunoCAP testing may be indicated to identify potential triggers.

MANAGEMENT OF ACUTE EXACERBATIONS

- Close monitoring of symptoms is needed, as they can change over time (**Table 2-4**).

TABLE 2-4	Classifying Asthma Severity in the Urgent Care Setting		
	Symptoms and Signs	Initial PEF or FEV_1 (% Predicted or Personal Best)	Clinical Course
Mild	Dyspnea only with activity (assess tachypnea in young children)	≥70%	• Usually, care at home • Prompt relief with inhaled SABA • Possible short course of OCS
Moderate	Dyspnea interferes with or limits usual activity	40–69%	• Usually needs office or ED visit • Relief from frequent SABA • OCS; some symptoms last for 1–2 days after treatment has begun
Severe	Dyspnea at rest; interferes with conversation	<40%	• Usually requires ED visit; likely admission • OCS; some symptoms last for >3 days after treatment has begun • Standing use of SABA often necessary
Subset: Life-threatening	Too dyspneic to speak; perspiring	<25%	• ED/admission; possibly intensive-care unit • Minimal or no relief from frequent SABA • IV corticosteroids • Adjunctive therapies helpful

ED = emergency department; FEV_1 = forced expiratory volume in 1 second; OCS = oral corticosteroids; PEF = peak expiratory flow; SABA = short-acting β_2-agonist.

Reproduced with permisison from National Asthma Education and Prevention Program Expert Panel Report 3: Guidelines for the Diagnosis and Management of Asthma. NIH Publication Number 08-5846. October 2007. US Department of Health and Human Services. National Institute of Health. National Heart Lung and Blood Institute.

- Escalation of care in the emergency, inpatient, and primary care setting is outlined in the CHOP Asthma clinical pathways.

    CHOP Asthma Pathways—Emergency (https://www.chop.edu/clinical-pathway/asthma-emergent-care-clinical-pathway by Zorc J, Scarfone R, Reardon A, et al)

    CHOP Asthma Pathway—Inpatient (https://www.chop.edu/clinical-pathway/asthma-inpatient-care-clinical-pathway by Kenyon C, Zorc J, Dunn M, et al)

    Asthma Medications:

- Albuterol: MDI, 4–8 puffs or nebulized 5 mg/dose (for those ≥20 kg) every 20 minutes × 3 doses

- Ipratropium bromide: 0.25–0.5 mg nebulized, every 20 minutes × 3 doses with initial albuterol treatments. Has additive effect with beta-agonists, and reduces likelihood of admission from emergency department (ED). Once hospitalized, no reduction in length of hospital stay has been demonstrated with ongoing therapy with this medication.

- Systemic corticosteroids (for moderate to severe exacerbations):
  ✓ Methylprednisolone 1–2 mg/kg IV, then 1 mg/kg/dose (maximum, 60 mg/day) every 6 hours; or
  ✓ Oral prednisone 2 mg/kg once then 1 mg/kg/dose (maximum, 60 mg); or
  ✓ Dexamethasone (weight-based) orally or IV initially and repeated 12–18 hours later
  ✓ Treatment is usually continued for at least 5 days.

If Severely Ill or Escalating Care, Consider

- Epinephrine 1:1000, 0.01 mg/kg or 0.01 mL/kg (maximum, 0.3 mg or 0.3 mL/dose) subcutaneously (SC) every 15 minutes. (Repeat doses of IM epinephrine can also be used if needed emergently.); or
- Terbutaline 0.01 mg/kg/dose (maximum, 0.4 mg) SC every 10–15 minutes for two doses. For an IV infusion, bolus with 10 mcg/kg (maximum, 750 mcg) over 5 minutes and then start an infusion at 0.4 mcg/kg/min (range, 0.4–3 mcg/kg/min)
- Magnesium sulfate: 25–50 mg/kg (maximum, 2 g) IV/intraosseous over 15–30 minutes. Pretreatment with an isotonic IV fluid bolus is often helpful to prevent hypotension due to vasodilation. Close monitoring of vital signs is recommended during and for 30 minutes after infusion.
- Positive-pressure ventilation with or without endotracheal intubation may be needed in the most extreme cases.

Further Testing

- Arterial blood gases (consider obtaining if there is concern for respiratory insufficiency/failure)
  ✓ Early or mild/moderate exacerbation: Elevated pH, low partial pressure of carbon dioxide (pCO_2), normal or low partial pressure of oxygen (pO_2) (respiratory alkalosis)
  ✓ Respiratory insufficiency is suggested by normal pH and pCO_2 with low pO_2.
  ✓ Respiratory failure is suggested by low pH with elevated pCO_2 (respiratory acidosis) and low pO_2.
- Chest x-ray (obtain only if there is concern for another diagnosis or complication)
  ✓ Typical findings include hyperinflation, peribronchial thickening, atelectasis
  ✓ Other diagnoses or complications may be identified, including pneumonia, aspirated foreign body, pneumothorax, and pulmonary edema due to a cardiac etiology.

Admission to Hospital

If respiratory distress is persistent, oxygen saturation persistently <90%, peak flow rate less than 50% of predicted levels, underlying high-risk factors (e.g., congenital heart disease, neuromuscular disease, cystic fibrosis), ED visit in previous 24 hours, or prior history of severe exacerbation.

Asthma Follow-up and Management

- Patients with uncontrolled asthma or exacerbation should schedule a follow-up appointment within 2 weeks (often helpful to have appointment scheduled prior to discharge).
- For exacerbations requiring ED visit or hospitalization, initiation of a controller medication or step-up therapy should be considered (**Figure 2-2**).
- Upon discharge:
  ✓ Prescribe/refill SABA inhaler with aero-chamber (spacer) and train patient/caregivers in its proper use. (Families should have in hand at time of discharge, if possible)
  ✓ Develop a written asthma action plan and adjust/review with patient/caregivers (see www.nhlbi.nih.gov/health/public/lung/asthma/asthma_actplan.pdf).

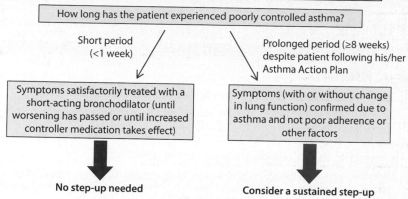

FIGURE 2-2 Consideration for Step-up Asthma Therapy. Reproduced with permission from Chipps BE, Bacharier LB, Farrar JR, et al: The pediatric asthma yardstick: Practical recommendations for a sustained step-up in asthma therapy for children with inadequately controlled asthma, Ann Allergy Asthma Immunol 2018 Jun;120(6):559–579.

✓ Educate patient/family about avoiding identified triggers (smoking, allergen, infections, irritants, pollutants, exercise).

✓ Treat comorbid conditions (allergic bronchopulmonary aspergillosis, GERD, obesity, obstructive sleep apnea, sinusitis, allergic rhinitis)

✓ Ensure that inactivated flu vaccination is up to date for all patients.

✓ For patients with concurrent allergy, consider referral to allergist for consultation. For patients with underlying lung pathology, consider referral to pulmonary specialist.

• Integrate changes to asthma care plan with all health care disciplines (primary care provider, pharmacists, community asthma educators).

Analgesia and Sedation

Arul M. Lingappan, MD
F. Wickham Kraemer III, MD
Melissa Desai Patel, MD, MPH

ANALGESIA

GENERAL PRINCIPLES

Analgesia is the diminution or elimination of pain in the conscious patient.

- Even neonates demonstrate behavioral and hormonal changes in response to painful procedures.
- Children do not have to understand the meaning of pain to communicate pain or to experience it.
- Preemptive analgesia may decrease postinjury opioid requirements

ASSESSMENT OF PAIN

Observational-Behavioral Measures

- Useful in infants and toddlers (who do have physiologic and behavioral responses to pain, such as increased heart rate, blood pressure, respiratory rate, crying, flushing, facial expressions, and body movements)
- Example: FLACC (Face, Leg, Activity, Cry, Consolability) Behavioral Pain Scale (Merkel SI, et al. The FLACC: a behavioral scale for scoring postoperative pain in young children. *Pediatr Nurs* 1997;23:293–297.)

Self-Report

- The OUCHER scale combines numeric and faces scales, making it appropriate for young children (available at https://oucherpainscalecuu.wordpress.com).
- Wong–Baker FACES scale: The child is asked to point to the face that best represents his/her own pain (available at http://www.wongbakerfaces.org).
- Verbal numeric pain rating: Useful in developmentally normal children 6–7 years of age (or older). Pain is rated from 0 to 10 (0 is no pain and 10 is the worst pain imaginable).

NONPHARMACOLOGIC METHODS OF ANALGESIA

- Distraction, music, play
- Acupuncture, massage, and hypnosis are other methods of analgesia; these usually require trained practitioners.

LOCAL ANESTHESIA

EMLA

- 2.5% lidocaine/2.5% prilocaine
- Apply to intact skin; complete anesthesia in 60–90 minutes
- Use for blood drawing/IV placement, bone marrow aspiration, lumbar puncture in nonemergent settings
- May use LMX, which is topical lidocaine only; it has a faster onset, with anesthesia in 30 minutes.
- Contraindications: Methemoglobinemia (avoid EMLA) in children less than 1 month of age

LET

- Used for dermal lacerations; may apply to open wound
- Contraindicated in areas supplied by end arteries (digits, pinna, nose, penis).

VISCOUS LIDOCAINE

- For older children who can expectorate
- Combine with diphenhydramine and aluminum hydroxide, magnesium hydroxide (e.g., Maalox) in equal parts (1:1:1) to create "magic mouthwash" (can exclude lidocaine if mouth sores create a concern for systemic absorption)
- Usual dose: 15 mL of undiluted mixture to "swish and spit" (not swallow); maximum dose is 4.5 mg/kg of body weight or 300 mg of lidocaine component (up to every 3 hours). Smaller amounts work well.

LIDOCAINE JELLY

- Used for nasogastric tube placement and urethral catheterizations

INJECTABLE LOCAL ANESTHETIC

- Buffer with 1 mL (1 meq/mL) sodium bicarbonate ($NaHCO_3$) per 9 mL lidocaine or 0.1 mL $NaHCO_3$ per 10 mL bupivacaine to reduce pain associated with injection.
- Enhance efficacy and duration by using in combination with epinephrine.
- Contraindicated in areas supplied by end arteries (digits, pinna, nose, penis).

NONNARCOTIC ANALGESICS

ACETAMINOPHEN

- Antipyretic; weak analgesic
- Usual dose: 10–15 mg/kg PO or rectally every 4–6 hours; adult dose: 325–650 mg/dose
- Maximum dose: 4 g/day (adults); 75 mg/kg/day (children)
- Acetaminophen should be administered in a separate formulation from an opioid to reduce the toxic potential of an acetaminophen overdose
- Side effects: Hepatic necrosis (overdosage)

NSAIDs

- Useful for inflammatory pain
- Ibuprofen: child dose, 5–10 mg/kg PO every 6–8 hours (maximum, 40 mg/kg/day); adult dose, 200–400 mg/dose (maximum, 1.2 g/day)
- Ketorolac: 0.5 mg/kg/dose IV/IM every 6 hours with maximum of 30 mg every 6 hours, which is the usual adult dose (avoid if postconceptual age is <44 weeks versus <6 months, depending on institutional protocol)
- Naproxen: child dose, 5–10 mg/kg/dose PO every 8–12 hours (maximum, 1000 mg/day); adult dose, 250–500 mg/dose (maximum, 1000 mg/day)
- Side effects: Platelet inhibition, gastrointestinal irritation, nephrotoxicity

ASPIRIN

- No longer routinely used for analgesia because of side effects, but continues to be utilized for its antiplatelet effects in specific situations (e.g., Kawasaki disease, vascular shunts, etc.)
- Side effects: Reye's syndrome (avoid in children with varicella or influenza)

KETAMINE

- Low-dose infusions of 0.1–0.2 mg/kg/hr may be utilized for analgesia (especially in patients who are on long-term opioids as part of a weaning regimen) and higher-dose infusions (e.g., 0.5–2 mg/kg/hr) or boluses (2 mg/kg IV or 4 mg/kg IM) may be used for sedation/anesthesia
- Side effects: Excessive salivary secretions (prevent with glycopyrrolate pretreatment), nystagmus, increased ICP (though cerebral perfusion pressure maintained given increased mean arterial pressure), emergence of delirium or hallucinations

DIAZEPAM

- 0.05–0.1 mg/kg/dose IV every 6–8 hours for muscle spasms and anxiolysis
- 0.1–0.2 mg/kg/dose PO every 6–8 hours (usual adult dosing, 2–10 mg)
- Prolonged half-life can lead to late onset of side effects (sedation, respiratory depression, and hypotension) and can be worsened by coadministration of opioids.

NARCOTIC ANALGESICS

- All doses referred to here are equianalgesic doses.
- All narcotics may have side effects of respiratory depression, sedation, nausea, vomiting, pruritus, and constipation.
- All opioid effects can be reversed with naloxone hydrochloride (Narcan) 0.01 mg/kg IV/IM/SC/ETT; naloxone can be repeated every 2 minutes as needed to a maximum of 10 mg (although lower doses may be considered in postsurgical patients to prevent excessive postoperative pain after reversal).

CODEINE

- Codeine is metabolized into morphine by cytochrome P450 2D6, but this enzyme is absent in up to 10% of the population.
- No longer recommended for use in children because of variable metabolism, where nonmetabolizers will have minimal to no analgesia, and ultrarapid metabolizers will be at risk for excessive sedation, respiratory depression, and death.

FENTANYL

- 0.001 mg/kg/dose IV (=1 mcg/kg/dose) with onset in 1–2 minutes; duration: 0.5–1 hour (repeat or higher dosing may result in increased context-sensitive half-life)
- 0.01 mg/kg/dose transmucosal with onset in 15 minutes (FDA-approved for cancer pain only)
- The transdermal patch is used in chronic pain management for opioid-tolerant patients with expected pain management needs of several weeks.
- Side effects: Use with caution, as chest-wall rigidity may occur with high doses and rapid IV push; reversible with naloxone or neuromuscular paralysis, which will also require endotracheal intubation.

HYDROMORPHONE

- 0.015 mg/kg/dose IV/SC (usual adult dose, 0.4–0.8 mg), with onset in 5–10 minutes; duration: 3–4 hours
- 0.02–0.08 mg/kg/dose PO (usual adult, dose 2–4 mg), with onset in 30–60 minutes; duration: 3–4 hours
- No active metabolites

MEPERIDINE

- Rarely used for analgesic purposes because of severe drug interactions (MAO inhibitors)
- Occasionally used to treat postoperative shivering or medication-induced shaking (e.g., amphotericin-related rigors)
- Side effects: Tachycardia, seizures, worsens bronchospasm, serotonin syndrome
- Active metabolite, normeperidine, may accumulate and induce seizures

METHADONE

- 0.1 mg/kg/dose IV, with onset in 15–30 minutes; duration: 12–24 hours
- 0.1 mg/kg/dose PO, with onset in 30–60 minutes; duration: 12–24 hours
- Rarely used to treat acute pain. Never used as first-line therapy
- Commonly used for sedation withdrawal, as part of an opioid taper
- Side effects: Because of drug accumulation with long half-life, respiratory side effects may not appear until days after drug initiation.
- Contraindications: Prolonged QT syndrome, obtain a baseline ECG, as methadone may prolong QT interval

MORPHINE

- 0.1 mg/kg/dose IV (usual adult dose, 2–4 mg), with onset in 5–10 minutes; duration: 3–4 hours
- 0.1–0.2 mg/kg/dose SC, with onset in 10–30 minutes; duration: 4–5 hours
- 0.3–0.5 mg/kg/dose PO, with onset in 30–60 minutes; duration: 4–5 hours
- Side effects: Nausea, sedation, pruritus, constipation, seizures (in neonates—due to decreased elimination of active metabolite morphine-3-glucuronide)
- Contraindications: Renal failure (active metabolites may accumulate to cause profound sedation and/or respiratory depression)

NALBUPHINE

- 0.1 mg/kg/dose (usual adult dose, 5 mg),with onset in 5–10 minutes; duration: 6 hours
- Partial opioid agonist, results in plateau of analgesic effects but also minimizes risk of respiratory depression
- May be used to treat opioid-related side effects (e.g., pruritus, nausea/vomiting) due to the partial opioid antagonism at the mu receptor
- Relative contraindications: Long-term opioids such as nalbuphine may precipitate acute opioid withdrawal

OXYCODONE

- 0.1 mg/kg/dose PO, with onset in 30–60 minutes; duration: 4–6 hours
- Active metabolite, oxymorphone, can accumulate in renal failure
- When oxycodone is available in combination with acetaminophen (Percocet), there is limited utility in young children because of the toxicity of acetaminophen.

PCA

- Indicated for acute/chronic pain of known etiology as well as preemptive pain management.
- Cardiorespiratory monitoring is required.
- Minimum developmental age of about 7 years to self-administer PCA
- Parents and nurses can also be trained to administer PCA to younger patients and those with developmental delay
- Route: IV or, rarely, SC

- Dosing for PCA:
  - ✓ Morphine: Basal dose, 10–20 μg/kg/hr; bolus dose, 10–20 μg/kg; lockout, 8–10 minutes, four to six boluses per hour; maximum total dose per hour, 100–150 μg/kg
  - ✓ Hydromorphone: Basal dose, 3–4 μg/kg/hr; bolus dose, 3–4 μg/kg/hr; lockout, 8–10 minutes, four to six boluses per hour; maximum total dose per hour, 15–20 μg/kg
  - ✓ Fentanyl: Basal dose, 0.25–1 μg/kg/hr; bolus dose, 0.25–1 μg/kg; lockout, 8–10 minutes, two to three boluses per hour; maximum total dose per hour, 2 μg/kg

SEDATION

SEDATION IS A CONTINUUM

- Minimal sedation (anxiolysis): A drug-induced state in which cognitive function and coordination may be impaired. Patients respond normally to verbal commands. Protective airway reflexes are maintained. Ventilatory and cardiovascular functions are unaffected.
- Moderate sedation: A drug-induced state of depressed consciousness. Patients respond purposefully to verbal commands, either alone or accompanied by light tactile stimulation. There is significant loss of orientation to environment, with moderate impairment of gross motor function. Protective airway reflexes are maintained. Able to maintain patent airway and cardiovascular function. There may be mild alterations in ventilatory responsiveness
- Deep sedation: A drug-induced state of depressed consciousness or unconsciousness from which a patient is not easily aroused. Patients may respond purposefully to painful stimulation. May be accompanied by a partial or complete loss of protective reflexes, which may include the inability to maintain a patent airway independently, and respond purposefully to physical stimulation or verbal command. Spontaneous ventilation may be inadequate. Cardiovascular function is usually maintained.
- General anesthesia: Drug-induced loss of consciousness with loss of protective reflexes, inability to maintain patent airway, and loss of purposeful response. Cardiovascular function may be impaired.

PREPARATION FOR SEDATION

Patient-Related Factors

- Presedation assessment (**Table 3-1** and **Figure 3-1**): Essential to identify high-risk patient populations to both anticipate and reduce adverse sedation events.
- NPO guidelines (American Society of Anesthesiology [ASA]):
  - ✓ No clear liquids for 2 hours before sedation
  - ✓ No breast milk for 4 hours prior to sedation
  - ✓ No formula, milk or light meals for 6 hours prior to sedation
  - ✓ No fatty foods or full meals for 8 hours prior to sedation
  - ✓ In an emergency situation: Delay sedation if possible or use lightest possible level of sedation. Consider elective intubation for airway protection.
- ASA classification:
  - I: Normal healthy patient
  - II: Mild systemic disease
  - III: Severe systemic disease
  - IV: Severe systemic disease associated with significant dysfunction and potential threat to life
  - V: Critical medical condition for which operative intervention is critical to survival

TABLE 3-1	Presedation Assessment

- History
  - ✓ Allergies and adverse reactions
  - ✓ Current medications
  - ✓ Indication for procedure
  - ✓ Previous sedation/anesthesia history
  - ✓ History of upper airway problems, obstructive sleep apnea, snoring
  - ✓ Prematurity and corrected gestational age (if applicable)
  - ✓ Major medical illnesses, physical abnormalities (e.g., facial dysmorphisms, scoliosis, syndromes, etc.), neurologic problems, developmental delays
  - ✓ Review of systems addressing active pulmonary, cardiac, renal, hepatic, and metabolic concerns
  - ✓ Current or recent illnesses (e.g., upper respiratory infection, fever, anemia, etc.)
  - ✓ Relevant family history (e.g., anesthesia-related complications)
- Examination
  - ✓ Age
  - ✓ Weight
  - ✓ Vital signs (including blood pressure, heart rate, respiratory rate, oxygen saturation)
  - ✓ Cardiovascular exam
  - ✓ Lung exam
  - ✓ Neurologic exam
  - ✓ Mental status
  - ✓ Airway status (see Figure 3-1 for Mallampati Classification)

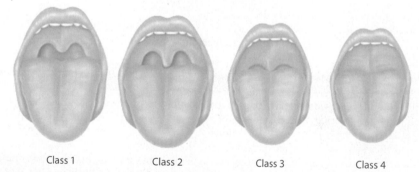

| Class 1 | Class 2 | Class 3 | Class 4 |

FIGURE 3-1 Mallampati classification of pharyngeal structures. Class 1, soft palate, fauces, uvula, pillars; class 2, soft palate, fauces, portion of uvula; class 3, soft palate, base of uvula; class 4, hard palate only. Reproduced with permission from Bruncardi FC, Anderson DK, Billar TR, et al: *Schwartz's Principles of Surgery*, 11th ed. New York, NY: McGraw Hill; 2019.

Procedural Considerations

- Duration of procedure
- Painful versus nonpainful
- Position for procedure
- Need for immobility
- Age and ability to cooperate with instructions

Provider-Related Factors
- At least two dedicated sedation providers are required—one to administer the sedation and the other to monitor it.
- When deep sedation/general anesthesia is administered, the sedation provider cannot also be the provider performing the procedure.
- Providers require airway skills and advanced life support skills. They must have experience in managing complications and the ability to rescue a patient from a level of sedation that is deeper than anticipated.
- Traditionally administered by anesthesiologists, intensivists, and emergency medicine physicians with support from registered nurse, certified registered nurse anesthetist, nurse practitioner, or physician assistant
- Increasing number of pediatric hospitalists perform sedation within a dedicated sedation program, with similar outcomes and complication rates. The dedicated sedation program includes a robust training program, as well as a credentialing maintenance program.

Equipment (can use SOAPME acronym)
- Suction—Apparatus including catheters (soft suction, Yankauer tip)
- Oxygen—Supply and age-appropriate–sized positive-pressure oxygen delivery system
- Airway—Size-appropriate equipment (nasopharyngeal and oropharyngeal airways, face-mask, bag–valve–mask, etc.)
- Pharmacy—Medications for sedation, sedative antagonists and resuscitation, IV fluids
- Monitors—Pulse oximeter, blood pressure, ECG, end-tidal CO_2 detector, stethoscope
- Equipment—Special equipment or drugs for the given case

Monitoring
- Continuous pulse oximetry, heart rate, and end-tidal monitoring
- Vital signs with blood pressure monitored every 15 minutes for minimal sedation and every 5 minutes for moderate or deep sedation
- Consider full cardiorespiratory monitoring for specific cases (e.g., ketamine)
- Backup system for emergencies: Highly trained and reliable staff (e.g., code team, 911)

OVERVIEW OF SEDATIVE DRUGS

- Providing adequate sedation often requires medications from various classes (i.e., analgesic and hypnotic) to achieve adequate levels of sedation. Keep in mind that polypharmacy is associated with higher rates of complications.
- Anxiolytics make patients more relaxed
  - ✓ Benzodiazepines (e.g., diazepam, midazolam, lorazepam): Provide anxiolysis and amnesia. Often used as premedication or as adjunct with analgesics. Administered PO, IV, IN, IM, or PR
  - ✓ Nitrous oxide: Anxiolytic with some analgesia effect. Administered via inhaled delivery system
- Analgesics—Achieve pain control
  - ✓ Lidocaine (e.g., LMX): Local analgesia at the procedure site. Administered topically or SC.
  - ✓ Opioid agonists (e.g., fentanyl, morphine, hydromorphone): Dose-dependent analgesia and sedation. Often used in conjunction with anxiolytics or hypnotics. Administered PO, IV, or IN.
  - ✓ Ketamine: Dissociative sedative with analgesic and amnestic properties. Administered PO, IV, or IM.

- Hypnotics—Achieve sleep/immobility, especially useful for noninvasive procedures
  - ✓ Chloral hydrate: Produces sleep with mild-to-moderate respiratory depression. Currently limited manufacturing resources. Administered PO or PR.
  - ✓ Barbiturates (e.g., pentobarbital): Potent sedative, hypnotic, and anesthetic properties. Administered PO, IV, or PR.
  - ✓ Central α_2-adrenergic agonists (e.g., clonidine, dexmedetomidine): Sedative, anxiolytic, and sometimes analgesic properties. Administered PO, IN, or IV.
  - ✓ Etomidate: Short-acting anesthetic and amnestic. Especially useful in settings of hemodynamic instability. Administered IV.
  - ✓ Propofol: Sedative, hypnotic, and anesthetic properties. Administered IV.
- Sedative antagonists
  - ✓ Flumazenil: Short-acting agent that reverses benzodiazepine-induced sedation. Use cautiously in patients with seizure disorders, as benzodiazepine reversal can induce seizures.
  - ✓ Naloxone: Short-acting agent that reverses opiate-induced sedation

SEDATION-RELATED COMPLICATIONS

- Airway obstruction
- Laryngospasm
- Hypoventilation and apnea
- Vomiting/aspiration
- Cardiovascular instability
- Emergence agitation/delirium

POSTSEDATION RECOVERY AND DISCHARGE

- Throughout recovery, the patient should be monitored with vital signs at regular intervals until patient is awake and interactive
- Patients should be discharged only after specific criteria have been met: Stable vital signs, adequate pain control, return to level of consciousness that is similar to baseline for that patient, adequate head control and muscle strength to maintain patent airway, adequate hydration (tolerates oral challenge), and nausea/vomiting should be controlled

PROCEDURE-SPECIFIC SEDATION

CT SCAN

- Need for relative immobility but not analgesia. CT scanning is of short duration.
- Young infants often can be swaddled and may not require sedation. Patients 6 months–3 years old are the most likely age group to require sedation
- Option 1: Pentobarbital 2–4 mg/kg PO 30 minutes before procedure; repeat half dose 20–30 minutes after initial dose if patient still moving. Maximum dose, 100 mg or 8 mg/kg. Works well in infants <10 kg who do not require an IV for the procedure. Can use in conjunction with IN Versed or fentanyl if additional sedation is needed.
- Option 2: Propofol 2 mg/kg IV push with additional increments of 0.5–1 mg/kg as needed to get patient still. Time to sedation is 1–2 minutes, and time to recovery is 15 min–1 hour.
- Midazolam and fentanyl are unreliable in producing sedation with immobility but can be used as an adjunct to hypnotics to decrease the total dose of longer-acting medications.

MRI

- Need for relative immobility but not analgesia. MRI typically lasts >45 minutes.
- Young infants can often be swaddled or placed in an immobilizer device and may not require sedation.
- Children 6–8 years of age often require sedation, but some older children, especially those with developmental delays, claustrophobia, attention-deficit/hyperactivity disorder (ADHD), and/or anxiety, may require sedation as teenagers
- Option 1: Pentobarbital 2–3 mg/kg IV (maximum dose, 100 mg/dose) with titration to response. Give in increments of 1–3 mg/kg. Can use in conjunction with IV midazolam (0.05–0.1 mg/kg [maximum, 2.5 mg/dose]) and fentanyl (1 µg/kg [maximum, 100 µg/dose]) to reduce total pentobarbital dose required
- Option 2: Propofol: 2 mg/kg IV (maximum, 100 mg/dose) with titration to response. Give in increments of 0.5–2 mg/kg. Will require an infusion of 150–250 µg/kg/min to maintain deep sedation for duration of imaging.

LUMBAR PUNCTURE

- Infants younger than 2 months are not routinely sedated for this procedure.
- Topical or local injection of lidocaine should be included as part of the analgesia for this procedure.
- Nitrous oxide: 50–70% nitrous titrated to effect. Can add 1 µg/kg fentanyl if patients have an IV in place.
- Midazolam 0.05–0.1 mg/kg IV given 3–5 minutes before lumbar puncture significantly decreases anxiety in older children. Repeat 0.1 mg/kg IV doses as needed to achieve adequate sedation (maximum, 2.5 mg/dose).
- Fentanyl 1–2 µg/kg IV given via slow push over 3–5 minutes can provide analgesia. Repeat 1 µg/kg IV doses as needed to achieve adequate sedation (maximum, 100 µg/dose)
- Can use midazolam and fentanyl together to achieve moderate to deep sedation as indicated. Can consider adding ketamine or pentobarbital as needed, depending on patient-specific characteristics (see options below)

PAINFUL PROCEDURES

Examples of painful procedures may include fracture reduction, incision and drainage, burn debridement, and placement of a central venous line.

- Option 1: Midazolam 0.05–0.1 mg/kg IV (maximum, 2.5 mg/dose) plus fentanyl 1–2 µg/kg IV (maximum, 100 µg/dose). Titrate additional doses as needed to achieve adequate sedation.
- Option 2: Ketamine 0.5–2 mg/kg slow IV push (maximum, 100 mg/dose). Titrate additional doses as needed to achieve adequate sedation. Consider atropine or glycopyrrolate premedication to decrease secretions. Can use midazolam and fentanyl adjuncts if needed to reduce total ketamine dose. In addition, midazolam may reduce side effects of hallucinations from ketamine.
- Option 3: Fentanyl 1 mcg/kg (maximum dose, 100 mcg) or ketamine 0.5 mg/kg (maximum dose, 50 mg) followed by propofol 1 mg/kg bolus. May repeat propofol 0.5 mg/kg bolus until desired effect is reached. Can start propofol infusion at 150 mcg/kg/min to maintain sedation for longer procedures.
- When using combination of sedatives/analgesics, start with lowest dose possible and give additional doses as needed to achieve desired depth of sedation.

WEANING NARCOTICS AND SEDATIVES

- Patients who have been taking narcotics, benzodiazepines, or other classes of medications for an extended duration may develop withdrawal symptoms if these medications are abruptly discontinued. Therefore, these medications should be gradually weaned (e.g., 10–20% dose reduction every other day) while watching for withdrawal symptoms.
- After decreasing the medication dose to a normal starting dose (e.g., oxycodone 0.1 mg/kg/dose), the dosing interval can be increased to every 8–12 hours as needed, then daily as needed before stopping
- Withdrawal symptoms from opioids include pupillary dilation, diarrhea, sweating, muscle aches, tachypnea, tachycardia, and hypertension.
- Withdrawal symptoms from benzodiazepines include tremor, agitation, tachypnea, tachycardia, and hypertension.
- There may be a delay (e.g., days) between the reduction of the analgesic or sedative medication and the onset of withdrawal symptoms. Consider administering a rescue dose of that class of medication to see if the patient's symptoms abate.
- For patients on both opioids and benzodiazepines, weaning the opioid first is usually better tolerated. By focusing on weaning one medication at a time, there is less confusion about the cause of any withdrawal symptoms.

Calculations

Robert P. Kavanagh, MD
Samuel A. Rosenblatt, MD, MSEd
Donald L. Boyer, MD, MSEd, FAAP

ALVEOLAR-ARTERIAL OXYGEN GRADIENT (A-a GRADIENT)

$$\text{A-a gradient} = PAO_2 - PaO_2$$
$$PAO_2 = F_iO_2(P_{atm} - P_{H_2O}) - (PaCO_2/R)$$

$PAO_2 = $ *Alveolar partial pressure of O_2 [mm Hg]*
$PaO_2 = $ *Arterial partial pressure of O_2 [mm Hg]*
$F_iO_2 = $ *Fraction of inspired O_2 (0.21 in room air)*
$P_{atm} = $ *Atmospheric pressure (about 760 mm Hg at sea level)*
$P_{H_2O} = $ *Partial pressure of water vapor (about 47 mm Hg at 37°C)*
$PaCO_2 = $ *Arterial partial pressure of CO_2 [mm Hg]*
$R = $ *Respiratory quotient, reflecting basal metabolic rate describing amount of CO_2 production for a given O_2 consumption (ranges from 0.7 to 1; usually 0.8 is used)*

- Measure of the efficiency of the oxygenation of blood
- The normal A-a gradient varies with age. A helpful calculation is [age(in years)/4] + 4
- Normal A-a gradient ranges from 5–10 mm Hg when breathing room air and 20–65 mm Hg when on 100% O_2. A higher A-gradient reflects impaired transfer of oxygen from the alveoli to the peri-alveolar capillaries
- Gradient is affected by V/Q or diffusion abnormalities but unaffected by hyperventilation or hypoventilation.
- If PaO_2 corrects with supplemental O_2, consider asthma or other conditions associated with V/Q mismatch.
- If PaO_2 does not correct with supplemental O_2, consider shunt.

ABSOLUTE NEUTROPHIL COUNT

$$ANC = WBC \times (PMN/100 + Bands/100)$$

$WBC = $ *White blood cell count [cells/mm³]*
$PMN = $ *Percentage of polymorphonuclear neutrophils*
$Bands = $ *Percentage of band neutrophils*

- Neutropenia is defined as an ANC less than 1500 cells/mm³.
- Severe neutropenia (ANC <500 cells/mm³) is associated with a high risk of infection.

ANION GAP (SERUM)

$$\text{Serum AG} = [Na^+] - ([Cl^-] + [HCO_3^-])$$

$[Na^+] = $ *Serum concentration of sodium ions [meq/L]*
$[Cl^-] = $ *Serum concentration of chloride ions [meq/L]*
$[HCO_3^-] = $ *Serum concentration of bicarbonate ions [meq/L]*

- Aids in classifying metabolic acidosis
- The normal anion gap is 8–12 meq/L.
- An elevated anion gap is caused by an increase in unmeasured anions, which may be any of the following:
  "MUD PILES": methanol; uremia; diabetic ketoacidosis; paraldehyde or phenformin; iron, infection, or isoniazid; lactic acidosis; ethanol or ethylene glycol; and salicylates
- Acidosis with a normal anion gap ("non–anion gap acidosis") is generally caused by a loss of HCO_3^-, which can be associated with multiple causes, including the following:
  "HARD-UP": hyperalimentation; acetazolamide; renal tubular acidosis; diarrhea; ureteroenteric fistula; pancreaticoduodenal fistula

  Note: Hypoalbuminemia leads to underestimation of the AG and requires the following correction: Corrected AG = AG + 0.25(40 − Alb)

ARTERIAL OXYGEN CONTENT (CaO₂)

$$CaO_2 = (Hgb \times 1.36 \times SaO_2) + (0.003 \times PaO_2)$$

Hgb: Hemoglobin concentration [g/dL]
SaO_2: Oxygen saturation of arterial blood (in decimal form, e.g. 99% = 0.99)
PaO_2: Arterial partial pressure of O_2 [mm Hg]
(1 g Hgb can carry 1.36 mL of oxygen [mL/g])
0.003: Oxygen solubility coefficient [O_2/dL/mm Hg]

- Directly reflects the total number of oxygen molecules in the arterial blood, both bound to hemoglobin and dissolved in plasma.
- The SaO_2 may be obtained by pulse oximetry and reflects the oxygen bound by hemoglobin.
- Note that the contribution of dissolved oxygen (as reflected in the latter portion of the equation [$0.003 \times PaO_2$]) is very small but becomes more clinically significant in cases of severe anemia, When the amount of bound oxygen is reduced due to lower hemoglobin levels.
- Normal CaO_2 range for healthy adults: 17–24 mL/dL

BIOSTATISTICS

	Disease	No Disease
Positive test	TP	FP
Negative test	FN	TN

FN = false negative; FP = false positive; TN = true negative; TP = true positive.

- Prevalence: Proportion of people with disease in an entire population
  {(TP + FN)/(TP + FP + FN + TN)}
  Remember that "incidence" is the number of new cases in a time frame (often a year) and prevalence is the number of people with disease in the total population at any one time.
- Sensitivity: Proportion of people with the disease who test positive.
  ✓ Sensitivity = {TP/(TP + FN)}
- Specificity: Proportion of people without the disease who test negative.
  ✓ Specificity = {TN/(FP + TN)}

- Positive predictive value (PPV): Proportion of people with a positive test result who actually have the disease
  - ✓ PPV = {TP/(TP + FP)}
- Negative predictive value (NPV): Proportion of people with a negative test result who do not have the disease
  - ✓ NPV = {TN/(FN + TN)}
- Odds ratio (OR): Evaluates whether the odds of a certain event or outcome is the same for two groups
  - ✓ OR = (TP × TN)/(FN × FP)
- Absolute risk reduction (ARR): The difference on outcome rates between the control and the treatment groups
  - ✓ ARR = CER − EER, where CER is the control group event rate and EER is the experimental event rate
- Relative risk reduction (RRR): Measures how much the risk (rate of some outcome) is reduced in the experimental group compared to the control group
  - ✓ RRR = (CER – EER)/CER
- Number needed to treat (NNT): The number of patients that would need to be treated to prevent one bad outcome
  - ✓ NNT = 1/ARR or 1/(CER − EER)
- Likelihood ratio for a test result is defined as the ratio between the probability of observing that result in patients with the disease in question, and the probability of that result in patients without the disease

$$\text{Positive likelihood ratio} = \text{sensitivity}/(1 - \text{specificity})$$
$$\text{Negative likelihood ratio} = (1 - \text{sensitivity})/\text{specificity}$$

BODY MASS INDEX (BMI)

$$\text{Body Mass Index} = \text{Weight/Height}^2$$

Weight [kg]
Height [m]
- Adult values [kg/m²]: Normal is 18.5–24.9; overweight is 25–30; obese is greater than 30
- Pediatric norms vary by age and according to growth charts

BODY SURFACE AREA (MOSTELLER METHOD)

$$\text{BSA} = \sqrt{\text{Weight} \times \text{Height}/3600}$$

BSA = Body surface area [m²]
Weight [kg]
Height [cm] (notice difference from BMI calculation which is in meters)
- Used to calculate dosages for certain medications (e.g., steroids, chemotherapeutic agents)
- Other formulas for BSA have been derived (Boyd, Dubois, and Haycock).

CARDIAC OUTPUT (CARDIAC INDEX)

$$CO = HR \times SV$$
$$CI = CO/BSA$$

CO = Cardiac output [L/min]
HR = Heart rate [beats/min]
SV = Stroke volume [L/beat]
CI = Cardiac index [L/min/m^2]
BSA = Body-surface area [m^2]

- Stroke volume is influenced by preload, contractility, and afterload
- Cardiac index is preferred in pediatrics to account for the size of the patient
- The normal range of the cardiac index at rest is 2.6–4.2 L/min/m^2

CEREBRAL PERFUSION PRESSURE

$$CPP = MAP - ICP$$

or

$$CPP = MAP - CVP$$

(choice of equation is determined by whichever "downstream" pressure is higher [ICP or CVP])
CPP = Cerebral perfusion pressure [mm Hg]
CVP = Central venous pressure (direct measure) [mm Hg]
MAP = Mean arterial pressure (calculated or direct measure) [mm Hg]
ICP = Intracranial pressure (direct measure) [mm Hg]

- ICP monitoring should be considered in comatose patients with severe traumatic brain injury.
- Maintenance of CPP may reduce cerebral ischemia after brain injury and improve outcomes
- Note that in a hypotensive patient, even small increases in ICP can have a detrimental effect on CPP.
- Generally, a goal ICP <20 mmHg is desired for patients recovering from a brain injury
- CPP goals may vary with age, ranging from >40 mmHg in infants to >60 mmHg in adolescents; excessively low CPP is associated with secondary hypoxic injury.
- MAP can be calculated by adding one-third the pulse pressure to the diastolic pressure (see MAP calculation).

CHANGE IN SERUM SODIUM (ΔSODIUM)

$$\Delta Sodium = (\text{Infusate Na}^+ + \text{Infusate K}^+ - \text{Serum Na}^+)/(TBW + 1)$$

ΔSodium [mmol/L] = Expected change in serum sodium for every 1 L of infused fluid
Infusate Na$^+$: Amount of sodium in infusion [mmol/L]
Infusate K$^+$: Amount of potassium in infusion [mmol/L]
Serum Na$^+$: Serum sodium [mmol]
TBW: Total body water (Liters)

TBW Watson Formula*:	Male TBW	$2.447 - (0.09 \times age) + (0.11 \times height) + (0.34 \times weight)$
	Female TBW	$-2.1 + (0.11 \times height) + (0.25 \times weight)$

*Generally estimated at 60% of total body weight (kg); age measured in years; height measured in centimeters; weight measured in kilograms; TBW is higher (about 70%) in neonates and infants.

- Equation predicts change in serum sodium associated with administration of 1 L of intravenous fluid. May be used to limit the risk of demyelinating encephalopathy due to rapid correction of hyponatremia or hypernatremia

CONVERSIONS OF UNITS

$°Fahrenheit = (1.8 × °Celsius) + 32$
1 inch = 2.54 centimeters (cm)
1 teaspoon = 5 milliliters (mL)
1 tablespoon = 15 milliliters (mL)
1 fluid ounce = 30 milliliters (mL)
1 deciliter (dL) = 0.1 liter (L)
1 dry ounce = 30 grams (g)
1 atmosphere = 760 mm Hg = 760 torr (1 torr = 1 mm Hg)
1 mm Hg = 1.36 cm H_2O
2.2 pounds = 1 kilogram (kg)
1 milligram (mg) = 0.001 gram (g)
1 microgram (mcg or μg) = 0.001 milligrams (mg)

CORRECTED SERUM CALCIUM (FOR HYPOALBUMINEMIA)

$$Corrected\ Calcium = [(Normal\ albumin - Measured\ albumin) × 0.8] + Ca$$

Normal *serum albumin concentration is about 4.0 g/dL*
Ca = *Measured serum calcium concentration [mg/dL]*
- Corrects the measured total serum calcium concentration to account for hypoalbuminemia
- Total calcium level reflects both bound and free (ionized) calcium levels.

CORRECTED SERUM SODIUM (FOR HYPERGLYCEMIA)

$$Corrected\ Sodium = Na^+ + (Gluc - 100) × 1.6/100$$

Na^+ = Serum *sodium concentration [mmol/L]*
$Gluc$ = Serum *glucose concentration [mmol/L]*

CREATININE CLEARANCE (FROM TIMED URINE SPECIMEN)

$$CrCl = (U_{Cr} × U_{vol})/(P_{Cr} × T_{min})$$

$$Corrected\ CrCl = CrCl × 1.73/BSA$$

$CrCl$ = *Creatinine clearance [mL/min]*
$Corrected\ CrCl$ = *Corrected to a body surface area (BSA) of 1.73 m² [mL/min/1.73 m²]*
U_{Cr} = *Urine creatinine [mg/dL]*
U_{vol} = *Urine volume [mL]*
P_{Cr} = *Plasma creatinine concentration [mg/dL]*
T_{min} = *Time of urine collection [minutes]*
- Represents the volume of plasma cleared of creatinine per unit time
- Creatinine is freely filtered, not reabsorbed, and minimally secreted by the kidneys. Thus, creatinine clearance is an estimate of glomerular filtration.
- CrCl is often normalized to a BSA of 1.73 m² in order to compare with reference values

CREATININE CLEARANCE (SCHWARTZ METHOD)

$$CrCl = K \times Height/P_{Cr}$$

CrCl = Creatinine clearance [mL/min]
K (age-dependent constant) = 0.33 for low birth weight infants; 0.45 for term infants; 0.55 for children; 0.55 for adolescent girls; 0.7 for adolescent boys
Height [cm]
P_{Cr} = Plasma creatinine concentration [mg/dL]

- The Schwartz equation provides a simple estimate of creatinine clearance (glomerular filtration rate [GFR]) in children based on height and serum/plasma creatinine.
- GFR can be used to screen for kidney disease, follow disease progression, confirm the need for definitive treatment (e.g., dialysis, transplantation), and help determine medication dose adjustments for patients with kidney injury or disease.

ENDOTRACHEAL TUBE SIZE

$$ETT\ size(mm) = [Age(yr)/4] + 4$$

ETT = Endotracheal tube (inner diameter size)
- Subtract 0.5 mm for cuffed tubes.
- Tube size correlates more reliably with height than with weight.

FRACTIONAL EXCRETION OF SODIUM (FE$_{Na}$)

$$FE_{Na} = 100 \times (U_{Na} \times P_{Cr})/(U_{Cr} \times P_{Na})$$

U_{Na} = Urine sodium concentration [meq/L]
P_{Cr} = Plasma creatinine concentration [mg/dL]
U_{Cr} = Urine creatinine concentration [mg/dL]
P_{Na} = Plasma sodium concentration [meq/L]

- FE_{Na} <1.0% suggests prerenal kidney injury
- FE_{Na} >2.0% suggests intrinsic or postrenal kidney injury

FRACTIONAL EXCRETION OF UREA (FE$_{UREA}$)

$$FE_{Urea} = 100 \times (U_{Urea} \times P_{Cr})/(U_{Cr} \times P_{Urea})$$

U_{Urea} = Urine urea concentration [mg/dL]
P_{Cr} = Plasma creatinine concentration [mg/dL]
U_{Cr} = Urine creatinine concentration [mg/dL]
P_{Urea} = Plasma urea concentration (blood urea nitrogen, BUN) [mg/dL]

- May be more accurate than FENa for patients receiving diuretic medications
- FE_{Urea} <35% suggests prerenal kidney injury
- FE_{Urea} >50% suggests intrinsic renal disease (acute tubular necrosis)

FREE WATER DEFICIT

$$FWD = Coefficient \times Weight \times (Na/140 - 1)$$

FWD = *Free water deficit [L]*
Weight [kg]
Na = Measured serum sodium concentration [meq/L]
Coefficient: 0.6 for children and nonelderly men; 0.5 for nonelderly women and elderly men; 0.45 for elderly women.
- In cases of hypernatremia, this formula is used to determine the volume of free water that would be required to correct the serum sodium to normal (usually given as 140 mEq/L, but may be adjusted for patients whose normal sodium levels are higher or lower).
- Overly rapid correction of hypernatremia may cause cerebral edema.

GLUCOSE INFUSION RATE (GIR)

$$GIR = [IV\ rate\ (mL/hr) \times Dextrose\ \% \times 1000(mg/g)] / [Weight\ (kg) \times 60(min/hr) \times 100(mL/dL)]$$

Glucose infusion rate (GIR) [mg/kg/min]
IV rate = Hourly IV fluid administration rate (mL/hr)
Dextrose % = Percent dextrose (glucose) in intravenous fluid (e.g., D10 = 10% dextrose = 10 g/dL dextrose = 100 g/L dextrose)
- Used in the management of hypoglycemia, especially in neonates
- Glucose utilization of healthy neonates is approximately 5–8 mg/kg/min

MEAN ARTERIAL PRESSURE (MAP)

$$MAP = \tfrac{1}{3}SBP + \tfrac{2}{3}DBP$$

or

$$MAP = DBP + \tfrac{1}{3}PP$$

SBP = Systolic blood pressure [mmHg]
DBP = Diastolic blood pressure [mmHg]
PP = Pulse pressure (SBP – DBP) [mmHg]
- Based on assumption that diastole lasts approximately twice as long as systole
- The MAP is considered to be the pressure that perfuses all the organs except the heart, which is perfused mostly during diastole.

OSMOLALITY (SERUM)

$$Serum\ Osm = (2 \times Na^+) + \frac{Gluc}{18} + \frac{BUN}{2.8}$$

Na^+ = Serum sodium concentration [meq/L]
Gluc = Serum glucose concentration [mg/dL]
BUN = Blood urea nitrogen concentration [mg/dL]
- Normal serum osmolality is approximately 285–295 mOsm/L.
- Osmolal gap = Measured Osm − Calculated Osm (normal ≤10 mOsm/L)
- If the measured serum osmolality is more than 10 mOsm/L above the calculated serum osmolality, consider causes for an osmolal gap due to unmeasured osmotically active substances such as mannitol, ethanol, methanol, and ethylene glycol.

OXYGENATION INDEX (OI)

$$OI = [P_{maw} \times FiO_2 \times 100]/PaO_2$$

P_{maw} = *Mean airway pressure [cm H_2O]*
FiO_2 = *Fraction of inspired oxygen (e.g., 21% = 0.21)*
PaO_2 = *Arterial partial pressure of O_2 [mm Hg]*
- A higher OI indicates more severe lung disease
- Used as part of the criteria for pediatric ARDS (PARDS):
     Normal <4, Mild 4–8, Moderate 8–16, Severe >16
- OI >25, mortality >40%
- OI >40 has been suggested as a threshold for considering extracorporeal membrane oxygenation (ECMO) support

P/F RATIO

$$P/F = PaO_2/FiO_2$$

PaO_2 = *Arterial partial pressure of O_2 [mm Hg]*
FiO_2 = *Fraction of inspired oxygen (e.g., 21% = 0.21)*
- Index of severity of hypoxemia; lower number indicates more severe lung disease.
- Used as part of the definition of pediatric acute respiratory distress syndrome (PARDS).
- For a patient with acute respiratory failure on positive end-expiratory pressure (PEEP) of ≥5 cmH$_2$O, bilateral lung disease, and the absence of left atrial hypertension:
✓ P:F 200-300 = mild ARDS
✓ P:F 100-200 = moderate ARDS
✓ P:F < 100 = severe ARDS

Q_p/Q_s RATIO

$$Q_p/Q_s = [S_{Ao}O_2 - S_{MV}O_2]/[S_{PV}O_2 - S_{PA}O_2]$$

Q_p = *Pulmonary blood flow [L/min]*
Q_s = *Systemic blood flow [L/min]*
$S_{Ao}O_2$ = *Oxygen saturation of aortic blood [%]*
$S_{MV}O_2$ = *Oxygen saturation of mixed venous blood [%]*
$S_{PV}O_2$ = *Oxygen saturation of pulmonary venous blood [%]*
$S_{PA}O_2$ = *Oxygen saturation of pulmonary arterial blood [%]*
- Q_p:Q_s is derived from the Fick principle and represents the ratio of pulmonary blood flow to systemic blood flow
- In a two-ventricle heart without shunts, Q_p:Q_s = 1
- With a left-to-right shunt, Q_p:Q_s >1; with a right-to-left shunt, Q_p:Q_s <1
- Central venous blood (e.g., right atrial sample) is often substituted for mixed venous blood
- $S_{PV}O_2$ is assumed to be 95–99% in the absence of lung disease
- For single-ventricle patients prior to stage II repair, $S_{PA}O_2 = S_{Ao}O_2$

QT INTERVAL CORRECTED (QT$_c$ [BAZETT])

$$QT_c = QT/\sqrt{RR}$$

QT = Measured QT interval [seconds]
RR = Preceding RR interval [seconds]
1 box width = 0.04 seconds (assuming 25 mm/sec)
- QT_c > 0.45 seconds is concerning for long QT syndrome
- Certain electrolyte abnormalities and medications may increase the QT_c

WINTER'S FORMULA

$$PaCO_2 = 1.5(HCO_3^-) + 8 \pm 2$$

$PaCO_2$ = Arterial partial pressure of CO_2 [mm Hg]
$[HCO_3^-$ = Serum concentration of bicarbonate ions [meq/L]
- Calculates the expected $PaCO_2$ in pure metabolic acidosis (respiratory compensation)
- The patient's actual (measured) $PaCO_2$ is then compared:
  ✓ If the two values correspond, respiratory compensation can be considered to be adequate.
  ✓ If the measured $PaCO_2$ is higher than the calculated value, there is also a primary respiratory acidosis.
  ✓ If the measured $PaCO_2$ is lower than the calculated value, there is also a primary respiratory alkalosis.

CHAPTER 5

Cardiology

Jill J. Savla, MD, MSCE
Matthew J. O'Connor, MD
Chitra Ravishankar, MD
Joseph W. Rossano, MD, MS

CONGENITAL HEART DISEASE

NEWBORN SCREENING FOR CONGENITAL HEART DISEASE (CHD)

Goal is to identify critical congenital heart defects after birth but before hospital discharge and before signs of illness develop.

EPIDEMIOLOGY

- Critical congenital heart defects occur in 1 of 4 infants born with any CHD.
- Screening is most likely to detect the following critical congenital heart defects: hypoplastic left heart syndrome, pulmonary atresia, tetralogy of Fallot, total anomalous pulmonary venous return, transposition of the great arteries, tricuspid atresia, and truncus arteriosus.

DIAGNOSTICS

- Perform pulse oximetry screening (also see https://www.cdc.gov/ncbddd/heartdefects/hcp.html).
  - ✓ Pulse oximetry complements but does not replace thorough history and physical exam.
  - ✓ Perform at 24–48 hours of age (to minimize false positive results) or just before discharge if age <24 hours at discharge.
  - ✓ Apply pulse oximeter to right hand and one foot.
- Failed screening definition
  - ✓ O_2 saturation <90%; OR
  - ✓ O_2 saturation <95% in right hand and foot on 3 measurements, each separated by 1 hour; OR
  - ✓ >3% absolute difference in O_2 saturation between right and foot on three measurements, each separated by 1 hour

MANAGEMENT

- Any infant who fails screening requires evaluation to identify cause of hypoxemia.
  - ✓ Consider echocardiography unless a reversible cause is identified and treated appropriately.
  - ✓ Consider cardiology consultation.

CONGENITAL HEART DISEASE—CYANOTIC LESIONS WITH LIMITED PULMONARY CIRCULATION

TRICUSPID ATRESIA

A form of cyanotic CHD in which there is no outlet from the right atrium (RA) to the right ventricle (RV) and the RV is hypoplastic. The entire systemic blood flow enters the left atrium (LA) via a patent foramen ovale (PFO) or an atrial septal defect (ASD).

EPIDEMIOLOGY

• 1% of congenital heart defects

PATHOPHYSIOLOGY

• A ventricular septal defect (VSD) is usually present. The pathophysiology in tricuspid atresia depends on whether the great arteries are normally-aligned or transposed and on whether there is any obstruction to pulmonary or systemic blood flow.

CLINICAL MANIFESTATIONS

• With pulmonary atresia or severe pulmonary stenosis, presentation is within 24–48 hours; most patients present by 2 months of age with cyanosis and tachypnea.
• Occasionally, patients with transposition of the great arteries (TGA) develop pulmonary overcirculation and present with CHF.
• Rarely, older patients present with cyanosis, dyspnea on exertion, polycythemia, and easy fatigability.
• On exam: May have holosystolic murmur at left sternal border or ejection systolic murmur at left upper sternal border; single S2; increased left ventricle (LV) impulse

DIAGNOSTICS

• Chest x-ray: May show pulmonary undercirculation or overcirculation
• ECG: Left-axis deviation, RA enlargement, LV hypertrophy
• Echocardiography: Usually sufficient to delineate anatomic features

MANAGEMENT

Medical

• prostaglandin (PGE1) infusion in severely cyanotic infants (e.g., pulmonary atresia or severe pulmonic stenosis and subpulmonic stenosis) maintains patency of ductus arteriosus and promotes pulmonary blood flow; rarely, in neonates with tricuspid atresia, transposed great arteries, and coarctation of the aorta, PGE_1 is used to maintain systemic blood flow.
• Treatment of CHF with diuretics may be necessary in patients with high pulmonary flow.

Surgical

• If pulmonary blood flow is diminished, initial palliative procedures may include balloon atrial septostomy, Blalock–Taussig shunt, or surgical septectomy.
• If pulmonary blood flow is increased, pulmonary arterial banding may be beneficial.
• Stage 1 Norwood operation is performed if there is tricuspid atresia, transposed great arteries, and coarctation of the aorta.
• Ultimate goal is staged single ventricle palliation to Fontan completion.

TETRALOGY OF FALLOT (TOF)

A form of CHD characterized by anterior deviation of the conal septum (or its fibrous remnant), narrowing or atresia of the pulmonary outflow, and a malalignment type of VSD. The classic pathognomonic features in the tetralogy are overriding aorta, right ventricular outflow tract obstruction, malalignment VSD, and RV hypertrophy.

EPIDEMIOLOGY

• 5–7% of CHD; incidence: 1 in 2700
• 15–20% of patients with TOF have 22q11.2 deletion syndrome

PATHOPHYSIOLOGY

- Pulmonary-valve annulus has variable size and helps determine degree of RV outflow-tract obstruction.
- Severity of symptoms is determined by degree of RV outflow-tract obstruction (related to subvalvar or valvar pulmonary stenosis) and right-to-left shunt; degree of shunt depends on pulmonary vascular resistance (PVR), systemic vascular resistance (SVR), and presence or absence of a patent ductus arteriosus (PDA).
- VSD is usually large and unrestricted.
- Mild cases may not be cyanotic (otherwise known as a "pink tet").

CLINICAL MANIFESTATIONS

- Paroxysmal hypercyanotic attacks ("tet spells")
  - ✓ Characterized by the sudden onset of increased cyanosis, dyspnea, and change in mental status (often with irritability)
  - ✓ A sudden increase in the ratio of pulmonary to systemic vascular resistances results in increased right-to-left shunting across the VSD and reduction in pulmonary blood flow.
  - ✓ May lead to severe hypoxemia, metabolic acidosis, and death
  - ✓ Onset generally between 2 and 9 months of age
- If TOF is untreated, cyanosis and dyspnea with exertion is observed in most patients by 1 year of age; clubbing and the tendency to assume a "knee-to-chest" or squatting position are seen in older children.
- On exam: prominent RV impulse, harsh systolic ejection murmur at left sternal border, and single second heart sound

DIAGNOSTICS

- Chest x-ray: "Boot-shaped" heart, clear lung fields, possible right aortic arch
- ECG: Right-axis deviation, RV hypertrophy, dominant R-wave or RSR′ pattern in precordial leads
- Echocardiography: Defines anatomy
- Cardiac catheterization: May rarely be required to delineate coronary artery anatomy or assess for major aorto-pulmonary collateral arteries in patients with pulmonary atresia.

MANAGEMENT

"Tet" Spells

- Calm or feed the baby.
- Place the patient in parent's lap in knee-to-chest position.
- Supplemental oxygen
- Sedative such as morphine or ketamine.
- Phenylephrine or IV beta-blocker is rarely required.

Medical

- Avoid stressors such as cold, fever, dehydration, or hypoglycemia in neonates.
- If RV outflow-tract obstruction is severe, infants may be dependent on a PDA for pulmonary blood flow and require a PGE_1 infusion.
- Oral propranolol may decrease frequency and severity of "tet" spells.

Surgical or Catheter-Based Interventions

- Palliative surgery: Systemic-to-pulmonary-artery shunt (e.g., modified Blalock–Taussig shunt) can augment pulmonary blood flow in severely cyanotic infants.
- Stent angioplasty: In the current era, stenting of the ductus arteriosus or the right ventricular outflow tract may be other options for palliation.
- Total surgical correction: Often done during infancy; involves relief of the pulmonary outflow-tract obstruction (typically with a transannular patch) and VSD closure.

CONGENITAL HEART DISEASE—CYANOTIC LESIONS WITH MIXING OF SYSTEMIC AND PULMONARY CIRCULATIONS

TRUNCUS ARTERIOSUS

A form of cyanotic CHD in which a single arterial trunk arises from the heart and supplies the coronary arteries, at least one pulmonary artery, and the systemic arterial circulation.

- One semilunar valve with two to six septal leaflets, which may be stenotic and/or regurgitant
- Large VSD

EPIDEMIOLOGY

- 1–3% of congenital heart defects
- May be associated with 22q11.2 deletion syndrome

PATHOPHYSIOLOGY

- Because blood leaves the heart through a single trunk, complete mixing of systemic and pulmonary venous return occurs and cyanosis may be minimal.
- The degree of arterial SaO_2 depends on the ratio of SVR to PVR.
- As PVR decreases postnatally, pulmonary blood flow increases and heart failure often develops.
- Associated anomalies may include truncal-valve stenosis, truncal-valve insufficiency, and interrupted aortic arch.

CLINICAL MANIFESTATIONS

- Neonates usually present with mild cyanosis and tachypnea in the first month of life.
- Neonates with truncus and interrupted aortic arch present within the first 24–48 hours when the ductus arteriosus constricts.
- Other clinical features of 22q11.2 deletion syndrome may be present.
- On physical exam: Bounding pulses; systolic ejection click; single S_2; harsh systolic murmur; diastolic decrescendo murmur if truncal insufficiency present

DIAGNOSTICS

- Chest x-ray: Cardiomegaly, boot-shaped heart, pulmonary congestion, possible right aortic arch
- ECG: LV hypertrophy, RV hypertrophy
- Echocardiography: Usually sufficient to delineate anatomy

MANAGEMENT
Medical

- PGE_1 for truncus arteriosus with interrupted aortic arch or isolated pulmonary artery that is supplied from the ductus arteriosus
- Surgery recommended in neonatal period

Surgical

- Patch closure of the VSD, placement of a conduit from the RV to the pulmonary arteries after separating them from the truncus
- In the past, surgical banding of the individual pulmonary arteries was used to limit pulmonary overcirculation; this strategy is no longer used owing to the high incidence of pulmonary hypertension.

TRANSPOSITION OF THE GREAT ARTERIES (TGA)

A form of cyanotic CHD in which the aorta arises from the morphological RV and the pulmonary artery arises from the morphological LV.

- The most common form is dextro-transposition of the great arteries with cardiac segments {S, D, D}, also called D-TGA, in which the morphologic right ventricle is D-looped and the aorta is anterior and to the right of the pulmonary artery.
- Associated abnormalities include VSD, pulmonary stenosis, and coarctation of the aorta.

EPIDEMIOLOGY

- 5% of CHD; male:female = 3:1

PATHOPHYSIOLOGY

- TGA results in two parallel circuits such that the oxygenated blood is carried by the pulmonary artery to the lungs and the deoxygenated blood is carried by the aorta to the body.
- To sustain life, mixing must occur through an associated PDA, VSD, or ASD, with the ASD being the most effective site of mixing.
- If untreated, TGA is usually fatal in the neonatal period.

CLINICAL MANIFESTATIONS

- Cyanosis immediately after birth is typical in TGA with intact ventricular septum.
- On exam: Often, no murmur is appreciated; however, murmur of VSD may be noted; single, loud S_2.

DIAGNOSTICS

- Hyperoxia test: 100% oxygen is administered via oxygen hood for 10 minutes. If PaO_2 increases above 100 mmHg, parenchymal lung disease is suspected, whereas a PaO_2 less than 50 indicates cyanotic heart disease.
- Chest x-ray: Mild cardiomegaly, "egg-on-a-string" appearance of cardiac silhouette, pulmonary vascular congestion
- ECG: Right-axis deviation, RV hypertrophy
- Echocardiography: Confirms anatomy and associated defects; helps estimate degree of mixing

- Cardiac catheterization: Primarily indicated for balloon atrial septostomy as initial palliative procedure for adequate mixing; angiography may also be used to define coronary anatomy.

MANAGEMENT

Medical

- PGE_1: Maintains patency of the ductus arteriosus in order to augment mixing
- Oxygen

Surgical or Catheter-Based Interventions

- Balloon atrial septostomy (Rashkind procedure): Increases interatrial mixing and is indicated in the presence of cyanosis and a restrictive ASD.
- Arterial switch operation (ASO): Restores LV as the systemic ventricle (anatomic correction)
- Atrial switch operation (Mustard or Senning technique): Risk of late RV failure and arrhythmias and rarely used in the current era (physiologic correction)

TOTAL ANOMALOUS PULMONARY VENOUS CONNECTION (TAPVC)

A form of cyanotic CHD in which the pulmonary veins drain anomalously and none of the pulmonary veins connect to the morphologic left atrium. There are four types of TAPVC:

1. Supracardiac: Pulmonary veins drain to a confluence that courses superiorly to a "vertical vein," which often drains into the innominate vein or superior vena cava, before returning to the right atrium.
2. Infracardiac: Pulmonary veins drain to a confluence that courses inferiorly through a descending vein, which travels below the diaphragm and often drains into the portal system. Blood then flows to the hepatic veins, inferior vena cava, and RA. Pulmonary venous obstruction occurs more frequently with the infracardiac type of TAPVC.
3. Cardiac: TAPVC directly to the morphologic right atrium or to the coronary sinus
4. Mixed: Combination of types of TAPVC (supracardiac, infracardiac, and/or cardiac)

EPIDEMIOLOGY

- 1–2% of congenital heart defects; male > female
- Most common supracardiac > infracardiac > cardiac > mixed

PATHOPHYSIOLOGY

- Because pulmonary venous return enters the systemic venous circulation, survival depends on mixing through an ASD or a patent foramen ovale.
- Right atrial, ventricular, and pulmonary artery dilation are common because of volume overload.
- If pulmonary venous obstruction exists (common with infracardiac TAPVC), pulmonary congestion and pulmonary hypertension develop. In this case, neonates will be profoundly cyanotic and show signs of respiratory distress immediately after birth.
- If there is no pulmonary venous obstruction and the ASD is not restrictive, then oxygen saturations above 90% are common. These patients are still at risk for right-sided heart failure.

CLINICAL MANIFESTATIONS

- If pulmonary venous obstruction exists, patients present at 24–48 hours of life with cyanosis, tachypnea, and tachycardia.
- If pulmonary venous obstruction does not exist, patients present with mild cyanosis, failure to thrive, dyspnea, and/or CHF.
- With pulmonary venous obstruction: Single, loud S_2; gallop; faint or no murmur
- Without pulmonary venous obstruction: Increased right ventricular impulse; S_2 widely split and fixed; 2/6 to 3/6 systolic ejection murmur at left upper sternal border; middiastolic rumble at left lower sternal border (LLSB)

DIAGNOSTICS

- Chest x-ray: If pulmonary venous obstruction exists, pulmonary edema is seen. If pulmonary venous obstruction does not exist, cardiomegaly is seen.
- ECG: RV hypertrophy
- Echocardiography: Large RV, compressed LV, ASD, or patent foramen ovale (with all right to left shunting) may be seen.
- MRI: May be used to confirm diagnosis and help define anatomy.
- Cardiac catheterization and angiography: Help define anatomy, ratio of pulmonary to systemic flow, and degree of pulmonary hypertension

MANAGEMENT

- Supplemental oxygen
- PGE_1 may decrease venous obstruction in infracardiac TAPVC by maintaining patency of the ductus venosus. However, PGE_1 carries a risk of worsening pulmonary congestion by increasing left to right shunt through a PDA.
- In obstructive type of TAPVC, emergency surgery will relieve pulmonary venous obstruction. In the absence of obstruction, surgery is generally recommended in infancy.
- The goal of surgery is to redirect/connect pulmonary venous return to the LA.

HYPOPLASTIC LEFT HEART SYNDROME (HLHS)

A form of cyanotic CHD characterized by underdevelopment of the left heart, including significant hypoplasia of the LV, ascending aorta, and aortic arch; the mitral and/or aortic valves may be hypoplastic, stenotic, or atretic. Systemic circulation is dependent on a PDA.

EPIDEMIOLOGY

- 1% of CHD, more common in males
- Most common cause of cardiac death in the first month of life
- Chromosomal abnormalities in up to 25% of patients

PATHOPHYSIOLOGY

- Blood returning from the lungs passes through a patent foramen ovale or an ASD into the RA and RV.
- If a VSD is present and the aortic valve is not completely stenotic, a small amount of blood may enter the aorta directly. Otherwise, there is complete mixing of systemic and

pulmonary blood, which enters the pulmonary artery and passes through a PDA into the systemic circulation, including retrograde flow in the ascending aorta.
- As the PDA closes, systemic output decreases and metabolic acidosis ensues.

CLINICAL MANIFESTATIONS

- Most present within 48–72 hours of life, as the ductus arteriosus closes
- Cyanosis, dyspnea, poor feeding, heart failure, hepatomegaly, poor perfusion, decreased peripheral pulses, shock
- A minority with a restrictive ASD or intact atrial septum present immediately after birth with profound cyanosis, respiratory failure, and circulatory collapse
- On exam: Right parasternal lift; single, loud S_2; soft, nonspecific systolic ejection murmur

DIAGNOSTICS

- Prenatal ultrasound: Allows for antenatal diagnosis, counseling, and time to consider treatment options; it is the increasingly predominant method for diagnosis in current era.
- Chest x-ray: Cardiomegaly, pulmonary venous congestion, pulmonary edema
- ECG: RV hypertrophy
- Echocardiography: Defines anatomy
- Cardiac catheterization: Rarely needed in the current era, except for treatment of a restrictive ASD with a balloon atrial septostomy

MANAGEMENT

Medical

- Without intervention, HLHS is usually fatal within the first month of life.
- PGE_1 maintains ductal patency and systemic perfusion.
- Ratio of PVR to SVR is actively managed to ensure adequate oxygenation and systemic output. Generally, oxygen saturation (SaO_2) greater than 70% is adequate and SaO_2 greater than 90% is undesirable because it indicates pulmonary overcirculation. Supplemental oxygen is usually *not* required

Surgical

- Stage 1 Norwood procedure: First in a three-stage surgical palliation of HLHS. While survival has improved, there is still a substantial risk of death during childhood.
- Hybrid: Consisting of bilateral pulmonary artery bands and stenting of the PDA; preferred neonatal palliation in some centers
- Orthotopic heart transplantation: Rarely utilized as primary therapy; requires lifelong immunomodulatory therapy; shortage of available donors

CONGENITAL HEART DISEASE—ACYANOTIC LESIONS AND OBSTRUCTION TO BLOOD FLOW

PULMONARY STENOSIS

A form of CHD in which obstruction of the RV outflow tract leads to a systolic pressure gradient between the right ventricle and the pulmonary artery.

- Valvar pulmonary stenosis: Most common form of pulmonary stenosis; often an isolated defect due to fused, rudimentary, or absent commissures on the pulmonary valve

- Dysplastic pulmonary valve: Pulmonary valve obstruction due to a thickened, irregular pulmonary valve with limited excursion or leaflet mobility; frequently associated with Noonan syndrome
- Subvalvar pulmonary stenosis: Often due to muscular obstruction from the infundibulum; may be associated with anterior malalignment VSD
- Supravalvar pulmonary stenosis: Least common form of pulmonary stenosis; may be associated with Williams syndrome

EPIDEMIOLOGY

- 8–10% of congenital heart defects

PATHOPHYSIOLOGY

- Critical pulmonary stenosis: Severe pulmonary stenosis in the neonatal period with pulmonary blood flow dependent on left to right flow through the ductus arteriosus to the pulmonary artery
- Pressure gradient across the pulmonary valve may be misleading in the presence of a patent ductus arteriosus.

CLINICAL MANIFESTATIONS

- Severe pulmonary stenosis presents in the neonatal period with decreased pulmonary blood, cyanosis due to right to left flow across the foramen ovale, and signs of right heart failure
- Physical examination: Widely split second heart sound that is variable and becomes wider during inspiration, systolic ejection murmur at the left upper sternal border

DIAGNOSTICS

- Chest x-ray: May show darkened lung fields due to the lack of pulmonary blood flow.
- ECG: RV hypertrophy or RV strain in severe disease
- Echocardiography: Defines anatomy, location, and severity of lesion
- Cardiac catheterization: Can establish the severity, measure pressure gradient across the pulmonary valve, and can be used for treatment of pulmonary stenosis

MANAGEMENT

Medical

- PGE_1 maintains patency of the ductus arteriosus to augment pulmonary blood flow in severely ill neonates with critical obstruction

Surgical or Catheter-Based Interventions

- Percutaneous balloon pulmonary valvuloplasty is the preferred approach for pulmonary stenosis.
- Surgical valvotomy or pulmonary valve replacement with a homograft RV–PA conduit are other options used in complex CHD lesions.

AORTIC STENOSIS

A form of acyanotic CHD in which obstruction of the LV outflow tract leads to a systolic pressure gradient between the left ventricle and the aorta.

- Valvar aortic stenosis: Most common form of aortic stenosis; frequently due to a bicuspid or bicommissural aortic valve; identified in up to 2% of adults
- Subvalvar stenosis: Due to fibromuscular ring or shelf below the aortic valve; may be associated with posterior malalignment VSD or aortic coarctation
- Supravalvar stenosis: Least common form of aortic stenosis; may be localized or diffuse; often associated with Williams syndrome

EPIDEMIOLOGY

- 3–6% of congenital heart defects; male:female = 4:1

PATHOPHYSIOLOGY

- Critical aortic stenosis: Severe aortic stenosis in the neonatal period with systemic blood flow dependent on right to left flow through the ductus arteriosus to the aorta; often associated with a unicuspid or unicommissural aortic valve
- Pressure gradient may increase as cardiac output increases with growth during childhood.
- Abnormal diastolic filling is due to LV hypertrophy.

CLINICAL MANIFESTATIONS

- Symptoms depend on severity and location of obstruction. Mild aortic stenosis is often asymptomatic in infancy, but it can present with irritability, paleness, tachycardia, tachypnea, retractions, and rales.
- Neonates with critical or severe aortic stenosis can present with low cardiac output and heart failure once the PDA closes; symptoms include hypotension, poor perfusion, pulmonary edema, respiratory distress, or cardiogenic shock.
- Ventricular arrhythmias and sudden death may occur
- Physical examination: Early systolic ejection click at the apex; harsh ejection systolic murmur at the base radiates to the neck; palpable left ventricular lift; precordial systolic thrill at base

DIAGNOSTICS

- Chest x-ray: May show cardiomegaly (evidence of LV hypertrophy) and pulmonary edema with critical obstruction.
- ECG: LV hypertrophy or LV strain in severe disease
- Echocardiography: Defines anatomy and hemodynamic severity of the lesion
- Cardiac catheterization: Can establish the severity, measure pressure gradient across the aortic valve, and sometimes used for treatment of aortic stenosis

MANAGEMENT

Medical

- PGE_1 maintains patency of the ductus arteriosus to augment systemic blood flow in severely ill neonates with critical obstruction.
- Inotropic support with dopamine or epinephrine may also be required to maintain adequate cardiac output both before and after the intervention.

Surgical or Catheter-Based Interventions

- Aortic valve stenosis: Percutaneous balloon aortic valvuloplasty is the preferred approach for aortic stenosis.

- Surgical valvotomy or aortic-valve replacement with prosthetic valve or pulmonary autograft (e.g., Ross procedure preferred in infants and young children) are other options.
- Subaortic stenosis: Surgical removal of fibromuscular shelf or membrane, myomectomy may be required for muscular tunnel-like obstruction (Konno procedure)
- Supravalvar stenosis: Surgery to widen or repair stenotic segment

COARCTATION OF THE AORTA

A form of CHD in which there is narrowing of the aorta, most commonly in the juxtaductal region just beyond the origin of the left subclavian artery.

- May occur in isolation or in association with other cardiac defects

EPIDEMIOLOGY

- 5–8% of congenital heart defects; male:female = 2:1
- Often associated with Turner syndrome

PATHOPHYSIOLOGY

- Degree of symptoms and timing of presentation depends on severity of coarctation
- Decreased blood flow to lower extremities and lower half of the body may occur, especially after closure of the ductus arteriosus.
- LV outflow-tract obstruction leads to LV hypertrophy and increased systolic pressures; eventually LV dysfunction may develop, causing low-output cardiac failure and pulmonary edema.
- Extensive collateral circulation may develop in older children and young adults who are not diagnosed early in life.

CLINICAL MANIFESTATIONS

- Neonates: May present in the first 3 weeks of life (especially after closure of the ductus arteriosus) with tachypnea, poor feeding, diaphoresis, decreased femoral pulses and/or cardiogenic shock.
- Infants: Presentation may be similar to dilated cardiomyopathy.
- Older children: Upper-extremity (i.e., right arm) hypertension and claudication
- On exam: Decreased or absent femoral pulses; systolic murmur at left sternal border between third and fourth intercostal space radiating to left infrascapular area; ejection click if bicuspid aortic valve present

DIAGNOSTICS

- Four-extremity BPs: BP differential in which right upper extremity blood pressure is >10 mmHg higher than in lower extremities
- Chest x-ray: Cardiomegaly and pulmonary edema is usually seen in neonates and infants, rib notching is noted in children over 6 years of age.
- ECG: LV hypertrophy and possible LA enlargement in older children; RV hypertrophy in neonates
- Echocardiography: Reveals segment of coarctation and associated anomalies.
- Cardiac catheterization: May be performed to delineate affected segment and potentially for treatment in older children, adolescents, and adults.
- MRI: May help define lesion and identify collateral vessels; used for serial follow-up.

MANAGEMENT

Medical

- PGE_1 maintains patency of ductus to help provide distal perfusion in severely affected neonates. Inotropic support may be required for those presenting in extremis.
- Rebound hypertension is common in the immediate postoperative period and may require antihypertensive medication, especially in older children.

Surgical

- Timing depends on age at diagnosis, severity of disease, and related defects.
- Surgery is usually preferred for neonates and infants. Techniques include end-to-end anastomosis, patch augmentation, and subclavian flap repair. Percutaneous balloon angioplasty or stent angioplasty for native coarctation is usually reserved for recurrent coarctation or primary therapy in older children, adolescents, or adults.

CONGENITAL HEART DISEASE—ACYANOTIC LESIONS AND SHUNTING OF BLOOD THROUGH HEART DEFECTS

ATRIAL SEPTAL DEFECT (ASD)

A form of acyanotic CHD characterized by an opening in the atrial septum at one of the following four locations:

- Ostium secundum ASD: A deficiency in septum primum; most common type of ASD
- Ostium primum ASD: A deficiency in the canal septum (near the tricuspid valve); associated with a common atrioventricular canal (CAVC)
- Sinus venosus ASD: An interatrial communication in which the superior vena cava, the inferior vena cava, and/or a pulmonary vein override the atrial septum
- Coronary sinus ASD: An interatrial communication at the ostium (mouth) of the coronary sinus due to total or partial unroofing of the coronary sinus. This results in blood shunting from the left atrium into the coronary sinus and then into the right atrium; least common type of ASD

EPIDEMIOLOGY

- 5–10% of CHD; male:female = 1:2; 1 in 1500 live births

PATHOPHYSIOLOGY

- Small defects may close spontaneously
- Direction and magnitude of shunt depends on size of the defect and relative compliance of the ventricles
- Chronic left-to-right shunt results in right atrial and right ventricular volume overload; if unrepaired, pulmonary vascular disease (i.e., pulmonary hypertension) can develop in adulthood

CLINICAL MANIFESTATIONS

- Often asymptomatic in childhood; cardiac evaluation is prompted by murmur; may not present until adulthood
- Occasionally presents in childhood with fatigue, dyspnea, respiratory infections, and CHF

- CHF is more common if the ASD is associated with obstructive lesions affecting the left heart, such as mitral valve abnormalities or mild coarctation
- Atrial dysrhythmias (such as atrial fibrillation and supraventricular tachycardia) are more common in adults
- Pulmonary hypertension is more common in adults
- Paradoxical emboli may occur
- Physical exam: S1 loud or normal; S_2 widely split and fixed; prominent right ventricular cardiac impulse; midsystolic pulmonary ejection murmur; diastolic murmur at LLSB may represent flow across the tricuspid valve if Qp:Qs greater than 2:1

DIAGNOSTICS

- Chest x-ray: Right atrial enlargement, right ventricular hypertrophy (RVH), dilated pulmonary artery, and increased pulmonary vasculature
- ECG: Right-axis deviation and RVH
- Echocardiography: Reveals location, size, and associated anomalies
- Cardiac catheterization: May be used to confirm presence of the defect and determine Qp:Qs and pulmonary vascular resistance in adults. In the current era, device closure in the catheterization laboratory is quite common.

MANAGEMENT

Medical

- Heart failure symptoms may be managed with digoxin and diuretics (e.g., furosemide)
- Secundum ASDs close spontaneously in about 40–50% of patients.

Surgical or Catheter-Based Interventions

- Usually recommended if pulmonary:systemic flow ratio (Qp:Qs is greater than 2:1 or the patient is symptomatic.
- Uncomplicated ASDs are often closed between 3 and 6 years of age to prevent pulmonary vascular disease in adulthood.
- Defect is primarily closed with a suture or a patch is applied, usually under cardiopulmonary bypass, though device closure in the cardiac catheterization laboratory is being increasingly used.

VENTRICULAR SEPTAL DEFECT (VSD)

A form of acyanotic CHD characterized by an opening in the ventricular septum at one of the following locations:

1. Central (conoventricular or perimembranous) VSD: Defect involving the interventricular part of the membranous septum, at the center of the base of the ventricular mass; most common type of VSD
2. Muscular (trabecular) VSD: Defect within the trabeculated component of the ventricular septum (subtypes include anterosuperior, midseptal, apical, and posteroinferior); can involve multiple, small defects which may be difficult to repair surgically
3. Outlet VSD: Defect above the limbs of the RV septal band; subtypes include conoseptal hypoplasia (i.e., doubly committed juxta-arterial) and malalignment defects (anterior vs. posterior)
4. Inlet or canal-type VSD: Defect in the inlet component of the right ventricle that extends beneath the full length of the tricuspid valve

EPIDEMIOLOGY

- 2 to 6 per 1000 live births; 25% of congenital heart defects
- Most common form of CHD (after bicuspid aortic valve)

PATHOPHYSIOLOGY

- Direction and magnitude of shunt depends on size of the defect and relative pulmonary and systemic vascular resistances
- Small defects (restrictive) are not usually hemodynamically significant.
- Large defects (unrestrictive) can allow significant left-to-right shunting as the PVR declines, causing pulmonary overcirculation and heart failure.
- Large, unrepaired defects can lead to pulmonary vascular disease (i.e., pulmonary hypertension) and Eisenmenger syndrome (reversal of VSD flow and right-to-left shunt).
- Complications include pulmonary vascular disease, RV muscle bundles (RV outflow-tract obstruction), subaortic membrane, aortic-valve prolapse (aortic regurgitation), and endocarditis.

CLINICAL MANIFESTATIONS

- May be asymptomatic and present with a murmur
- Symptomatic VSDs often present with dyspnea, poor growth, feeding difficulties, sweating, and fatigue at 4–6 weeks of age as PVR decreases.
- Physical exam findings vary depending on size and location of the VSD, may include loud, harsh, blowing holosystolic murmur at LLSB; palpable thrill at LLSB with parasternal lift and apical thrust; S_3 and a middiastolic rumble may be present in large unrestrictive VSDs. Smaller defects can be associated with louder murmurs

DIAGNOSTICS

- Chest x-ray: May be normal or may reveal cardiomegaly and increased pulmonary vasculature
- ECG: May be normal or may reveal evidence of LV hypertrophy, LA hypertrophy, and biventricular hypertrophy
- Echocardiography: Reveals size and location of VSD
- Cardiac catheterization: Rarely indicated in the current era

MANAGEMENT

Medical

- Small VSDs are often well tolerated.
- Approximately 70% of VSDs close spontaneously. Small, muscular defects are most likely to close spontaneously, and inlet or outlet defects are the least likely to close spontaneously.
- If signs of pulmonary overcirculation or heart failure, consider administering diuretics, ACE inhibitors, or digoxin.

Surgical

- Indications for surgery include uncontrolled heart failure from pulmonary overcirculation, development of aortic regurgitation, RV outflow tract obstruction, and endocarditis.
- Surgical closure with a Dacron or Gortex patch
- Palliative pulmonary artery banding is usually reserved for complicated cases and premature infants

COMMON ATRIOVENTRICULAR CANAL (CAVC)

A form of CHD in which both atria connect to one common AV valve annulus.

- Complete AV canal: Has both an atrial component (i.e., primum ASD) and a large (unrestrictive) ventricular component (i.e., canal-type VSD).
- Transitional AV canal: Has both an atrial component and a small (restrictive) ventricular component.
- Incomplete (partial) AV canal: Has only an atrial component (i.e., primum ASD) and no ventricular component; often associated with a cleft in the mitral valve.

EPIDEMIOLOGY

- 4–5% of congenital heart defects; 0.2 to 0.3 in 1000 live births
- 30% of children with CAVC have trisomy 21 (i.e., Down syndrome); 20–25% of children with trisomy 21 have CAVC.

PATHOPHYSIOLOGY

- Varying degrees of left-to-right shunt result in CHF and recurrent pneumonia. The hemodynamic effect of the lesion depends on the specific type of the defect, the degree of shunting, and valvular incompetence.

CLINICAL MANIFESTATIONS

- Usually present within the first few weeks of life with failure to thrive, tachypnea, tachycardia, respiratory infections, and/or heart failure due to pulmonary overcirculation
- Untreated defects may lead to Eisenmenger syndrome (irreversible pulmonary arterial hypertension resulting from long-standing excessive pulmonary blood flow).
- Physical exam findings depend on the extent of the lesion and may include hyperdynamic precordium with palpable thrill at LLSB; accentuated pulmonic component of S_2; variable systolic murmur may be inaudible or grade 2/6 to 3/6 and holosystolic; signs of heart failure.

DIAGNOSTICS

Findings depend on the extent of the lesion and may include:

- Chest x-ray: Cardiomegaly, pulmonary vascular congestion, prominent main pulmonary artery
- ECG: Counterclockwise loop, left or superior deviation of QRS axis (-40 to -150 degrees), ventricular hypertrophy (right and/or left)
- Echocardiography: Used to define size of the defects, size of the ventricles, and valve anatomy.
- Cardiac catheterization: May be used to evaluate for pulmonary hypertension, particularly in patients with trisomy 21 (i.e., Down syndrome).

MANAGEMENT

Medical

- When pulmonary overcirculation and/or heart failure occurs, diuretics, digoxin, and ACE inhibitors are used.

Surgical

- Definitive surgical treatment is usually recommended before 6 months of age, particularly in infants with trisomy 21.

- Palliative pulmonary artery banding is usually reserved for cases in which more definitive surgical options are challenging (e.g., prematurity or small for gestational age).

PATENT DUCTUS ARTERIOSUS (PDA)

A form of acyanotic CHD defined as persistence of the ductus arteriosus beyond the normal age of spontaneous closure (about 2–3 months).

EPIDEMIOLOGY

- 5–10% of congenital heart defects; male:female = 1:2; 2 to 4 in 1000 live births
- Occurs more frequently in premature infants

PATHOPHYSIOLOGY

- The ductus arteriosus is a normal structure in fetal life that is formed from the embryonic sixth aortic arch.
- In utero, the ductus arteriosus serves to shunt or divert blood away from the collapsed, fluid-filled lungs with high resistance; therefore, blood flows from the pulmonary artery through the ductus arteriosus to the aorta.
- The ductus arteriosus normally closes in the first 1 to 2 weeks after birth.
- Similar to a VSD, the direction and magnitude of the shunt depends on size of the PDA and the relative pulmonary and systemic vascular resistances.
- Chronic left-to-right shunt results in pulmonary overcirculation and left heart dilation and can lead to the development of pulmonary vascular disease (i.e., pulmonary hypertension).

CLINICAL MANIFESTATIONS

- May be asymptomatic and present with a murmur
- Similar to VSDs; often present a few months after birth, when the PVR decreases, with difficulty feeding, poor weight gain, tachycardia, tachypnea, increased work of breathing, frequent respiratory infections, or diaphoresis.
- Preterm infants with PDA may have difficulty weaning from the ventilator and are at risk for necrotizing enterocolitis
- Physical exam: Continuous murmur, which is present through systole and diastole, is heard at the left upper sternal border and radiates to the back, hyperactive precordium, bounding peripheral pulses are present due to the diastolic runoff and widened pulse pressure.

DIAGNOSTICS

- Chest x-ray: Enlarged cardiac silhouette and pulmonary vascular congestion
- ECG: Left atrial enlargement (broad, notched P waves)
- Echocardiography: Confirms the presence, size, and direction of shunting.

MANAGEMENT

Medical

- Symptoms of heart failure due to pulmonary overcirculation may be managed with digoxin and diuretics such as furosemide.
- For the preterm infant, medical closure is often attempted with indomethacin or naproxen.

Surgical or Catheter-Based Interventions

- Usually recommended in premature infants for whom medical therapy has failed, infants who fail to wean from the ventilator, older children with persistent heart failure symptoms, or asymptomatic patients with an audible murmur.
- Surgical PDA ligation can be done via lateral thoracotomy.
- Transcatheter device occlusion of PDAs is now the treatment of choice in older infants and children.

Silent PDA

- A small PDA is considered "silent" when no murmur is heard on physical exam, the patient is asymptomatic, and it is hemodynamically insignificant (i.e., no left heart dilation); silent PDAs can be monitored and do not require surgical closure or catheter-based intervention.

SURGERIES FOR CONGENITAL HEART DISEASE

ARTERIAL SWITCH OPERATION (ASO)

- Indication: Transposition of the great arteries
- Definition: The coronary arteries are reimplanted into the pulmonary artery (neoaorta). The pulmonary artery and aorta are transected above the sinus of Valsalva, the pulmonary artery is usually brought in front of the neoaorta (LeCompte maneuver), and reattached.

MODIFIED BLALOCK–TAUSSIG (BT) SHUNT

- Indication: Tetralogy of Fallot, tricuspid atresia, pulmonary atresia
- Definition: A Gortex tube graft connects the subclavian artery to the ipsilateral pulmonary artery, thereby creating a systemic to pulmonary shunt.

NORWOOD PROCEDURE

- Indication: Usually first stage for single ventricle heart disease (e.g., HLHS)
- Reconstruction of the hypoplastic ascending aorta and the aortic arch using the main pulmonary artery and homograft patch, placement of a BT shunt or shunt from RV to the pulmonary artery (Sano modification), and removal of the atrial septum.

BIDIRECTIONAL GLENN OR HEMI-FONTAN (3–6 MONTHS) PROCEDURE

- Indication: Usually second stage for single ventricle heart disease (e.g., HLHS, tricuspid atresia)
- Definition: Direct connection of the superior vena cava to undivided right pulmonary artery, allowing blood flow to both lungs

FONTAN PROCEDURE (2–4 YEARS)

- Indication: Usually third stage for single ventricle heart disease
- Definition: Connection of the inferior vena cava to the right pulmonary artery. Modifications include lateral tunnel Fontan and extracardiac Fontan conduit with or without fenestration.

MUSTARD OR SENNING PROCEDURE

- Indication: This atrial switch operation was historically used to treat TGA prior to the advent of the arterial switch operation.
- Definition: Use of prosthetic baffles or native atrial septal tissue to divert pulmonary venous blood to the RV and systemic venous blood to the LV

PULMONARY ARTERY (PA) BANDING

- Indication: Single ventricle heart disease with increased pulmonary blood flow, complicated VSD
- Definition: Constriction of the pulmonary artery to reduce pulmonary blood flow

ROSS PROCEDURE

- Indication: Aortic stenosis, aortic regurgitation, or mixed aortic-valve disease
- Definition: Replacement of diseased aortic valve and root with patient's own pulmonary valve and root (autograft). A homograft is placed into the position of the pulmonary valve, and the coronary arteries are reimplanted into the autograft.

ACQUIRED HEART DISEASE

KAWASAKI DISEASE

A vasculitis of medium and small-sized arterioles, of unknown etiology, Kawasaki disease is the most common cause of acquired heart disease in children. See Chapter 29, on Rheumatology, for further details.

MYOCARDITIS

Myocarditis is inflammation of the myocardium with myocellular necrosis.

EPIDEMIOLOGY

- Typically sporadic, but occasionally epidemic
- Infants usually have more acute and fulminant course.
- Has been implicated in sudden infant death syndrome

ETIOLOGY

- Viral form is most common (e.g., parvovirus, coxsackievirus, adenovirus).
- Other infectious agents: Bacterial, fungal, parasitic, *Borrelia burgdorferi*
- *Trypanosoma cruzi* (Chagas disease) and *Clostridium diphtheriae* are common outside the United States
- Collagen vascular disease
- Immune-mediated: Kawasaki disease, rheumatic fever
- Toxin-induced (e.g., cocaine)
- Giant-cell myocarditis: Rare, but often severe and fatal

PATHOPHYSIOLOGY

- Involves damage to the myocardium from the initial infection, as well as the subsequent immune response
- May result in dilated cardiomyopathy

CLINICAL MANIFESTATIONS

- Often preceded by a flu-like illness
- May present with new-onset CHF or arrhythmias
- Dyspnea, exercise intolerance, fevers

- May be acute and fulminant or chronic
- On exam: Fever, tachycardia, tachypnea, gallop, signs of CHF, murmur of mitral insufficiency

DIAGNOSTICS

- Chest x-ray: Cardiomegaly with or without pulmonary edema
- ECG: Tachycardia, low QRS voltages, ST/T-wave changes, arrhythmias
- Echocardiography: Enlarged chambers, impaired LV function, mitral regurgitation
- Laboratory studies: ESR, CRP, cardiac enzymes, serum viral titers
- Endomyocardial biopsy: Gold standard for diagnosis. Viral PCR on biopsy sample is more sensitive than serum PCR
- MRI: Increasingly utilized for the diagnosis. Can demonstrate myocardial inflammation and quantify function.

MANAGEMENT

Medical

- Heart failure: Afterload reduction and diuretics are first-line therapies. Inotropic agents should be used with caution, as the damaged myocardium is more sensitive to arrhythmias and is reserved for patients with poor perfusion.
- Immunosuppression may be appropriate depending on etiology: intravenous immunoglobulin (IVIG; 2 g/kg) and occasionally corticosteroids
- Outcome: Approximately 60% recover completely with normalization shown by echocardiography, 20% either undergo heart transplantation or die, and 20% have residual dysfunction; there is a good prognosis for the fulminant presentation.

Surgical

- LVAD and ECMO may be used as a bridge to recovery or transplantation.
- Transplantation may be necessary.

PERICARDITIS

Inflammation of the pericardium.

EPIDEMIOLOGY

- Infectious type more common in younger children
- Incidence slightly higher in males

ETIOLOGY

- Viral: Echovirus and coxsackie B virus most common
- Bacterial, including *Mycoplasma tuberculosis*
- Collagen vascular: Rheumatoid arthritis, systemic lupus erythematosus
- Uremia
- Neoplastic or radiation induced
- Drug-induced (e.g., procainamide, hydralazine)
- Postpericardiotomy syndrome: Seen in about 10% of children 1–4 weeks after cardiac surgery; most commonly seen after ASD repair.

PATHOPHYSIOLOGY

- Deposits of infectious material or an inflammatory infiltrate results in an immune response and leads to changes in pericardial membrane function
- A pericardial effusion may result if altered hydrostatic and/or oncotic pressure leads to fluid accumulation
- Tamponade: An increase in intrapericardial pressure results in restriction of ventricular filling and a decrease in cardiac output
- Constrictive pericarditis is the late result of earlier pericarditis and is characterized by a thick, fibrotic, calcified pericardium
- Postpericardiotomy syndrome: A nonspecific hypersensitivity reaction after manipulation of the pericardial space

CLINICAL MANIFESTATIONS

- Fever, dyspnea
- Chest pain often radiates to the back or left shoulder, is worse with lying down, and is alleviated by leaning forward.
- On exam: Fever, tachypnea, tachycardia, friction rub, muffled heart sounds (if an effusion is present)
- With tamponade, may have signs of CHF, pulsus paradoxus (exaggerated decrease in systolic BP by greater than 10 mm Hg on inspiration), or Kussmaul sign (paradoxical rise in jugular venous pressure during inspiration).

DIAGNOSTICS

- Chest x-ray: Cardiomegaly with "water bottle" appearance if effusion present
- ECG: Tachycardia, diffuse ST elevation, T-wave inversion; may see electrical alternans if effusion present (variation of QRS axis with each beat due to movement of the heart within the pericardial fluid).
- Echocardiogram: With effusion, will see fluid in the pericardial space. In tamponade: RV collapse in early diastole, atrial collapse in end diastole and early systole.

MANAGEMENT

- Viral: Usually self-limited. Treatment includes rest, analgesia, and anti-inflammatory medications.
- Bacterial: Open drainage and aggressive antibiotic therapy
- Collagen vascular: Steroids and salicylates often used
- Postpericardiotomy: Rest, nonsteroidal anti-inflammatory agents
- Constrictive pericarditis: Pericardial stripping
- Pericardiocentesis: Indications include for hemodynamic compromise, for bacterial pericarditis, and as a diagnostic aid; send pericardial fluid for cell count, culture, and cytology; complications can include arrhythmias and hemopericardium.

ENDOCARDITIS

Infection/inflammation of the cardiac endothelium with associated immunologic response.

EPIDEMIOLOGY

- Incidence is increasing because of the increase in the numbers of IV drug users, survivors of cardiac surgery, and patients taking immunosuppressants and the increase in the long-term use of IV catheters.
- More common with CHD associated with a steep pressure gradient: PDA, restrictive VSD, left-sided valvular disease, systemic–pulmonary communications

ETIOLOGY

- Common organisms: *Streptococcus viridans* group (about 50%); *Staphylococcus aureus* (about 30%)
- Other organisms: For example, fungal, HACEK (*Haemophilus* spp., *Actinobacillus actinomycetemcomitans*, *Cardiobacterium hominis*, *Eikenella corrodens*, *Kingella* spp.) group.
- Common bacterial etiologies associated with various conditions:
  ✓ CHD: *S. aureus*
  ✓ Dental procedures: *S. viridans* group
  ✓ bowel/GU surgery: group D *Streptococcus*
  ✓ IV drug use: *Pseudomonas* spp., *Serratia* spp.
  ✓ Cardiac surgery: *Candida* spp.

PATHOPHYSIOLOGY

- Turbulent blood flow damages the endothelium.
- Damaged site serves as nidus for adherence of bacteria.
- Platelets and fibrin form a vegetation that may embolize.
- Immune response produces systemic symptoms.

CLINICAL MANIFESTATIONS

- Fevers, chills, night sweats, dyspnea, arthralgias, central nervous system manifestations, chest/abdominal pain
- On exam: Tachycardia; new or changing murmur; splenomegaly; manifestations of heart failure; Roth spots (pale retinal lesions surrounded by hemorrhage); Janeway lesions (flat, painless, on palms and soles); Osler nodes (painful nodes on pads of fingers and toes)

DIAGNOSTICS

- Multiple blood cultures obtained from separate blood draws (fill culture bottle to maximum permitted)
- Elevated ESR and CRP
- Leukocytosis, anemia, hypogammaglobulinemia
- Hematuria may result from immune complex glomerulonephritis with hypocomplementemia and positive rheumatoid factor (10–70%)
- Echocardiography: Can detect vegetations greater than 2–3 mm; may detect valvular dysfunction; transesophageal echocardiography is more sensitive.

Modified Duke Criteria

- Major criteria: Positive blood culture (typical microorganism from two different blood cultures; enterococcus without primary focus; positive serology for Q fever) or echocardiographic evidence of vegetations

- Minor criteria: Predisposing condition, temperature greater than 38.0°C, vascular or immunologic phenomena on physical exam, laboratory studies suggestive of infection
- Definite endocarditis: Pathologic diagnosis, 2 major, 1 major and 3 minor, or 5 minor
- Possible endocarditis: 1 major and 1 minor or 3 minor
- Rejected: Alternative diagnosis accounts for symptoms, resolution of manifestations with ≤4 days of antibiotic therapy, or no pathologic evidence at surgery

MANAGEMENT

Empiric therapies based on American Heart Association guidelines (therapy may be tailored based on susceptibilities):

- *S. viridans* group: Penicillin G for 4–6 weeks
- *S. aureus:* Nafcillin for 6–8 weeks
- HACEK group: Third-generation cephalosporin for 4 weeks
- Culture-negative: Ceftriaxone and gentamycin (add nafcillin or vancomycin if high level of suspicion for staphylococcal endocarditis) for 4–6 weeks
- Fungal: Amphotericin B; surgery often indicated
- Indications for surgery: Intracardiac abscess, severe valvular regurgitation, recurrent embolic disease, heart failure, infected prosthetic material
- Outcome: Most relapses occur in 1–8 weeks after therapy; mortality is 20–25% with antibiotics; serious morbidity (e.g., heart failure, systemic, or pulmonary emboli) in 50–60% of patients

ENDOCARDITIS PROPHYLAXIS

Adapted from Wilson W, Taubert KA, Gewitz M, et al. Prevention of infective endocarditis: Guidelines from the American Heart Association: A guideline from the American Heart Association Rheumatic Fever, Endocarditis, and Kawasaki Disease Committee, Council on Cardiovascular Disease in the Young, and the Council on Clinical Cardiology, Council on Cardiovascular Surgery and Anesthesia, and the Quality of Care and Outcomes Research Interdisciplinary Working Group. *Circulation* 2007;116:1736–1754.

Infective endocarditis prophylaxis for dental procedures is reasonable only for patients with underlying cardiac conditions associated with the highest risk of adverse outcome from infective endocarditis from dental procedures (listed below). Antibiotic prophylaxis is also reasonable for high-risk patients who undergo an invasive procedure of the respiratory tract that involves incision, biopsy, or drainage of the respiratory mucosa (e.g., tonsillectomy and adenoidectomy). The administration of prophylactic antibiotics solely to prevent endocarditis is no longer recommended for patients who undergo genitourinary or gastrointestinal tract procedures, including diagnostic esophagogastroduodenoscopy or colonoscopy.

High-Risk Patients

- Prosthetic cardiac valve or prosthetic material used for cardiac valve repair
- Previous infectious endocarditis
- Cardiac transplantation recipients with cardiac valvular disease
- Congenital heart disease only in the following categories:
  - ✓ Unrepaired cyanotic congenital heart defect, including palliative shunts and conduits
  - ✓ Completely repaired congenital heart defect with prosthetic material or device, whether placed by surgery or by catheter intervention, during the first 6 months after the procedure
  - ✓ Repaired CHD with residual defects at the site or adjacent to the site of a prosthetic patch or prosthetic device (which inhibit endothelialization)

PROPHYLAXIS RECOMMENDATIONS

Dental and Oral Procedures

- Regimen: Single dose 30–60 minutes before procedure
- Oral: Amoxicillin 50 mg/kg (children) or 2 g (adult)
- Cephalexin, clindamycin, or azithromycin are acceptable alternatives for penicillin-allergic patients.

CARDIOMYOPATHIES

Broadly defined as diseases of the heart muscle.

The common cardiomyopathies encountered in childhood are dilated cardiomyopathy, hypertrophic cardiomyopathy, restrictive cardiomyopathy, and left ventricular noncompaction.

DILATED CARDIOMYOPATHY (DCM)

EPIDEMIOLOGY

- Most common cardiomyopathy of childhood
- Characterized by an enlarged (dilated) ventricle with depressed ventricular function.
- Incidence is 0.6–0.7 per 100,000 children

ETIOLOGY

- Most cases are idiopathic; multiple possible etiologies, including genetic mutations, cytoskeletal protein abnormalities, metabolic diseases, myocarditis, and endocrinopathies.

CLINICAL MANIFESTATIONS

- Often leads to heart failure and need for heart transplantation. Transplant-free survival is only about 50% at 5 years in pediatric patients with dilated cardiomyopathy (worse than myocarditis).

MANAGEMENT

- Medical treatment often includes inhibition of the renin–angiotensin–aldosterone system (e.g., ACE inhibitors, angiotensin-receptor blockers, and aldosterone antagonists), β-adrenergic receptor blockade, diuretics, and digoxin.
- Device therapy may include implantable cardioverter–defibrillators with or without the ability to perform cardiac resynchronization therapy, and ventricular assist devices.

HYPERTROPHIC CARDIOMYOPATHY

EPIDEMIOLOGY

- The second most common cardiomyopathy diagnosed in childhood.
- Characterized by a thickened (hypertrophied) non-dilated LV, with the observed hypertrophy not occurring secondary to another disease (e.g., aortic valve stenosis).
- The incidence is 1 in 500 (many cases not diagnosed).

ETIOLOGY

- Most cases caused by a mutation of genes encoding for sarcomeric proteins. However, other etiologies, including glycogen storage diseases, Noonan syndrome, and mitochondrial diseases can also lead to the hypertrophic cardiomyopathy phenotype.

CLINICAL MANIFESTATIONS

- LV outflow-tract obstruction can occur from subaortic hypertrophy and systolic anterior motion of the mitral valve.
- The most common disease leading to sudden death with athletics in the United States.
- Symptoms can include chest pain, palpitations, arrhythmias, and heart failure. However, many patients are asymptomatic.

OTHER CARDIOMYOPATHIES

EPIDEMIOLOGY

- Restrictive cardiomyopathy
  - ✓ Least common cardiomyopathy encountered in childhood, with an estimated incidence of 0.03–0.04 per 100,000 children
- Left ventricular noncompaction
  - ✓ Increasingly recognized cardiomyopathy characterized by prominent trabeculations in the LV giving a characteristic "spongy" appearance to the myocardium,
  - ✓ True incidence and prevalence of left ventricular noncompaction is unknown and may be associated with other disorders such as Barth syndrome, chromosomal abnormalities, and mitochondrial disorders,

CLINICAL MANIFESTATIONS

- Restrictive cardiomyopathy
  - ✓ Characterized by a severe abnormality in the diastolic function of the myocardium. Systolic function is usually preserved.
  - ✓ Poor prognosis, with most children not surviving 2–3 years after the diagnosis unless they undergo heart transplantation. There is a high risk of sudden death, pulmonary hypertension, and thromboembolism.
- Left ventricular noncompaction
  - ✓ Wide variability in disease, ranging from coexisting with complex CHD, associated with a dilated or hypertrophied ventricle, to normal LV size and function
  - ✓ Prognosis is variable, but arrhythmias, dilation, hypertrophy, and dysfunction portend a worse prognosis.

MANAGEMENT

- Restrictive cardiomyopathy
  - ✓ No known effective medical therapies; heart transplantation is often recommended in newly diagnosed patients

HEART FAILURE

Heart failure is a clinical diagnosis that occurs when there are signs or symptoms from any structural or functional impairment of ventricular filling or ejection of blood.

There are several classification systems that exist to categorize the severity of the heart failure.

- American Heart Association/American College of Cardiology (AHA/ACC) heart failure staging—based on risk, symptoms, and treatment
- New York Heart Association (NYHA) functional classification—based on symptoms and physical activity alone

- Ross criteria—specific to pediatric heart failure based on the child's developmental status

ETIOLOGY

- Congenital cardiac causes of heart failure (symptoms generally arise from excessive blood flow to the lungs in left to right shunting lesions or from low cardiac output due to left heart obstructive lesions): VSD, complete AV canal, PDA, critical pulmonary or aortic stenosis, coarctation of the aorta, tricuspid atresia, TGA, truncus arteriosus, HLHS
- Primary heart muscle disease causes of heart failure: dilated cardiomyopathy, hypertrophic cardiomyopathy, restrictive cardiomyopathy, other congenital/genetic defects (metabolic disorder or muscular dystrophy)
- Acquired cardiac causes of heart failure: Arrhythmias, viral myocarditis, Kawasaki disease, rheumatic heart disease, chemotherapy (e.g., doxorubicin)
- Noncardiac causes of heart failure: Acute hypertension, anemia, hyperthyroidism and hypothyroidism, obstructive sleep apnea

CLINICAL SUBTYPES

- Conceptually, children with heart failure can be placed into one of four categories based on the presence/absence of venous congestion (i.e., wet or dry) and the presence/absence of adequate systemic output (i.e., warm or cool)
  1. Warm and dry: Represents a patient with asymptomatic ventricular dysfunction (normal filling pressures and adequate perfusion).
  2. Warm and wet: Most common presentation, characterized by venous congestion such as pulmonary edema due to elevated ventricular filling pressures with adequate perfusion.
  3. Cold and wet: Characterized by venous congestion such as pulmonary edema due to elevated ventricular filling pressures and poor perfusion.
  4. Cold and dry: Normal ventricular filling pressures, but poor perfusion

CLINICAL MANIFESTATIONS

- Infants: Failure to thrive, increased work of breathing, tachypnea, dyspnea, feeding difficulties, fussiness, irritability, excessive perspiration or diaphoresis, decreased urine output
- Children and adolescents: Shortness of breath, reduced exercise tolerance, wheezing, cough, orthopnea, nausea, vomiting, abdominal pain, peripheral edema
- On exam ("wet"): Peripheral edema, hepatomegaly, rales, tachypnea, tachycardia, gallop rhythm
- On exam ("cold"): weak peripheral pulses, cool extremities, delayed capillary refill, mottling, mental status changes
- Criteria for hospitalization: Respiratory distress, inability to tolerate feeding, failure to tolerate or poor clinical response to outpatient oral therapy, severe illness or acute decompensated heart failure (evidenced by hypotension, poor perfusion, or mental status changes)

DIAGNOSTICS

- Chest x-ray: Helps assess degree of cardiomegaly and pulmonary edema
- ECG: May demonstrate sinus tachycardia, increased voltages, abnormal ST segments, T-wave flattening or inversions, Q waves, and/or rhythm disturbances. The ECG is rarely normal in advanced cardiomyopathy or heart failure.
- Echocardiography: Helps define congenital heart defects, ventricular size, ventricular function, shortening fraction, ejection fraction, and evidence of diastolic dysfunction.
- Laboratory values: Blood gas (with lactate), mixed venous saturation, B-type natriuretic peptide (BNP), troponin-I, complete blood count (CBC), complete metabolic panel

(CMP) including electrolytes and liver-function tests, consider viral or other infectious studies

MANAGEMENT

- General measures: Treatment of precipitating factors such as fluid overload, fever, anemia, infection, hypertension, and arrhythmias
- Diuretics:
  - ✓ Loop diuretics (e.g., furosemide) are considered first-line therapy for heart failure symptoms. Electrolyte abnormalities (e.g., hypokalemia, hypochloremia) are common.
  - ✓ Thiazide diuretics (e.g., chlorothiazide, hydrochlorothiazide) work at the distal tubule and are often used to complement loop diuretics
  - ✓ Spironolactone is a potassium-sparing diuretic and is often used in combination with loop or thiazide diuretics.
- Digoxin increases cardiac contractility; toxicities include bradycardia, heart block, and ventricular arrhythmias.
- Afterload-Reducing Agents:
  - ✓ Reduction in afterload results in increased stroke volume and improved cardiac output.
  - ✓ ACE inhibitors (e.g., captopril, enalapril): Reduce PVR by blocking the conversion of angiotensin I to angiotensin II. ACE inhibitors are also thought to have a positive effect on myocardial remodeling,
  - ✓ IV afterload-reducing agents (and vasodilators): Milrinone, nitroprusside, and hydralazine are usually reserved for ICU patients with decompensated heart failure and low cardiac output,
- IV inotropic agents: Dopamine, dobutamine, and milrinone are generally reserved for ICU patients with decompensated heart failure and evidence of life-threatening low cardiac output

ELECTROCARDIOGRAPHY

PRECORDIAL LEAD PLACEMENT (FIGURE 5-1)

V1: 4th ICS, RSB
V2: 4th ICS, LSB
V3: Equidistant between V2 and V4
V4: 5th ICS, left MCL
V5: Horizontal to V4, left AAL
V6: Horizontal to V4, left MAL
V3R, V4R, V5R, V6R: Mirror image to V3, V4, V5, and V6 on the right side of the chest.

RATE

- On a standard ECG, paper moves at 25 mm/sec.
- Each small square is 1 mm (0.04 second) and each large square is 5 mm (0.2 second) (Figure 5-2).
- Heart rate can be estimated by counting the number of large boxes between QRS intervals where 1 box = 300 bpm, 2 boxes = 150 bpm, 3 boxes = 100 bpm, 4 boxes = 75 bpm, 5 boxes = 60 bpm, and 6 boxes = 50 bpm.

RHYTHM

- The cardiac rhythm may be determined by examining the rhythm strip that appears at the bottom of a standard 12-lead ECG

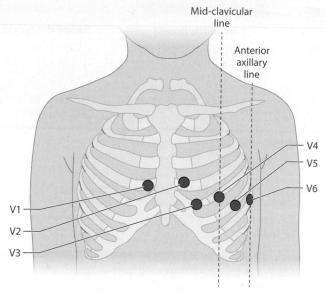

FIGURE 5-1 Precordial lead placement for ECG.

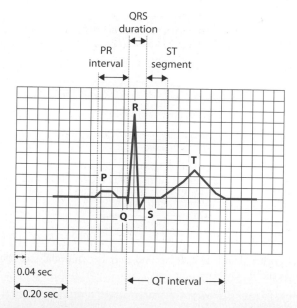

FIGURE 5-2 Segments and intervals. (Reproduced with permission from Ewtry EH, Jeon C, Ware MG: *Blueprints Cardiology*, 2nd ed. Philadelphia, PA: Lippincottt Williams & Wilkins; 2006.)

TABLE 5-1	Normal QRS Axis by Age	
Age	**Mean (Degrees)**	**Range (Degrees)**
1 week–1 month	+110	+30 to +180
1–3 months	+70	+10 to +125
3 months–3 years	+60	+10 to +110
>3 years	+60	+20 to +120
Adult	+50	−30 to +105

Reproduced with permission from Park MK: *Pediatric Cardiology for Practitioners*, 4th ed. St. Louis, MO: Mosby; 2002.

AXIS

- The QRS axis represents the net direction of electrical activity during ventricular systole (**Figure 5-2** and **Table 5-1**).

P WAVE

- Represents sinus node depolarization (**Figure 5-1**)
- Best seen in leads II and V_1
- In children, the P wave is normally less than 2.5 mm tall and 0.10 second in duration.
- Tall P waves may represent right atrial enlargement, whereas wide P waves may represent left atrial enlargement

PR INTERVAL

- From beginning of P wave to beginning of QRS complex
- Refer to **Table 5-2** for interval norms for PR.

QRS COMPLEX

- Represents ventricular depolarization (see **Table 5-2**)

QT INTERVAL

- Measured from beginning of QRS complex to end of T wave
- QT interval varies with heart rate and is corrected by the Bazett formula as follows:

$$QT_c = \frac{QT}{\sqrt{RR \text{ preceding}}}$$

- A QTc interval greater than 0.44–0.46 second may be abnormal (see section below on "Long-QT Syndrome")

ST SEGMENT

- Segment between the end of the QRS complex and beginning of the T wave
- Displacement by more than 1–2 mm from the isoelectric line may represent myocardial injury, pericarditis, or a repolarization abnormality.

TABLE 5-2   QRS Duration Norms and PR Interval Norms in Seconds

Age	QRS Duration Norms		PR Interval Norms	
	Mean	**Upper Limit**	**Mean**	**Upper Limit**
0–1 month	0.05	0.065	0.09–0.10	0.11–0.12
1–6 months	0.05	0.07	0.09–0.11	0.11–0.14
6 months–1 year	0.05	0.07	0.10–0.11	0.11–0.14
1–3 years	0.06	0.07	0.10–0.12	0.12–0.15
3–8 years	0.07	0.08	0.12–0.15	0.14–0.17
8–12 years	0.07	0.09	0.14–0.16	0.15–0.18
12–16 years	0.07	0.10	0.15–0.16	0.16–0.19
Adult	0.08	0.10	0.15–0.17	0.17–0.21

Modified with permission from Park M, Guntheroth WG: *How to Read Pediatric ECGs*, 3rd ed. St. Louis, MO: Mosby; 1992.

TABLE 5-3   R and S Voltage Norms in V_1 and V_6: Mean (Upper Limit) in Millimeters

Age	R in V_1	R in V_6	S in V_1	S in V_6
0–1 month	15 (25)	6 (21)	10 (20)	4 (12)
1–6 months	11 (20)	10 (20)	7 (18)	2 (7)
6 months–1 year	10 (20)	13 (20)	8 (16)	2 (6)
1–3 years	9 (18)	12 (24)	13 (27)	2 (6)
3–8 years	7 (18)	14 (24)	14 (30)	1 (5)
8–12 years	6 (16)	14 (24)	16 (26)	1 (4)
12–16 years	5 (16)	14 (22)	15 (24)	1 (5)
Young adult	3 (14)	10 (21)	10 (23)	1 (13)

Modified with permission from Park M, Guntheroth WG: *How to Read Pediatric ECGs*, 3rd ed. St. Louis, MO: Mosby; 1992.

T WAVE

- Represents ventricular repolarization
- Normally upright in leads I and II and inverted in lead aVR
- Abnormalities may represent ischemia or electrolyte abnormalities.

LEFT VENTRICULAR HYPERTROPHY, ECG SIGNS

- Left-axis deviation (**Table 5-3**)
- R wave in leads I, II, III, aVL, V5, or V6 greater than upper limit of normal
- S wave in V1 or V2 greater than upper limit of normal
- Signs of volume overload: Q wave in V5 and V6 ≥5 mm and tall, symmetric T waves
- Signs of strain: Inverted T waves in leads I or aVF and V5–V6

RIGHT VENTRICULAR HYPERTROPHY, ECG SIGNS

- Right-axis deviation
- R wave in V1, V2, or aVR greater than upper limit of normal

- S wave in I or V6 greater than upper limit of normal
- Q wave in V1
- Signs of strain: T axis outside normal range (0 to −90 degrees), inverted in V1

ARRHYTHMIAS

ATRIAL FIBRILLATION

An ectopic atrial focus leads to an extremely fast atrial rate (350–600 bpm). The ventricular response is usually fast (>100 bpm) and "irregularly irregular." The fast, disorganized ventricular response may lead to decreased cardiac output. Atrial fibrillation is much more common in adults than in children.

ETIOLOGY

- Structural heart disease, dilated atria, myocarditis, digitalis toxicity, cardiac surgery

MANAGEMENT

- For sustained atrial fibrillation (>48 hours), consider anticoagulation with warfarin or heparin and echocardiography to look for thrombus.
- Digoxin with or without beta-blockers may control the ventricular rate.
- Termination of atrial fibrillation may be achieved through direct-current cardioversion (especially in unstable patients) or with antiarrhythmic medications (e.g., amiodarone).

ATRIAL FLUTTER

An intraatrial reentrant circuit leads to a rapid atrial rate—around 300 bpm—with a characteristic sawtooth pattern on ECG. Because the ventricles cannot respond at 300 bpm, there is often a 2:1, 3:1, or 4:1 block.

ETIOLOGY

- Structural heart disease, myocarditis, digitalis toxicity, cardiac surgery, dilated atria with mitral insufficiency

MANAGEMENT

- To prevent thromboembolism, consider anticoagulation with warfarin or heparin and TEE before cardioversion.
- Vagal maneuvers or adenosine may produce a temporary slowing of the heart rate, but do not terminate the rhythm.
- Procainamide or amiodarone may terminate the rhythm.
- Digoxin slows the ventricular rate by increasing the AV block.
- Direct current cardioversion often restores normal sinus rhythm

ATRIOVENTRICULAR BLOCK

AV block ("heart block") occurs when conduction through the atrioventricular node is impaired.

FIRST-DEGREE AV BLOCK

- Definition: Indicates that the PR interval is above the upper limit of normal for age
- Etiology: Rheumatic fever, cardiomyopathy, ASD, Ebstein anomaly, infectious diseases, ischemic heart disease, hyperkalemia, digitalis toxicity, other medications
- Management: Generally asymptomatic and does not require treatment.

SECOND-DEGREE AV BLOCK, MOBITZ TYPE I (WENCKEBACH)

- Definition: Progressive lengthening of PR interval with eventual dropped beat
- Etiology: Myocarditis, cardiomyopathy, myocardial infarction, congenital heart defect, cardiac surgery, digitalis toxicity, other medications
- Management: Usually does not progress and does not require treatment

SECOND-DEGREE AV BLOCK, MOBITZ TYPE II

- Definition: Normal PR intervals are followed by episodes of heart block (i.e., P-wave is not conducted to the ventricles)
- Etiology: Myocarditis, cardiomyopathy, myocardial infarction, congenital heart defect, cardiac surgery, digitalis toxicity, other medications
- Management: May progress to complete heart block; may require pacemaker.

THIRD-DEGREE AV BLOCK

- Definition: Complete dissociation of atrial and ventricular activity (i.e., no relationship between P wave and QRS complex)
- Etiology: Isolated anomaly, maternal SLE, Sjögren syndrome, congenital heart defect, cardiac surgery, myocarditis, endocarditis, Lyme carditis, acute rheumatic fever, cardiomyopathy, myocardial infarction, certain drug overdoses
- Management: Patients are often unstable and may require transcutaneous pacing, atropine, or isoproterenol. A transvenous or permanent pacemaker is often required.

LONG-QT SYNDROME

A cardiac repolarization abnormality characterized by prolongation of the QT interval, which can result in torsades de pointes and sudden cardiac death.

- Corrected QT interval is calculated by the Bazett formula (see section on "QTc Interval").

ETIOLOGY

Hereditary Causes of Long-QT Syndrome

- Jervell–Lange-Nielsen syndrome: Autosomal recessive, congenital deafness
- Romano–Ward syndrome: Autosomal dominant transmission, normal hearing
- Sporadic mutations in potassium and sodium channels

Acquired Causes of a Prolonged QT Interval

- Electrolyte abnormalities: Hypokalemia, hypomagnesemia, hypocalcemia
- Drugs: Antiarrhythmics, tricyclic antidepressants, erythromycin, antihistamines, phenothiazine, cocaine, organophosphates
- Other: Stroke, subarachnoid hemorrhage, myocardial ischemia, liquid protein diets

PATHOPHYSIOLOGY

- Lengthening of ventricular repolarization leads to R-on-T phenomena and precipitation of torsades de pointes
- Congenital long-QT syndrome may result from a variety of mutations that affect transmembrane ion channels responsible for cardiac repolarization.

CLINICAL MANIFESTATIONS

- Often presents with unexplained syncope or sudden cardiac death brought on by exercise or fright
- May present with presyncope, seizures, dizziness, and palpitations

DIAGNOSTICS

- Family History: Long-QT syndrome or unexplained sudden cardiac death
- ECG: Increased QTc, torsades de pointes, T-wave alternans, notched T waves, low resting heart rate
- Corrected QT interval: QTc >440 msec is suspicious and QT_c >460 msec is worrisome.
- Exercise stress test: Prolongation of QTc seen with exercise
- 24-hour Holter monitor: May reveal arrhythmia.

MANAGEMENT

Short Term

- Immediate cardioversion if torsades de pointes is present
- Magnesium bolus and infusion
- Maintain high normal level of potassium
- Temporary cardiac pacing
- Withdrawal of offending drugs
- Correction of electrolyte abnormalities
- Isoproterenol in cases of acquired long-QT syndrome

Long Term

- Beta-blockers
- Left thoracic sympathectomy
- Permanent pacemaker and cardioverter–defibrillator
- May have to avoid sports and stressful activities
- Avoid combining multiple medications with QT-prolonging side effects

PREMATURE ATRIAL CONTRACTION (PAC)

An atrial beat arising from an ectopic stimulus in the left or right atrium, which occurs before the next normal sinus beat is due.

- The P wave has a different shape than the normal sinus P wave.
- If the PAC is conducted, the QRS complex is generally the same as the QRS complex of preceding beats.
- Occasionally, the PAC is conducted aberrantly through the ventricles causing a wide QRS complex.
- If the PAC reaches the AV node while it is still refractory, the PAC may not be conducted to the ventricles.

ETIOLOGY

- PACs are very common in healthy people and do not necessarily indicate the presence of disease.
- Other causes: Emotional stress, hyperthyroidism, caffeine, structural heart disease, medications (epinephrine, theophylline)

MANAGEMENT

- Medical management generally not required if PACs are an isolated finding.

PREMATURE VENTRICULAR CONTRACTION (PVC)

A ventricular beat arising from an ectopic ventricular stimulus, which occurs before the next normal sinus beat is due.

- Wide QRS complex (greater than 0.08 second in infants, greater than 0.12 second in children)
- Two PVCs in a row are called a "couplet" or a "pair."
- Three PVCs in a row define ventricular tachycardia.
- PVCs may be uniform, indicating that they arise from a single focus.
- Multiform PVCs may arise from different foci or from the same focus and often signify underlying heart disease
- R-on-T phenomenon: When PVCs occur during the T wave of the preceding beat, they may precipitate ventricular tachycardia or ventricular fibrillation.

ETIOLOGY

- PVCs often occur in normal hearts.
- Other causes: Anxiety, caffeine, hypoxemia, sympathomimetics, myocardial infarction, electrolyte abnormalities, and structural heart disease

MANAGEMENT

- PVCs are often benign and usually do not require treatment.
- Correction of underlying abnormalities (e.g., electrolyte abnormalities) may reduce the frequency of PVCs.
- Medications such as beta-blockers or antiarrhythmics are occasionally considered.

SUPRAVENTRICULAR TACHYCARDIA (SVT)

A reentrant supraventricular rhythm may occur when there are two conducting pathways, unidirectional block in one pathway, and slow conduction in the other pathway. SVT may also be due to an automatic atrial rhythm. The two most common forms of reentrant SVT are

- Atrioventricular nodal reentry tachycardia: The AV node consists of a slow, posterior pathway and a fast, anterior pathway. Onset may be triggered by a premature atrial impulse, which reaches the AV node when the fast pathway is still refractory. The premature impulse conducts antegrade through the slow pathway and then retrograde through the fast pathway. AV nodal reentry tachycardia is more common in teens and young adults
- A reentry tachycardia: An accessory pathway exists outside of the AV node. Antegrade conduction typically occurs via the AV node and retrograde conduction

via the accessory pathway (orthodromic). This results in a normal QRS complex. Antegrade conduction occasionally occurs via the accessory pathway and retrograde conduction via the AV node (antidromic). This results in a wide QRS complex, which may be difficult to differentiate from ventricular tachycardia. AV reentry tachycardia is common in Wolff–Parkinson–White syndrome and is more common in infants and toddlers

CLINICAL MANIFESTATIONS

- Rapid, regular heart rate, usually 150–250 bpm
- Palpitations, syncope, near-syncope, lightheadedness, shortness of breath

DIAGNOSTICS

- Laboratory studies: Consider electrolytes
- Chest x-ray: May show infection, cardiomyopathy, pulmonary edema
- Echocardiogram: If structural heart defect suspected
- ECG during SVT: Heart rate 150–250 bpm, P wave may be within or after QRS, typically narrow QRS, occasionally wide QRS
- ECG after termination of the SVT: May show a delta wave (upsloping QRS complex) in WPW syndrome.
- Adenosine: May terminate the arrhythmia.

MANAGEMENT

Short Term

- If unstable, direct-current cardioversion: (0.5 J/kg increased in steps to 2 J/kg)
- Vagal maneuvers: Ice to face, Valsalva, carotid-sinus massage
- Adenosine by rapid IV push (initial dose, 0.1 mg/kg [maximum, 6 mg], increase by 0.05 mg/kg if unsuccessful to maximum of 0.35 mg/kg, or 12 mg)
- Calcium-channel blockers (avoid in infants younger than 1 year), class IC agents, digoxin (controversial), and amiodarone may also be effective.

LONG TERM

- Antiarrhythmic drug therapy: Propranolol, verapamil, amiodarone, procainamide, quinidine, flecainide, digoxin
- Radiofrequency catheter ablation is often successful in ablating the accessory pathway.
- No treatment is sometimes an acceptable alternative.
- Digoxin and calcium-channel blockers are contraindicated in WPW syndrome.

VENTRICULAR FIBRILLATION

An uncoordinated, chaotic ventricular rhythm with QRS complexes of varying size and shape. Ventricular fibrillation is a pulseless rhythm without effective cardiac output and is fatal unless effectively treated.

ETIOLOGY

- Hyperkalemia, severe hypoxia, surgery, myocarditis, myocardial infarction
- Drugs and toxins: Digitalis, quinidine, catecholamines, anesthetics

MANAGEMENT

- CPR, airway, oxygen, IV or IO access
- Defibrillate up to three times (2 J/kg, 4 J/kg, 4 J/kg) and then with 4 J/kg 30–60 seconds after each medication
- Epinephrine (first dose: 0.1 mL/kg of 1:10,000 IV/IO or 0.1 mL/kg of 1:1000 via ETT; subsequent doses 0.1 mL/kg of 1:1000 IV/IO/ETT)
- Amiodarone (5 mg/kg IV/IO)
- Lidocaine (1 mg/kg IV/IO)

VENTRICULAR TACHYCARDIA (VT)

Defined as at least three premature ventricular beats in a row at a rate above 120 bpm (varies by age) characterized by wide QRS complexes.

- Sustained VT lasts longer than 30 seconds

ETIOLOGY

- Cardiomyopathy, myocarditis, cardiac surgery, electrolyte abnormalities, drugs and toxins, long-QT syndrome, anomalous left coronary artery

MANAGEMENT

Ventricular Tachycardia with Pulses

- Early cardiology consultation is recommended
- Consider amiodarone (5 mg/kg IV over 20–60 minutes), procainamide (15 mg/kg over 30–60 minutes), or lidocaine (1 mg/kg over 2–4 minutes).
- If signs of shock are present, immediate synchronized cardioversion is indicated (0.5–1 J/kg initially, up to 2 J/kg).
- Magnesium (25 mg/kg over 10–20 minutes) is indicated if torsades de pointes is suspected.

Pulseless Ventricular Tachycardia

- CPR, airway, oxygen, IV or IO access
- Defibrillate up to three times (2 J/kg, 4 J/kg, 4 J/kg) and then with 4 J/kg 30–60 seconds after each medication.
- Epinephrine (first dose: 0.1 mL/kg of 1:10,000 IV/IO or 0.1 mL/kg of 1:1000 via ETT; subsequent doses 0.1 mL/kg of 1:1000 IV/IO/ETT)
- Amiodarone (5 mg/kg IV/IO)
- Lidocaine (1 mg/kg IV/IO)
- Magnesium (25 mg/kg over 10–20 minutes) is indicated if torsades de pointes is suspected

WOLFF–PARKINSON–WHITE (WPW) SYNDROME

A form of ventricular preexcitation in which an accessory pathway bypasses the AV node, leading to a variety of supraventricular tachyarrhythmias.

EPIDEMIOLOGY

- Affects 0.1–3% of general population
- Occasionally inherited in an autosomal dominant pattern
- May be associated with Ebstein anomaly of the tricuspid valve or levo-transposition of the great arteries (i.e., congenitally corrected transposition)

PATHOPHYSIOLOGY

- Atrial impulses bypass the AV node through the accessory pathway, causing preexcitation.
- Paroxysmal SVT in WPW usually results from antegrade conduction through the AV node and retrograde conduction through the accessory pathway (orthodromic).
- Paroxysmal SVT may result from antegrade conduction through the accessory pathway and retrograde conduction through the AV node (antidromic). In this case, the QRS complex is wide and the rhythm may be difficult to distinguish from VT.
- Patients are also at risk for atrial fibrillation, atrial flutter, and ventricular fibrillation (rare).

CLINICAL MANIFESTATIONS

- Palpitations, dizziness, syncope, chest discomfort, shortness of breath

DIAGNOSIS

- Family history: WPW, SVT, sudden cardiac death, unexplained early death (e.g., car accidents, drownings)
- ECG: Shortening of the PR interval, widening of the QRS complex, slurred upstroke of the QRS complex (delta wave)

MANAGEMENT

- Vagal maneuvers such as ice to face, Valsalva, carotid sinus massage (hemodynamically stable patients)
- Adenosine: Initial drug of choice (initial dose, 0.1 mg/kg IV; maximum, 6 mg)
- Other potential agents: Beta-blockers, digoxin, calcium channel antagonists (contraindicated in infants and young children), procainamide; however, caution should be used with digoxin and calcium-channel blockers, which may increase the ventricular rate during atrial fibrillation and can lead to ventricular fibrillation
- Radiofrequency catheter ablation is the treatment of choice in symptomatic and high-risk patients

SYNCOPE

Transient loss of consciousness and postural tone due to inadequate cerebral perfusion.

EPIDEMIOLOGY

- 15% of children and adolescents between ages 8 and 18 experience syncope.
- Unusual under age 6 except in the setting of seizure disorders, breath-holding, and cardiac abnormalities.

ETIOLOGY

- Neurocardiogenic syncope (vasodepressor, vasovagal):
  - ✓ Most common type of syncope; may be provoked by increased vagal tone during micturition, defecation, cough, or hair brushing; may be provoked by peripheral vasodilation during fight-or-flight response, warm temperature, anxiety, or blood drawing.
  - ✓ Decreased cardiac filling leads to increased cardiac contractility and activation of stretch receptors. A reflex increase in vagal tone further compromises cardiac output, resulting in syncope.

- Cardiac syncope:
  ✓ Dysrhythmias may include SVT, VT, heart block, WPW, long-QT syndrome
  ✓ Outflow-tract obstruction: HCM, pulmonary hypertension
  ✓ Inflow obstruction: Restrictive cardiomyopathy, effusion
  ✓ May be accompanied by brief seizure (Stokes–Adams syndrome)
- Neuropsychiatric syncope: Seizures, migraines, hypoglycemia, "hysterical" syncope, hyperventilation (e.g., panic attack)
- Presyncope due to POTS: Characterized by ≥30-bpm increase in heart rate with standing upright (≥40 bpm for adolescents 12–19 years old), the absence of orthostatic hypotension (systolic blood pressure does *not* drop more than 20 mmHg), and symptoms. Predominantly affects females between ages 13 and 25 years.

CLINICAL MANIFESTATIONS

- Symptoms of presyncope may include diaphoresis, dizziness, lightheadedness, palpitations, nausea, abdominal pain, headache, blurred or tunnel vision, weakness, and fatigue.
- Cardiac symptoms may include palpitations, shortness of breath, chest pain, and color changes.
- Family history may be notable for sudden death, arrhythmias, congenital heart defects, seizures, metabolic disorders, and psychiatric history.
- Significant physical exam findings are uncommon in children.
- Vital signs may demonstrate orthostasis.
- Systolic ejection murmur that increases with Valsalva maneuver or standing leads to concern for HCM.
- Loud second heart sound may indicate pulmonary hypertension.

DIAGNOSTICS

- History: Perform a thorough review of systems to ask about associated symptoms, potential triggers, modifying factors, and impact on daily activities. Include diet and exercise history.
- Vitals: Obtain orthostatic vital signs (i.e., check vitals while supine, sitting, and standing).
- 12-lead ECG recommended regardless of cardiac symptoms.
- If concern for seizure activity or trauma: Neurology referral, EEG, head CT
- If concern for cardiac disease: ECG, chest x-ray, echocardiography, exercise stress test, Holter monitor
- Tilt-table testing may help diagnose neurocardiogenic syncope, but has poor sensitivity and specificity.

MANAGEMENT

Acute Management

- Keep patient supine until fully recovered
- For an arrhythmia, consider pharmacologic treatment, defibrillation, or cardioversion as per Pediatric Advanced Life Support protocols

Cardiac Syncope

- Congenital heart disease present: Treat underlying cause
- Arrhythmia present: May need internal defibrillator, medication, radiofrequency ablation in catheterization laboratory (e.g., WPW syndrome)
- Exercise stress test and electrophysiologic testing in catheterization laboratory may aid in diagnosis.

Presyncope Due to Postural Tachycardia Syndrome (POTS)

- Nonpharmacologic treatments (first-line therapy): Increase fluid and salt intake to increase blood volume (at least 2–3 liters of water per day and 10–12 grams of dietary salt intake per day); use compression stockings to decrease venous pooling; encourage regular exercise.
- Nonpharmacologic treatments (second-line therapy): Prescribe salt tablets or fludrocortisone (Florinef) to boost sodium retention; midodrine metabolites are $alpha_1$-agonists that constrict vessels and increase venous return; for severe symptoms, administer IV fluids with 1–2 liters of normal saline (repeated IV infusions are not recommended for routine care); invasive electrophysiology studies and radiofrequency ablation procedures are not recommended for the sinus tachycardia seen in patients with POTS.

Neurocardiogenic (Vasovagal) Syncope

- Volume expansion: Encourage fluid and salt intake.
- Mineralocorticoids (e.g., Florinef) increase circulating volume and help maintain cerebral perfusion pressure. Efficacy is approximately 60–80%.
- Beta-blockers modify the abnormal feedback loop and prevent increased vagal output.

Dermatology

Kara N. Shah, MD, PhD

BLISTERING DISORDERS

NECROTIZING FASCIITIS

An acute, rapidly progressive, necrotizing, life-threatening infection of the subcutaneous tissues, often associated with septic shock or streptococcal toxic shock syndrome.

- Can be rapidly fatal if not recognized and treated promptly and appropriately

EPIDEMIOLOGY

- Rare in children; estimated 500–1500 cases per year in the United States
- Can be seen at any age, including neonates
- Most children with invasive group A β-hemolytic *Streptococcus* (GABHS) infection are otherwise healthy; more than 50% of children with non-GABHS necrotizing fasciitis have at least one risk factor.
- Risk factors: Antecedent varicella infection (with GABHS-related cases); recent surgery or trauma; intramuscular injection; chronic medical conditions (diabetes mellitus, malnutrition, obesity, immunosuppression). In neonates, circumcision, omphalitis, history of scalp electrode placement, necrotizing enterocolitis

ETIOLOGY

- Inoculation of bacteria into the subcutaneous tissues with resultant proliferation and release of destructive enzymes and exotoxins results in extensive tissue necrosis, thrombosis of blood vessels, and rapid progression along fascial planes.
- Common: GABHS. Typically involves the groin or lower extremities.
- Less common: Aerobic and nonaerobic organisms, including *Staphylococcus aureus*, anaerobic streptococci, group B *Streptococcus*, *Proteus vulgaris*, *Escherichia coli*, *Pseudomonas aeruginosa*, and *Bacteroides fragilis*. May be polymicrobial. Usually involves the abdominal wall, perianal or genital area, or a postoperative wound.

DIFFERENTIAL DIAGNOSIS

- Cellulitis, erysipelas, pyoderma, staphylococcal scalded skin syndrome, toxic shock syndrome, burns

CLINICAL MANIFESTATIONS

- Initial symptoms may be nonspecific and include localized pain, fever, chills, vomiting, pharyngitis, malaise, altered mental status, and myalgias.
- Skin manifestations are toxin-mediated, are typically seen with GABHS-related necrotizing fasciitis, and present with erythematous ill-defined patch(es) or plaque(s).
- Associated signs and symptoms include severe pain out of proportion to clinical findings, extreme tenderness involving both affected and clinically unaffected areas, numbness, edema, and murky dishwater-like discharge.
- Rapid progression to purpuric patch(es) or plaque(s) with or without blistering, followed by the development of ulceration and gangrene. Crepitus may be appreciated in non-GABHS-related necrotizing fasciitis.

- This systemic toxicity may include features of septic shock or, in the case of invasive GABHS, toxic shock syndrome with hypotension and multisystem organ failure.
- Fournier's gangrene: Involvement of the genital and perianal area; typically polymicrobial

DIAGNOSTICS

- Clinical diagnosis requires high level of suspicion.
- Cultures of blood, wound, and deep tissue (incisional biopsy)
- Histologic examination of incisional biopsy reveals tissue necrosis.
- CBC: Leukocytosis
- CRP, ESR: Elevated
- Metabolic panel: Hyponatremia, elevated blood urea nitrogen, metabolic acidosis, hypocalcemia, elevated serum creatine phosphokinase
- Ultrasonography may show fascial thickening and fluid collections.
- MRI is more sensitive than CT but may overestimate involvement; a negative MRI can exclude necrotizing fasciitis

MANAGEMENT

- Prompt surgical consultation and surgical exploration with wide excision of necrotic tissue; delay results in higher mortality. Surgical reexploration and repeat debridement may be required 24–48 hours later.
- Wound care: Vacuum-assisted wound closure, flap reconstruction, and split-thickness skin grafting may be required.
- Pain management
- Empiric therapy should include a beta-lactam (e.g., ceftriaxone) plus clindamycin; vancomycin, ceftaroline, or daptomycin should be added if MRSA is a concern. Antibiotics should be modified if organisms are identified. For GABHS-related cases, use penicillin plus clindamycin. If anaerobes are suspected (e.g., presence of gas) then either metronidazole or clindamycin should be used).
- IVIG may benefit patients with GABHS-related necrotizing fasciitis and toxic shock syndrome.
- Hyperbaric oxygen therapy may be helpful when available.
- In children, mortality is about 5%; it is highest in those with comorbid medical conditions, non–GABHS-related disease, septic shock, multisystem organ failure, and young age.
- The risk of secondary invasive GABHS infection is significantly elevated in household contacts and approaches 200 times that of the general population; therefore, chemoprevention should be considered for close contacts

STAPHYLOCOCCAL SCALDED SKIN SYNDROME

A bacterial toxin-mediated exfoliative rash characterized by areas of erythema and superficial desquamation, resembling a superficial burn.

EPIDEMIOLOGY

- Generally occurs in children who lack neutralizing antibodies to staphylococcal toxins, including neonates and children younger than 5 years or older children and adults with renal impairment or immunosuppression.
- Outbreaks of SSSS may occur in nurseries and neonatal units as a result of asymptomatic carriage by staff.
- Occult or apparent infection or colonization with *Staph. aureus* strains harboring exfoliative exotoxin, typically belonging to phage group II.

ETIOLOGY

- Exfoliative toxins A and B are produced by certain strains of *Staph. aureus* and act as serine proteases that degrade a specific keratinocyte cell adhesion molecule, desmoglein-1, resulting in the formation of a superficial, substratum corneum blister at the stratum granulosum.
- Nidus of infection typically involves head or neck or circumcision site (neonates) but may not be clinically apparent.
- Exotoxin dissemination via the bloodstream results in generalized blistering and may result in part from delayed renal clearance of exotoxin and/or lack of antiexotoxin antibodies.

DIFFERENTIAL DIAGNOSIS

- Thermal burn, toxic epidermal necrolysis, Kawasaki disease, toxic shock syndrome, toxin-mediated perineal erythema, erythema multiforme, Stevens-Johnson syndrome (SJS), epidermolysis bullosa

CLINICAL MANIFESTATIONS

- Prodrome of fever (low-grade), malaise, irritability, rhinorrhea, pharyngitis, and/or conjunctivitis
- Tender, erythematous patches develop initially in intertriginous zones and on face; may become more generalized.
- Superficial, flaccid bullae develop in involved areas and often rupture spontaneously, revealing moist, denuded areas resembling burns.
- Nikolsky sign: Extension of blister with applied lateral pressure along its edge
- Perioral, periocular, and perinasal erythema and crusting are characteristic.
- Involved areas eventually desquamate and heal without scarring within 2–3 weeks.

DIAGNOSTICS

- Bacterial gram stain and culture: Nares/nasopharynx, perianal/perineum, conjunctivae, umbilicus (neonates), blood (rarely positive); rarely, source may be osteomyelitis, septic arthritis, pyomyositis, pneumonia, or other noncutaneous infection. Toxin-induced blisters or areas of exfoliation are generally culture-negative.
- Skin biopsy: Rarely necessary but can differentiate SSSS from TEN, skin biopsy for frozen section can be performed rapidly to differentiate superficial split within granular layer of epidermis (SSSS) from deeper, full-thickness epidermal involvement (TEN).

MANAGEMENT

- Most patients have an excellent prognosis if condition is identified and treated promptly.
- Parenteral antibiotics are recommended. Use oxacillin, nafcillin, or cefazolin for empiric therapy. Methicillin resistance is rare in exotoxin-producing strains of *Staph. aureus*. Clindamycin may be added to decrease exotoxin production.
- Localized or limited involvement may respond to oral antibiotics such as clindamycin, penicillinase-resistant penicillin, or first- or second-generation cephalosporin.
- Topical and/or systemic corticosteroids are contraindicated.
- Therapy should be continued for a minimum of 7–10 days.
- Wound care: Leave bullae intact. Denuded areas may be covered with petrolatum gauze or other nonadherent contact-layer dressing. Minimize friction. Monitor for secondary infection.

- Cool compresses applied to areas of facial crusting and application of ophthalmic antibiotic ointment may be helpful.
- Patients require supportive therapy with pain management, nutrition, temperature control, and hydration.

STEVENS–JOHNSON SYNDROME (SJS) AND TOXIC EPIDERMAL NECROLYSIS (TEN)

Rare hypersensitivity reactions within the spectrum of severe cutaneous adverse reactions. Predominantly drug-related, they share a common pathophysiology. They are dermatologic emergencies with significant morbidity and mortality.

- SJS manifests as atypical targetoid lesions associated with erosions involving two or more mucous membranes. Bullous lesions may be present. Skin involvement is limited to 10% or less of BSA
- SJS/TEN overlap shares features of SJS and TEN with involvement of 10–30% BSA in association with mucous membrane involvement.
- TEN manifests as extensive skin erythema, pain, and sloughing involving >30% BSA, usually in association with mucous membrane erosions.

EPIDEMIOLOGY

- Estimated incidence of 2 per 1 million general population

ETIOLOGY

- Proposed pathogenesis involves activation of cytotoxic T cells by drug antigens and elaboration of inflammatory cytokines and circulating proapoptotic factors, including Fas ligand and granulysin, which leads to keratinocyte apoptosis, skin necrosis, and skin detachment.
- Genetic susceptibility has been demonstrated in some populations in association with specific HLA alleles, including HLA-B*1502 and carbamazepine-induced SJS.
- Most common drugs implicated: Antibiotics (aminopenicillins, sulfonamides), allopurinol, NSAIDs of the oxicam type, and aromatic anticonvulsants (phenobarbital, phenytoin, carbamazepine). Other drugs: antibiotics (cephalosporins, tetracyclines, macrolides, quinolones) and NSAIDs of the acetic acid type
- SJS may also occur with *Mycoplasma pneumoniae* infection or other respiratory virus infection, including influenzae; the clinical presentation often manifests as mucositis without significant cutaneous manifestations (*M. pneumoniae* respiratory infection–induced rash and mucositis (MIRM)).
- In some cases, no clear etiology can be identified.

DIFFERENTIAL DIAGNOSIS

- Exanthematous erythematous macules and papules: Viral exanthems, morbilliform/exanthematous drug eruption, urticarial hypersensitivity, urticarial vasculitis, DRESS/DIHS
- Targetoid lesions: Annular urticaria, erythema multiforme
- Bullous lesions: Bullous impetigo, linear IgA disease (chronic bullous dermatosis of childhood), childhood bullous pemphigoid, childhood pemphigus vulgaris, generalized bullous fixed drug eruption
- Skin peeling and sloughing: SSSS, toxic shock syndrome, Kawasaki disease, paraneoplastic pemphigus, acute generalized exanthematous pustulosis acute cutaneous graft-versus-host disease

• Mucositis: Herpetic gingivostomatitis, aphthous stomatitis, pemphigus vulgaris, acute genital ulceration/idiopathic vulvar aphthosis

CLINICAL MANIFESTATIONS

• Generally develops within 2 months of drug initiation, and often within first 1–4 weeks.
• Prodrome of fever, malaise, pharyngitis, and eye pain may be noted.
• Cutaneous manifestations typically begin on the torso and face and may rapidly generalize.
• SJS: Primary lesions are discrete, atypical targetoid lesions, often violaceous and/or blistered. Lesions may coalesce, in particular on the face and torso.
• TEN: Primary lesions are tender, erythematous patches and plaques that develop large bullae that coalesce and rapidly slough, leaving large denuded areas of skin. Positive Nikolsky sign: extension of blister with applied lateral pressure along edge of blister.
• Mucositis (oropharyngeal, conjunctivae, urethral, genital, perirectal) often results in pain, poor oral intake, and dehydration.
• Ocular manifestations include conjunctivitis, eyelid edema, blepharitis, corneal erosions, symblepharon, and corneal scarring, which is a major cause of long-term morbidity and may result in blindness.
• Rarely, gastrointestinal and respiratory epithelia may become involved.
• Severe cutaneous involvement may result in cutaneous dyschromia and scarring. Nail dystrophy and alopecia may occur. Areas of mucous membrane involvement, including the oropharynx, vagina, urethra, and esophagus, are at risk for scarring, adhesions, and strictures. Long-term sequelae are reported in approximately 50% of children.

DIAGNOSTICS

• Usually a clinical diagnosis, but skin biopsy can be helpful if the diagnosis is uncertain. SJS presents with an intense interface reaction along the dermal–epidermal junction with central necrosis or blister formation. TEN can be diagnosed with a frozen section that reveals full-thickness epidermal necrosis and a subepidermal split.
• Consider evaluation for associated infection, including bacterial culture and HSV PCR from lesional skin and oropharyngeal swab for *M. pneumoniae* PCR.

MANAGEMENT

• Dermatology consultation recommended.
• Promptly discontinue all possible inciting medications.
• Initiate treatment of etiologic underlying infection, if appropriate.
• Supportive care: Pain management, nutritional support, maintain isothermia, maintain hydration and electrolyte balance (hyponatremia, hypokalemia, and hypophosphatemia are common).
• Close surveillance is required for infection/sepsis and impending respiratory failure, which increase the risk of death. Hypovolemia and septicemia may result in shock and multisystem organ failure.
• Wound care: Bullae should be left intact but may be drained via sterile technique. Aggressive debridement should be avoided. Apply petrolatum gauze or other nonadherent contact layer. Use topical antibiotics judiciously. Use of specialized mattress to minimize pressure can be helpful. Frequently apply bland emollients/lubricating ointments to involved mucosa. Oral hygiene may be assisted by use of an oral disinfectant rinse such as chlorhexidine.

- Appropriate consultation for mucous membrane involvement: Eyes (ophthalmology); urethral (urology); gastroesophageal, intestinal, rectal (gastroenterology); tracheobronchial (pulmonology)
- Systemic corticosteroids are of uncertain benefit. Short-term early use may moderate disease progression, but prolonged use is contraindicated.
- Use of IVIG may be effective at arresting progression of the disease for both SJS and TEN. For progressive disease, especially if recognized early, within first 2–3 days of presentation, consider IVIG 1 mg/kg/day for 3–4 days. Other therapeutic agents that have been used with variable response include cyclosporine and infliximab.

EXANTHEMS

DRUG REACTION WITH EOSINOPHILIA AND SYSTEMIC SYMPTOMS (DRESS)/DRUG-INDUCED HYPERSENSITIVITY SYNDROME (DIHS)

A distinct and potentially life-threatening severe adverse drug reaction characterized by a morbilliform cutaneous eruption with fever, lymphadenopathy, hematologic abnormalities, and multiorgan manifestations.

EPIDEMIOLOGY

- Incidence is unknown but some report overall population risk ranging from 1 in 1000 to 1 in 10,000 drug exposures.
- Incidence may be as high as 10–50 per 100,000 individuals on anticonvulsants such as phenytoin and carbamazepine and 1 per 100 children on lamotrigine.
- Individuals with specific HLA haplotypes are predisposed; HLA alleles are necessary but not sufficient to elicit a drug response.

ETIOLOGY

- Considered a severe systemic hypersensitivity reaction to a medication and its reactive drug metabolites; although specific pathophysiology is not known, appears to be mediated by activation of CD4-positive and CD8-positive T lymphocytes.
- Eosinophilia may play a role in visceral complications.
- Aromatic anticonvulsants (phenobarbital, carbamazepine, phenytoin, and lamotrigine), minocycline, and sulfonamide antibiotics are the most common causes but antibiotics, including ampicillin, cefotaxime, streptomycin, and vancomycin have also been implicated.
- Antivirals such as abacavir and nevirapine, antidepressants such as bupropion and fluoxetine, antihypertensives such as amlodipine and captopril, nonsteroidal antiinflammatory drugs (NSAIDs) such as celecoxib and ibuprofen, as well as miscellaneous medications such as allopurinol, ranitidine, epoetin alfa, and mexiletine have also been implicated.
- Most often occurs between 2 and 6 weeks after initiation of a medication but reaction can occur more quickly upon reexposure to a medication.
- HLA-B*5701 allele has been associated with abacavir-induced DRESS.
- HLA-A*3101 is associated with carbamazepine drug reactions including DRESS and SJS/TEN syndrome
- HLA-DR3 and HLA-DQ2 are associated with carbamazepine-induced DRESS.
- HLA-B*5801 is associated with allopurinol-induced DRESS.
- Primary activation or reactivation of herpesviruses, including HHV-6 infection, cytomegalovirus infection, EBV, and HHV-7, have also been implicated.

DIFFERENTIAL DIAGNOSIS

• SJS, TEN, toxic-shock syndrome, Kawasaki disease, exfoliative dermatitis, acute generalized exanthematous pustulosis, viral exanthema, acute cutaneous lupus erythematosus

CLINICAL MANIFESTATIONS

• There is no reliable standard for diagnosis, though several scoring systems have been proposed. Diagnostic criteria include acute onset of exanthema with fever, suspicion of drug reaction, hospitalization, lymphadenopathy, involvement of at least one internal organ, and hematologic abnormalities, including lymphopenia, lymphocytosis, atypical lymphocytosis, eosinophilia >10%, or thrombocytopenia.
• Often a prodrome of fever, pharyngitis, and malaise 2–3 days before onset of rash
• Characteristic cutaneous features include a morbilliform exanthem with accentuation on the face, upper trunk, and proximal extremities, but may progress to erythroderma. Pruritus is common. Other morphologies that are less common can occur; these include vesicles, atypical targetoid plaques, purpura, and sterile pustules.
• Facial edema is common, especially periorbital.
• Diffuse lymphadenopathy occurs in 30–60% of patients.
• Associated mucosal involvement includes cheilitis and pharyngeal erythema; erosions are rare.
• Desquamation develops several days to weeks after the initial eruption and may last for several weeks.
• Multiple organ systems can be involved; hepatic (hepatitis), renal (tubulointerstitial nephritis), and pulmonary complications are the most common.
• Shortness of breath, tachypnea, and nonproductive cough may occur; more severe pulmonary manifestations are rare but more common with minocycline-induced DRESS and may include interstitial pneumonitis and pulmonary edema.
• Myocarditis and pericarditis may occur but are rare in children. Myocarditis can occur months after withdrawal of the offending medication.
• Severe, atypical cases can have neurologic (encephalitis, meningitis, polyneuritis) or gastrointestinal (diarrhea, pancreatitis, gastrointestinal mucosal hemorrhage) involvement.
• Neurologic manifestations are rare and typically occur weeks after the onset of the rash; they are thought to be related to reactivation of HHV-6.
• Autoimmune complications, especially autoimmune thyroiditis (Graves' disease), can be seen as delayed sequelae. Development of type 1 diabetes mellitus and autoimmune hemolytic anemia have also been reported.
• Rash and other abnormalities typically resolve over 1–2 months after discontinuation of the offending medication.
• Avoidance of the causative medication as well as any cross-reacting medications is mandatory; family members may also be at risk and should be counseled appropriately.

DIAGNOSTICS

• CBC: Lymphocytosis, atypical lymphocytosis, eosinophilia, and/or thrombocytopenia may be seen.
• Liver-function tests: Elevated liver transaminases, in particular ALT, elevated alkaline phosphatase; markedly elevated ALT and serum bilirubin with jaundice are important predictors of acute liver failure and death.
• Metabolic panel: Elevated serum creatinine may be seen.
• Urinalysis: Proteinuria and eosinophilic sediment may be seen.
• Lactate dehydrogenase level may be elevated.

- Evaluation of HHV-6, HHV-7, EBV, and/or CMV by serum PCR.
- Evaluation of hepatitis A IgM antibody, hepatitis B surface antigen, hepatitis B core IgM antibody, hepatitis C viral RNA may help exclude viral hepatitis.
- Consider ANA testing if systemic lupus erythematosus is being considered.
- Thyroid-function testing should be performed at baseline (TSH, free thyroxine) and then approximately 6 weeks after presentation.

MANAGEMENT

- Dermatology consultation is recommended.
- Consider consultation with other specialists as appropriate, depending on severity of other organ involvement.
- Identify and withdraw causative medication.
- Fluid replacement and correction of electrolyte abnormalities
- For cases of mild, predominantly cutaneous involvement, initiation of a mid- to high-potency topical corticosteroid is appropriate.
- Antihistamines may help with associated pruritus.
- For cases with significant systemic involvement, initiation of systemic corticosteroids such as prednisone or methylprednisolone at a dose of 1–2 mg/kg/day is recommended. Tapering gradually over weeks to months after clinical examination have shown improvement in laboratory abnormalities; rapid tapering may precipitate relapse.
- IVIG at a dose of 1 g/kg per dose once daily can be considered in severe cases that do not respond to corticosteroids.
- Plasmapheresis and immunosuppressive drugs such as cyclophosphamide, cyclosporine, mycophenolate mofetil, and rituximab may also be considered for corticosteroid- and/or IVIG-resistant cases,

ACUTE URTICARIAL HYPERSENSITIVITY

An acute cutaneous reaction characterized by pruritic, transient annular, and polycyclic urticarial plaques that resemble erythema multiforme.

ETIOLOGY

- Acute urticaria results from degranulation of mast cells and basophils and release of vasoactive substances, including histamine, bradykinin, and prostaglandin D_2, which cause extravasation of plasma into the dermis.
- Acute urticaria may be immune-mediated, either by IgE (most medication- and food-related urticaria), cytotoxic T cells, or immune complex formation; or may be non–immune-mediated such as occurs with complement-mediated urticaria (radiocontrast agents, bacterial and viral infections, opioids) or physical urticaria.
- In children, acute urticaria usually occurs in response to medications (most commonly penicillin and related antibiotics) or infection, most commonly respiratory viruses, gastrointestinal viruses, or streptococcal infection, although in some cases, no clear etiology can be identified.

EPIDEMIOLOGY

- Acute urticaria is very common and occurs in up to 10% of children by adolescence.
- Acute urticaria occurs more commonly in infants and younger children but may be seen at any age.

TABLE 6-1	Comparison of Acute Urticarial Hypersensitivity and Erythema Multiforme	
Acute Urticarial Hypersensitivity		**Erythema Multiforme**
Annular, polycyclic urticarial lesions (centers are often pale)		Targetoid lesions (dusky centers with pale rim of edema and peripheral erythema)
Lesions range from small to giant		Lesions are often small to medium-sized
Evanescent lesions (resolve within 24 hours)		Fixed lesions (persist for up to 1 week)
Acral edema of hands, feet, and face common		Acral edema not typically seen
Pruritus common		Pruritus uncommon
Response to antihistamines and corticosteroids		Possible response to corticosteroids; no response to antihistamines

DIFFERENTIAL DIAGNOSIS

- Serum sickness, serum-sickness–like reaction, erythema multiforme, arthropod bites/papular urticarial, annular/gyrate erythema, viral exanthema, cutaneous mastocytosis, autoimmune disease, urticarial vasculitis (**Table 6-1**)

CLINICAL MANIFESTATIONS

- Primary lesions: Generalized annular and polycyclic urticarial papules and plaques that typically are evanescent, lasting less than 24 hours. Occasionally, lesions may resolve with a residual ecchymosis or hyperpigmentation
- Angioedema of hands, feet, and face is common and resolves more slowly than urticaria.
- Dermatographism: Stroking of the skin results in urtication at the site.
- Associated symptoms may include fever and specific symptoms suggestive of associated infection but are often absent.
- Progression to anaphylaxis is rare.
- By definition, acute urticaria resolves within 6 weeks, but it often resolves within several days.

DIAGNOSTICS

- No specific diagnostic tests are indicated unless necessary for the identification of a specific associated infection.
- Skin biopsy may be performed if the diagnosis is uncertain and manifests dermal edema; dilatation of blood and lymphatic vessels, and a sparse perivascular mononuclear infiltrate with variable numbers of eosinophils and neutrophils.

MANAGEMENT

- Discontinue potential causative medications.
- H_1-antagonist antihistamines may be administered at regularly scheduled intervals. As acute urticaria is self-limiting, therapy is rarely needed for more than 1–2 weeks. Use of nonsedating second-generation antihistamines (loratidine, cetirizine) or third-generation antihistamines (levocetirizine, desloratadine, fexofenadine) are typically better tolerated than sedating antihistamines (diphenhydramine, hydroxyzine).
- Consider adjunct H_2-antagonist antihistamines (cimetidine, ranitidine)
- The cutaneous urticarial reaction typically responds rapidly to antihistamines; the edema may respond more slowly.

- Topical corticosteroids are not indicated.
- Rarely, a short course of a systemic corticosteroid may be indicated in the case of a severe, persistent reaction that is unresponsive to antihistamine therapy.
- Treat associated infection as indicated, although will not hasten resolution of urticaria.

ERYTHEMA MULTIFORME

An acute, self-limited, and sometimes recurrent immunologically mediated mucocutaneous eruption characterized by target lesions with an acral predilection. The oral mucous membranes are commonly affected. The use of the terms erythema multiforme minor and erythema multiforme major should be avoided.

EPIDEMIOLOGY

- Overall incidence is reportedly 1–6 per million.
- Most commonly affects older children and young adults.

ETIOLOGY

- Erythema multiforme is a hypersensitivity reaction seen in response to a plethora of inciting agents, including infectious agents, medications, vaccinations, inflammatory conditions, and environmental agents. It is believed to be a cell-mediated delayed-type hypersensitivity reaction (**Table 6-2**).
- Infectious agents, including numerous bacterial, viral, and fungal microorganisms, appear to be the most common inciting agents, although many cases have no clearly identifiable cause.
- Recurrent erythema multiforme is strongly associated with HSV infection and may occur a few days to a few weeks after HSV infection or recurrence.
- Drug-induced erythema multiforme appears to be related to impaired metabolism of the causative drug, which results in the production of reactive and/or toxic drug metabolites that may serve as haptens.

DIFFERENTIAL DIAGNOSIS

- Exanthematous erythematous macules and papules: Viral exanthems, urticaria, urticarial vasculitis, secondary syphilis
- Targetoid lesions: Annular urticaria, fixed drug eruption, annular/figurate erythema
- Mucositis: Herpetic gingivostomatitis, aphthous stomatitis, pemphigus vulgaris

CLINICAL MANIFESTATIONS

- Primary lesions: Classic target lesions present as erythematous papules that rapidly evolve over 1–2 days to manifest a central violaceous macule, which may blister, surrounded by an intermediate ring of pallor and a peripheral erythematous rim. Pruritus or a burning sensation may be reported. Target lesions favor extremities, including hands and feet
- Köbner phenomenon: Lesions may present at sites of recent trauma.
- Target lesions typically present over several days and then remain fixed in location and morphology for at least 1 week, after which time they slowly resolve. May resolve with postinflammatory hyperpigmentation.
- Mucositis: Typically mild and limited to one mucous membrane (usually the oral mucosa); rarely involves conjunctival or, urogenital mucosa.
- Systemic symptoms are uncommon but may include low-grade fever, cough, and rhinorrhea.

TABLE 6-2 Evaluation and Management of Cutaneous Drug Hypersensitivity

Primary Lesion	Clinical Features	Common Causes	Management
Urticaria	Evanescent, pruritic wheals lasting <24 hours; angioedema of hands, feet, face	Penicillin-based antibiotics	Discontinue drug; start antihistamines (consider combination of H_1- and H_2-antihistamines)
Morbilliform eruptions	Symmetrical "measles-like" exanthem with erythematous macules and papules; may be pruritic	Antibiotics (e.g., penicillins and sulfonamides)	Discontinuation of drug advised, although in some patients, reaction may resolve even if drug continued; antihistamines for pruritus; topical corticosteroids
Erythema multiforme	Target lesions (dusky center, pale edematous rim with erythematous border) lasting >24 hours; mild mucositis (one mucous membrane, usually oral); may be mildly pruritic	Usually occurs with infections (e.g., herpes simplex) rather than drugs	Self-limited; supportive care
Stevens–Johnson syndrome	Atypical target lesions; mucositis (2 or more mucous membranes)	Antibiotics (e.g., penicillins, sulfonamides); anticonvulsants (e.g., phenobarbital, phenytoin, carbamazepine); M. pneumoniae (may present with marked mucosal involvement with limited to no cutaneous involvement)	Prompt discontinuation of drug. Early initiation of systemic corticosteroids may be of benefit but use is controversial. Severe cases may respond to IVIG. Supportive care.
Toxic epidermal necrolysis	Extensive areas of tender, erythematous skin associated with skin sloughing and denudation; mucositis often present; patients typically appear ill	Antibiotics (e.g., penicillins, sulfonamides); anticonvulsants (e.g., phenobarbital, phenytoin, carbamazepine, lamotrigine)	Prompt discontinuation of drug. Early initiation of systemic steroids may be of benefit but use is controversial. Severe cases may be successfully treated with IVIG. Supportive care. Monitor for systemic complications.
DRESS (also known as DIHS)	Exanthematous eruption associated with liver toxicity, fever, lymphadenopathy, eosinophilia, atypical lymphocytosis, although not all features may be present early in course	Aromatic anticonvulsants (e.g., phenytoin, phenobarbital, carbamazepine); sulfonamide antibiotics; minocycline	Discontinuation of drug; systemic corticosteroids; supportive care; monitor for systemic complications.

DIAGNOSTICS

- Usually a clinical diagnosis by means of skin biopsy may help in atypical cases. Histology demonstrates a vacuolar interface dermatitis with vacuolar changes and dyskeratotic basal keratinocytes; a mild-to-moderate superficial perivascular lymphocytic infiltrate may be seen.
- HSV PCR from an oropharyngeal specimen may be performed if there is clinical suspicion for HSV-associated erythema multiforme.

MANAGEMENT

- Erythema multiforme is a self-limited phenomenon, often requiring only supportive care.
- Bland emollients or topical antibiotics may be applied to eroded areas.
- Patients with mucositis and poor oral intake may require intravenous rehydration or hyperalimentation.
- Antihistamines (diphenhydramine, hydroxyzine, cetirizine) may be used to treat associated pruritus.
- In patients with HSV-associated erythema multiforme, treatment with acyclovir may be indicated early in the course of the rash.
- Ophthalmologic consultation is recommended for ocular involvement.

VASCULAR PHENOMENA

COMPLICATED HEMANGIOMAS

Hemangiomas of infancy are common vascular tumors that undergo a typical growth pattern of proliferation, stabilization (plateau), and gradual involution. Most hemangiomas require no therapy beyond active nonintervention and appropriate anticipatory guidance. Complications may arise with hemangiomas occurring near vital structures, in certain anatomic locations, or in patients with multiple hemangiomas (Table 6-3).

EPIDEMIOLOGY

- Occur in approximately 10% of infants
- More common in female infants, preterm infants, multiple gestations, and in association with chorionic villus sampling and amniocentesis
- Most complications arise during the proliferative phase, during the first 3–6 months of life.

ETIOLOGY

- Most cases are sporadic and have no clear genetic predisposing factors.
- Hemangiomas of infancy share many similar cellular markers with placental tissue and may have a common precursor.

DIFFERENTIAL DIAGNOSIS

- Vascular malformations: Venous malformation, arteriovenous malformation, lymphatic malformation, capillary malformation
- Kaposiform hemangioendothelioma
- Rapidly involuting congenital hemangioma: A congenital hemangioma that involutes rapidly (during the first year) and may result in cutaneous atrophy

TABLE 6-3	Complications Related to Hemangiomas
Predisposing Factor	**Complication**
Periocular location	Amblyopia
Nasal tip, ear	Cosmetic disfigurement
Beard distribution	Airway involvement
Orolabial	Ulceration
Large facial, segmental distribution	PHACES syndrome
Large pelvic and/or buttocks, segmental distribution	PELVIS/SACRAL syndrome
Midline prevertebral location	Spinal dysraphism
Perineal or perianal site	Ulceration
Multiple ($\geq$6)	Visceral hemangiomatosis
Large hemangiomas	Mild thrombocytopenia; *not* Kasabach–Merritt phenomenon

PELVIS/SACRAL = perineal/buttock segmental hemangioma, external genitalia anomalies, lipomeningocele, vesicorenal anomalies, imperforate anus, and skin tags (perianal); PHACES = posterior fossa abnormalities, large segmental facial hemangioma, cerebrovascular arterial anomalies, coarctation of the aorta, eye abnormalities, and midline sternal anomalies.

- Noninvoluting congenital hemangioma: A congenital hemangioma with overlying telangiectasia that does not involute
- Vascular tumor mimics: Lipoblastoma, fibrosarcoma, or other soft-tissue sarcomas; often large, congenital lesions showing rapid growth, ulceration, and fixation to underlying tissue; dermoid cyst; myofibroma

CLINICAL MANIFESTATIONS

- Hemangiomas are often not visible at birth and typically manifest within the first 2–8 weeks of life, frequently as faint areas of macular erythema that rapidly increase in size.
- Superficial hemangiomas have a "strawberry" appearance. Deep hemangiomas may appear soft and bluish without much superficial change. Mixed hemangiomas may have features of both superficial and deep morphology,
- Hemangiomas undergo proliferation and may grow rapidly during the first 3–5 months of life; the growth phase then typically slowly plateaus or stabilizes until approximately 1 year of age. After 1 year of age, hemangiomas undergo slow, gradual involution over 5–8 years.
- Most involute significantly, but residual telangiectasia or fibrofatty tissue may remain.
- Complications prompting treatment may include rapidly growing periocular hemangiomas that threaten vision, symptomatic airway hemangiomas, extensive ulcerated hemangiomas with secondary infection or sepsis, symptomatic visceral hemangiomatosis resulting in congestive heart failure, PHACES syndrome, and sacral/pelvis syndrome
- PHACES syndrome: posterior fossa abnormalities, large segmental facial hemangioma, cerebrovascular arterial anomalies, coarctation of the aorta, eye abnormalities, and midline sternal anomalies
- PELVIS/SACRAL syndrome

DIAGNOSTICS

- MRI of the orbits or neck, respectively, may help delineate anatomic extent of orbital or airway hemangiomas.
- MRI of the brain is recommended to evaluate for associated anomalies as seen in PHACES syndrome. MRA of head and neck is also important for delineating the cerebrovascular arterial anomalies of PHACES syndrome.
- MRI of the lumbosacral spine and renal ultrasound are recommended to evaluate suspected cases of PELVIS/SACRAL syndrome.
- ECG and echocardiography are recommended when PHACES is suspected
- Skin biopsy for atypical lesions may help confirm the diagnosis of a hemangioma and exclude a diagnosis of fibrosarcoma, other vascular tumor, or vascular malformation.

MANAGEMENT

- Dermatology consultation is recommended for complicated hemangiomas.
- Consultation with other subspecialists, including ophthalmology, otolaryngology, plastic surgery, and cardiology, as appropriate, should be considered when complications are present or suspected.
- The following are indications for systemic treatment: Periocular hemangiomas threatening vision; symptomatic airway involvement; ulcerated hemangiomas unresponsive to conservative management; congestive heart failure due to coarctation of the aorta or hepatic hemangiomatosis; large segmental hemangiomas such as seen in PHACES syndrome and PELVIS/SACRAL syndrome; proliferating hemangiomas with risk for significant cosmetic disfigurement.
- Consider propranolol therapy 2–3 mg/kg/day divided every 8–12 hours. Propranolol is now considered as first-line therapy. Monitor for propranolol-related side effects, including bradycardia, hypotension, and hypoglycemia
- Consider systemic steroid therapy (2–3 mg/kg/day of prednisone or prednisolone) if propranolol is contraindicated or as adjunctive therapy if response to propranolol is suboptimal. If initiating corticosteroids, consider gastrointestinal prophylaxis with ranitidine or cimetidine.
- Management of ulcerated hemangiomas should include evaluation for infection; soaks with tap water, saline, or acetic acid twice daily; topical antibiotic therapy (topical mupirocin or topical metronidazole); and daily to twice-daily dressing changes with non-adherent dressing (Telfa, petrolatum gauze, or Mepilex). Consider timolol 0.5% solution applied topically twice daily or pulsed dye laser therapy.
- If response to propranolol and/or corticosteroids is suboptimal, consider surgical intervention or interventional radiologic embolization of selected hemangiomas.
- Patients with six or more hemangiomas are at increased risk for visceral hemangiomatosis (although visceral hemangiomas may be seen in the absence of cutaneous hemangiomas); the liver is the most common extracutaneous site, although almost any organ may be involved. Hepatomegaly, splenomegaly, congestive heart failure, and hypothyroidism are potential complications. Abdominal ultrasonography or MRI, MRI of the brain, MRI of the chest, and/or MRI of the spine may help delineate the extent of involvement where appropriate,
- Uncomplicated hemangiomas with little to no risk for complications may be managed with active nonintervention or initiation of topical timolol 0.5% solution, as appropriate.

ATOPIC DERMATITIS

A chronic, relapsing inflammatory skin disease characterized by pruritus, erythema, scaling, oozing, and crusting. Impaired skin-barrier function and abnormalities in the immune response lead to a predilection for recurrent bacterial and/or viral skin infections. Associated with other atopic diseases: asthma, allergic rhinosinusitis and conjunctivitis, food allergy, eosinophilic gastrointestinal disorders.

• Infectious complications, namely bacterial superinfection with *Staph. aureus* and eczema herpeticum, are associated with acute flares.

EPIDEMIOLOGY

• Atopic dermatitis affects approximately 20% of the pediatric population.
• Age at onset is typically within the first 2 years of life, and while many children will "outgrow" their atopic dermatitis, a small but significant minority will develop persistent and/or progressively worsening disease.
• Eczema herpeticum is seen in 10–20% of patients with atopic dermatitis and is associated with early onset atopic dermatitis and more severe disease.
• Bacterial colonization and superinfection with *Staph. aureus* is very common, and systemic infection such as osteomyelitis and septicemia may also occur. Staphylococcal superantigens promote inflammation
• Secondary bacterial infection with *S. pyogenes* may also be seen, either alone or in combination with *Staph. aureus* infection.
• In addition, patients with atopic dermatitis may develop other cutaneous infections, including widespread viral infection with molluscum contagiosum, coxsackievirus, vaccinia or papillomavirus, and fungal infections with dermatophyte molds or pityrosporum.

ETIOLOGY

• Atopic dermatitis is a complex disease in which genetic and environmental factors contribute to chronic skin inflammation; allergic sensitization to food and environmental allergens and the production of specific IgE antibodies predicts more severe, persistent disease.
• Impaired skin barrier results from decreased expression of proteins involved in the formation of the cornified cell envelope, including filaggrin, and dysfunction of both innate and adaptive immunity lead to increased susceptibility to microbial colonization of the skin and cutaneous infections.
• Bacterial superantigens and toxins contribute to inflammation and disease flares.

DIFFERENTIAL DIAGNOSIS

• Seborrheic dermatitis, scabies, contact dermatitis, nummular dermatitis, immunodeficiency

CLINICAL MANIFESTATIONS

• Colonization of the skin in patients with atopic dermatitis is common and must be distinguished from infection.
• Acute flares of atopic dermatitis manifest as erythematous, scaling patches and plaques, often with excoriations and crusting when secondary bacterial infection is present.
• Systemic symptoms such as fever or malaise may be present but are often absent unless *Strep. pyogenes* infection or eczema herpeticum is present or a systemic infection has developed.

- Complications of secondary bacterial infection include acute poststreptococcal glomerulonephritis.
- Eczema herpeticum presents acutely with the development of grouped, monomorphous, round, "punched out" erosions; crusting may be present. If herpes keratoconjunctivitis is present, there may be associated ocular pain, tearing, erythema, blurry vision, and/or photophobia. Secondary bacterial infection is common.
- Other complications of eczema herpeticum include meningitis, encephalitis, and bacterial sepsis, which have the potential for significant morbidity and mortality.

DIAGNOSTICS

- Wound culture for bacterial Gram stain and culture may be performed from any crusted area.
- HSV PCR should be performed if eczema herpeticum is suspected.
- Enterovirus PCR can also be performed from vesicles or from stool if coxsackievirus superinfection is suspected.

MANAGEMENT

- Initiate use of topical corticosteroids of appropriate potency based on the age of the patient, the site(s) involved, and the severity (**Table 6-4**). In general, topical corticosteroids should not be withheld during the treatment of bacterial superinfection and eczema herpeticum.

TABLE 6-4	Topical corticosteroid potencies
Class 1 (super potent)	
Clobetasol (Temovate) 0.05% ointment, cream, gel, solution	
Clobetasol (Olux) 0.05% foam	
Clobetasol (Clobex) 0.05% shampoo, spray	
Halobetasol (Ultravate) 0.05% ointment, cream	
Betamethasone dipropionate augmented (Diprolene) 0.05% ointment, gel	
Fluocinonide (Vanos) 0.1% cream	
Class 2 (potent)	
Fluocinonide (Lidex) 0.05% ointment, cream, gel	
Desoximetasone (Topicort) 0.25% ointment, cream	
Desoximetasone (Topicort) 0.05% gel	
Betamethasone dipropionate (Diprosone) 0.05% ointment	
Betamethasone dipropionate augmented (Diprolene) 0.05% cream, lotion	
Mometasone (Elocon) 0.1% ointment	
Class 3 (potent)	
Fluticasone (Cutivate) 0.005% ointment	
Betamethasone dipropionate (Diprosone) 0.05% cream	
Betamethasone valerate (Valisone) 0.1% ointment	
Fluocinonide (Lidex) 0.05% cream	
Desoximetasone (Topicort) 0.05% cream	

TABLE 6-4	Topical corticosteroid potencies *(Continued)*
Mometasone (Elocon) 0.1% ointment	
Triamcinolone (Kenalog) 0.1% ointment	

Class 4 (mid-potent)

Hydrocortisone valerate (Westcort) 0.2% ointment

Mometasone (Elocon) 0.1% cream

Prednicarbate (Dermatop) 0.1% ointment

Triamcinolone (Kenalog) 0.1% cream

Fluocinolone (Synalar) 0.025% ointment

Desoximetasone (Topicort LP) 0.05% cream

Betamethasone (Luxiq) 0.12% foam

Clocortolone (Cloderm) 0.1% cream

Class 5 (mid-potent)

Hydrocortisone valerate (Westcort) 0.2% cream

Betamethasone valerate (Valisone) 0.1% cream

Hydrocortisone butyrate (Locoid) 0.1% cream, ointment, solution

Betamethasone (Diprosone) 0.05% lotion

Triamcinolone (Kenalog) 0.1% lotion

Fluticasone (Cutivate) 0.05% cream

Fluocinolone (Synalar) 0.025% cream

Prednicarbate (Dermatop) 0.1% cream

Class 6 (mild)

Alclometasone (Aclovate) 0.05% ointment, cream

Desonide (Desowen) 0.05% cream

Betamethasone valerate (Valisone) 0.1% lotion

Fluocinolone (Synalar) 0.01% cream, solution

Desonide (Verdeso) 0.05% foam

Desonide (Desonate) 0.05% hydrogel

Fluocinolone (Dermasmoothe FS) 0.01% scalp oil

Class 7 (mild)

Hydrocortisone 2.5% ointment, cream

Hydrocortisone 1% ointment, cream

Reproduced with permission from Shah SS, Kemper AR, Ratner AJ: *Pediatric Infectious Diseases: Essentials for Practice*. New York, NY: McGraw Hill; 2019.

- In cases of suspected bacterial superinfection, parenteral antibiotics should be started empirically and adjusted based on culture results. Use of recent prior skin culture results may help guide antibiotic choice. In the absence of a history of methicillin-resistant *Staph. aureus* infection, use of a first- or second-generation cephalosporin for 7–10 days is recommended. For the treatment of *S. pyogenes* use of either a first- or second-generation cephalosporin or amoxicillin/clavulanate for 10 days is recommended.

- In the absence of clinical features suggestive of infection, mupirocin ointment or retapamulin ointment should be applied to eroded or crusted areas to minimize bacterial colonization.
- In cases of suspected eczema herpeticum, acyclovir should be started empirically. In patients with periocular involvement, ophthalmology consultation is recommended and use of antiviral ophthalmic medications such as 1% trifluridine or 3% vidarabine should be considered.
- Wet wraps performed once or twice a day is helpful for acute flares. Apply topical corticosteroids to affected areas, followed by damp gauze or pajamas; should be left in place for at least 1-2 hours. Apply bland emollients after wet wraps are removed. Use of tubular gauze such as Tubifast simplifies the regimen.
- Atopic skin care consisting of frequent application of bland emollients, limiting bathing to less than 10 minutes, and use of a gentle nonsoap cleanser is recommended.
- Use of a sedating antihistamine such as diphenhydramine or hydroxyzine may be helpful in reducing pruritus and facilitating sleep at bedtime and naptime.
- For patients with recurrent bacterial superinfection, initiation of bleach baths or use of an antibacterial skin cleanser such as chlorhexidine 2-3 times weekly in addition to use of mupirocin ointment to any eroded or crusted skin areas may be helpful.
- For patients with recurrent eczema herpeticum, initiation of oral acyclovir at prophylactic dosing may be considered.

CHAPTER 7

Emergency Medicine

James Dodington, MD
Paul L. Aronson, MD, MHS

INITIAL APPROACH TO THE SICK CHILD

Emergency evaluation differs from a standard inpatient history and physical in that less background information is available about the child and evaluation and intervention steps often need to happen at the same time. Figure 7-1 outlines some of the early steps in the evaluation of the sick child, as well as interventions to consider at each stage.

EMERGENT AIRWAY AND CERVICAL SPINE STABILIZATION

- Open airway with head-tilt/jaw-thrust maneuver (use jaw thrust alone for trauma patients).
- Clear debris using large-bore suction catheter (e.g., Yankauer).
- Immobilize cervical spine with collar (with attention to proper pediatric sizing).
- Establish airway (apply oxygen, assist ventilation, place advanced airway if needed for airway protection or for apnea).

BREATHING/VENTILATION

- Assess breath sounds, chest rise, and respiratory rate.
- Assess need for needle decompression or chest-tube placement (e.g., absent breath sounds in one lung).

CIRCULATION

- Establish IV access with a maximum of three IV placement attempts in emergency evaluation then consider intraosseous access (if <8 years old) or central venous access.
- Consider 20 mL/kg of normal saline administered as fast as possible (typically over 5 minutes) if there are signs of severe dehydration or shock.
- Initiate chest compressions if patient is in cardiopulmonary arrest.

DISABILITY (RAPID NEUROLOGIC EVALUATION) AND DEXTROSE

- Assess mental status via Glasgow Coma Scale score (**Table 7-1**) or classify as AVPU: alert, responds to verbal stimuli, responds to painful stimuli, or unresponsive.
- Obtain bedside dextrose sample, replace dextrose if indicated.

EXPOSURE/DECONTAMINATION

- Fully undress patient to evaluate for hidden injury with attention to possible contamination and safety of patient and staff.
- Maintain normothermia to decrease metabolic needs.

OBTAIN BRIEF HISTORY

- The initial history is brief and can be recalled by the mnemonic AMPLE (allergies, medications, past medical history, last meal, events prior to presentation).

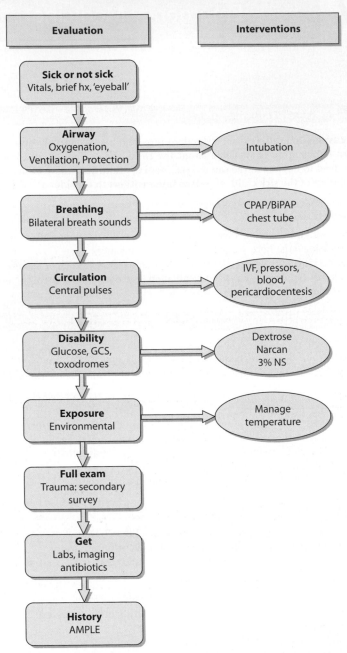

FIGURE 7-1 Emergency evaluation and interventions. AMPLE = allergies, medications, past medical history, last meal, and events; BiPAP = bilevel positive airway pressure; CPAP = continuous positive airway pressure; GCS = Glasgow Coma Scale; IVF = intravenous fluid; NS = normal saline.

TABLE 7-1	Pediatric Glasgow Coma Scale		
Component	**Score**	**Infant Response**	**Child Response**
Eye opening	4	Spontaneous	Spontaneous
	3	To voice	To voice
	2	To pain	To pain
	1	No eye opening	No eye opening
Verbal	5	Coos, babbles	Oriented, appropriate words
	4	Irritable, cries only	Confused
	3	Cries with pain	Inappropriate words
	2	Moans with pain	Incomprehensible sounds
	1	No response	No response
Motor	6	Spontaneous/purposeful movement	Obeys commands
	5	Localizes pain	Withdraws from touch with localization
	4	Withdraws from pain	Withdraws from pain
	3	Flexion response to pain	Flexion response to pain
	2	Extension response to pain	Extension response to pain
	1	No movement	No movement

BRIEF RESOLVED UNEXPLAINED EVENT (BRUE)

DEFINITION

Previously known as apparent life-threatening event (ALTE), BRUE is not a specific diagnosis but rather a term used to describe an event in an infant <1 year old when the observer reports an acute, brief (<1 minute), and resolved episode after which the infant has returned to baseline, there is no explanation for the event after taking the history and performing the physical examination, and at least one of the following was present:

1. cyanosis or pallor
2. absent, decreased, or irregular breathing
3. marked change in tone (hypertonia or hypotonia)
4. altered level of responsiveness.

EPIDEMIOLOGY

• Incidence: Approximately 0.2–0.4%; peaks between 1 and 3 months

PATHOPHYSIOLOGY

BRUEs by definition have no identifiable cause after history taking and physical examination. The presence of fever or respiratory symptoms, for example, would preclude the diagnosis of BRUE. Similarly, BRUE does not include events of choking or gagging with feeding. While most of these diagnoses are unlikely in the absence of specific symptoms or physical examination findings, the following can be considered infants who experience a BRUE:

- Normal physiologic variation: Normal infants may exhibit pauses in breathing of up to 10–20 seconds during sleep.
- Apnea of infancy: Unexplained pauses in breathing that last longer than 20 seconds or are accompanied by cyanosis, pallor, hypotonia, or bradycardia. These events usually cease by 43 weeks post-conception
- Gastroesophageal reflux
- Infections: Respiratory viral infections including respiratory syncytial virus (RSV), pertussis, pneumonia, sepsis, urinary tract infection, bacterial meningitis
- Metabolic derangements: Inborn errors of metabolism, hypoglycemia, hypocalcemia
- Hematologic issues: Anemia
- Cardiovascular disorders: Conduction disorders (prolonged QT), congenital heart disease, cardiomyopathy
- Respiratory conditions: Airway anomalies, foreign-body aspiration, breath-holding spells
- Neurologic: Seizures, intracranial hemorrhage, increased intracranial pressure
- Child abuse: Nonaccidental head trauma, poisoning, suffocation, caregiver-fabricated illness

DIAGNOSIS

- Thorough history and physical examination are critical to identifying concerning causes in infants who experience a BRUE.
- History: Exact details of the event, including duration, preceding circumstances, relationship to feeding, location of the infant, any interventions, and state of the infant after the event. Presence of respiratory effort, color change, choking, gasping, emesis, limpness, stiffness, rhythmic movements, eye movements, nasal congestion, and fever. Comprehensive past medical, family, and social histories. Talk to all caregivers and eyewitnesses.
- Physical examination: Comprehensive exam to assess for abnormalities in any organ system. Focus on general appearance, vital signs, and neurologic, respiratory, and cardiac exams.
- If patient has symptoms (e.g., fever, respiratory), is ill-appearing, or has an abnormal physical examination, the event is not a BRUE and the infant should be treated according to the likely diagnoses (e.g., evaluation for sepsis in a febrile young infant, neuroimaging and skeletal survey if child abuse is suspected).
- If the diagnosis of BRUE is made, apply risk-stratification criteria per the American Academy of Pediatrics guideline [Pediatrics 2016;137(5)]:
  - ✓ Low-risk: Age >60 days; ≥32 weeks' gestational age with corrected gestational age ≥45 weeks; no CPR performed by medical personnel; event duration <1 minute; first event
  - ✓ Higher-risk: One or more of the low-risk criteria not met
- Laboratory, imaging, and other testing
  - ✓ Low-risk: May consider pertussis testing (e.g., repeated apnea or cyanosis, particularly in infants <2 months old) and 12-lead ECG (rarely abnormal, but a noninvasive test). Should not routinely obtain other laboratory testing, chest radiography, neuroimaging, EEG, echocardiogram, or studies for gastroesophageal reflux
  - ✓ Higher-risk: No specific testing recommendations; consider targeted testing based on history and physical examination.

MANAGEMENT

- Low-risk: Briefly monitor infants with continuous pulse oximetry and serial examinations in the ED. Educate parents/caregivers about BRUEs, offer resources for CPR training, and

engage parents in shared decision-making about disposition. The infant does not need to be hospitalized solely for cardiorespiratory monitoring in the absence of parents' preference for admission. Home cardiorespiratory monitoring and prescriptions for antireflux medications (e.g., ranitidine) are not recommended

- Higher-risk: Consider hospitalization and treat the infant based on most likely diagnoses.

BURNS

DEFINITION

- Acute injury due to transfer of thermal energy

EPIDEMIOLOGY

- Death from fire and burns is a leading cause of unintentional death for U.S. children <14 years of age.
- Mechanisms changes with age: Scalds, contact burns, fire, chemical, electrical radiation
  ✓ Infants: Bathing-related scalds, abuse
  ✓ Toddlers: Scalds by hot liquid spills
  ✓ School-age: Fire (playing with matches)
  ✓ Adolescents: Volatile agents and high-voltage electric lines

PATHOPHYSIOLOGY

- Superficial: Redness and mild inflammatory response confined to epidermis; heals in 3–6 days
- Superficial Partial-thickness: Blistering; pink-red color; blanches with pressure; heals in 7–21 days
- Deep partial-thickness: Wet or waxy appearance; perceptive to pressure only owing to destruction of cutaneous nerves; healing in >3 weeks and usually involves surgical treatment
- Full thickness or fourth-degree: Full-thickness involving underlying fascia, muscle, or bone; requires surgical treatment for healing

DIAGNOSIS

- Always evaluate airway patency/inhalational injury.
  ✓ Look for soot in nares or throat.
  ✓ Low threshold to intubate as airway edema can be rapidly life-threatening.
- Evaluate for any circumferential burns that may need surgical fasciotomy.
- Describe burn by thickness (see "Pathophysiology") and BSA affected (**Table 7-2**).

TABLE 7-2	Percent Body-Surface Area by Age		
	Neonate	**Toddler**	**Adolescent/Adult**
Head	18	15	9
One arm	8	8	9
Front torso	20	20	18
Back	20	20	18
One leg	13	15	18

MANAGEMENT

- Analgesia
  - ✓ IV opioids
    - 1 mcg/kg fentanyl
    - 0.1 mg/kg morphine (Consider dosing in aliquots of 2-mg maximum in children.)
  - ✓ Consider covering or draping with clean, dry bandage (decreased air exposure can decrease pain).
- IV Fluids
  - ✓ Start with 20 cc/kg lactated Ringer's or normal saline bolus.
  - ✓ Parkland fluid resuscitation formula: 4 mL/kg/% BSA
    - Give half in the first 8 hours and half in the next 16 hours.
    - Parkland formula may underestimate evaporative loss and maintenance needs of young children.
- Td (Tetanus vaccination) as needed (see "Lacerations")
- Admit or transfer to burn center for pediatric patients
  - ✓ Superficial partial-thickness >10% BSA or any deep partial-thickness or full thickness burns
  - ✓ Significant burns to hands, face, feet, genitalia, perineum
  - ✓ Electrical/chemical/inhalational injury
  - ✓ Circumferential burns
  - ✓ Previously ill children
  - ✓ Significant associated injuries or suspected nonaccidental or intentional injury
  - ✓ Family inability to care for patient
- Wound care
  - ✓ Superficial and superficial partial-thickness burns that do not need surgical management/burn center transfer
    - Remove sloughing epidermis with gauze and sterile water
    - Do not rupture blisters
    - Cover with a topical antimicrobial agent and wound dressing
      ▷ Bacitracin
      ▷ Sterile petroleum gauze (Xeroform) dressing; cut to cover burn area
    - Daily wound dressing changes; consider premedication before wound care
    - Follow-up with burn center or with primary care provider within 2 days
- Consider carbon monoxide or cyanide poisoning
  - ✓ Administer 100% O_2
  - ✓ Hyperbaric oxygen if significantly elevated CO level or symptoms (e.g., altered mental status)
    - Consult with poison control/hyperbaric oxygen service.
    - Carboxyhemoglobin levels: 20–60% is toxic; >60% is potentially lethal.
  - ✓ Evaluate for neurologic symptoms or signs, signs of ischemia, or metabolic acidosis.
  - ✓ Cyanide antidotes if burning plastics/enclosed fire/elevated lactate
    - Cyanokit
    - Hydroxycobalamin

CARDIAC ARREST

DEFINITION

- Cardiac arrest: Abrupt loss of heart function
- Cardiopulmonary resuscitation: Attempt to restore vital functions after apparent death

EPIDEMIOLOGY

- Incidence of out-of-hospital nontraumatic cardiac arrest in children approximately 8 in 100,000 person-years overall, but 73 in 100,000 person-years in infants <1 year of age
- Asystole most common rhythm (>75%); ventricular fibrillation or pulseless ventricular tachycardia in only 5–15% of arrests
- 8.3% survival to discharge from out-of-hospital cardiac arrest; lowest survival rates in infants
- Up to 39% survival if in-hospital arrest

PATHOPHYSIOLOGY

- Respiratory distress with progression to respiratory failure leads to bradycardia and asystole is the most common etiology for cardiac arrest in children.
- Circulatory compromise leading to circulatory failure occurs less commonly.

DIAGNOSIS

- Sudden unexplained infant death is the most common etiology.
- Other etiologies include drowning, trauma, congenital heart disease, hypertrophic cardiomyopathy, long-QT syndrome or other ion channelopathies
- Consider evaluation for potentially reversible causes if unclear etiology of cardiac arrest (evaluation not necessary in most infants with sudden unexplained infant death):
  - ✓ Hypovolemia
  - ✓ Hypoxia
  - ✓ Hydrogen (acidosis)
  - ✓ Hypoglycemia
  - ✓ Hypothermia or hyperthermia
  - ✓ Tension pneumothorax
  - ✓ Tamponade
  - ✓ Toxins
  - ✓ Thrombosis (pulmonary or cardiac)

MANAGEMENT

- PALS algorithms
- Key points:
  - ✓ Initiate immediate CPR using CAB sequence
  - ✓ With two providers, use a ratio of 15 chest compressions to 2 breaths if there is no definitive airway; with only one provider, use 30 chest compressions to 2 breaths.
    - Compressions at a rate of 100–200
    - 4 cm depth in infants; 5 cm in children (i.e., at least 1/3 diameter of the chest)
    - Change compressors every 2 minutes
  - ✓ Determine whether rhythm is shockable (defibrillate at 2 J/kg then 4 J/kg; maximum, 10 J/kg or adult dose).
    - Asystole/ PEA: nonshockable; epinephrine every 3–5 minutes (0.01 mg/kg IV or IO)
    - Ventricular fibrillation/pulseless ventricular tachycardia: shockable; defibrillate: 2 J/kg then 4 J/kg; maximum, 10 J/kg or adult dose
  - ✓ Heart rate <60 bpm with poor perfusion is also an indication for CPR and epinephrine in infants and children.

DROWNING

DEFINITION

- According to the WHO, drowning is defined by respiratory impairment from submersion or immersion in a liquid.
- Outcomes are classified as either death, survival with morbidity, or survival with no morbidity. (*Note:* WHO does not recognize "Dry Drowning" as an entity.)

EPIDEMIOLOGY

- Second leading cause of injury death in children from 1 to 14 years
- Most prevalent in toddlers/teenagers

PATHOPHYSIOLOGY

- Hypoxemia (laryngospasm or aspiration) leads to loss of consciousness
- CNS damage begins after 4–6 minutes of hypoxemia.
  ✓ Fear/cold may trigger diving reflex, which shunts blood to brain/heart.
- Patients are at risk for sepsis due to breakdown of protective mucosal barriers.

DIAGNOSIS

- Risk stratification based on low-risk and high-risk clinical scenarios.
- Low-risk: If event involved immediate rescue without CPR or rescue breaths, and child presents without respiratory distress, hypoxia, or tachypnea, chest x-ray on arrival may be the only intervention indicated.
- If event involved unclear mechanism prior to submersion, CPR, rescue breaths, and/or the child presents with any hypoxia, tachypnea or respiratory distress, the following diagnostic tests should be obtained:
  ✓ Chest x-ray on arrival: May reveal pulmonary edema with bilateral diffuse alveolar pattern or signs of aspiration (can be delayed finding and may need repeat in 4–8 hours after initial x-ray if symptoms persist or progress).
  ✓ Serum electrolytes including glucose
    ▪ Diabetes insipidus or syndrome of inappropriate antidiuretic hormone may occur as a result of CNS injury.
    ▪ Elevated creatinine occurs with hypoxic end organ injury.
  ✓ Arterial or venous blood gas: Hypoxemia and metabolic acidosis
  ✓ ECG: Risk for bradycardia, ventricular fibrillation, and ventricular tachycardia
  ✓ CNS imaging if CNS ischemia is suspected
  ✓ Comprehensive metabolic panel (CMP): Hypoxic–ischemic injuries to kidney (elevated creatinine), liver (elevated hepatic transaminases), or pancreas (elevated amylase or lipase)

MANAGEMENT

- Immediate management
  ✓ Initiate immediate CPR if needed (CAB, as above)
  ✓ Evaluate core temperature for evidence of hypothermia.
  ✓ Consider continuous ECG monitoring.
  ✓ Prophylactic antibiotics are generally not recommended unless there is systemic toxicity, hemodynamic instability, or signs or symptoms of pneumonia; piperacillin–clavulanate provides broad empiric coverage if necessary.
- If low-risk clinical scenario and no respiratory distress, observe for 6–12 hours.
  ✓ If normal vital signs, physical examination. and x-ray, discharge home.

- If mild respiratory distress:
  ✓ Evaluate carefully in children, for whom tachypnea may be only sign.
  ✓ Chest x-ray: Often normal or mild pulmonary edema.
  ✓ Monitor for hypoglycemia: obtain initial blood glucose level and repeat levels for symptoms of hypoglycemia (e.g., altered mental status).
  ✓ Monitor; administer supplemental oxygen as needed.
  ✓ Admit to hospital.
- If significant respiratory distress:
  ✓ Chest x-ray is usually abnormal.
  ✓ Monitor as for mild respiratory distress.
  ✓ Administer supplemental oxygen, intubate, or administer positive end-expiratory pressure, as needed.
  ✓ Admit/transfer to intensive care unit.

HEAD INJURY

DEFINITION

- Traumatic brain injury (TBI): Disruption of normal brain function that occurs because of trauma directly to the head or elsewhere on the body with force transmitted to the head.
- Mild: GCS score 13–15
  ✓ Concussion is a type of mild TBI.
- Moderate: GCS 9–12
- Severe: GCS ≤8

EPIDEMIOLOGY

- TBI is a leading cause of death and disability in children.
- Falls account for >50% of ED visits for TBI in children.
- Other mechanisms: Struck by or against objects, MVCs, sports-related, child abuse (infants)
- >300,000 annual ED visits for children/adolescents due to sports- or recreation-related TBI, with increasing numbers over the last 20 years

PATHOPHYSIOLOGY

- Primary brain injury: Neuronal damage from traumatic injury
- Secondary: Injury to brain cells not injured by initial event
  ✓ Hypoxia
  ✓ Hypoperfusion
  ✓ Metabolic derangements

DIAGNOSIS

- Mild TBI: Risk stratification according to PECARN Head Injury Prediction Rule (**Table 7-3**)
- Balance low risk of missing a clinically important TBI with low risk of malignancy with CT of brain
  ✓ Clinically important TBI: Death, neurosurgery, intubation >24 hours, or hospitalization ≥2 nights
- Age <2 years
  ✓ With GCS 13 or 14, altered mental status, or palpable skull fracture, obtain CT.
  ✓ With more than one other risk factor or

TABLE 7-3 Low-risk components of the PECARN Head Injury Prediction Rule	
Age <2 years	**Age ≥2 years**
Normal mental status	Normal mental status
No palpable skull fracture	No signs of basilar skull fracture
No LOC/LOC <5 seconds	No LOC
Severe mechanism of injury not present*	Severe mechanism of injury not present*
None or frontal scalp hematoma	Vomiting
Acting normally per parents	No severe headache

*MVC with patient ejection, death of a passenger, or rollover; pedestrian/unhelmeted bicyclist vs. automobile; high-impact object to head; fall >3 feet (age <2 years) or >5 feet (age ≥2 years).
LOC = loss of consciousness; PECARN = Pediatric Emergency Care Applied Research Network.
Data from Kuppermann N, Holmes JF, Dayan PS, et al: Identification of children at very low risk of clinically-important brain injuries after head trauma: a prospective cohort study, *Lancet* 2009 Oct 3;374(9696):1160–1170.

✓ With only one risk factor, such as occipital, parietal, temporal hematoma in infant >6 months; LOC ≥5 seconds; severe mechanism of injury; not acting normally, CT versus observation in ED for ~4 hours after injury; opportunity for shared decision-making with parents.
✓ With none of the above present, CT not recommended
• Age ≥2 years
  ✓ GCS 13 or 14; altered mental status; signs of basilar skull fracture, obtain CT.
  ✓ With more than one other risk factor, consider CT versus observation in ED for ~4 hours after injury; opportunity for shared decision-making with parents.
  ✓ History of LOC; vomiting; severe mechanism of injury; severe headache, consider CT versus observation in ED for ~4 hours after injury; opportunity for shared decision-making with parents.
  ✓ With none of the above present, CT not recommended.
• Moderate or severe TBI, obtain CT.
• Symptoms and signs of concussion
  ✓ Historical: LOC, amnesia
  ✓ Physical: Headache, vomiting
  ✓ Cognitive: Feeling as though in a fog, difficulty concentrating, confusion
  ✓ Behavior: Irritability, emotionally labile
  ✓ Sleep disturbance: Insomnia, excess sleeping

MANAGEMENT

• If CT is negative or there is no progression of symptoms after observation in the ED, discharge home with detailed return instructions.
• If CT is positive: Neurosurgery consultation, hospitalization
• Elevated ICP:
  ✓ Airway protection (before CT if GCS ≤8 or declining)
  ✓ Head of bed elevated to 30 degrees
  ✓ Avoid hyperventilation; goal PCO_2 30–35
  ✓ Maintain normothermia and euglycemia
  ✓ 3% NS preferred over mannitol
    ▪ 3–5 ml/kg of 3% NS saline
    ▪ 0.5–1 g/kg mannitol

✓ Consider seizure prophylaxis, neurosurgical decompression
- Concussion management
  ✓ Goal is to protect the brain during healing period by avoidance of activities that divert energy or stress the brain.
  ✓ Cognitive "brain rest" and slow return to activities.
    - 24-hour period of rest prescribed from the ED (avoid texting/videogames, school-work, physical activities)
    - If asymptomatic at rest after 24 hours, slowly return to school and to play, advancing activities every 24 hours. May need frequent breaks at school.
  ✓ Follow-up exam with primary physician or concussion specialist prior to return to play.
  ✓ Return to play guidelines available at https://www.cdc.gov/headsup/index.html

HYPOGLYCEMIA

DEFINITION

- No consensus definition
- One definition:
  ✓ Infants blood sugar <40 mg/dL
  ✓ Children/adolescents/adults <60 mg/dL

EPIDEMIOLOGY

- Most commonly a result of an infection or other acute metabolic stress
- Children with certain chronic conditions at higher risk during metabolic stress (e.g., inborn error of metabolism) or because of medications (e.g., insulin therapy in diabetes mellitus).

PATHOPHYSIOLOGY

- Occurs when glucose utilization exceeds available glucose in the blood
- Differential diagnosis
  ✓ Decreased intake/increased losses: Diarrhea/vomiting, fasting/poor oral intake
  ✓ Increased utilization/cellular uptake: Sepsis, ingestions, hyperthermia, hyperinsulinism
  ✓ Decreased production/availability: Adrenal insufficiency, glycogen storage diseases, galactosemia, fatty acid oxidation disorders, other inborn errors of metabolism, liver failure

DIAGNOSIS

- Symptoms/signs (may or may not be present)
  ✓ Infants: Fussiness/irritability, decreased responsiveness, hypothermia, seizure
  ✓ Children/adolescents/adults: Sweating, tremor, confusion, tachycardia, seizure, stupor
- Diagnostic Testing:
  ✓ Finger stick glucose
  ✓ Urine/serum ketones
    - Differentiates ketotic (most common; fasting, poor intake, some inborn errors of metabolism) from nonketotic hypoglycemia (adrenal insufficiency, fatty acid oxidation disorders, hyperinsulinism)
  ✓ Critical draw: obtain in an infant with unclear etiology after history and physical examination (e.g., no source of infection, adequate intake)
    - Obtain when infant is hypoglycemic
    - Includes insulin level, beta-hydroxybutyrate, testing for inborn errors of metabolism

TABLE 7-4	Rule of 50s for Glucose Correction*	
Age	**Correction**
Infants	5 mL/kg of D10
Children	2 mL/kg of D25
Adolescents/adults	1 mL/kg of D50 (maximum, 1 ampule)

*Product of the mL/kg and the dextrose strength should equal "50"

MANAGEMENT

- Dextrose 0.5 g/kg IV bolus
- Need larger-bore IV for higher dextrose concentrations
  ✓ Peripheral IV: use D10 solution
- Rules of 50s mnemonic for glucose correction (**Table 7-4**)
- Continuous glucose infusion may be required for inadequate oral intake, excess insulin, inborn errors of metabolism.

HYPOTHERMIA

DEFINITION

- Mild: Between ≥32 and ≤35°C core temperature
- Moderate: Between ≥28 and <32°C core temperature
- Severe: <28°C core temperature

EPIDEMIOLOGY

- Neonates, physical disability, drug, or alcohol use/ingestion increase risk
- Mortality range, 30–80%

PATHOPHYSIOLOGY

- Physiologic mechanisms to conserve heat: Increased muscle tone and shivering
- If reflexes fail to maintain normal range, basal metabolic rate decreases, tissue hypoxia begins, and lactic acidosis occurs.
- In moderate-to-severe hypothermia, impaired mental status, including "paradoxical undressing" (patient paradoxically removes their clothes) and cold-induced bronchorrhea (failure to protect airway)
- Severe hypothermia: Increased myocardial irritability
- Can get cold-induced diuresis, DIC, decreased liver function and cardiac arrest

DIAGNOSIS

- Consider with environmental exposures, trauma patients, infants, sepsis, burns
- Severe hypothermia mimics death; if hypothermia or rapid cooling is the primary event, resuscitation with rewarming should be attempted

MANAGEMENT

- ABCs; CPR if needed
- In the presence of moderate-to-severe hypothermia with either an organized cardiac rhythm or PEA, but without a clear pulse, if there are cardiac contractions on bedside ECG: There is limited evidence but consensus that chest compressions can be held during active rewarming.

- If patient develops asystole, begin chest compressions.
- Correct electrolyte abnormalities
- Fluid replacement
- Warming method depends on core temperature
  - ✓ 32–35°C:
    - Passive rewarming: Simple external rewarming (e.g., warm blankets) with removal of any wet clothing
  - ✓ <32°C:
    - Active rewarming: Direct heating pads, bear hugger, warming lights; rewarm the trunk first to reduce after drop of temperature during rewarming
  - ✓ <28°C:
    - Active core rewarming: Warm normal saline infusion (40–42°C); surgical consultation the need for irrigation of thorax with warm saline through chest tubes and potential ECMO

SEPSIS

DEFINITION

- Systemic inflammatory response syndrome (SIRS) criteria
  - ✓ Fever
  - ✓ Leukocytosis
  - ✓ Tachycardia (outside of age-normal range) (**see Appendix A**)
  - ✓ Tachypnea (outside of age-normal range) (see Appendix A)
- Sepsis: SIRS plus infection
- Severe sepsis: Sepsis plus organ dysfunction (This criterion is now used this in adults to define sepsis.)
- Septic shock: Sepsis plus cardiovascular dysfunction
- Hypotension not required, as it is often a late sign in children with severe sepsis.
- Children, particularly young infants, with sepsis may also present with hypothermia and/ or bradycardia.

EPIDEMIOLOGY

- Rising incidence; approximately 0.89 cases per 1000 children
- ~10% mortality for severe sepsis

PATHOPHYSIOLOGY

- Usually pathogenic bacteria entering the bloodstream
- Releasing toxic products (such as endotoxin) into circulation leading to a cascade of inflammatory mediators
- Warm shock: Peripheral vasodilation
- Cold shock: Peripheral vasoconstriction

DIAGNOSIS

- Heart rate, respiratory rate, temperature, or systolic blood pressure outside of age-normal values and temperature correction
- Warm shock (more common in older children and adults)
  - ✓ Flash (<1 second) capillary refill (measure on chest or forehead, i.e., centrally)
  - ✓ Bounding pulses
  - ✓ Wide pulse pressure
  - ✓ Altered mental status

- Cold shock (more common in infants and young children)
  - ✓ Prolonged (>2 seconds) capillary refill
  - ✓ Cold extremities
  - ✓ Decreased pulses
  - ✓ Altered mental status
- Bacterial cultures looking for source and laboratory studies looking for end-organ dysfunction
  - ✓ Blood culture (peripheral and from central line if present)
  - ✓ Urine culture (all infants <6 months, consider in older infants and children)
  - ✓ CSF culture (if patient stable for procedure; often empirically treat and obtain later)
  - ✓ CBC with differential (elevated WBC or cell line suppression), procalcitonin (elevated in sepsis, may be used for risk stratification in the PICU)
  - ✓ iStat (evaluate for electrolyte disturbance, hypoglycemia)
  - ✓ CMP (renal or liver dysfunction)
  - ✓ Lactate (elevation corroborates diagnosis of sepsis, may predict septic shock)
  - ✓ Coagulation studies (disseminated intravascular coagulation)
  - ✓ Urinalysis, CSF cell count

MANAGEMENT

- Early recognition and treatment of septic shock improves outcomes
- Goal-directed stepwise management (**Figure 7-2**)

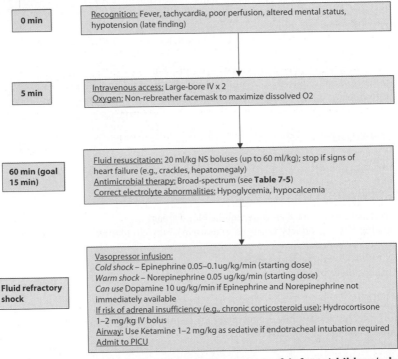

FIGURE 7-2 Initial management/hemodynamic support of infants/children/adolescents with septic shock. Adapted with permission from Davis AL, Carcillo JA, Aneja RK, et al: American College of Critical Care Medicine Clinical Practice Parameters for Hemodynamic Support of Pediatric and Neonatal Septic Shock, *Crit Care Med* 2017 Jun;45(6):1061–1093.

TABLE 7-5	Empiric Antimicrobial Therapy in the Child with Suspected Sepsis
Characteristics	**Antimicrobial Therapy**
Healthy, no central line	Vancomycin plus ceftriaxone
Immunocompromised, recent hospitalization, chronic medical condition, central line	Vancomycin plus cefepime (or ceftazidime if cefepime not available)
Oncology	Vancomycin + cefepime (or ceftazidime) + gentamicin
Suspected intraabdominal source	Piperacillin/tazobactam or ceftriaxone plus metronidazole; consider addition of vancomycin

- Antimicrobial therapy (**Table 7-5**)
- Bundled care
  - ✓ Sepsis recognition/management pathways often integrated into the electronic health record
    - Recognition bundle: Trigger based on vital signs with or without past medical history and with or without clinician assessment
    - Resuscitation bundle: Rapid IV access, fluid resuscitation, antimicrobial therapy, vasopressor initiation within 60 minutes
    - Stabilization bundle: Optimization of therapy in the ED and PICU
    - Performance bundle: Quality improvement to measure pathway adherence and outcomes

TRAUMA

DEFINITION

- Injury extent:
  - ✓ Example—Multiple trauma: Significant injury to two or more body areas
- Injury type:
  - ✓ Example—MVC vs. penetrating trauma from stabbing

EPIDEMIOLOGY

- Leading cause of death among patients <18 years of age
- Joint ED–surgical management is the standard of care, as is transfer to a pediatric trauma center for any significantly injured child

PATHOPHYSIOLOGY

- Predominant mechanism in children is blunt trauma.
- Need to avoid triad of hypothermia, acidosis and/or coagulopathy during initial evaluation (can lead to secondary injury/worse outcomes).

DIAGNOSIS

- Goal is to identify life-threatening injuries (and address them).
- Primary survey
  - ✓ Airway: Patent or not; cervical spine protection in place
  - ✓ Breathing: Breath sounds present bilaterally (or not)
  - ✓ Circulation: Central pulses

✓ Disability: GCS, moves all four extremities, pupil assessment
✓ Exposure: Removal of clothing and environmental control (e.g., warm blankets)
- Secondary survey
  ✓ Protocolized detailed head-to-toe exam to find other injured areas
- Laboratory studies: Some centers routinely obtain lab studies in all trauma activations; consider strongly for any trauma patient with high-risk mechanism (e.g., pedestrian struck by an automobile, MVC with ejection), altered mental status, suspected intraabdominal or pelvic injury based on abdominal tenderness or seatbelt sign, multiple traumas, or hemodynamic instability/severe injury.
  ✓ CBC, CMP (with LFTs), lipase, type and screen, UA; consider toxicology screens in adolescents.
- Imaging
  ✓ For most trauma activations, obtain chest x-ray in trauma bay; consider pelvic x-ray for same indications for obtaining laboratory studies
  ✓ Increasing use of bedside ultrasound (FAST) to assess for intraabdominal hemorrhage and pericardial effusion
  ✓ Imaging of the cervical spine:
    - Limited data available for children <8 years of age:
      ▷ General guidelines: Obtain x-ray of cervical spine for GCS <15, neurologic deficit, high-risk mechanism (e.g., MVC with ejection, death of passenger), persistent midline cervical spine tenderness or pain on range of motion, anatomical predisposition to injury (e.g., Trisomy 21), multiple trauma; consider in all trauma activations for preverbal children (as difficult to assess spinal tenderness)
    - For children ≥8 years of age, some suggest use of the NEXUS criteria for cervical spine imaging (If all five criteria below are met, then the cervical spine is considered clinically clear without imaging; if one or more are present, obtain cervical spine imaging.)
      ▷ No midline tenderness
      ▷ Normal level of alertness
      ▷ No evidence of intoxication
      ▷ No abnormal neurologic findings
      ▷ No painful distracting injuries
    - Generally start with cervical spine x-ray
    - If clinical concern continues (persistent pain or tenderness) or any abnormality is shown on x-ray, proceed to cervical MRI without contrast in consultation with neurosurgery.
    - CT of the cervical spine can be used in a patient with multiple injuries who is too unstable to undergo MRI.
  ✓ CT
    - For head CT recommendations, see "Head Trauma" section.
    - Chest and/or abdominal/pelvic CT obtained for suspected injury (e.g., abdominal tenderness), hemodynamic instability, multiple trauma

MANAGEMENT

- Management of ABCs as needed
  ✓ Airway: Bag-valve mask ventilation, endotracheal intubation
  ✓ Breathing: Oxygen, needle decompression
  ✓ Circulation: Large-bore IVs × 2, normal saline bolus (up to 2) followed by rapid PRBC transfusion if persistent hemodynamic instability

✓ Disability: See "Head Trauma" section for management of increased ICP.
- Surgical management as needed for injuries identified
  ✓ Nonsurgical management (e.g., bed rest, interventional radiology for embolization) of intraabdominal injuries is the standard of care except for persistent hemodynamic instability or bleeding disorder with inability to control hemorrhage.

FOREIGN-BODY INGESTIONS

EPIDEMIOLOGY AND PATHOPHYSIOLOGY

- High-risk ingestions include button batteries, detergent pods, magnet toys, and expanding toys
- Button batteries:
  ✓ Increasing number of objects are powered by button batteries (toys, remote controls, children's books with musical push buttons), resulting in an increase in ingestions.
  ✓ Injury occurs primarily from direct electrical current and caustic alkaline injury with liquefactive necrosis; direct pressure can also be a factor.
  ✓ Increasing number of fatal cases in recent years, most of which are associated with 20 mm 3V lithium disc battery
- Detergent pods:
  ✓ Agents thought to contribute to symptoms include propylene glycol, ethoxylated alcohols, and highly concentrated detergents.
- Magnet toys:
  ✓ Number of magnets is important as ingestion of >1 magnet represents significant increase in risk of injury because magnets can attract and cause intestinal obstruction, necrosis, and perforation.
- Expanding toys:
  ✓ Commonly balls made of superabsorbent polymers that expand when exposed to water
  ✓ Generally attractive to toddlers because of their size and color; easy to swallow.
  ✓ Superabsorbent polymer technology more common now in household products and gardening supplies in addition to toys

DIAGNOSIS

Clinical Manifestations

- Button battery ingestions may be asymptomatic or might cause respiratory symptoms, pain, drooling, or dysphagia
- Detergent pods:
  ✓ Detergent pods may cause drooling, coughing or gagging, respiratory distress, vomiting, and mental status changes that may be profound.
- Magnet toys:
  ✓ Number of magnets is important as ingestion of 1 magnet represents significant increases in risk of injury because magnets can attract and cause intestinal obstruction, necrosis, and perforation.
  ✓ Magnet ingestions are often asymptomatic but may cause abdominal obstruction or fistulas.
- Expanding toys:
  ✓ Ingestion of expanding toys may also be initially asymptomatic but can rapidly cause symptoms of gastrointestinal tract obstruction, including nausea/vomiting, abdominal distention, and pain

Diagnostic Studies

- Plain x-ray of the chest and abdomen; however, does not rule out foreign body, as many toys are radiolucent.
- For detergent pods: blood gas, CMP, glucose, ECG, and CBC should be obtained if child has altered mental status, tachypnea, or respiratory distress.

MANAGEMENT

- Supportive care, including close airway monitoring
  - ✓ In patients with worsening respiratory distress or mental status changes, early placement of an advanced airway may be indicated.
- For esophageal foreign bodies involve gastrointestinal/otolaryngology consultation to discuss removal.
  - ✓ Emergent removal is indicated for button batteries in the esophagus and multiple magnets anywhere in the gastrointestinal tract; also highly recommended for expanding toys.
  - ✓ Urgent removal is indicated for other foreign bodies in the upper esophagus (e.g., at the thoracic inlet); foreign bodies in the distal third of the esophagus may spontaneously pass into the stomach, and admission with repeat x-ray in 8–12 hours is an option.
- Most gastric foreign bodies will pass through the gastrointestinal tract spontaneously. Discuss removal with gastrointestinal consultation for button batteries and for sharp (e.g., a needle) or large (>5 cm in length or >2 cm in width) foreign bodies.

NONACCIDENTAL TRAUMA (NAT)/CHILD ABUSE EVALUATION IN THE ACUTE CARE SETTING

DEFINITION

- Physical child abuse may be broadly defined as injury inflicted on a child by a parent or caretaker.

EPIDEMIOLOGY

- Approximately 4.4 million reports of child maltreatment per year involving an estimated 7.9 million children. Of those reports substantiated, ~17% involve physical abuse

DIAGNOSIS

- Approaches to identifying abuse, especially in children less than 24 months, rely on careful history taking and identification of possible "red flag" or sentinel injuries (i.e., oral injuries, bruising as described below, or fractures associated with the occurrence of abuse).
- Careful history with attention to possible traumatic injuries or nonspecific symptoms that may represent inflicted injuries/trauma
- Assess the developmental stage of the patient and compare to history obtained, with attention to whether the injury is implausible (e.g., bruising or frenulum injury in 3-month-old infant, extremity fracture in a preambulatory child), timeline, and possible delay in seeking medical care
- For children under 24 months of age, who represent the highest risk of missed abusive injuries, assess if exam represents suspicious injuries that are associated with the occurrence of child abuse:
  - ✓ Any bruising or oral/frenulum injury in infants younger than 5 months of age
  - ✓ Bruises located on the torso, ear, neck, or buttocks
  - ✓ Bruises with a pattern of the striking object (e.g., hand slap, belt or loop marks, or other objects)
  - ✓ Burns without clear accidental history

✓ Intracranial injuries without clear traumatic history
✓ Abdominal injuries without clear traumatic history
✓ Human bite marks

- Laboratory testing and imaging for diagnosis is complicated and usually assisted by consultation with a child abuse specialist. General guidelines for children age ≤6 years with suspected abusive injuries (in children >6 years of age, obtain based on clinical suspicion):
  ✓ CBC for anemia and to assess for bleeding disorder
  ✓ CMP with AST and ALT for occult abdominal trauma/liver injury
  ✓ Lipase for pancreatic injury
  ✓ Urinalysis
  ✓ Consider laboratory testing for rickets or bleeding disorder based on presence of fractures or hemorrhage, respectively.
  ✓ X-ray site of suspected injuries.
  ✓ For children ≤24 months, skeletal survey should be obtained to evaluate for occult fractures but should be ordered in conjunction with child abuse specialist.
  ✓ Head CT for infants ≤12 months if external head injuries or clinical symptoms/signs of intracranial hemorrhage; head MRI as inpatient if infant is asymptomatic and physical abuse is suspected.

MANAGEMENT

- If available, contact multidisciplinary team with pediatric specialists and social workers trained in child abuse and neglect assessment for consultation, especially in cases involving young children.
- Familiarize yourself with state agencies involved in child protection and reporting procedures as a mandated reporter,
- In cases of severely ill children, stabilize and remember to consider NAT as a possible mechanism of injury, with attention to head imaging and abdominal injury evaluation that could be a source of significant injuries.
- Consider further evaluation and social work involvement for any unexplained traumatic injuries or worrisome injuries as above.

Endocrinology 8

Marissa Kilberg, MD, MSEd
Katherine Lord, MD

GLUCOSE HOMEOSTASIS

DIABETES MELLITUS

A heterogeneous group of disorders characterized by fasting and postprandial hyperglycemia that affects approximately 2.5 per 1000 children under 20 years of age.

EPIDEMIOLOGY

- Type 1 DM: Onset is usually in childhood, but may occur at any age; accounts for 85% of diabetes cases in children.
- Type 2 DM: Most prevalent in obese children during puberty; more frequent in children who identify as African American, Hispanic, Pacific Islander, Asian, and Pima Indian; accounts for 12% of diabetes cases in children.
- MODY: Autosomal dominant inheritance; onset usually between 9 and 25 years of age; accounts for 1–2% of diabetes cases in children.
- Neonatal diabetes: De novo or inherited; onset usually <6 months of age; accounts for 1% of diabetes cases in children.

ETIOLOGY

- Type 1 DM: Autoimmune-mediated destruction of β cells in predisposed individuals (certain HLA haplotypes), trigger(s) unknown, but thought to be environmental
- Type 2 DM: Progressive insulin secretory defect on the background of insulin resistance
- MODY: Genetic defects in enzymes or nuclear transcription factors involved in the regulation of insulin secretion or pancreatic islet development
- Neonatal diabetes: Genetic defects in KATP channel, insulin, or transcription factors involved in the regulation of insulin secretion or in pancreatic-islet development
- Other: Pancreatectomy, exocrine pancreatic disease (cystic fibrosis, hemochromatosis); other endocrinopathies (acromegaly, Cushing disease, pheochromocytoma); medications (glucocorticoids, beta-blockers, phenytoin, asparaginase, cyclosporine, tacrolimus, pentamidine, diazoxide, nicotinic acid, thiazides); infections (cytomegalovirus, congenital rubella); genetic syndromes (Prader–Willi, trisomy 21, Turner, Klinefelter)

PATHOPHYSIOLOGY

- Insulin deficiency and/or impaired insulin action results in the abnormal metabolism of carbohydrate, protein, and fat.
- Type 1 DM: Destruction of pancreatic β-cells leads to absolute insulin deficiency. Lack of insulin results in excessive hepatic glucose production and impaired glucose utilization in muscle and fat, leading to hyperglycemia, glycosuria, and osmotic diuresis. Lipolysis and impaired lipid synthesis lead to elevated lipids, cholesterol, triglycerides, and free fatty acids, which are converted into ketones. Impaired utilization of glucose, excessive caloric and water losses in urine, and increasing catabolism all lead to weight loss.

- Type 2 DM: Insulin resistance and inadequate insulin secretion result in relative insulin deficiency. Most patients have sufficient insulin to suppress lipolysis and ketogenesis, although this is not always the case in the pediatric population where patients do present with ketoacidosis.
- MODY: Each of the MODY gene defects result in very unique clinical features spanning mild, not progressive, fasting hyperglycemia to more profound insulin dependent DM. There are also genes that initially cause a hyperinsulinism picture with hypoglycemia in infancy and progress to later diabetes. Monogenic diabete are also often associated with other non-endocrine manifestations such as developmental delay, cardiomyopathy and hepatic dysfunction.
- Neonatal Diabetes: Similar to other types of diabetes, these patients present in infancy with polyuria, poor weight gain and high risk of diabetic ketoacidosis. Individuals that have pancreatic aplasia may also present with diarrhea due to insufficiency of the exocrine pancreas.

CLINICAL MANIFESTATIONS

- Type 1 DM: Polyuria, polydipsia, polyphagia, weight loss, fatigue, weakness, blurred vision, increased risk of infection; frequently presents with ketosis with or without acidosis.
- Type 2 DM: Overweight or obese; acanthosis nigricans (velvety hyperpigmented patches in skin folds of neck and axillae); wide spectrum of presentation in adolescents from detection on routine screening to diabetic Ketoacidosis (DKA); may already have long-term complications at diagnosis.

DIAGNOSTICS

- Criteria for diagnosis of DM: Fasting plasma glucose $\geq$126 mg/dL, HbA_{1c} $\geq$6.5%, 2-hour plasma glucose $\geq$200 mg/dL during oral glucose-tolerance test using a glucose load of 1.75 g/kg (up to 75 g) or random plasma glucose $\geq$200 mg/dL in the presence of symptoms of diabetes.

Other Tests

- Urinalysis for glucose
- HbA_{1c} reflects average blood glucose over previous 3 months; used as an index of long-term glycemic control; $\geq$6.5% generally indicates diabetes. HbA_{1c} inaccurately reflects glycemia with red-cell transfusions, severe hypertriglyceridemia, uremia, lead poisoning, asplenia, splenomegaly, certain anemias and hemoglobinopathies. In general, conditions with increased erythrocyte lifespan will have falsely elevated HbA_{1c} while conditions with shortened erythrocyte lifespan will have falsely low HbA_{1c}.
- Fasting insulin and C-peptide is low in type 1 DM and can be low, normal, or elevated in type 2 DM.
- β-cell autoantibodies are positive in >90% of patients with type 1 DM and are negative in most patients with type 2 DM.

MANAGEMENT

- Seek consultation from a pediatric endocrinologist. The following recommendations are general guidelines used at the authors' institution (also see "Diabetic Ketoacidosis" section).
- All patients on insulin therapy should wear a medic-alert bracelet

Long Term

- Type 1 DM: Daily requirement for exogenous insulin to match carbohydrate intake. Most effective insulin regimen is basal-bolus with long-acting basal insulin given once or twice daily and rapid-acting bolus insulin given with meals to cover carbohydrate consumption and to correct hyperglycemia.

✓ For newly diagnosed patients, calculate the TDD of insulin: 0.4 unit/kg/day for all patients, then, if necessary, add 0.2 units/kg/day (up to 1.2 units/kg/day) for each indicator of insulin resistance: ketones, obesity, puberty, acidosis.

✓ Calculating basal-bolus doses: Basal insulin dose is 40% of the TDD; carbohydrate ratio is 400/TDD (equals the grams of carbohydrate covered by 1 unit of rapid-acting insulin) if ≥8 years of age, 300/TDD if <8 years; and hyperglycemia correction factor is 1800/TDD (equals expected decrease in blood glucose (mg/dL) from 1 unit of fast-acting insulin).

✓ Insulin pumps deliver rapid-acting insulin as a continuous subcutaneous infusion plus boluses with meals (see **Table 8-1**)

✓ An alternative is to use an NPH/bolus or premixed insulin regimen if patients are unable to adhere to basal-bolus regimen.

  ▪ NPH is given as 50% of the TDD with breakfast, 10% with dinner, and 10% at bedtime; 15% of the TDD is given as rapid-acting insulin with breakfast and another 15% with dinner.

  ▪ Premixed insulin is dosed as 70% of TDD with breakfast and 30% with dinner. Patients must adhere to a carbohydrate-restricted diet and eat at specified times. **Table 8-1** outlines the pharmacokinetics of the various insulin analogs

• Type 2 DM: Weight management, increase daily physical activity, decrease sedentary activity, decrease caloric and fat intake; most require insulin or oral hypoglycemic agents.

✓ Metformin is the only oral hypoglycemic agent approved for use in children ≥10 years of age. Goal dose is 1000 mg twice daily; generally, the dose is titrated up over several weeks to avoid significant GI side effects.

TABLE 8-1	Subcutaneous Insulin Pharmacodynamics			
Type	**Name**	**Onset (hour)**	**Peak (hour)**	**Duration (hour)**
Rapid-acting*	Lispro (Humalog, Admelog)	0.25	0.75	3–4
	Aspart (Novolog, Fiasp†)			
	Glulisine (Apidra)			
Short-acting	Regular	0.5	2–5	5–8
Intermediate-acting	NPH	2–4	6–9	10–12
Long-acting‡	Glargine (Lantus, Basaglar, Toujeo§)	1–2	None	12–24
	Detemir (Levemir)			
Ultra Long-acting	Degludec (Tresiba)	1–4	None	Up to 48 hours
Premixed	70/30	70% NPH, 30% regular or rapid-acting		
	75/25	75% NPH, 25% regular or rapid-acting		

*Usually given just before meal. Also used in insulin pumps.
†Fiasp is the newest pediatric approved rapid-acting insulin formulation and it has a faster time of onset but similar peak and duration.
‡No peak; relatively constant concentration.
§Toujeo is an ultraconcentrated form of insulin glargine for individuals, formulated to have a smaller injection volume for those on very high insulin doses, and may have slightly different pharmacodynamics with duration of action just over 24 hours

✓ Insulin, as described above, should be started in patients with HbA_{1c} >8.5% but may be able to be decreased with increased insulin sensitivity resulting from dietary modification, increased physical activity and metformin.

✓ Normalize glucose, self-monitoring; normalize HgA_{1c}—check every 3 months.

• Monitor for long-term complications:

✓ Small vessels: Retinopathy (regular ophthalmologic screening); nephropathy (regular screening for hypertension and microalbuminuria); peripheral neuropathy

✓ Large vessels: Atherosclerosis (regular screening for hyperlipidemia)

Management of Ketosis without Acidosis (Sick-Day Rules)

• If ill or hyperglycemic (>240 mg/dL), check for presence of ketones (urine or blood)
• Encourage oral hydration: 1 oz/hr/year of age (up to 16 oz); if glucose <200 mg/dL, drink carbohydrate-containing fluids, if glucose >200 mg/dL, drink sugar-free fluids.
• If patient is not tolerating oral hydration, use IVF management similar to that used in DKA (see "Diabetic Ketoacidosis" section).
• Provide extra-rapid-acting insulin (ketone dose), 10% of TDD every 2 hours until ketosis resolves.
• Monitor blood glucose and urine ketones every 2 hours.
• Patients remaining on insulin pumps should use subcutaneous injections for ketone doses.
• If ketones are not clearing, consider increasing insulin dose.
• If signs and symptoms persist or worsen, consider the possibility of DKA.

Management in Setting of InterCurrent Illness without Ketosis

• If vomiting, initiate IVF with dextrose, omit any standing rapid-acting insulin doses, give usual long-acting insulin dose, and use sliding scale insulin correction every 4 hours, or start insulin infusion (0.02–0.05 units/kg/hr), and monitor serum electrolytes and glucose.
• May require additional insulin (110–120% TDD) due to insulin resistance seen during illness.

Management of Hypoglycemia

• May occur because of honeymoon phase, insulin dose error, reduced oral intake, or increased activity.
• Give simple carbohydrates (juice, sugar-containing soda, cake icing, or glucose tablets); recheck glucose 20 minutes later, repeat as necessary until >70 mg/dL.
• If vomiting, combative, seizing, or losing consciousness, give glucagon 1 mg intramuscularly.

DIABETIC KETOACIDOSIS

PATHOPHYSIOLOGY

• Lack of insulin results in hyperglycemia, ketosis, and metabolic acidosis with compensatory respiratory alkalosis (rapid deep breathing, Kussmaul respirations). Ketones include acetoacetate, which is converted to acetone, causing fruity breath. Glycosuria and ketonuria cause urinary water and electrolyte losses, resulting in dehydration. Dehydration, acidosis, and hyperosmolality all contribute to altered mental status. All of these symptoms can be exacerbated by concomitant trauma or infection

DIAGNOSTICS

• Criteria for diagnosis of DKA: Glucose >200 mg/dL, pH <7.3, and HCO_3^- <15 mmol/L. There is associated glycosuria, ketonuria, and ketonemia.

Other Tests

• Blood gas; electrolytes, including sodium, potassium, bicarbonate, BUN, creatinine, glucose, calcium, magnesium, phosphorus; blood or urine ketones

- Leukocytosis and elevated serum amylase are common.
- If sepsis is suspected, check blood and urine cultures.

MANAGEMENT

- Consult pediatric endocrinology. Consider admission to intensive care unit if pH <7.0, age <3 years, blood glucose >1000 mg/dL, or altered mental status. Replete intravascular volume first, then correct fluid deficit, electrolytes, and acid–base status.
- Fluids: Replace fluid deficit, as well maintenance requirements and monitor ongoing losses from osmotic diuresis. Most patients are about 10–20% dehydrated. Within the first hour, give 0.9% NS bolus of 10 mL/kg; reassess and repeat as necessary to prevent hypovolemic shock. Give NS at 1.5–2 times maintenance rate for 24–48 hours.
- Electrolytes: Monitor glucose every 1 hour, other electrolytes every 2–4 hours.
  ✓ Use a two-bag system to lower glucose by 50–100 mg/dL/hr until in goal range of 100–180 mg/dL. The two-bag system consists of one bag of IV fluids with no dextrose and another with 10% dextrose, both with the same saline and electrolyte concentrations. By varying the rate of fluid given with each bag, one can vary the dextrose infusion rate without changing electrolytes or total volume. When glucose is >300 mg/dL, use only bag without dextrose unless glucose is decreasing too quickly; when glucose is 200–300 mg/dL, use each bag at half of the total rate; when glucose is <200, use only bag containing 10% dextrose.
  ✓ Potassium: Patients are initially hyperkalemic because of acidosis; however, their total body K^+ is low, and they become hypokalemic as acidosis improves and insulin and glucose are given. Potassium should be added to IV fluids when urine output is confirmed and there is no significant hyperkalemia. Potassium should be provided as equal parts potassium chloride and potassium phosphate: If serum K^+ is <4 mEq/L, add 30 mEq/L KCl and 20.4 mM KPhos; if K^+ is 4–5.4 mEq/L, add 20 mEq/L KCl and 13.6 mM KPhos. If K^+ 5.5–6 mEq/L, add 10 mEq/L KCl and 6.8 mM KPhos. If K^+ is >6.0 mEq/L, do not add potassium to fluids, and obtain ECG to evaluate for arrhythmia.
  ✓ Phosphorus: Hyperosmolar diuresis results in phosphate loss, and hypophosphatemia can result in lactic acidosis. Phosphorus should be provided in IV fluids as KPhos.
  ✓ Sodium: Hyperglycemia causes a pseudohyponatremia. Rapid changes in serum Na^+ should be avoided. Corrected Na^+ = serum Na^+ + (1.6 × [(glucose − 100)/100]).
  ✓ Bicarbonate: Metabolic acidosis corrects with insulin therapy, although it can be exacerbated by hyperchloremia in some patients treated with NS, in which case IV fluids should be changed to half NS. Administration of bicarbonate should be avoided because of increased risk of cerebral edema.
- Insulin: Regular insulin should be given IV at 0.1 units/kg/hr. When acidosis resolves (HCO_3^- ≥15 mM or pH >7.3) and patient is tolerating oral intake, transition to subcutaneous insulin. The first dose of rapid-acting subcutaneous insulin should be given 15–30 minutes before stopping the IV infusion to allow adequate time for absorption. It is optimal to convert to a subcutaneous regimen just before a meal. For patients in DKA, it is best, when possible, to give long-acting basal insulin while still on infusions in order to help with the transition to subcutaneous insulin. Follow sick day rules as described above until ketones are negative
- Cerebral edema: Occurs in 1% of patients with DKA, but mortality rate is 40–90%. Risk factors include age <5 years, new diagnosis of diabetes, high serum osmolality, severe acidosis, and severe dehydration. Treatment includes 3% saline 5–10 mL/kg over 30 minutes or mannitol 10–20 g/m² (0.5–1 g/kg) IV every 2–4 hours.

HYPOGLYCEMIA

Hypoglycemia is defined as signs or symptoms of brain dysfunction resulting from low plasma glucose. After the first 3 days of life, infants and children should be able to maintain glucose >70 mg/dL. Capillary and venous glucose levels are 10–15% lower than arterial glucose.

ETIOLOGY

- Neonates: Transitional hypoglycemia, sepsis, polycythemia, panhypopituitarism, congenital hypoglycemic disorder
- Drugs: Alcohol, salicylate, beta-blockers, sulfonylureas
- Ketotic hypoglycemia: A diagnosis of exclusion and of unknown etiology; normal fasting mechanisms, but impaired fasting tolerance. Occurs in setting of prolonged fasting or during times of illness. Typically presents at 1–5 years of age; usually resolves by 8–10 years of age.
- Hyperinsulinemia: Infant of a diabetic mother; hyperinsulinism (congenital or perinatal stress-induced); Beckwith–Wiedemann syndrome; congenital disorders of glycosylation; factitious hyperinsulinism/surreptitious insulin administration (Munchausen syndrome, factitious disorder imposed by another [Munchausen by proxy syndrome]); sulfonylurea ingestion; insulinoma.
- Counterregulatory hormone deficiency: GH deficiency; primary or central adrenal insufficiency (see "Adrenal Insufficiency").

Inborn Errors of Metabolism

- Disorders of gluconeogenesis: GSD 1a (glucose-6-phosphatase deficiency); GSD 1b (glucose 6-phosphate transporter deficiency); fructose-1,6-diphosphatase deficiency; hereditary fructose intolerance, galactosemia
- Disorders of glycogen storage: GSD 0 (glycogen synthase deficiency); GSD 3 (debrancher enzyme deficiency); GSD 6 (glycogen phosphorylase deficiency); GSD 9 (phosphorylase kinase deficiency)
- Disorders of fatty acid oxidation and ketone utilization
- Other: Postprandial hypoglycemia (dumping syndrome), liver disease, severe diarrhea, severe malnutrition, malabsorption, severe malaria, Jamaican vomiting sickness (from eating unripe ackee fruit of *Blighia spaida* tree), and Reye syndrome

PATHOPHYSIOLOGY

- Normal fasting mechanisms include hepatic glycogenolysis, hepatic gluconeogenesis, adipose tissue lipolysis, fatty acid oxidation and ketogenesis, counterregulatory hormone response, and insulin suppression. Defects in these metabolic pathways can result in hypoglycemia.

CLINICAL MANIFESTATIONS

- Activation of the autonomic nervous system results in diaphoresis, shakiness, tachycardia, anxiety, weakness, hunger, nausea, and vomiting. Neuroglycopenia results in irritability, restlessness, headache, confusion, poor speech, poor concentration, altered level of consciousness, seizure, hypothermia, behavior and personality changes, and a sense of impending doom. Newborns may have no clinical symptoms or may exhibit cyanosis, apnea, respiratory distress, refusal to feed, or brief myoclonic jerks.

DIAGNOSTICS

- Critical laboratory tests: When blood glucose is below 50 mg/dL, obtain the following labs: glucose, comprehensive metabolic panel, lactate, beta-hydroxybutyrate, FFA, insulin, C-peptide, IGF-BP1, ammonia, acylcarnitine profile, free and total carnitine, GH, cortisol,

urine organic acids, and urine ketones. A sulfonylurea panel should be sent if factitious hyperinsulinism is suspected.

- Glucagon stimulation test: After obtaining the critical laboratory tests, when blood glucose is below 50 mg/dL, administer glucagon 1 mg IM/IV, measure glucose at 0, +10, +20, +30, and +40 minutes. If blood glucose does not rise by 20 mg/dL in 20 minutes, use dextrose for rescue. A positive response is a rise in blood glucose by 30 mg/dL in 40 minutes.

Biochemical Profiles for the Different Causes of Hypoglycemia

- Ketotic hypoglycemia: Acidosis, elevated serum and urine ketones; undetectable insulin; negative glycemic response to glucagon
- Hyperinsulinism: Detectable insulin and/or C-peptide, low IGF-BP1; suppressed ketones, suppressed FFA; positive glycemic response to glucagon. Undetectable or low insulin does not rule out hyperinsulinism. Diagnosis is made on the basis of markers of insulin action (suppressed ketones and FFA, positive response to glucagon).
- GH deficiency: Elevated ketones; GH <7–10 ng/mL; abnormal GH stimulation tests
- ACTH/cortisol deficiency: Elevated ketones; cortisol <18 mcg/dL; abnormal stimulation tests (see "Adrenal Insufficiency")
  ✓ GH and cortisol values at the time of hypoglycemia have poor specificity for a hormone deficiency; the diagnosis of GH deficiency or adrenal insufficiency cannot be made on the bas is of these results alone.
- GSD 1abs: Lactic acidosis, hyperlipidemia, hyperuricemia, hypophosphatemia, anemia, microalbuminuria; abnormal fed glucagon stimulation test (increase in lactate with no rise in glucose); GSD 1b also has neutropenia
- GSD Types 0, 3, 6, 9: Elevated ketones, normal lactate in fasting hypoglycemic state
- Fatty acid oxidation disorders: Suppressed ketones, low serum carnitine, abnormal acylcarnitine profile, and urine organic acids
- Factitious hyperinsulinism due to surreptitious insulin administration: Suppressed ketones, suppressed FFAs, increased insulin levels with inappropriately low C-peptide levels relative to the insulin level. With administration of sulfonylurea drugs, levels of both insulin and C-peptide will be elevated,

MANAGEMENT

- If awake and alert, give glucose orally. If impaired consciousness, give D10 or D20 as a 2–4 mL/kg IV bolus then start continuous glucose (NG or IV). Consult a pediatric endocrinologist and/or metabolism specialist.
- Hyperinsulinism: Glucagon 1 mg IM/IV in emergency; glucagon 1 mg/24 hr continuous infusion as temporizing measure; diazoxide; octreotide SC in infants > 2 months (due to risk of fulminant necrotizing entercolitis); continuous enteral dextrose; pancreatectomy. Referral to a hyperinsulinism center.
- GSD: Frequent or continuous feeds; uncooked cornstarch may extend feeding interval. For type 1, avoid galactose, lactose, fructose, and sucrose.
- GH deficiency: Subcutaneous GH replacement in divided twice daily doses
- ACTH/cortisol deficiency: Glucocorticoid replacement (see "Adrenal Insufficiency")
- Postprandial hypoglycemia (late-dumping syndrome): Acarbose (if >1 year of age); if acarbose fails, continuous feedings.

HYPOTHALAMIC–PITUITARY–ADRENAL (HPA) AXIS

ADRENAL INSUFFICIENCY

Cortisol deficiency due to disorders of the hypothalamus, pituitary, or adrenal gland.

ETIOLOGY

- Primary adrenal insufficiency: Autoimmune adrenalitis, autoimmune polyglandular syndromes; tuberculosis, HIV, fungal infections; Waterhouse–Friderichsen syndrome (adrenal hemorrhage associated with meningococcemia); adrenal thrombosis, infarction, or necrosis; CAH; adrenoleukodystrophy; triple A syndrome; primary xanthomatosis; hereditary resistance to ACTH; metastatic carcinoma or lymphoma
- Secondary adrenal insufficiency: Long-term glucocorticoid therapy, pituitary or hypothalamic structural abnormalities, tumors, surgery, head trauma, cranial irradiation, infectious or inflammatory processes

PATHOPHYSIOLOGY

- Primary adrenal insufficiency: Inability of the adrenal gland to produce cortisol results in elevated ACTH and MSH, leading to hyperpigmentation. May also be associated with deficiency or excess of other adrenal hormones. Mineralocorticoid (aldosterone) deficiency causes hyponatremia, hyperkalemia, metabolic acidosis, dehydration, and hypotension. Androgen deficiency results in absent secondary sexual characteristics. In some forms of CAH, there are increased levels of mineralocorticoid and/or androgen due to specific enzymatic defects. Mineralocorticoid excess causes hypertension. Androgen excess results in virilization, accelerated growth, advanced bone age, increased muscle mass, acne, hirsutism, and deep voice.
- Secondary adrenal insufficiency: Inability of the hypothalamus to secrete CRH or of the pituitary to secrete ACTH, resulting in cortisol deficiency, but not mineralocorticoid deficiency

CLINICAL MANIFESTATIONS

- Signs and symptoms of adrenal insufficiency include fatigue, apathy, listlessness, weakness, anorexia, weight loss, nausea, vomiting, diarrhea, abdominal pain, dizziness, orthostatic hypotension and tachycardia, salt craving, hyperpigmentation (in primary adrenal insufficiency), decreased axillary and pubic hair, and hypovolemia. Acute adrenal crisis is characterized by fever, confusion, hypotension, shock, and death; it is often precipitated by severe stress such as significant illness, surgery, or trauma,

DIAGNOSTICS

- Initial evaluation: Hyponatremia, hyperkalemia, hypochloremia, metabolic acidosis, hypoglycemia, morning cortisol (6–8 a.m.) <10 mcg/dL or a cortisol level less than 18 mcg/dL drawn during acute illness
- Diagnostic confirmation: Elevated ACTH, low cortisol in primary adrenal insufficiency
  - ✓ ACTH stimulation test: ACTH normally stimulates adrenal gland production of cortisol >18 mcg/dL. In primary adrenal insufficiency, there is minimal to no response to standard/high ACTH dose of 250 mcg (125 mcg for infants) given IV, with cortisol measured at 0, 30, 60 minutes. In secondary adrenal insufficiency, there may be some response until the adrenal glands atrophy over time, so a low ACTH dose (1 mcg) is used.
  - ✓ Metyrapone test: Metyrapone inhibits 11β-hydroxylase, which converts 11-deoxycortisol to cortisol, and thereby inhibits cortisol production, leading to increased ACTH and 11-deoxycortisol if HPA axis is intact. Give metyrapone 30 mg/kg PO (maximum, 3 g); measure ACTH, cortisol, and 11-deoxycortisol at 0, 120, 180, 240 minutes.
  - ✓ CRH stimulation test: Preferred test for secondary adrenal insufficiency when CRH is available. Give CRH 1 mcg/kg IV and measure ACTH and cortisol at 15, 30, 60, and 90 minutes after administration.

✓ Insulin-tolerance test: Insulin-induced hypoglycemia stimulates counterregulatory hormones, including ACTH and cortisol. Use with caution because of risk of hypoglycemic seizure.

- Other studies: Plasma renin activity is elevated in patients with mineralocorticoid deficiency. Abdominal ultrasound or CT may visualize adrenal hypertrophy or hemorrhage in patients with primary adrenal insufficiency. Brain/pituitary MRI should be obtained in patients with secondary adrenal insufficiency to assess for CNS lesions.

MANAGEMENT

- If adrenal insufficiency is suspected, consult endocrinology. In stable patients, send studies to confirm diagnosis before starting steroids (cortisol level at a minimum). Steroid treatment will interfere with the interpretation of test results and will lead to secondary adrenal insufficiency if used long term. Patients with confirmed diagnosis should wear a medical alert bracelet.
- Fluids: Correct hypovolemia with NS boluses as needed.
- Glucocorticoids: Hydrocortisone is 4 times less potent than prednisone, 5 times less potent than methylprednisolone, and 25–30 times less potent than dexamethasone.
  ✓ Maintenance therapy: Hydrocortisone 6–12 mg/m²/day PO divided TID
  ✓ Stress dosing: For physiologic stress (fever, vomiting, dental procedures) give hydrocortisone 50 mg/m²/day PO divided every 8 hours (or IV divided every 4 hours). For severe stress (surgery, trauma, severe illness, or repeated emesis) give hydrocortisone 100 mg/m² IV/IM once followed by 100 mg/m²/day IV divided every 4 hours.
  ✓ Secondary adrenal suppression: Patients without previously diagnosed adrenal insufficiency who are treated with glucocorticoids for ≤10 days can discontinue treatment without weaning. Patients treated for >10–14 days may have HPA axis suppression, so glucocorticoids should be tapered and stress dose coverage should be provided until the HPA axis recovers.
- Mineralocorticoid replacement: Patients with primary adrenal insufficiency with mineralocorticoid deficiency and salt-wasting forms of CAH require fludrocortisone 0.05–0.2 mg PO daily. Some patients require NaCl replacement.

CONGENITAL ADRENAL HYPERPLASIA (CAH)

Autosomal recessive mutations of adrenal steroidogenesis enzymes result in altered glucocorticoid, mineralocorticoid, and androgen production.

EPIDEMIOLOGY

- 21-hydroxylase deficiency: Incidence is 1:14,000 (accounts for 90–95% of cases).
- 11β-hydroxylase deficiency: Incidence is 1:100,000 (accounts for 5–8% of cases).
- 3β-HSD deficiency: Accounts for <5% of cases.
- 17α-hydroxylase/17,20-lyase deficiency: Incidence is rare (125 reported cases).
- StAR deficiency (lipoid CAH): Incidence is rare (<100 reported cases).

PATHOPHYSIOLOGY

- Adrenal steroidogenic enzyme deficiency results in excess accumulation of precursors and deficiency of end products. Certain precursors and products have glucocorticoid (cortisol, corticosterone), mineralocorticoid (aldosterone, DOC), and androgenic (dehydroepiandrosterone, androstenedione, testosterone, DHT) properties.

CLINICAL MANIFESTATIONS OF 21-HYDROXYLASE DEFICIENCY

- Classic salt-wasting CAH: Absent 21-hydroxylase activity results in complete cortisol and aldosterone deficiency, causing salt-wasting crisis in first 2–3 weeks. This manifests with lethargy, poor feeding, vomiting, diarrhea, dehydration, hyponatremia, hyperkalemia, metabolic acidosis, hypotension, shock, and death if untreated. Absence of cortisol feedback inhibition to pituitary leads to increased ACTH production, causing adrenal hyperplasia and accumulation of 17OHP and testosterone, resulting in virilization or ambiguous genitalia in females (clitoromegaly, fusion of labioscrotal folds), and accelerated skeletal maturation.
- Simple virilizing CAH: Decreased 21-hydroxylase activity results in virilization in females, premature puberty in males (pubic, axillary, and facial hair; phallic growth with prepubertal testes), and advanced bone age. There is no salt wasting.
- Nonclassic CAH: Mild 21-hydroxylase defects result in premature pubarche, mild-to-moderate hirsutism, menstrual irregularities, and decreased fertility in females.

DIAGNOSTICS

- Newborn screen: Diagnosis of 21-hydroxylase deficiency is suggested by elevated 17OHP on newborn screen (standardized for term neonates ≥24 hours old; elevated in premature, severely ill, and normal newborns <24 hours old). Confirm 17OHP level with serum sample, do not repeat newborn screen. Diagnosis should be suspected in infants with a salt-wasting episode, ambiguous genitalia, or elevated ACTH with low cortisol.
- Diagnostic confirmation: Diagnosis is confirmed by standard/high-dose ACTH stimulation testing. Salt-wasting and simple virilizing CAH have significantly elevated basal and stimulated 17OHP levels with an inadequate rise in cortisol, while nonclassic CAH has normal to mildly elevated basal 17OHP level, moderately elevated stimulated 17OHP level, and a normal cortisol response.
- Other studies: Include electrolytes (hyponatremia, hyperkalemia in salt-wasting CAH), plasma renin activity (elevated in mineralocorticoid deficiency), measurement of baseline and ACTH-stimulated levels of other adrenal steroids (pregnenolone, progesterone, DOC, corticosterone, 18-hydroxycorticosterone, 17-hydroxypregnenolone, 11-deoxycortisol, DHEA, androstenedione, and testosterone) to distinguish from other forms of CAH and for adrenal or testicular tumors, and lastly, genetic analysis for the presumed defective enzyme

MANAGEMENT

- If CAH is suspected, consult endocrinology (see "Adrenal Insufficiency"). Obtain BMP, 17OHP, androstenedione, testosterone, and plasma renin activity. Monitor BMP regularly for concern for salt wasting until diagnosis ruled out. If the patient has ambiguous genitalia, seek consultation from pediatric surgery/urology, genetics, and psychology.

CUSHING SYNDROME

Results from chronic glucocorticoid excess.

ETIOLOGY

- Iatrogenic: Long-term exposure to supraphysiologic doses of glucocorticoids
- Cushing disease: ACTH-secreting pituitary adenoma
- Ectopic ACTH Syndrome: ACTH-secreting nonpituitary tumor (neuroblastoma, pheochromocytoma, thymoma, bronchial and pancreatic carcinoma)

- Adrenal tumors: Cortisol-secreting adrenal adenoma or carcinoma
- Nodular adrenal hyperplasia: Secretes both cortisol and adrenal androgens, can be associated with McCune–Albright syndrome.

EPIDEMIOLOGY

- Iatrogenic is the most common cause in pediatric patients. Cushing disease has a higher incidence in patients older than 7 years, whereas adrenal tumors have a higher incidence in patients younger than 7 years. Ectopic ACTH syndrome and nodular adrenal hyperplasia are rare in pediatric patients.

CLINICAL MANIFESTATIONS

- Weight gain, truncal obesity, round facies, buffalo hump, hypertension, fatigue, plethora, headache, acne, hirsutism, menstrual irregularities, precocious or delayed puberty, linear growth retardation, osteopenia, weakness, proximal muscle wasting, violaceous striae, easy bruising, psychological disturbances. Hyperpigmentation with excess ACTH.

DIAGNOSTICS

- Cortisol: 24-hour urinary free cortisol (>4 times the upper limit of normal), nighttime salivary cortisol (>1 mcg/dL at bedtime or >0.27 mcg/dL at midnight), midnight plasma cortisol (>2 mcg/dL)
- Overnight dexamethasone-suppression test: Dexamethasone 15 mcg/kg (maximum, 1 mg) PO at 10 p.m., checking an 8 a.m. plasma cortisol (>5 mcg/dL is diagnostic, normal is suppression to <1.8 mcg/dL)
- Other studies: 8 a.m. cortisol and ACTH, combination low-dose/high-dose dexamethasone-suppression test, CRH stimulation test, inferior petrosal sinus sampling
- Imaging: Brain/pituitary MRI, adrenal CT or MRI, chest and/or abdominal CT or MRI

MANAGEMENT

- Cushing disease is treated with a transsphenoidal adenomectomy. Ectopic ACTH syndrome requires surgical excision of the tumor; if tumor not resectable, consider treatment with steroidogenesis inhibitors or bilateral adrenalectomy. Adrenal tumors require unilateral adrenalectomy, whereas a bilateral adrenalectomy is indicated for nodular adrenal hyperplasia.

THYROID DISEASE

CONGENITAL HYPOTHYROIDISM

Most common congenital endocrine disorder (1 in 1600 to 1 in 2800 newborns); leading cause of preventable mental retardation.

PATHOPHYSIOLOGY

- Thyroid dysgenesis: Defects in follicular-cell differentiation or survival results in thyroid-gland hypoplasia, complete agenesis, or ectopic location; accounts for approximately 85% of cases and is more common in females.
- Thyroid dyshormonogenesis: Due to defects in thyroid hormone biosynthesis; accounts for approximately 15% of cases.

CLINICAL MANIFESTATIONS

- Birth: Mild phenotype, postmaturity, macrosomia, large fontanels

- Early infancy: Decreased tone, lethargy, poor feeding, prolonged jaundice, hoarse cry
- Childhood: Delayed linear growth, delayed bone age, fatigue, constipation, dry skin, cold intolerance, goiter in two thirds of patients

DIAGNOSTICS

- TSH is elevated and T_4 is low. Newborn screening is now routine, preferably at 48–72 hours of life; threshold TSH is 20–25 mcIU/mL.

MANAGEMENT

- Levothyroxine 37.5–50 mcg/day in term normal-sized infants, or 10–15 mcg/kg/day. Only tablets should be used, even in neonates and infants.
- Monitor TSH (goal is lower end of normal, 0.5–2 mU/L) and T_4

CONGENITAL HYPERTHYROIDISM

Usually due to maternal Graves disease

EPIDEMIOLOGY

- Occurs in <2% of infants of mothers with Graves disease, due to low incidence of thyrotoxicosis in pregnancy. Affects males and females equally.

PATHOPHYSIOLOGY

- Transplacental passage of maternal TRSAb or TSI leads to excessive thyroid hormone production in the offspring. Concomitant transplacental passage of TRBAb or TBII and/or antithyroid medications can affect the onset, severity, and course.

CLINICAL MANIFESTATIONS

- Prenatal: Fetal tachycardia, intrauterine growth retardation, goiter
- Postnatal: Irritability, hyperactivity, anxiety, flushing, diaphoresis, voracious appetite, decreased subcutaneous fat, goiter, exophthalmos, elevated temperature, elevated blood pressure, elevated heart rate, elevated respiratory rate, advanced bone age, craniosynostosis, frontal bossing, triangular facies, microcephaly, ventriculomegaly. In severe cases, hepatosplenomegaly, jaundice, cardiac failure, and death may occur.
- Long-term effects: Growth retardation, intellectual and developmental impairments, secondary central hypothyroidism

DIAGNOSTICS

- TRAb (may be blocking or stimulatory), T_4, and T_3 are elevated; TSH is low. If TRAb is negative but suspicion is high, TSI can be ordered.

MANAGEMENT

- Admission to a neonatal/newborn intensive care unit with endocrinology consult
- Methimazole or PTU (see "Graves Disease" section for dosing)
- SSKI 1 drop (48 mg iodide)/day or Lugol solution (1–3 drops/day) accelerates decline in circulating thyroid hormone.
- β-blockers
- If decompensation, consider digoxin, IV fluids, corticosteroids.
- Monitor TSH, T_4, and T_3 frequently. Remission is gradual as maternal TRAb is degraded; usually euthyroid by 3–4 months of age.

ACQUIRED HYPOTHYROIDISM

EPIDEMIOLOGY

- Hashimoto thyroiditis, or autoimmune hypothyroidism, is the most common cause of acquired hypothyroidism in children. The presentation is variable, as the child may be hypothyroid, euthyroid, or transiently hyperthyroid at diagnosis. Autoimmune hypothyroidism has a female predominance (2:1) and 40–50% of patients will have a positive family history of autoimmune thyroid disease. It can be associated with other autoimmune disorders and is more common in patients with certain chromosomal disorders, such as Down syndrome and Turner syndrome.

PATHOPHYSIOLOGY

- Autoimmune hypothyroidism is the consequence of antibody-mediated (antithyroglobulin antibody, antithyroid peroxidase (anti-TPO) antibody) destruction of thyroid tissue resulting in low thyroid hormone levels. Absence of thyroid hormone feedback on the hypothalamus and pituitary results in increased levels of TRH and TSH. TSH stimulation of the thyroid gland results in goiter.

CLINICAL MANIFESTATIONS

- Fatigue, cold intolerance, constipation, nontender goiter, bradycardia, delayed deep tendon reflexes, proximal muscle weakness, irregular menses, linear growth failure with preservation of normal weight gain

DIAGNOSTICS

- Elevated TSH; low T_4 and free T_4; positive Tg and TPO antibodies. In subclinical primary hypothyroidism, there will be a mildly elevated TSH with normal T_4 levels. In contrast, a child with central hypothyroidism can have a low, normal, or even elevated TSH combined with low T_4 levels.

MANAGEMENT

- Thyroid hormone replacement with levothyroxine tablets, not suspension; initial dose recommendations based on age, as follows:
  - ✓ 0–3 months: 10–15 mcg/kg/day
  - ✓ 3–6 months: 8–10 mcg/kg/day
  - ✓ 6–12 months: 6–8 mcg/kg/day
  - ✓ 1–5 years: 5–6 mcg/kg/day
  - ✓ 6–12 years: 4–5 mcg/kg/day
  - ✓ >12 years: 2–3 mcg/kg/day
  - ✓ Adult: 1.6 mcg/kg or 75–200 mcg/day
- TSH, T_4, and free T_4 should be checked 6–8 weeks after initiating treatment or with dose adjustments. Thyroid function should be monitored every 6 months until growth is complete and then yearly. The goal of treatment is to keep the TSH and T_4 within the normal range.

GRAVES DISEASE

EPIDEMIOLOGY

- Graves disease is an autoimmune disease that affects the thyroid, orbital tissue, and skin. It is the most common cause of hyperthyroidism in children, with peak incidence in adolescence. More common in females (5:1). Often associated with other autoimmune disorders and a family history of autoimmune thyroid disease

PATHOPHYSIOLOGY

- TRSAb/TSI bind to and stimulate TSH receptors in the thyroid gland, resulting in excessive thyroid hormone synthesis and release, as well as follicular-cell hyperplasia. These effects may be counterbalanced by TRBAb/TBII.

CLINICAL MANIFESTATIONS

- Hyperthyroidism: Goiter of varying degrees, exophthalmos, lid lag, tachycardia, palpitations, heat-intolerance, cardiomegaly, systolic hypertension, widened pulse pressure, tachypnea, diarrhea, tremors, proximal muscle weakness, tongue fasciculations, emotional lability, hyperactivity, difficulty concentrating, difficulty sleeping, increased appetite without change in weight or with weight loss, linear growth acceleration, bone maturation
- Thyroid storm: Acute onset of hyperthermia and severe tachycardia that can progress rapidly to delirium, coma, and death

DIAGNOSTICS

- Elevated T_4, free T_4, T_3, free T_3, Tg; low TSH; positive TSI or TRAb, presence of positive TPO or TgAb does not rule out Graves disease.

MANAGEMENT

- Medical management: Antithyroid/thionamide drugs: methimazole and PTU inhibit TPO, which oxidizes iodide into iodine so that it can be incorporated into Tg tyrosine residue, thereby inhibiting thyroid hormone synthesis. PTU also inhibits 5'-deiodinase in peripheral tissues, thus inhibiting T_4-to-T_3 conversion. Methimazole 0.25–1.0 mg/kg/day divided 1–3 times daily; PTU 5–10 mg/kg/day divided 2–3 times daily. Rare side effects of these medications include hypersensitivity reactions and agranulocytosis. PTU is only used as a second-line treatment because of a black box warning about liver dysfunction and death.
- β-blockers: Propranolol is generally used for acute thyrotoxicosis. Atenolol is used for symptomatic relief of catecholamine-mediated symptoms until patient is euthyroid and is generally dosed 25–50 mg daily.
- Radioiodine (I-131) thyroid ablation: Used as an alternative or adjuvant to medical or surgical therapy. Complete effects may not be seen for 2–3 months. Results in hypothyroidism, necessitating lifelong thyroid hormone replacement. Failure rate of approximately 20%.
- Surgical management (total thyroidectomy): Indicated if there is failure of medical therapy or concern for a coexisting carcinoma. Should be performed only after a euthyroid state has been achieved medically, in order to decrease surgical risks. This can be achieved using iodide drops (SSKI) or Lugol solution prior to surgery.
- Monitoring: TSH, T_4, T_3, TSI (disappearance predicts remission)

SALT AND WATER HOMEOSTASIS

CEREBRAL SALT WASTING

- CNS insult resulting in renal sodium loss, polyuria, hypovolemia, and hyponatremia

ETIOLOGY

- Head trauma, neurosurgery, CNS tumor, meningitis, hydrocephalus, stroke, brain death

PATHOPHYSIOLOGY

- Unclear but thought to be due to increased atrial or brain-derived natriuretic factor

TABLE 8-2	Distinguishing Features of SIADH and CSW	
Feature	**SIADH**	**CSW**
Serum sodium	Low	Low
Serum osmolality	Low	Low
Serum BUN and creatinine	Low	Normal or High
Serum aldosterone and renin	Low	Low
Serum uric acid	Low	Normal
Urine output	Low	High
Urine sodium*	High	High
Urine osmolality	High	High
Volume status	Euvolemic or hypervolemic	Hypovolemic
Treatment	Fluid restriction	Volume repletion with salt and water

*Generally higher in CSW compared to SIADH. Can be difficult to interpret in patients on sodium-containing IV fluids or supplements.
CSW = Cerebral Salt Wasting. SIADH, Syndrome of Inappropriate Antidiuretic Hormone

CLINICAL MANIFESTATIONS

• Polyuria, hypovolemia, evidence of dehydration (tachycardia, poor skin turgor, dry mucous membranes), hypotension, nausea, vomiting, weakness, headache, lethargy, psychosis, coma, seizures. There is generally an associated CNS insult within the past week.

DIAGNOSTICS

• See **Table 8-2**. Other studies include atrial natriuretic peptide (high), anti-diuretic hormone (ADH) (normal or low), creatinine clearance (normal or low), body weight (stable or decreased)

MANAGEMENT

• The underlying disorder should be treated if possible. Intravascular volume should be repleted with NaCl and water (initially may need NaCl 150–450 meq/L).
• Acute hyponatremia: Correct rapidly with 3% saline 12 mL/kg over 1 hour to increase sodium by 10 mM.
• Chronic hyponatremia: Correct serum sodium by 0.5 mM/hr or 12 mM/day; increased risk of central pontine myelinolysis if corrected too quickly.
  ✓ Sodium deficit = total body water × wt in kg × (desired Na − patient Na)
• Monitoring: Vital signs, weight, intake/output, neurologic exam, serum and urine electrolytes
• Prognosis: Generally resolves within 2–4 weeks; however, patients are at risk for developing other salt/water disorders (DI, SIADH) and must be reevaluated with any change in clinical status.

SYNDROME OF INAPPROPRIATE ANTIDIURETIC HORMONE (SIADH)

Inappropriately elevated ADH (vasopressin) results in expanded intravascular volume and low serum osmolality.

ETIOLOGY

- CNS: Meningitis, encephalitis, brain tumor, brain abscess, head trauma/surgery, hypoxic-ischemic encephalopathy, hydrocephalus, CNS leukemia, Guillain–Barré syndrome
- Infections: Pneumonia, HIV/AIDS, tuberculosis, herpes zoster, respiratory syncytial virus, aspergillosis, infantile botulism
- Pulmonary: Asthma, cystic fibrosis, empyema, bacterial pneumonia, abscess
- Neoplasms: Oat-cell carcinoma; bronchial carcinoid; lymphoma; Ewing sarcoma; tumors of pancreas, duodenum, thymus, bladder, ureter
- Drugs: Carbamazepine, lamotrigine, chlorpropamide, vinblastine, vincristine, tricyclics
- Other: Postictal state, prolonged nausea, acute intermittent porphyria

PATHOPHYSIOLOGY

- Inappropriate secretion of ADH by hypothalamus or ectopic secretion of ADH or ADH-like peptide stimulates renal collecting ducts to resorb water, leading to volume expansion, dilutional hyponatremia, and decreased serum osmolality. Hypo-osmolality may lead to cellular swelling and cerebral edema

CLINICAL MANIFESTATIONS

- Anorexia, nausea, vomiting, headache, weakness, irritability, personality changes, change in mental status, seizures. In contrast to CSW, is clinically euvolemic or hypervolemic.

DIAGNOSTICS

- See **Table 8-2**. Other studies include ADH (high), serum potassium (low), serum chloride (low), and body weight (stable or increased). Must rule out adrenal insufficiency, hypothyroidism, renal insufficiency, and diuretic use.

MANAGEMENT

- The underlying disorder should be treated, if possible. Fluid restriction is key. Salt administration is not effective for long-term management.
- Symptomatic hyponatremia (seizures or coma): Correct rapidly with 3% saline 1–2 mL/kg/hr to increase sodium by 10 mM; increased risk of central pontine myelinolysis if chronic hyponatremia is corrected too quickly.
- Chronic hyponatremia: Correct serum sodium by 0.5 mM/hr via fluid restriction (below)
- Long-term management: Fluid restriction to 1 L/m²/day (accounts for obligatory renal solute load of 500 mOsm/m²/day excreted in 500 mL/m²/day and insensible losses of 500 mL/m²/day). Demeclocycline induces nephrogenic DI and may be helpful in infants for whom fluid restriction will not supply enough calories for growth.
- Monitoring: Vital signs, weight, intake/output, neurologic exam, serum and urine electrolytes and osmolality

DIABETES INSIPIDUS

Inability to produce or respond to ADH/vasopressin results in excess urinary water loss.

ETIOLOGY

Central DI

- CNS neoplasm, congenital midline brain lesions, head trauma (basal skull fracture, fracture of sella turcica), neurosurgery in region of hypothalamus or pituitary, intraventricular hemorrhage, brain death

- Genetic mutation in ADH gene (generally autosomal dominant, less commonly autosomal recessive)
- Infiltrative disease: Langerhans-cell histiocytosis, lymphocytic hypophysitis, sarcoidosis
- Infectious disease: Viral encephalitis, bacterial meningitis, cryptococcus, toxoplasmosis, congenital cytomegalovirus, tuberculosis, actinomycosis, Guillain–Barré syndrome
- Increased vasopressin metabolism by vasopressinase made by placenta
- DIDMOAD/Wolfram syndrome
- Other: Autoimmune diseases, drug-induced (ethanol, phenytoin, halothane), idiopathic

Nephrogenic DI

- Drug-induced is most common: Lithium, demeclocycline, foscarnet, clozapine, amphotericin, methicillin, rifampin
- X-linked mutation in vasopressin V2 receptor; accounts for 95% of congenital cases
- Autosomal recessive mutation in aquaporin 2
- Other: Ureteral obstruction, chronic pyelonephritis, polycystic kidney disease, medullary cystic disease, renal dysplasia, chronic renal failure, hypercalcemia, hypokalemia, sickle cell disease, Sjögren syndrome, sarcoidosis, amyloidosis, primary polydipsia (mild)

CLINICAL MANIFESTATIONS

- Polyuria, nocturia, polydipsia (crave cold fluids, especially water), dehydration, hypernatremia, altered mental status, seizure, coma
- Hypothalamic tumors: Growth failure, precocious puberty, cachexia or obesity, fever, sleep disturbance, behavioral changes, symptoms of increased intracranial pressure
- Nephrogenic DI: Infants exhibit irritability, poor feeding, water preference, vomiting, growth failure, and intermittent high fevers. Repeated episodes of dehydration result in brain damage, mental retardation, and abnormal behavior.

DIAGNOSTICS

- Initial studies: Serum osmolality, urine osmolality, and serum sodium checked as an outpatient after the longest period of fasting the patient is known to safely tolerate. DI is unlikely if serum osmolality <270 mOsm/L or urine osmolality >600 mOsm/L. If patient does not meet criteria to rule out or to diagnose DI (see criteria below), a water-deprivation test is necessary.
- Water-deprivation test: Admit patient, withhold fluid, and frequently monitor serum sodium, serum osmolality, urine osmolality, urine output, urine sodium, vital signs, and body weight.
  - ✓ Normal result is urine osmolality >1000 mOsm/L or >600 mOsm/L and stable.
  - ✓ DI is diagnosed if serum osmolality >300 mOsm/L and urine osmolality <600 mOsm/L. Give vasopressin to determine whether central (urine output decreases and urine osmolality increases) or nephrogenic (no change in urine output or urine osmolality)
- Other studies: Serum potassium, calcium, glucose, BUN; urine glucose and amino acids if suspect another cause for diuresis; MRI of pituitary and hypothalamus; ultrasound if suspect urinary tract anomaly; evaluation of anterior pituitary hormones; β-hCG test for germinoma.

MANAGEMENT

Initial

- Correct free water deficit, replace ongoing excessive urinary water loss, replace vasopressin, monitor intake and output, check frequent serum sodium.
- If hypotensive, give NS bolus. For fluid replacement, use enteral water when possible; otherwise, half NS is generally preferred.

✓ Free water deficit (L) = (0.6 × (wt in kg)) × (1 − (desired Na / patient Na))
✓ Correct chronic hypernatremia slowly (0.5 mM/h) to avoid cerebral edema.
✓ Correct acute or symptomatic (seizure) hypernatremia rapidly (3–4 mM/h)r.
- Use IV vasopressin to decrease urine output. Can be administered continuously and has a short half-life so can be titrated frequently.

Chronic

- Patients with intact thirst mechanism should be allowed free access to fluids (especially in nephrogenic DI). Patients without intact thirst or unable to take in water spontaneously (infants, postoperative patients) should be given maintenance fluid requirement of 1 L/m²/day or 40 mL/m²/hr with enteral formula or IV D5 1/4 NS, in addition to replacing urine output >40 mL/m²/hr or >3–5 mL/kg/hr with enteral water or IV D5W 1/4 NS.
- In central DI, treatment is with desmopressin (DDAVP: a modified form of vasopressin with extended half-life) which can be administered by various routes (enteral, intranasal, subcutaneous).
- Infants with central DI can be treated with the addition of free water to formula or given between feedings; goal daily volume should be titrated in the inpatient setting and should be based on frequent serum sodium monitoring. Chlorothiazide combined with a low renal solute formula may also be used.
- Patients who are without intact thirst and are taking DDAVP should be given a fixed daily intake volume to avoid both hyponatremia and hypernatremia.
- In nephrogenic DI, patients generally require 300–400 mL/kg/day of fluids. Salt and protein restriction minimize renal solute load and thus diuresis; choose foods with a high ratio of calories to osmotic load in order to ensure adequate growth. Hydrochlorothiazide 1–3 mg/kg/day, alone or in combination with indomethacin (2 mg/kg/day) and/or amiloride is commonly used.

CALCIUM HOMEOSTASIS

HYPOCALCEMIA

Serum calcium <7 mg/dL or ionized calcium <1.2 mM due to an imbalance of calcium absorption, excretion, or distribution that can be seen in a variety of disorders.

ETIOLOGY

- Hypoparathyroidism: 22q11 deletion/DiGeorge syndrome, surgery, hypomagnesemia, autoimmune polyglandular syndrome, PTH mutations, CaSR activating mutations, pseudohypoparathyroidism
- Nutritional: Vitamin D deficiency, calcium deficiency, magnesium deficiency
- Drugs: Loop diuretics, chemotherapy (cisplatin, asparaginase), transfusions
- Other: Hyperphosphatemia, hypoalbuminemia, organic acidemias, renal insufficiency

CLINICAL MANIFESTATIONS

- Constipation, paresthesia, Chvostek sign (facial muscle twitch when tapping facial nerve), Trousseau sign (carpopedal spasm with blood pressure cuff inflation), prolonged QTc, arrhythmia, seizure

DIAGNOSTICS

- Serum calcium, magnesium, phosphorus, BUN, creatinine, albumin, alkaline phosphatase; ionized calcium; PTH at time of hypocalcemia; 25-hydroxyvitamin D, 1,25-dihydroxyvitamin D; urine calcium, creatinine, phosphorus, magnesium, and ECG (see **Table 8-3**)

TABLE 8-3   Laboratory Findings in Major Causes of Rickets

Cause	Ca	Phos	PTH	25-(OH)D	1,25-(OH)₂D	Alk Phos	Urine Ca	Urine Phos
Calcium deficiency	↓, NL	↓	↑	NL	↑	↑	↓	↑
Phosphorus deficiency	NL, ↑	↓	NL, ↓	NL	↑	↑	↑	↓
Vitamin D deficiency	↓, NL	↓,	↑	↓	↓, NL, ↑	↑	↓	↑
VDDR, type 1*	↓, NL	↓	↑	NL	↓	↑	↓	↑
VDDR, type 2†	↓, NL	↓	↑	NL	↑	↑	↓	↑
25-hydroxylase deficiency	↓, NL	↓	↑	↓	↓	↑	↓	↑
Familial hypophosphatemic rickets	NL	↓	NL	NL	↓, NL	↑	NL	↓, NL
Chronic renal failure	↓, NL	↑	↑	NL	↓	↑	↓, NL	↓

*Due to deficiency of 1α-hydroxylase. Also called pseudovitamin D–deficient rickets.
†Due to mutation of the vitamin D receptor. Also called vitamin D–resistant rickets.
NL = normal; PTH = parathyroid hormone; VDDR = vitamin D–dependent rickets.

MANAGEMENT

- Acute symptomatic hypocalcemia: Calcium gluconate 100 mg/kg IV bolus run over 4 hours or continuous IV calcium infusion with 1–3 mg/kg/hr elemental calcium; central access is preferred given risk of soft tissue damage with extravasation.
- Maintenance: Oral calcium supplementation (50–75 mg/kg/day elemental calcium divided TID and administered with meals, may be higher in neonates); depending on etiology, treatment may also include vitamin D, calcitriol, and/or magnesium.
- Monitoring: Serum calcium, phosphorus, magnesium; urine calcium, creatinine, phosphorus; PTH; alkaline phosphatase; 25-hydroxyvitamin D

HYPERCALCEMIA

- Total serum calcium >11 mg/dL or ionized calcium >1.4 mM

ETIOLOGY

- Transient neonatal: Maternal excess vitamin D intake, maternal hypocalcemia
- Syndromes: Williams syndrome, Bartter syndrome
- Hyperparathyroidism: Primary (isolated parathyroid adenoma, MEN syndrome, homozygous inactivating mutation of CaSR; secondary (renal failure, chronic hyperphosphatemia); ectopic PTHrP production
- Drugs: Thiazide diuretics, lithium, vitamin A, calcium, alkali, aminophylline
- Other: Excessive calcium or vitamin D intake, immobilization, neoplasia, inflammation, juvenile rheumatoid arthritis, and subcutaneous fat necrosis

CLINICAL MANIFESTATIONS

- Constipation, abdominal pain, polyuria, renal stones, failure to thrive, confusion, bony pain, hypertension, shortened QTc, arrhythmia

DIAGNOSTICS

- Serum calcium, magnesium, phosphorus, BUN, creatinine, albumin; ionized calcium; PTH at time of hypercalcemia, PTHrP; 25-hydroxyvitamin D, 1,25-dihydroxyvitamin D; urine calcium, creatinine, phosphorus, and ECG

MANAGEMENT

- Severe symptomatic hypercalcemia: IV fluids, calcitonin, glucocorticoids, IV loop diuretics, bisphosphonates, surgery for parathyroid adenoma
- Moderate hypercalcemia and maintenance: Increased fluid intake, high sodium diet, limited calcium and vitamin D intake
- Monitoring: Serum calcium, phosphorous, magnesium; urine calcium, creatinine, phosphorous; PTH; 25-hydroxyvitamin D

RICKETS

- Decreased or defective bone matrix mineralization due to decreased phosphorus availability (a result of secondary hyperparathyroidism in response to hypocalcemia) for deposition of hydroxyapatite, usually involving the epiphysis and newly formed trabecular and cortical bone

ETIOLOGY

- Rickets of prematurity: 30% of affected infants have birth weight <1000 g

Vitamin D Abnormalities

- Nutritional deprivation: Low vitamin D intake with decreased sunlight exposure; malabsorption (celiac disease, biliary obstruction, gastric resection, pancreatic-insufficient cystic fibrosis); medications that affect vitamin D metabolism (cholestyramine, phenytoin, phenobarbital)
- Metabolic errors: Defects in hepatic vitamin D metabolism (rare); renal 25-hydroxyvitamin D-1α-hydroxylase deficiency (pseudovitamin D-deficient rickets or vitamin D-deficient rickets type I); inactivating mutations in vitamin D receptor (vitamin D-resistant rickets or vitamin D-deficient rickets type 2); 25-hydroxylase deficiency
- Calcium deficiency: Nutritional deprivation, hypercalciuria
- Phosphorus deficiency: Nutritional deprivation: low birth weight infants, use of aluminum-containing antacids
  - ✓ FHR: Defective renal tubular phosphorus resorption; most common form of congenital rickets in North America; usually X-linked dominant, autosomal dominant and autosomal recessive forms are less common.
  - ✓ Kidney: Chronic renal failure leading to renal osteodystrophy; renal tubular acidosis (primary, Fanconi syndrome, tyrosinemia type 1)
  - ✓ Other: Oncogenic hypophosphatemic osteomalacia, cadmium and lead excess
- Drugs: Aluminum, bisphosphonates, and fluoride inhibit bone mineralization.
- Hypophosphatasia: Autosomal recessive mutations in the liver/bone/kidney alkaline phosphatase gene result in accumulation of pyrophosphate, which prevents formation of hydroxyapatite that is necessary for bone mineralization. Vitamin D supplementation should be avoided because of increased risk of secondary hypercalcemia.

CLINICAL MANIFESTATIONS

- Craniotabes, frontal bossing, cranial suture widening, metaphyseal flaring, rachitic rosary (enlargement of the costochondral junctions), Harrison grooves, genu varum (bow-leg) in early childhood, genu valgum (knock-knee) in late childhood, bone pain, seizures, dental abnormalities, muscle weakness, hypotonia, atelectasis, pneumonia, anemia

DIAGNOSTICS

- Calcium, ionized calcium, phosphorus, magnesium, alkaline phosphatase, 25-hydroxyvitamin D, 1,25-dihydroxyvitamin D; urine calcium, creatinine, phosphorus; x-rays can show osteopenia with pseudofracture lines; widening, flaring, cupping, or fraying of long bone metaphyses; rachitic rosary; flaring of the lower thoracic rib cage; and rachitic changes of the iliac crest in adolescents (last to fuse). See **Table 8-3.**

MANAGEMENT

- Vitamin D deficiency: Vitamin D_2 (ergocalciferol) or D_3 (cholecalciferol) 1000–5000 IU PO daily (depending on age); can also be given in larger once-weekly doses; decrease to 400–1000 IU daily maintenance dose when vitamin D level and other biochemical markers have normalized; for severe vitamin D deficiency, a loading dose of 25,000–50,000 IU is generally recommended.
- Elemental calcium: 50–100 mg/kg/day prevents hypocalcemia secondary to bone matrix re-mineralization ("hungry bone" syndrome).
- Calcitriol (1,25-dihydroxyvitamin D): 20–100 ng/kg/day until serum calcium normalizes
- Vitamin D-deficient rickets type 1: Calcitriol 10–20 ng/kg/day
- Vitamin D-deficient rickets type 2: High doses of calcitriol (100–600 ng/kg/day) and elemental calcium (1–3 g/day) should be tried in all patients. Patients with refractory disease

may require continuous IV or intracaval elemental calcium 0.4–1.4 g/m²/day. After rickets has resolved, maintain with elemental calcium 3.5–9 g/m²/day.

- Familial hypophosphatemic rickets: Elemental phosphorus 40–100 mg/kg/day divided 4–6 times/day (<3 g/day); calcitriol 20–60 ng/kg/day. If rickets recurs and/or nephrocalcinosis develops, consider adding amiloride and thiazide diuretic to increase renal tubular calcium absorption.
- Chronic renal disease, renal osteodystrophy: Limit phosphorus intake to <1200 mg/day.
  ✓ Oral elemental calcium 500–1000 mg/m²/day to decrease dietary phosphorus absorption.
  ✓ Calcitriol 10–50 ng/kg/day to maintain PTH within normal limits.
  ✓ Occasionally requires parathyroidectomy if PTH levels do not normalize.
  ✓ Avoid aluminum-containing medications.
- Calcium deficiency: Elemental calcium 25–100 mg/kg/day
- Hypophosphatasia: Enzyme replacement (asfotase alfa) is available. Phosphate administration may heal rickets in mild cases. Vitamin D should be avoided.
- Monitoring: Serum calcium, phosphorus, creatinine, alkaline phosphatase, PTH; urine calcium, creatinine; skeletal x-rays; renal ultrasound to evaluate for nephrocalcinosis.

Fluids and Electrolytes

Selasie Q. Goka, MD
Stephanie L. Clark, MD, MPH

BODY COMPOSITION

- Total body water (TBW): 60% of total body weight (higher in newborns, up to 70%)
- Intracellular Fluid (ICF): Two-thirds of TBW or 40% of total body weight
- Extracellular Fluid (ECF): One-third of TBW or 20% of total body weight
- Interstitial space: 75% of ECF
- Vascular space or plasma: 25% of ECF
- Predominant electrolytes in intracellular fluid compartment: Potassium and magnesium
- Predominant electrolytes in ECF compartment: Sodium, chloride, and bicarbonate

FLUID THERAPY

MAINTENANCE FLUID THERAPY

Maintenance fluid requirements can be estimated by the Holliday–Segar method. Daily water requirements are calculated on the basis of body weight and the assumption that each kilocalorie of energy metabolized results in the net consumption of 1 mL of water (Table 9-1). Water requirements form the basis for the estimated needs for sodium and potassium (Table 9-2). This method is not recommended for premature infants or term infants younger than 2 weeks of age.

- While several studies argue strongly against the use of hypotonic maintenance fluids across all pediatric populations, limitations in the evidence include the populations studied, study heterogeneity, and paucity of data on potential adverse events from an increased solute load.
- It is equally likely that the administration of an inappropriately high fluid administration rate in the context of nonosmotic antidiuretic hormone release is responsible for most cases of iatrogenic hyponatremia.
- The focus on tonicity of maintenance fluid without adequate study of the rate or volume contributes to wide practice pattern variation.
- Holliday–Segar maintenance therapy is based on the assumptions that all daily water losses occur as the result of either insensible or urine losses and that all homeostatic mechanisms are intact.
- Insensible losses in the absence of conditions leading to increased fluid loss (e.g., fever, hyperventilation, prematurity and low birth weight, skin defects, burns) are usually 400–700 mL/m² of BSA (higher in neonates, up to 1150 mL/m² of BSA).

TABLE 9-1	Estimate of Maintenance Fluid Requirements Based on Body Weight	
	Water Requirement	
Body Weight	**Daily**	**Hourly**
First 10 kg	100 mL/kg/day	4 mL/kg/hr
Second 10 kg	50 mL/kg/day	2 mL/kg/hr
Weight above 20 kg	20 mL/kg/day	1 mL/kg/hr

TABLE 9-2	Basic Electrolyte Requirements
Electrolyte	**Estimated Need (mEq/100 mL water)**
Sodium	3
Potassium	2
Chloride	2

- The Holliday–Segar method may not be appropriate in children with urine outputs that are abnormally high (e.g., due to adrenal failure or diuretic exposure) or low (e.g., due to hypovolemia, SIADH secretion, renal failure, heart failure, nephrotic syndrome, or cirrhosis).
- Fever increases the metabolic rate; therefore, maintenance requirements go up (add about 10% for every degree Celsius increase >38°C for the duration of the febrile episode).
- Burns: Needs are increased based on the percent BSA involved.
- Oliguria/anuria in a euvolemic/hypervolemic child (e.g., established kidney injury): Maintenance fluid should be prescribed by calculating insensible losses and replacing urine output every few hours.
- Dextrose-containing IVFs are used to supply a portion of the caloric needs, to prevent hypoglycemia and starvation ketosis.
- Stock solutions containing D5 are appropriate for most situations, but D10 or higher is also available.
- Dextrose concentrations above 12.5% are usually reserved for central catheters because the increased osmolality is irritating to peripheral veins.

MAINTENANCE ELECTROLYTE CALCULATION

- Sodium requirement: 3 mEq/100 mL/day
- Potassium requirement: 2 mEq/100 mL/day

Sample Maintenance Fluid and Electrolyte Calculation:

Maintenance fluid, sodium, and potassium requirements for an otherwise healthy 37-kg child:

Water Requirement:

First 10 kg, give 100 mL/kg/day:	10 kg × 100 mL/kg/day = 1000 mL/day
Second 10 kg, give 50 mL/kg/day:	10 kg × 50 mL/kg/day = 500 mL/day
>20 kg give, 20 mL/kg/day:	17 kg × 20 mL/kg/day = 340 mL/day
Total:	37 kg 1840 mL/day

OR

First 10 kg, give 4 mL/kg/hr:	10 kg × 4 mL/kg/h = 40 mL/hr
Second 10 kg, give 2 mL/kg/hr:	10 kg × 2 mL/kg/h = 20 mL/hr
>20 kg give, 1 mL/kg/hr:	17 kg × 1 mL/kg/h = 17 mL/hr
Total:	37 kg 77 mL/hr

Sodium Requirement:

3 mEq/100 mL/day × 1840 mL/day = 55 mEq/day

$$\frac{55 \text{ mEq/day}}{1840 \text{ mL/day}} = \frac{Na^+}{1000 \text{ mL}}$$

$$Na^+ = 30 \text{ mEq/L}$$

- *Note:* Normal saline (NS) contains 0.9% NaCl or 154 mEq/L. In this case, a stock solution containing 0.22% NaCl (1/4 NS) would provide 34 mEq NaCl/L

Potassium Requirement:

2 mEq/100 mL/day $\times$ 1840 mL/day = 37 mEq/day

$$\frac{37 \text{ mEq/day}}{1840 \text{ mL/day}} = \frac{K^+}{1000 \text{ mL}}$$

$$K^+ = 20 \text{ mEq/L}$$

- The addition of 20 mEq/L of KCl would provide the approximate needs for potassium

Therefore, an order for routine maintenance fluids for this child would be:

D5/0.2% NaCl with 20 mEq KCl/L to run at 77 mL/hr.

- It can also be written as: D5/1/4 NS + 20 mEq KCl/L @ 77 mL/hr.
  Standard (Stock) Solutions for Routine Maintenance Intravenous Fluids (**Table 9-3**)
- It is important to note that the above calculations for maintenance fluids were derived using healthy, non-hospitalized children. Many hospitalized children, however, will have elevated ADH concentrations and are at risk of developing iatrogenic hyponatremia when given hypotonic fluid. As a result, while D5/0.2% NS with 20 mEq KCl/L provides a good theoretical starting point for choice of maintenance IVF solutions, each patient's fluid plan should be individualized based on their clinical scenario and comorbidities.
- The following are some general recommendations for maintenance fluid therapy:
- In accordance with the 2018 American Academy of Pediatrics guidelines, we suggest D5/0.9%NS as a good choice for most children >28 days and <18 years old without significant comorbidities.
- If electrolytes are checked at presentation and there is hyponatremia or the patient is at risk for SIADH (postoperative, trauma, severe stress or pain, CNS disease, pulmonary disease, etc.), consider running D5/0.9% at two-thirds maintenance rate. This allows for lower solute load and decreased total volume infused to the patient to avoid causing iatrogenic hyponatremia or worsening hyponatremia.
- The maximum maintenance rate for most patients is 100–120 ml/hour.
- KCl should be withheld from the IVFs until after the child's first void or if the patient is hyperkalemic (assuming electrolytes are checked). At least 10mEq of potassium per liter of

TABLE 9-3	Terminology and Conversions for Stock Intravenous Solutions		
Stock Solution	**Common Terminology**	**Dextrose Content (g/dL)**	**Sodium Chloride Content (mEq/L)**
Dextrose 5% in water	D5W	5	0
Dextrose 10% in water	$D_{10}W$	10	0
Dextrose 5% in 0.9% NaCl	D_5 NS	5	154
Dextrose 5% in 0.45% NaCl	D_5 ½NS	5	77
Dextrose 5% in 0.22% NaCl	D_5 ¼NS	5	34
Dextrose 5% in 0.22% NaCl	D_5 ¼NS	5	34
NaCl with 20 mEq KCl/L	+20 mEq KCl/L		
3% saline	Hypertonic saline	0	513

NS = normal saline.

fluid is needed to provide maintenance requirements in a patient who is NPO and prevent the risk of hypokalemia.

- D5 lactated Ringer's can be used as an alternative to D5/0.9% NS in patients who are not hyperkalemic and have voided as it contains potassium.
- For hypernatremic patients, D5/0.45% NS is an appropriate starting place but you should also proceed with the appropriate calculations.
- D10 should be substituted for D5 in premature infants and neonates because of their increased glucose requirements and diminished glycogen stores.
- Close monitoring of patient weight, intake and output while on IVF allows for adjustment of the fluid strategy as needed. There are no clear guidelines on electrolyte monitoring, however, it is advisable to monitor electrolytes regularly in patients who remain on IVF for prolonged periods. This will vary by institution but at the very least should be checked after 24–48 hours of IVF so that changes can be made to the fluid composition as needed.
- Patients who require ICU level care or have significant medical comorbidities such as heart failure, renal dysfunction, liver failure, oncologic diagnosis etc. will need a more individualized approach than the recommendations given above.
- Common stock IVFs are listed in **Table 9-3**

EXPLORATION OF BALANCED CRYSTALLOIDS VERSUS NORMAL SALINE

- Increased focus in past decade on what has been termed "balanced" crystalloids, such as lactated ringers solution, which have lower chloride concentrations and strong ion differences that more closely approximate plasma.
- Theorized benefits include decreased risk of hyperchloremic metabolic acidosis and acute kidney injury and overall improved outcomes for critically ill patients.
- Initial small studies showed mixed results, including improved mortality outcomes versus no change as compared to 0.9% saline; however, more recent larger randomized trials have shown improved hospital mortality and lower rates of acute kidney injury.
- More studies need to be performed; however, it is important to understand the shift that is occurring in the ICU setting with regard to maintenance fluid options for critically ill patients.
- Note that normal saline or lactated ringers may not be appropriate for every critically ill patient in the ICU (e.g., for those with significant hypertension, acute kidney injury, or chronic kidney disease).

REPLACEMENT FLUID THERAPY

Replacement therapy corrects preexisting deficits (dehydration) and ongoing losses.

DEHYDRATION

Consider both the extent of the dehydration and the overall balance of water and sodium that is created.

- If pre-illness weight is available, then calculate percent dehydration:

  % dehydration = [(Pre-illness weight − Current weight)/Pre-illness weight] × 100

- If pre-illness weight is not available, percent dehydration can be clinically assessed:
  - ✓ Mild dehydration (up to 3% in older children, 5% in infants): Thirst, normal exam, flat fontanelle, reduced urine output
  - ✓ Moderate dehydration (3–6% in older children, 5–10% in infants): Tachycardia, dry mucosa, sunken eyes, sunken fontanelle, delayed capillary refill, irritable, oliguria

✓ Severe dehydration (>6% in older children, >10% in infants): Thready pulses, low blood pressure, anuria, cold and mottled, lethargy
- In acute dehydration (<72 hours), mainly ECF volume (80% of total losses) is lost. In prolonged dehydration, fluid loss is more evenly lost from both extracellular (60%) and intracellular (40%) compartments
- Laboratory findings in dehydration:
  ✓ Elevation of serum creatinine and urea
  ✓ Alteration of serum sodium, potassium, and bicarbonate
  ✓ Increase in urine-specific gravity (except with impaired renal concentration)
  ✓ Elevation of blood cell counts (hemoconcentration)
- Type of dehydration
  ✓ Isonatremic (serum Na^+ 135–145 mEq/L): Loss of Na^+ and water in a balance that does not exceed the body's ability to maintain isonatremia
  ✓ Hyponatremic (serum Na^+ <135 mEq/L): Retention or replacement of free water in the face of Na^+ and water losses
  ✓ Hypernatremic (serum Na^+ > 145 mEq/L): Loss of free water in excess of Na^+-containing fluid

ONGOING LOSSES

- The gastrointestinal tract is a common source of ongoing losses from illness or postoperative drainage. These ongoing losses are replaced with parenteral fluids in volumes equivalent to the losses at a frequency that will avoid significant depletions (e.g., every 1–8 hours)
- The replacement fluid should contain electrolytes in concentrations that approximate the lost fluid. Some recommendations are listed in **Table 9-4**.

ORAL REHYDRATION

- Consider oral rehydration if patient is hemodynamically stable and if there is no impairment of swallowing function.
- ORS are best, with concentrations of electrolytes and carbohydrates that approximate the World Health Organization/UNICEF ORS product
- Small volumes (e.g., 5–10 mL) frequently (e.g., every 5–10 minutes) are initiated, and increased slowly as tolerated.

PARENTERAL REHYDRATION

Phase I: Initial stabilization
- Administer 20 mL/kg IVF bolus (NS) and repeat as needed. This will restore intravascular volume and stabilize hemodynamics.
Phase II: After initial stabilization
- IVF choice is dependent on nature/tonicity of dehydration (see below) and the degree of fluid deficit. Increased maintenance requirements (e.g., fever) may warrant further increases in the IVF rate.

TABLE 9-4	Replacement of Ongoing Fluid Losses
Source	**Replacement (1 mL:1 mL)**
Gastric secretions	0.45% NS + 10 mEq KCl/L
Diarrhea	0.2% NS + 25 mEq KCl/L + 20 mEq $NaHCO_3$/L
Small intestine	0.45% NS + 20 mEq KCl/L + 20 mEq $NaHCO_3$/L

NS = normal saline.

- Significant ongoing losses (e.g., continued vomiting and/or diarrhea) will require additional fluid replacement.
- Modifications to the rate and nature of the IVF should be guided by:
  ✓ Urine output: goal = 1–2 mL/kg/hr
  ✓ Weight, vital signs, clinical appearance
  ✓ Repeat serum electrolytes: If needed

Phase III: Resolution

- Trials of oral/gastric feeds usually begin with clear liquids if vomiting is present.
- If vomiting is resolved, or not a factor, prompt advancement to a regular diet is encouraged (including breast milk or infant formula).
- Avoid foods high in simple sugars (e.g., juices, sodas), which can worsen or prolong diarrheal symptoms.
- Wean IVF rate or hold IVF for short periods to encourage oral intake.

ISONATREMIC DEHYDRATION

- Fluid lost has sodium concentration similar to that of blood.
- Although the entire fluid deficit must be corrected, sodium repletion should be considered only for fluid lost from the ECF (intracellular fluid sodium concentration is negligible).
- In acute dehydration (illness <72 hours), 80% of the fluid lost is from the ECF while in chronic dehydration (illness >72 hours) 60% of the fluid lost is from the ECF.
- Do not forget that maintenance fluid should also be included in total fluid calculations.
- In general, the ideal IVF solution in isonatremic dehydration will usually approximate D5/0.45% NaCl.
- Some clinicians prefer to use D5/0.9% NaCl in this circumstance because of the risk of hyponatremia in a subset of patients with high circulating antidiuretic hormone levels. This approach must be used cautiously in patients with acute kidney injury/oligoanuria. Alternatively, D5/0.45% NaCl at two-thirds maintenance rate may be considered.

Example:

One-year-old with 10% dehydration, with current weight 9 kg, presents with 5 days of diarrhea. Serum sodium concentration is 140 mEq/L.

Pre-illness weight: (Current weight (kg) × 100)/100 − % dehydration
   = (9 × 100)/100 − 10 = 900/90 = 10 kg

Calculation of fluid deficit:

Fluid deficit = Pre-illness weight (kg) − Current weight (kg)

10 kg − 9 kg = 1 kg or 1 L

Calculation of sodium deficit from ECF losses:

- Sodium deficit = Fluid deficit (L) × Percentage of fluid loss from ECF (>72 hours of dehydration) × Average ECF sodium concentration (145 mEq/L)
- Sodium deficit = 1 L × 0.6 × 145 mEq/L = 87 mEq

Calculation of maintenance fluid and sodium requirements:

- Fluid: 10 kg × 100 mL/kg = 1000 mL
- Sodium: 1000 mL × 3 mEq/100 mL = 30 mEq

Total fluid and sodium requirement:

- Fluid: Deficit + Maintenance = 1000 mL + 1000 mL = 2000 mL
- Sodium: Deficit + Maintenance = 87 mEq + 30 mEq = 117 mEq

Optimal fluid: Fluid containing 117 mEq Na/2000 mL = 58.5 mEq/L
Available fluid: D_5/0.45% NaCl (77 mEq/L) at a rate of 83 mL/hr (2000 mL/24 hr)

HYPONATREMIC DEHYDRATION

- Sodium deficit in excess of water deficit
- Start calculations as if the patient had isonatremic dehydration and then calculate the additional sodium deficit.
- Sodium is freely distributed throughout the TBW (60% of the patient weight); therefore, the volume (factor) of distribution of sodium is 0.6 of the total body weight.
- **In general, the ideal IVF solution in hyponatremic dehydration will usually range between D5/0.45% and D5/0.9% NaCl**

Example:
One-year-old with 10% dehydration with current weight 9 kg, presents with 2 days of diarrhea. Serum sodium concentration is 123 mEq/L.
Pre-illness weight: (Current weight × 100)/100 – % dehydration
    = (9 × 100)/100 – 10 = 900/90 = 10 kg
Calculation of fluid deficit:
Fluid deficit = Pre-illness weight (kg) – Current weight (kg)
10 kg – 9 kg = 1 kg or 1 L
Calculation of sodium deficit from ECF losses (identical to isonatremic example):

- Sodium deficit = Fluid deficit (L) × Percentage of fluid loss from ECF (<72 hours of dehydration) × Average ECF sodium concentration (145 mEq/L)
- Sodium deficit = 1 L × 0.8 × 145 mEq/L = 116 mEq

Calculation of additional sodium deficit (specific to the hyponatremic patient):
(sodium [mEq] desired – sodium [mEq] actual) × volume (L) of distribution

- Example: Sodium = 123 mEq/L, weight = 10 kg, assumed volume of distribution of 0.6
Sodium deficit = (135 – 123) × 0.6 × 10 = 72 mEq sodium

Calculation of maintenance fluid and sodium requirements:

- Fluid: 10 kg × 100 mL/kg = 1000 mL
- Sodium: 1000 mL × 3 mEq/100 mL = 30 mEq

Total fluid and sodium requirement:

- Fluid: Deficit + Maintenance = 1000 + 1000 = 2000 mL
- Sodium: Deficits + Maintenance = 116 mEq + 72 mEq + 30 mEq = 218 mEq

Optimal fluid: Fluid containing 218 mEq Na/2000 mL = 109 mEq/L
Available fluid: May alternate between D5/0.45% (77 mEq/L) NaCl and D5/0.9% (154 mEq/L) NaCl every 12 hours at a rate of 83 mL/hr (2000 mL/24 hr); could also consider D5/0.75% (115.5 mEq/L) NaCl if your pharmacy is able to make it.

HYPERNATREMIC DEHYDRATION

FWD in excess of salt deficit
- Assumption: FWD = 0.6 × weight (kg) × [(actual sodium/140) – 1]
- **In general, the ideal IVF solution in hypernatremic dehydration will usually range between D5W and D5/0.2% NaCl**

Example:
One-year-old with 10% dehydration, with current weight 9 kg, presents with 5 days of diarrhea. Serum sodium concentration is 155 mEq/L.
Pre-illness weight: (Current weight × 100)/100 – % dehydration
    = (9 × 100)/100 – 10 = 900/90 = 10 kg

Calculation of fluid deficit:
Fluid deficit = Pre-illness weight − Current weight
10 kg − 9 kg = 1 kg or 1 L
Calculation of free water deficit:

- FWD = 0.6 × weight (kg) × [(actual sodium/140) − 1]
- Example: Sodium = 155 mEq/L, weight = 10 kg; FWD = 0.6 × 10 kg × [(155/140) −1]/ 140) − 1] = 0.64 L = 640 mL

Calculation of sodium deficit from ECF losses:

Total fluid deficit is 1000 mL: 640 mL should be replaced as free water and the remaining 360 mL should be replaced as in isonatremic dehydration.

Calculation of sodium deficit in remaining 360 mL of ECF losses:

- Sodium deficit = Fluid deficit (L) × Percentage of fluid loss from ECF × Average ECF sodium concentration (145 mEq/L)
- 0.36 (L) × 0.6 × 145 mEq/L = 32 mEq

Calculation of maintenance fluid and sodium requirements:

- Fluid: 10 kg × 100 mL/kg = 1000 mL
- Sodium: 1000 mL × 3 mEq/100 mL = 30 mEq

Total fluid and sodium requirement:

- Fluid: Deficit + Maintenance = 1000 + 1000 = 2000 mL
- Sodium: Deficit + Maintenance = 32 + 30 = 62 mEq

Optimal fluid: Fluid containing 62 mEq Na/2000 mL = 31 mEq/L
Available fluid: D_5/0.2% NaCl (34 mEq/L) at a rate of 83 mL/h (2000 mL/24 hr)

ELECTROLYTE ABNORMALITIES

TABLE 9-5	Pediatric Electrolyte Reference Ranges by Age		
		mg/dL	**Mmol/L**
Calcium (total)*	0−10 days	7.6−10.4	1.9−2.6
	10 days−24 mo	9−11	2.25−2.75
	24 mo−12 yr	8.8−10.8	2.2−2.7
	12−18 yr	8.4−10.2	2.1−2.55
Potassium*	Newborn	3.7−5.9	3.7−5.9
	Infant	4.1−5.3	4.1−5.3
	>1 yr	3.4−4.7	3.4−4.7
Phosphorus*	0−9 days	4.5−9	1.45−2.91
	10 days−24 mo	4−6.5	1.29−2.10
	3−9 yr	3.2−5.8	1.03−1.87
	10−15 yr	3.3−5.4	1.07−1.74
	>15 yr	2.4−4.4	0.78−1.42
Magnesium*		1.6−2.4	
Sodium*	< 1 yr	130−145 mEq/L	130−145
	>1 yr	135−147 mEq/L	135−147

*Note that local laboratory values might differ.
Data from Engorn B, Flerlage J: *The Harriet Lane Handbook, 20th ed.* Philadelphia, PA: Saunders: 2015.

HYPONATREMIA

Serum sodium concentration less than normal value for age (see Table 9-5)

ETIOLOGY

- Euvolemic: SIADH, hypothyroidism, psychogenic polydipsia, dilute infant formula
- Hypervolemic: Congestive heart failure, nephrotic syndrome, cirrhosis, renal failure, pregnancy
- Hypovolemic: Vomiting, diarrhea, poor intake, third-space losses (burns, pancreatitis, trauma), renal losses (diuretics, osmotic diuresis), adrenal insufficiency

CLINICAL MANIFESTATIONS

- Anorexia, headache, nausea, vomiting, lethargy, muscle cramping
- CNS: Seizures, altered mental status, decreased reflexes
- Brainstem herniation and respiratory arrest are possible

MANAGEMENT

- Rapid correction of hyponatremia (especially if chronic hyponatremia) can lead to pontine myelinolysis. In general, correct serum sodium at a rate 0.5 mEq/L/hr or less or 10–12 mEq/L in 24 hours
- For hyponatremia with symptomatic hypovolemia: Start with reexpansion of ECF volume with IV isotonic saline (e.g., NS 20 mL/kg over 30–60 minutes; may repeat).
- If patient has symptomatic hyponatremia (e.g., seizures): Consider IV hypertonic saline (e.g., 2–6 mL/kg of 3% NaCl over 1 hour) and repeat until seizures stop.
- SIADH: Water restriction (25–50% of daily maintenance requirement) with monitoring of serum sodium
- Definitive management requires establishing the underlying etiology. Compare urine and serum osmolality to differentiate between SIADH and water intoxication. Withhold offending medications.

IATROGENIC HYPONATREMIA IN HOSPITALIZED CHILDREN

- Hospitalized children may have various nonosmotic triggers for ADH release, including nausea, emesis, pain, stress, postoperative state, CNS disorders (e.g., meningitis, encephalitis, tumors, head injury), pulmonary diseases (e.g., pneumonia, asthma, bronchiolitis), malignancies and medications (e.g., morphine, cyclophosphamide, etc.).
- Isotonic IVFs (0.9% NaCl) are a reasonable option in children at risk for developing hyponatremia, although there is risk of hypernatremia. Can also consider D5/0.45% NaCl at two-thirds maintenance rate.
- Slight fluid restriction may also be considered, once the patient is euvolemic and hemodynamically stable.

HYPERNATREMIA

Serum sodium concentration greater than normal value for age (see Table 9-5)

ETIOLOGY

- Hypovolemic: Diabetes insipidus (central or nephrogenic), insensible free water losses (burns), decreased water intake, diarrhea and rehydration with inappropriately

hyperosmolar formula, nonintact thirst mechanism in the context of inappropriately low free water administration
- Hypervolemic: Salt poisoning (sodium bicarbonate, NaCl tablets, seawater ingestion), hyperaldosteronism, Cushing syndrome

CLINICAL MANIFESTATIONS

- Irritability, muscle weakness, lethargy, restlessness, muscle twitching
- CNS: Altered mental status, seizures, coma

MANAGEMENT

- Rapid correction of pronounced hypernatremia (especially if chronic hypernatremia) can result in life-threatening cerebral edema. In general, aim to lower serum sodium by 10–12 mEq/L per 24 hours.
- If patient is severely dehydrated, start with isotonic saline bolus (e.g., NS 20 mL/kg over 1 hour; may repeat) to restore circulation regardless of serum sodium level.
- Free water deficit (FWD) should be corrected over 24–48 hours. Free water deficit can be estimated by 4 mL FW/kg needed to reduce serum Na^+ by 1 mEq/L. Choose a solution that is hypotonic but that will not lower serum sodium too quickly. Remember to also give maintenance fluid as required.
- Follow serum Na^+ levels frequently (e.g., every 2–4 hours), until stable.

HYPOKALEMIA

Serum potassium concentration less than normal value for age (see Table 9-5)

ETIOLOGY

- Decreased intake: Anorexia, low dietary intake, IVFs without potassium
- Renal losses: Medications (diuretics, amphotericin B, penicillins), renal tubular acidosis type 1, Fanconi syndrome, osmotic diuresis (e.g., diabetic ketoacidosis), mineralocorticoid excess (hyperaldosteronism, licorice abuse), Bartter syndrome, Gitelman syndrome, Liddle syndrome, hypomagnesemia
- Extrarenal losses: Gastrointestinal losses (diarrhea, vomiting, fistulas), sweat losses (cystic fibrosis)
- Transcellular shift (into intracellular fluid): Alkalosis, insulin/glucose, beta agonists, familial hypokalemic periodic paralysis

CLINICAL MANIFESTATIONS

- Muscle: Weakness, paresthesias, hyporeflexia, paralysis, rhabdomyolysis
- Renal: Polyuria, polydipsia
- Cardiac: Bradycardia, prolonged QT, flattened T wave, appearance of U wave, AV block, premature beats, paroxysmal atrial or junctional tachycardia, ventricular arrhythmias

MANAGEMENT

- Determine etiology: Electrolytes, magnesium, arterial blood gas, creatine phosphokinase, urine electrolytes (potassium, osmolarity, or creatinine).
- Obtain ECG; consider continuous ECG monitoring.
- Replace potassium orally if mild or asymptomatic or in IVFs as potassium chloride or potassium bicarbonate (up to 40 mEq/L through peripheral IV and up to 80 mEq/L through central IV).

- For life-threatening hypokalemia, can give up to 1 mEq/kg/hr of IV potassium.
- Correct underlying acid–base disorder or other etiology.

HYPERKALEMIA

Serum potassium concentration greater than normal value for age (see Table 9-5)

ETIOLOGY

- Increased intake/production: Excessive acute IV administration, hemolysis, rhabdomyolysis
- Decreased excretion: Renal failure, hypoaldosteronism, type IV RTA, medications (potassium-sparing diuretics, beta-blockers)
- Acidosis causing transcellular shift
- Pseudohyperkalemia: Hemolyzed specimen, extreme leukocytosis or thrombocytosis

CLINICAL MANIFESTATIONS

- Paresthesias, weakness, decreased reflexes, hyporeflexia
- Cardiac manifestations can be life-threatening:
  ✓ ECG changes: Peaked T wave, depressed ST segment, widened PR interval, loss of P wave, wide QRS complex, sine-wave pattern
  ✓ Arrhythmias: Ventricular fibrillation, asystole

MANAGEMENT

- Discontinue potassium intake (think TPN, fluids, foods, medications, etc.); discontinue potassium-sparing diuretics; angiotensin-converting enzymes/angiotensin-receptor blockers.
- Perform ECG.
- Determine etiology: Electrolytes, arterial blood gas, creatine phosphokinase, urinalysis, urine electrolytes (potassium, osmolarity)
- If there are ECG changes other than peaked T wave or serum potassium greater than 8 mEq/L, consider the following interventions:
  ✓ Continuous ECG monitoring
  ✓ Calcium (e.g., 10% calcium gluconate 0.5 mL/kg IV over 2–5 minutes) in order to protect the myocardium from the deleterious effect of hyperkalemia
  ✓ Sodium bicarbonate (e.g., 2–3 mEq/kg IV over 30–60 minutes)
  ✓ Insulin (0.1–0.3 U/kg) plus glucose (1 g/kg)
  ✓ β-agonist (nebulized or IV): Controversial because it may cause arrhythmia.
  ✓ Sodium polystyrene (Kayexalate): Decreases total body potassium. Not recommended for use in infants.
  ✓ Furosemide if not in renal failure and has urine output
  ✓ For renal failure or if refractory to treatment, consider dialysis.

HYPOCALCEMIA

Serum total calcium or serum ionized calcium level less than normal for age (see Table 9-5)

ETIOLOGY

- Hypoparathyroidism: Familial, DiGeorge syndrome, idiopathic, surgical
- Vitamin D deficiency: Dietary deficiency, lack of sunlight, malabsorption
- Vitamin D resistance: Familial hypophosphatemic rickets
- Other: Chronic kidney disease, acute pancreatitis, magnesium deficiency, autosomal dominant hypocalcemic hypercalciuria

CLINICAL MANIFESTATIONS

- Vomiting, muscle weakness, irritability
- Severe: Tetany, seizures, laryngospasm, prolonged QT interval
- Rickets: Craniotabes, rachitic rosary, limb deformities (genu varum and genu valgum), splaying of wrists and ankles

MANAGEMENT

- Management depends on underlying etiology. Initial diagnostics include:
  - ✓ Serum: Electrolytes, calcium (total and ionized), BUN, creatinine, magnesium, phosphorus, protein, albumin, alkaline phosphatase, vitamin D levels, parathyroid hormone
  - ✓ Urine: Calcium, phosphorus, pH, protein, glucose
  - ✓ Hand/wrist x-ray
  - ✓ Consider ECG.
- If patient is hypoalbuminemic, correct total calcium (increase serum calcium by 0.8 mg/dL for each 1.0 g/dL that albumin is below normal) or measure ionized calcium level.

  Calculation: [(Normal serum albumin (4 g/dL) – Patient serum albumin) × 0.8] + Patient serum calcium = Corrected calcium
- For severe symptoms, consider IV calcium (e.g., calcium gluconate) replacement with cardiac monitoring.
- Once patient is stable, consider oral calcium replacement (e.g., calcium carbonate, calcium citrate).
- If patient is hypomagnesemic, replace magnesium (may be given IM).
- Depending on etiology, patient may need vitamin D replacement

HYPERCALCEMIA

Serum total calcium or serum ionized calcium level greater than normal for age (see Table 9-5)

ETIOLOGY

- Hyperparathyroidism, malignancy (bony metastases, ectopic parathyroid hormone production), immobilization, vitamin D intoxication, familial hypocalciuric hypercalcemia, hyperthyroidism, sarcoidosis, thiazide diuretics, milk-alkali syndrome, Williams syndrome, idiopathic hypercalcemia of infancy

CLINICAL MANIFESTATIONS

- Neurologic: Headache, weakness, lethargy, change in mental status, coma, hyporeflexia, seizures
- Gastrointestinal: Constipation, nausea, vomiting, anorexia, abdominal pain
- Renal: Nephrocalcinosis, nephrolithiasis, polyuria, polydipsia, kidney injury
- Cardiovascular: Bradycardia, short QT interval, hypertension

MANAGEMENT

- Attempt to identify and treat underlying etiology
- For severe hypercalcemia, consider IVFs (e.g., NS at two to three times maintenance rate) followed by furosemide every 6–8 hours.
- Consider bisphosphonates with or without calcitonin in refractory hypercalcemia.
- Steroids may be effective in specific cases (e.g., malignancy, sarcoidosis).

HYPERPHOSPHATEMIA

Serum phosphate level concentration greater than normal for age (see Table 9-5)

ETIOLOGY

- Acute phosphate load: Exogenous (phosphate-containing laxatives, fosphenytoin), endogenous (tumor-lysis syndrome, rhabdomyolysis, hemolysis)
- Cellular shift: Lactic acidosis, diabetic ketoacidosis
- Reduced GFR: Acute kidney injury, chronic kidney disease
- Increased reabsorption: Hypoparathyroidism, vitamin D toxicity, bisphosphonates, Familial tumoral calcinosis
- Pseudohyperphosphatemia: Hyperglobulinemia, hyperlipidemia, hemolysis, hyperbilirubinemia, liposomal amphotericin, sample contamination with tPA or heparin

CLINICAL MANIFESTATIONS

- Effects of symptomatic hypocalcemia due to calcium–phosphate precipitation
  ✓ Vomiting, muscle weakness, irritability
  ✓ Severe: Tetany, seizures, laryngospasm, prolonged QT interval

MANAGEMENT

- Primary cause for chronic hyperphosphatemia will be renal disease, if unable to treat renal disease directly, can manage hyperphosphatemia with decreased intake of phosphorus and/or use of oral phosphate binders. Can also consider use of renal replacement therapy if there is no improvement.
- If patient with normal renal clearance:
  ✓ Treat underlying etiology and/or remove exogenous source of phosphate
  ✓ Can consider IVF for dilution but may also decrease serum calcium worsening symptomatic hypocalcemia,

HYPOPHOSPHATEMIA

Serum phosphate level less than normal for age (see Table 9-5).

ETIOLOGY

- Cellular shift: Insulin secretion, respiratory alkalosis, hungry bone syndrome, refeeding syndrome
- Decreased intestinal absorption: Poor intake, chronic diarrhea, medications (antacids, niacin)
- Increased urinary excretion: Hyperparathyroidism, vitamin D deficiency/resistance, Fanconi syndrome, renal phosphate wasting

CLINICAL MANIFESTATIONS

- Bone mineral metabolism: Rickets, osteomalacia
- Neurologic: irritability, paresthesias, delirium, generalized seizures, coma
- Cardiac: Impaired myocardial contractility, ventricular arrhythmias
- Muscle: Proximal myopathy, dysphagia, ileus
- Hematologic: Hemolysis, thrombocytopenia

MANAGEMENT

- If etiology not obvious, can use urine phosphate level to elucidate:
  - ✓ A 24-hour urine phosphate concentration less than 100 mg indicates appropriate renal excretion of phosphate. Likely cellular shift or intestinal losses.
  - ✓ A 24-hour urine phosphate concentration greater than 100 mg indicates inappropriately high renal excretion of phosphate or renal phosphate wasting.
- Use oral phosphate for mild cases of hypophosphatemia or IV phosphate supplementation for severe or symptomatic cases.

HYPERMAGNESEMIA

Serum magnesium level greater than upper limit of normal (see reference table)

ETIOLOGY

- Decreased renal function
- Increased intake of magnesium
  - ✓ Oral load: Epsom salts, laxatives
  - ✓ Magnesium-based enemas
- Other
  - ✓ Hyperparathyroidism, familial hypocalciuric hypercalcemia, diabetic ketoacidosis, tumor lysis syndrome, lithium ingestion, milk-alkali syndrome, adrenal insufficiency

CLINICAL MANIFESTATIONS

- Nausea, vomiting, sedation, muscle weakness, decreased deep tendon reflexes
- Severe: Hypotension, muscle paralysis, bradycardia, cardiac arrest

MANAGEMENT

- If normal renal clearance:
  - ✓ Remove magnesium source, give IV fluids, can consider loop or thiazide diuretics (increase magnesium excretion).
- If moderate/severe renal clearance:
  - ✓ Remove magnesium source, administer hemodialysis or peritoneal dialysis, can consider intravenous fluids or diuretics (if patient not anuric) while preparing for renal replacement therapy.

HYPOMAGNESEMIA

Serum magnesium level less than lower limit of normal (see Table 9-5)

ETIOLOGY

- Gastrointestinal losses
  - ✓ Diarrhea (acute or chronic), malabsorption, small bowel bypass, acute pancreatitis
  - ✓ Proton-pump–inhibitor use
- Renal losses
  - ✓ Medication induced: Loop and thiazide diuretics, aminoglycosides, amphotericin B, cisplatin, pentamidine, EGF-receptor antibodies, digoxin, calcineurin inhibitors
  - ✓ Volume expansion
  - ✓ Diabetic ketoacidosis
  - ✓ Posttransplantation patients
  - ✓ Hypercalcemia

✓ Renal magnesium wasting: Bartter and Gitelman syndromes, EAST syndrome
• Refeeding syndrome

CLINICAL MANIFESTATIONS

• Neuromuscular: Tremor, tetany, convulsions, weakness, apathy, delirium, coma
• Cardiac:
  ✓ Moderate magnesium depletion: Widened QRS interval and peaked T waves
  ✓ Severe magnesium depletion: Widened PR interval, atrial and ventricular arrhythmias
• Calcium metabolism abnormalities: Hypocalcemia, hypoparathyroidism, PTH resistance, decreased calcitriol
• Electrolytes: Hypokalemia

MANAGEMENT

• Treat underlying disease
  ✓ Can give amiloride to patients with renal magnesium wasting.
• If etiology not obvious, can use urine magnesium level to elucidate:
  ✓ A 24-hour urine magnesium concentration less than 10 mg, indicates appropriately low renal excretion of magnesium. Likely GI losses.
  ✓ A 24-hour urine magnesium concentration greater than 10–30 mg, indicates inappropriately high renal excretion of magnesium or renal magnesium wasting.
• If patient has severe symptoms with IV repletion of magnesium.
  ✓ IMPORTANT to have cardiac monitoring of these patients
• If patient asymptomatic, give oral replacement therapy
  ✓ IMPORTANT to monitor for GI disturbances including abdominal pain and diarrhea

Máire Conrad, MD, MS
Amanda Muir, MD
Joseph Picoraro, MD

ESOPHAGUS AND STOMACH

GASTROESOPHAGEAL REFLUX DISEASE

Gastroesophageal reflux (GER) is a physiologic process of stomach contents regurgitating into the esophagus. Gastroesophageal reflux disease (GERD) occurs when GER is accompanied by disturbing symptoms or complications such as esophagitis, respiratory disease, failure to thrive, and/or neurobehavioral manifestations. (See PMID 29470322 for clinical practice guidelines published in *J Pediatr Gastroenterol Nutr* 2018;66:516–554.)

EPIDEMIOLOGY

- In infants, most GER is physiologic and benign.
- Functional GER occurs in more than half of all infants.
- Most common esophageal disorder

PATHOPHYSIOLOGY

- Transient LES relaxation allows gastric contents to flow in a retrograde direction up into the esophagus.
- Decreased gastric compliance in infants as compared with adults

CLINICAL MANIFESTATIONS

- Functional/simple GER in infancy: Silent oral regurgitation, effortless spitting, or forceful vomiting; symptoms peak at 1–4 months and resolve by 12–18 months of age; usually benign
- Gastroesophageal reflux disease: Significant complications develop in about 10% of untreated children.
  - ✓ Esophagitis: Crying, irritability, food aversion, heartburn, epigastric or chest pain, dysphagia/odynophagia, hematemesis, anemia, and/or guaiac-positive stools
  - ✓ Respiratory: Laryngospasm, bronchospasm, microaspiration pneumonia
  - ✓ Failure to thrive
  - ✓ Neurobehavioral manifestations: Sandifer syndrome (opisthotonic posturing, head tilting, seizure-like activity), arching, excessive irritability
- GERD in older children and adolescents: heartburn, regurgitation

DIFFERENTIAL DIAGNOSIS

- Infant: pyloric stenosis (forceful emesis), malrotation (bilious emesis), allergic proctocolitis of infancy (accompanied by bloody stools), eosinophilic esophagitis, colic
- Older children: Eosinophilic esophagitis, functional dyspepsia, *Helicobacter pylori* infection, peptic ulcer, achalasia, rumination, hiatal hernia

---

Note: Medication recommendations in this chapter may be off label based on patient age or specific disease. Consult product inserts for further information.

DIAGNOSTICS

- With uncomplicated GER, no diagnostic tests are warranted.
- GERD is a clinical diagnosis but several tests may be situationally helpful to consider:
  - ✓ Upper gastrointestinal series: Defines anatomy; useful to exclude malrotation, pyloric stenosis, webs, atresias, or other anatomic causes; not diagnostic for reflux
  - ✓ Scintigraphy or "milk scan": Detects delayed gastric emptying and/or pulmonary aspiration; not diagnostic for reflux
  - ✓ pH probe: Gold standard to quantify acid reflux; helps establish causal relationship between reflux and other symptoms
  - ✓ Impedance probe: Uses electrical impedance (resistance) to measure movement of air, fluid, and solids in the esophagus. Can detect nonacid contents and can be combined with pH probe monitoring. Particularly useful in correlating symptoms with reflux events in patient on acid-suppression therapy or in postprandial period, when stomach contents are likely to be nonacid.
  - ✓ Upper endoscopy: Allows direct visualization of the mucosa and the pathologic diagnosis of mucosal disease related to reflux; basal-cell hyperplasia, papillary elongation, and an inflammatory cellular infiltrate seen in esophagitis.

MANAGEMENT

- *Conservative therapy:* Appropriate as a component of treatment for all GER, and may be sole therapy for uncomplicated GER.
  - ✓ Thicken formula with rice cereal (½–1 tablespoon per ounce) (may improve overt regurgitation)
  - ✓ Smaller-volume feeds (goal is to avoid overfeeding but still maintain appropriate total daily amount of formula or breast milk)
  - ✓ Hold upright during and after feeding
  - ✓ Sleep with head elevated 30 degrees
    - Prone positioning may mitigate GER symptoms; however, the association of SIDS with prone positioning of young infants precludes a recommendation of prone positioning as a routine strategy.
  - ✓ Formula changes: 2–4 weeks of hydrolyzed or amino acid–based formula or maternal elimination of cow's milk in breast-fed babies is warranted if other conservative approaches fail.
- *Medical therapy:*
  - ✓ Antacid (magnesium hydroxide/aluminum hydroxide preparations; e.g., Maalox, Mylanta): 2.5 mL three times daily (weight <5 kg), 5 mL three times daily (weight >5 kg); separate from other medications by 1 hour
  - ✓ Acid suppression (H2-receptor antagonists (H2RAs) [e.g., ranitidine, famotidine] and PPI [e.g., omeprazole, lansoprazole, esomeprazole]): No evidence that PPI or H2RAs reduce crying or irritability associated with infant GERD. PPIs are superior to H2RAs in healing erosive esophagitis.
  - ✓ Prokinetics (metoclopramide, erythromycin, bethanechol, domperidone, and cisapride): Metoclopramide and low-dose erythromycin (3–5 mg/kg/dose) are available in the United States but are not currently recommended for treatment of GERD because of insufficient evidence and potential for side effects. Domperidone and cisapride are available only in clinical trials. No evidence that prokinetics improve crying and irritability associated with infant GERD.
- Postpyloric feedings via feeding tube (nasojejunal or gastrojejunal) may be especially beneficial in setting of aspiration events.

- *Surgical therapy:*
  - ✓ Fundoplication: Indicated for severe complicated GERD with failure of maximal medical therapy; may result in other long-term complications such as gas-bloat syndrome, chronic retching, and dumping syndrome. Dumping syndrome is a cluster of symptoms resulting from rapid transit of food or formula from stomach into small intestine, including abdominal pain, nausea, vomiting, diarrhea, dizziness, flushing, fatigue, and palpitations. Symptoms are the result of stretching of the intestinal wall and release of hormones leading to alterations in blood pressure and serum glucose levels.
    - Procedure that involves wrapping the gastric fundus around the lower esophagus. Many forms of this surgery exist based on the degree to which the stomach is wrapped. Efficacy is related in part to increased baseline tone of the LES and decreased transient LES relaxations.
      - ▷ Increased fundoplication failure rate has been observed in early infancy and children with neurologic impairment or following esophageal atresia repair.
      - ▷ Fundoplication surgery is associated with fewer hospitalizations for respiratory illness for children <4 years; older children do not experience a similar reduction in hospitalizations for respiratory illness.

PEPTIC ULCER DISEASE

Histologic inflammation and ulceration of the mucosa of the stomach and/or duodenum

EPIDEMIOLOGY

- In childhood, typically occurs after 8 years of age.
- Accounts for 15% of abdominal pain seen in specialty practice.

ETIOLOGY

- Primary PUD: Typically gastritis and duodenal ulcers. Tends to have a chronic relapsing and remitting course. It may be *H. pylori*–associated, non–*H. pylori*–associated, or idiopathic.
- Secondary PUD: Typically gastric ulcers. Tends to be acute, and with therapy, recovery is usually complete. Causes include physiologic stress, illness, burns, sepsis, shock, head injury, trauma (e.g., retching, nasogastric tube), drugs (e.g., NSAIDs, corticosteroids, alcohol, valproate, chemotherapy, KCl), allergic or eosinophilic gastritis, infectious, iron overdose, diabetes mellitus, Crohn's disease, Zollinger–Ellison syndrome, hyperparathyroidism, cystic fibrosis, vascular insufficiency (sickle cell disease, Henoch–Schönlein purpura), and radiation gastropathy.

PATHOPHYSIOLOGY

- Imbalance between cytotoxic factors (acid, pepsin, aspirin/NSAIDs, bile acids, *H. pylori* infection) and cytoprotective factors (mucous layer, local bicarbonate secretion, mucosal blood flow)
- Role of *H. pylori*: Gram-negative rod; causes chronic active gastritis and duodenal ulcers; spread by human-to-human transmission; *H. pylori* infection is often acquired during childhood but does not often lead to PUD.

CLINICAL MANIFESTATIONS

- Abdominal pain: Often epigastric but may not be localized in children; often postprandial and nocturnal.

- Anorexia, weight loss, early satiety, nausea, recurrent vomiting, upper gastrointestinal bleeding, anemia
- On physical exam, may note oral ulcers (e.g., Crohn's disease), wheezing (may imply GERD), abdominal tenderness.
- Consider rectal exam to look for perianal disease (e.g., Crohn's disease) and occult blood in stool.

DIAGNOSTICS

- Endoscopy: Biopsies of the upper intestinal tract is the gold standard for diagnosis for peptic ulcer disease. *H. pylori* may be detected on biopsies, but can be patchy; 6 biopsies from stomach body and antrum are recommended to increase sensitivity in making the diagnosis. Gastric tissue for *H. pylori* culture and sensitivity is recommended for recurrence. Numerous noninvasive tests are available with variable sensitivities and specificities.
- Blood and saliva antibody tests: NOT recommended in pediatric patients because of low sensitivity and specificity.
- Stool antigen test for *H. pylori:* Useful to diagnose *H. pylori* in conjunction with endoscopic biopsy and to test for eradication of infection (4–8 weeks after treatment completion). Recommend 2 weeks off of PPI and 4 weeks off of antibiotics to avoid false negative results. Some tests have sensitivity >95% for detection of *H. pylori* before and after treatment. This is the highest-yield noninvasive test available.
- Urea breath test: Useful for the initial diagnosis of *H. pylori* when combined with endoscopic biopsy and to test for eradication after therapy. Has limited availability as compared with stool antigen testing.

MANAGEMENT

Acid suppression:
- Use alone for non–*H. pylori* PUD or in conjunction with antibiotics for *H. pylori* PUD.
- H2RA: Ranitidine, famotidine; less effective in mucosal healing than PPI
- PPI: Omeprazole, esomeprazole, lansoprazole
- IV pantoprazole 1 mg/kg/day up to 40 mg/day for inpatient treatment

H. pylori therapy:
- Treatment options: See **Table 10-1**. Strict compliance is necessary. Treatment success should be validated by noninvasive testing (stool antigen or urease breath te.st) to monitor eradication of the organism 4–8 weeks after completion of therapy.

TABLE 10-1	Treatment Regimens for *H. pylori* Peptic Ulcer Disease	
Susceptibility	**Regimen**	**If penicillin allergy**
Unknown, first-line	PPI + amoxicillin + metronidazole	PPI + metronidazole + clarithromycin + bismuth salt
Known susceptibility to clarithromycin	PPI + amoxicillin + clarithromycin	PPI + metronidazole + clarithromycin
Resistance to metronidazole and clarithromycin	PPI + amoxicillin + metronidazole + bismuth salt	PPI + tetracycline + metronidazole + bismuth salt (age >8 years)

Note: All regimens are 14 days' duration.

SMALL AND LARGE INTESTINES

CELIAC DISEASE

Autoimmune disorder of the small intestine characterized by a permanent intolerance to gluten that results in mucosal damage and malabsorption

EPIDEMIOLOGY

- Prevalence: 1 in 300 worldwide
- More common in persons of European descent.
- Associated with juvenile-onset diabetes mellitus, selective IgA deficiency, dermatitis herpetiformis, autoimmune thyroid disease, Down syndrome, Turner syndrome, and Williams syndrome.
- Increased prevalence in children with first-degree relatives with celiac disease
- Increased risk of small bowel lymphoma

PATHOPHYSIOLOGY

- Gut exposure to grain proteins in wheat, rye and barley results in an autoimmune reaction that is toxic to enterocytes and leads to a flattened mucosal lining and impaired small intestinal absorptive capacity.

CLINICAL MANIFESTATIONS

- Symptoms are variable and can present at any age.
- Classically presents around age 1–3 years, but this is changing as more children are identified by increased screening practices
- Diarrhea, foul-smelling bulky greasy stools, abdominal distention, and pain
- Poor growth, anorexia, malaise, muscle wasting, irritability, unexplained iron deficiency anemia
- Elevated liver enzymes
- Symptoms can be subtle, with only mild diarrhea or recurrent abdominal pain or constipation
- Physical exam: Weight loss, short stature, edema, abdominal distention, rectal prolapse, muscle wasting, dental erosion, angular stomatitis, aphthous lesions, osteopenia, rickets

DIAGNOSTICS

- All testing needs to be performed on gluten-containing diet to avoid false negative results.
- Serology testing: Serum IgA and TTG-IgA are the standard screening tests (**Table 10-2**).

TABLE 10-2	Celiac Serology Testing		
Antibody Test	**Sensitivity**	**Specificity**	**Considerations**
TTG-IgA	92–98%	96–100%	For all ages; for screening
			Send with total serum IgA (reliable if serum IgA >20 mg/dL)
Deamidated anti–gliadin peptide IgA and IgG	Moderate	Low	For age <2 years, in addition to TTG-IgA
Anti-endomysial IgA	90–95%	98–100%	Not for screening; less reliable in age <2 years

- Antibody tests are good for initial screen but endoscopy required for definitive diagnosis.
- May present with elevated hepatic transaminases
- Endoscopy: Small bowel biopsies while eating a gluten-containing diet help make diagnosis; increased epithelial lymphocytes, villous atrophy, crypt hyperplasia, infiltration of lamina propria with inflammatory cells are consistent with celiac disease; resolution of abnormalities on gluten-free diet confirms diagnosis. Because of patchy nature of disease, biopsies from both duodenal bulb and distal duodenum should be obtained.
- Recommend annual testing of asymptomatic patients with diabetes mellitus, Turner syndrome, trisomy 21, Williams syndrome, select IgA deficiency, autoimmune thyroiditis. Testing should begin after diagnosis or after gluten introduced into diet for congenital conditions.
- First-degree relatives of patient with celiac disease should have annual screening starting at age 2 years.

MANAGEMENT

- Permanent gluten-free diet leads to full clinical and histologic remission; strict avoidance of wheat, rye, and barley; corn, oats and rice are permitted.
- Dietary counseling and careful attention to all food and medicinal products that may contain traces of gluten.
- Multivitamin/fat-soluble vitamins
- Medical therapy for iron deficiency and rickets, if present
- Very close follow-up of growth parameters and symptoms
- Periodic monitoring of dietary compliance with antibody profile; antibodies usually undetectable within 3–6 months after initiation of appropriate diet.
- Screening of all first degree relatives

CONSTIPATION

Abnormal defecation characterized by infrequent stooling, incomplete evacuation of the rectum, passage of large painful stools, involuntary soiling, or the inability to pass stool

EPIDEMIOLOGY

- Occurs in more than 10% of all children
- Majority of constipation in older children is functional
- Encopresis occurs in 1–2% of all children

ETIOLOGY

- Anatomic: Hirschsprung disease, imperforate anus, anal stenosis, malpositioned anus, ileal atresia, meconium ileus, colonic stricture, abdominal mass, hydrometrocolpos
- Physiologic: Hypothyroidism, celiac disease, lumbosacral spinal-cord defect, infant botulism, muscular diseases, cystic fibrosis, diabetes, lead poisoning, postinfectious "ileus," prune-belly syndrome, ascariasis, medications, excessive cow's milk ingestion, inadequate fluid intake, malnutrition, anorexia nervosa, functional constipation

PATHOPHYSIOLOGY

- Functional constipation: Cycle typically begins with voluntary withholding of stool. Stool returns from anal canal to rectum. Sensation of urge to defecate is decreased. Stool bolus becomes larger and harder, which perpetuates more withholding. Over time, rectal vault distends and normal sensation diminishes.

- Retentive encopresis: Involuntary soiling of liquid stool around solid stool, which results from chronic constipation
- Grunting baby syndrome: An infant with grunting, straining, and turning red while passing a soft stool has immature coordination of the stooling process and not true constipation.

CLINICAL MANIFESTATIONS

- Abdominal pain
- Stool consistency may be hard, soft, or even diarrheal.
- Stool frequency can be daily or infrequent.
- On physical exam, note abdominal tenderness/distention, stool on abdominal palpation, anal wink, anal tone, stool in rectal vault, width of rectal vault; conduct neurologic and lumbrosacral exams
- Signs of possible anatomic abnormalities: Blood in stool, failure to thrive, emesis, abdominal distention
- Signs of functional constipation: Retentive posturing; infrequent passage of large, hard bowel movements; involuntary soiling

DIAGNOSTICS

- The vast majority of cases of constipation in children is functional and does not require diagnostic workup.
- Laboratory testing: thyroid-stimulating hormone/free thyroxine (hypothyroid), total IgA/TTG-IgA (celiac), lead level (lead toxicity)
- One-view abdominal x-ray: Most useful to diagnose fecal impaction in the rectum. Limited use in correlating colonic stool burden with degree of constipation.
- Unprepped contrast enema/rectal biopsy: To evaluate for Hirschsprung disease
- Lumbar spine MRI: To evaluate for suspected spinal cord abnormality
- Anorectal manometry: To evaluate for Hirschsprung disease or internal anal sphincter achalasia

MANAGEMENT

- Clinical pathway: https://www.chop.edu/clinical-pathway (search "constipation")
    Authors: E. Kane, MD; M. Mittal, MD; K. Wagenman, RN; K. Fiorino, MD; C. Jacobstein, MD; R. Verma, MD; X. Morgan, CRNP; S. Peck, APN; C. McIntyre, PharmD; J. Crawford, CNS; A. Shah, MD; L. Utidjian, MD; J. Lavelle, MD
- Treat underlying medical disorders
- Surgical correction of anatomic defects
- Treatment of functional constipation may take months to years
    ✓ Bowel clean-out: Enemas, suppositories, lubricants, hyperosmolar agents
    ✓ Maintenance: Dietary fiber and fluids, hyperosmolar agents
    ✓ Toilet sitting: Twice-daily stooling attempts
    ✓ Diary/journal: Positive reinforcement
    ✓ Educate patient and parents. Frequent follow-up is critical to success
- Medications used to treat constipation:
    ✓ Enema: Mineral oil (rectally); sodium biphosphate (Fleet); or saline; all in children ≥2 years of age. Larger-volume enemas such as polyethylene glycol enemas to relieve rectal fecal impaction may be necessary.
    ✓ Suppositories: Glycerin, bisacodyl
    ✓ Lubricants: Mineral oil (orally)
    ✓ Osmotic laxatives: PEG 3350 (Miralax), lactulose, PEG with electrolytes (Go-Lytely)

✓ Stimulant laxatives: Senna, bisacodyl, magnesium citrate, magnesium hydroxide
✓ Fiber/bulk forming agents: Benefiber, Citrucel, Metamucil, Maltsupex
• Typical clean-out regimen:
✓ Enemas to clean out rectal vault
✓ Hyperosmotic and/or stimulant therapy: May require nasogastric tube for administration. Continue until clear effluent. Monitoring serum electrolytes appropriate when using large volumes

GASTROINTESTINAL BLEEDING

Loss of blood via the gastrointestinal tract

• Hematemesis: Bloody emesis due to active bleeding proximal to the ligament of Treitz
• Hematochezia: Bright red or maroon stool due to active bleeding in the colon or brisk bleeding from a more proximal site
• Melena: Dark, tarry stool often due to bleeding proximal to the ligament of Treitz

DIFFERENTIAL DIAGNOSIS

• Upper intestinal bleeding
✓ Infant: Swallowed maternal blood, esophagitis, gastric ulcer, vascular malformation, duplication cyst, vitamin K deficiency, hemophilia, trauma, maternal NSAID use
✓ Older child: Esophagitis, Mallory–Weiss tear, esophageal varices, foreign body with mucosal erosion, pill esophagitis, duplication cyst, Dieulafoy lesion, gastritis, gastric or duodenal ulcer, vascular malformation, duodenitis, portal hypertension gastropathy, NSAID injury, hemobilia, swallowed blood from oral/nasal pharynx, pulmonary bleeding (hemoptysis)
• Lower intestinal bleeding
✓ Infant: Anal fissure, swallowed maternal blood, milk-protein allergic colitis, infectious enterocolitis, vascular malformation, necrotizing enterocolitis, Hirschsprung disease with enterocolitis, Meckel diverticulum (rule of 2s: 2% of population, 2 feet from ileocecal valve, 2% become symptomatic, usually in children <2 years), intussusception, intestinal duplication, infantile inflammatory bowel disease
✓ Older child: Anal fissure, infectious enterocolitis/Clostridium difficile colitis, intussusception, inflammatory bowel disease, Meckel diverticulum, intestinal polyp, eosinophilic colitis, vascular malformations, intestinal duplication, Henoch–Schönlein purpura, hemolytic uremic syndrome, vasculitis, perianal strep cellulitis, solitary rectal ulcer, hemorrhoids, rectal trauma, sexual abuse

CLINICAL MANIFESTATIONS

• Variable presentation from hemodynamically stable to shock
• Note prior use of NSAIDs, steroids, indomethacin, antibiotics.
• Note history of trauma, liver disease, umbilical-vein catheterization (history of umbilical-vein catheterization is associated with portal-vein thrombosis and development of portal hypertension predisposing to esophageal varices).
• May present with vomiting, retching, regurgitation of bloody fluid, abdominal pain, anorexia, fever, weight loss, sepsis, asphyxia, recent surgery, mental status changes
• Inspect mouth, nares, pharynx for trauma.
• Abdomen: Hepatomegaly, splenomegaly, prominent abdominal vessels, right-lower-quadrant mass or tenderness
• Rectal: Blood, erythema, fissure, fistula, skin tag, polyp, hemorrhoid, rectal prolapse
• Stool: Blood or mucus within or surrounding stool

- Extremities: Capillary refill, digital clubbing, palmar erythema, purpura, or petechiae
- Skin: Pallor, jaundice, facial petechiae, pigmented freckles on lips/buccal mucosa, excoriations, hemangiomas, other vascular-appearing lesions
- Meckel diverticulum has been associated with cleft palate, bicornuate uterus, and annular pancreas
- For breastfeeding infant, inspect mother's nipple (dry, cracked, bleeding nipples suggest swallowed maternal blood).

DIAGNOSTICS

- Stool guaiac: False positive results may be due to rare meat, horseradish, turnips, tomatoes, fresh red cherries; false negative results may be due to vitamin C, expired assay card or developing solution, storage of stool for longer than 4 days
- Nasogastric lavage: Use normal saline at room temperature; absent blood does not exclude an upper gastrointestinal source; present blood does not identify the exact origin.
- Laboratory studies: CBC to assess for anemia, thrombocytopenia, PT/PTT to assess for coagulopathy particularly in setting of suspected liver disease, LFTs to assess for suspected liver disease—elevated transaminases, hypoalbuminemia, elevated conjugated/direct bilirubin, electrolytes to assess for abnormalities related to dehydration/volume shift, type and screen to prepare PRBC for possible transfusion of severe anemia or ongoing brisk bleeding and hemodynamic instability
- Stool bacterial culture and stool *Clostridioides difficile* toxins
- Abdominal x-ray: Free air, toxic megacolon, pneumatosis, small-bowel dilation
- Air or Gastrografin contrast enema: For suspected intussusception
- Meckel diverticulum scan: Technetium-99m pertechnetate scintigraphic study. Test has high specificity (95–100%) but lower sensitivity (50–92%). Use of H_2-receptor antagonist (ranitidine) prior to test may increase yield with a sensitivity of 62.5% with conventional study and a sensitivity of 87.5% when pretreated with ranitidine.
- Upper gastrointestinal series: Structural abnormality, tumor, polyp, signs of IBD
- CT/MR angiography: Useful in both slower and brisk bleeding to localize lesion. CTA with oral contrast (CT enterography) is the most sensitive test if patient can tolerate oral contrast.
- Tagged red blood cell bleeding scan and angiography: Reserved for brisk bleeding without clear localization on imaging studies
- Endoscopy or colonoscopy: Direct visual inspection, biopsy, culture
- Wireless video capsule endoscopy: For small-bowel obscure gastrointestinal bleeding

MANAGEMENT

- Initial management of all gastrointestinal bleeding: Identify and treat shock with IV access, isotonic fluids, oxygen, blood products.
- Nonvariceal upper gastrointestinal bleeding: IV acid reduction (ranitidine, pantoprazole); discontinue NSAIDs; fluid resuscitation, endoscopic hemostasis therapy if bleeding persists (bipolar electrocoagulation, heater probe, clips, injection therapy)
- Variceal upper gastrointestinal bleeding:
  ✓ Fluid resuscitation; transfuse red cells to maintain hemoglobin above 8 g/dL (avoid overtransfusion); transfuse platelets to greater than 50,000/mm³; FFP to correct coagulopathy
  ✓ Octreotide (bolus 1–2 mcg/kg over 2–5 minutes, then 1–2 mcg/kg/hr infusion): Reduces splanchnic arterial blood flow to decrease portal pressure
  ✓ Endoscopic band ligation, sclerotherapy

✓ Emergent surgical therapy for unresponsive severe bleeding: Portosystemic shunt, TIPS, Sengstaken–Blakemore tube occlusive balloon therapy, liver transplantation
- Lower gastrointestinal bleeding in an infant:
  ✓ Surgical evaluation for suspected intussusception, necrotizing enterocolitis, toxic megacolon, Hirschsprung disease
  ✓ If otherwise healthy and has blood-streaked mucus in stool without evidence of fissure, send stool culture and consider changing to elemental formula for presumptive milk-protein allergy.
  ✓ Flexible sigmoidoscopy for persistent bloody stools despite elemental formula and negative stool culture
  ✓ Anal fissures heal without intervention
- Lower gastrointestinal bleeding in an older child:
  ✓ Treat according to underlying cause if known.
  ✓ Treat constipation if present.
  ✓ Perform flexible sigmoidoscopy or colonoscopy for recurrent or persistent bleeding to detect colitis, intestinal polyps, IBD.
  ✓ Polyp removal by endoscopic snare electrocautery
  ✓ Meckel scan if no source identified by endoscopy
  ✓ Surgical evaluation if severe bleeding of unidentified source

INFLAMMATORY BOWEL DISEASE

An idiopathic chronic disease of the gastrointestinal tract resulting in inflammation, gastrointestinal tissue ulceration, diarrhea, protein-losing enteropathy, gastrointestinal bleeding, abdominal pain, and various extraintestinal manifestations. IBD is broadly divided into Crohn's disease (CD), ulcerative colitis (UC), and IBD, unspecified (IBD-U).

EPIDEMIOLOGY

- Family history can predispose to IBD.
- 20–30% of new IBD presents in persons younger than 20 years of age.
- 8% of pediatric IBD presents in children younger than 5 years of age.
- More common in developed countries

ETIOLOGY

- Interaction between environmental, gut microbial, immunologic, and genetic factors
- Dysregulation of mucosal immune system partially driven by abnormal intestinal flora

PATHOPHYSIOLOGY

- CD:
  ✓ May involve any segment of the gastrointestinal tract, mouth to anus
  ✓ Commonly involves small intestine and terminal ileum, but isolated colonic disease is also common in pediatric populations
  ✓ Transmural inflammation with thickened nodular bowel, noncaseating granulomas, strictures, fistulas, abscesses, adhesions
  ✓ Skip lesions, discontinuous disease
  ✓ Perianal disease (15%)
  ✓ Malabsorption of iron, zinc, folate, and vitamin B_{12}
  ✓ Carcinoma (risk of lymphoma, skin cancers, colon cancer increased over general population)

- UC:
  - ✓ Limited to the colon; starts in rectum and ascends continuously
  - ✓ Nonspecific gastritis and/or duodenitis common
  - ✓ Diffuse mucosal involvement/submucosal sparing
  - ✓ Can progress to toxic megacolon (<5%)
  - ✓ Carcinoma (significant increased risk of lymphoma, skin cancers, colon cancer over general population)
  - ✓ Colectomy is curative
- Indeterminate colitis:
  - ✓ Term used when macroscopic disease is localized to colon but without definitive features of UC or CD

CLINICAL MANIFESTATIONS

Intestinal Manifestations

- CD: Abdominal pain, diarrhea, rectal bleeding, aphthous oral lesions, perianal fissures/tags/fistulas, abdominal abscesses, anorexia, weight loss, linear growth deceleration
- UC: Bloody mucoid diarrhea, lower abdominal pain/tenderness, urgency to defecate, nausea/vomiting associated with defecation

Extraintestinal Manifestations

Occur in approximately 30% of patients with IBD, more typically after IBD diagnosis is made. A minority will manifest extraintestinal symptoms prior to intestinal symptoms.

- Systemic: Fever, malaise, anorexia, weight loss, growth delay/linear growth deceleration, delayed puberty
- Skin: Erythema nodosum, pyoderma gangrenosum, perianal disease
- Joints: Arthritis, arthralgia, enthesitis, clubbing, ankylosing spondylitis, sacroiliitis
- Eyes: Uveitis, episcleritis, keratitis, retinal vasculitis
- Hepatobiliary: Primary sclerosing cholangitis (more common in UC than in CD), autoimmune hepatitis, chronic active hepatitis, fatty liver, cholelithiasis
- Bone: Osteopenia, delayed bone age
- Renal: Nephrolithiasis, hydronephrosis, enterovesical fistula
- Vascular: Thrombophlebitis, vasculitis
- Heme: Anemia (iron, vitamin B_{12}, folate deficiency, hemolysis, marrow suppression from medications, anemia of chronic disease), thrombocytosis, neutropenia
- Oncologic: Lymphoma, acute myelogenous leukemia, colon cancer

DIAGNOSTICS

- CBC (low hemoglobin, low mean corpuscular volume, high platelets), ESR (high), C-reactive protein (high), albumin (low), alkaline phosphatase (low), iron studies (ferritin is acute-phase reactant so can be difficult to interpret in setting of inflammation and iron deficiency), folate, vitamins B_{12} and D levels, electrolytes, calcium, magnesium, phosphorus, zinc
- Unique IBD-related antibody serologies are sometimes used to aid the differentiation of CD and UC when unclear. anti-*Saccharomyces cerevisiae* antibody and p-ANCA are most well described, although other antibodies are now available. These antibodies are not used as screening tests to evaluate for IBD.
- Stool guaiac: Positive
- Stool for culture, *C. difficile* toxins A and B, ova and parasites, *Cryptosporidium* and *Giardia*

- Fecal calprotectin is highly sensitive and specific for gastrointestinal tract inflammation, especially colitis. Valuable in distinguishing between IBD and IBS.
  - ✓ When a combination of the above tests raise suspicion for IBD, the gold standard test to rule out the disease is upper endoscopy and colonoscopy. A radiology study (see below) may be chosen before endoscopy/colonoscopy depending on presenting symptoms (concern for obstruction, abscess, perforation).

Radiology

There is no one perfect imaging study to evaluate the small bowel in patients with IBD. Each study has its benefits and limitations. The optimal initial study depends on the patient and the symptoms and course of illness.

- Upper gastrointestinal with small bowel follow-through: Useful to evaluate for strictures. False negative results common for superficial mucosal disease and involves radiation exposure.
- Abdominal CT: Useful to assess for complications of CD such as intraabdominal abscess or phlegmon
- MR enterography: MRI of bowel with IV and oral contrast. No ionizing radiation. Useful to assess transmural disease. Typically requires laying still ~1 hour. Requires enteral contrast, therefore typically must be done unsedated.
- MRI pelvis: Frequently used to assess perianal disease and fistulae
- Wireless video capsule endoscopy: Useful to assess the mucosal surface, unable to assess disease beyond bowel lumen. Risk of capsule retention at site of narrowing/stricture. A test capsule is available for those considered at higher risk.
- Bone age: X-ray of wrist for delayed bone maturation
- DXA scan: Assesses bone mineral density, which may be low in chronic inflammatory diseases such as IBD. Normal range: Z score +2 to −2. Below Z score of −2, patients may be at risk for fracture; consider referral to bone health team.

Endoscopy

- Gold standard for diagnosis
- Mucosa may appear erythematous, edematous, friable, ulcerated
- Loss of normal vascular pattern and/or haustra
- Well-established diagnostic histopathologic criteria; chronic inflammation, crypt abscesses, architectural mucosal abnormalities, noncaseating granulomas (CD only), Paneth-cell metaplasia

MANAGEMENT

Medical

Choice of therapy for a given patient depends on many factors, including disease phenotype, location of disease, severity of symptoms, growth status, and age of patient, among other factors. Goal of pediatric IBD therapy is to achieve mucosal healing with the lowest number of adverse effects from medication and to optimize growth, nutrition, and quality of life. "Bottom up" (salicylates, steroids, antibiotics first), "top down" (biologics, immunomodulators), or use of enteral nutrition therapy at time of newly diagnosed IBD may be appropriate depending on the above factors.

- Salicylates: Sulfasalazine, oral mesalamine (Pentasa, Delzicol), balsalazide (Colazal), mesalamine enemas (Rowasa), and mesalamine suppositories (Canasa)
- Antibiotics: Metronidazole, ciprofloxacin, rifaximin, oral vancomycin
  - ✓ Antibiotics are indicated in setting of penetrating (fistulizing) luminal or perianal disease as well as in comorbid C. difficile infection.

✓ Use in active luminal CD and UC as adjunctive therapy is patient-specific. Metronidazole and ciprofloxacin have each been shown to improve symptoms in some studies while lacking significant benefit in others.

✓ Antibiotic salvage triple/quadruple therapy to rescue severe colitis refractory to steroids includes amoxicillin, doxycycline or ciprofloxacin (based on age), metronidazole, with or without vancomycin.

- Steroids: Prednisone, IV methylprednisolone, budesonide (Entocort: ileal release with less systemic absorption), budesonide MMX (Uceris: Multimatrix system technology; colonic release with less systemic absorption), hydrocortisone enema/rectal foam.

- Immunomodulators: 6-mercaptopurine, azathioprine, methotrexate, cyclosporine, tacrolimus
  ✓ To reduce steroid dependency or as adjunct to infliximab
  ✓ Associated with cases of pediatric IBD in which malignancy or hemophagocytic lymphohistiocytosis developed

- Biologic agents: anti-TNFα: infliximab (Remicade), adalimumab (Humira), certolizumab pegol (Cimzia), anti-integrin (vedolizumab [Entyvio])

- Anti-TNF
  ✓ To address moderate to severe CD or UC, fibrostenotic or fistulizing CD, steroid refractory UC, perianal disease, IBD-associated osteopenia/osteoporosis
  ✓ Obtain PPD/CXR to rule out latent TB infection before initiation.
  ✓ Ensure that vaccination series has been completed.

- Anti-integrin
  ✓ To address moderate to severe CD or UC, steroid refractory UC

- Enteral nutritional therapy: Nutrition-based therapy for CD, typically of the small intestine with delivery of semi-elemental formula via NG tube. May modulate gut microbiota to favor antiinflammatory response. Given as 80–100% of daily caloric intake to induce remission of disease. Shown to be better for inducing remission than systemic steroids.

- In acute severe UC, use of the Pediatric Ulcerative Colitis Activity Index scoring system of symptoms can guide clinical judgment regarding response to therapy and need to escalate therapy. The scoring includes abdominal pain, rectal bleeding, stool consistency, number of stools per day, nocturnal bowel movements, and activity level. For acute fulminant ulcerative colitis, refer to Clinical Pathway: https://www.chop.edu/pathways (Ulcerative Colitis, Acute Severe, Inpatient).

- Management of an acute IBD flare that requires hospitalization often includes reevaluation of disease severity and location, with objective determination of symptoms through accurate documentation of pain pattern and stool consistency and frequency.
  ✓ Medication adherence should be determined.
  ✓ If disease has worsened from previous baseline, escalation or change of therapy is strongly considered.
  ✓ If immunosuppressed with acute worsening, consider ruling out infectious causes including C. difficile and CMV colitis

- Discharge criteria following acute flare include improvement of presenting symptoms (e.g., tolerating oral intake without severe pain, minimal gross blood in stool and maintaining stable hemoglobin level, fewer diarrheal stools, gaining weight if admitted with weight loss, resolution of emesis, resolution of obstruction).

Surgical

- Indicated in uncontrolled bleeding (requiring frequent PRBC transfusions), bowel perforation, bowel obstruction, intractable disease, persistent growth failure, and intractable perianal disease

- CD:
  - ✓ Local resection (such as ileocecectomy or hemicolectomy), diverting ileostomy or colostomy, abscess/fistula management
  - ✓ Incision and drainage of perirectal abscesses with or without drain placement
  - ✓ Seton: A suture is placed through the fistulous tract forming a loop, to allow for continuous draining and healing from lumen to skin. Without seton, fistulous tracts tend to heal at the skin side first, and pus may be trapped creating an abscess.
- UC: Total colectomy with ileoanal anastomosis for medically refractory disease

MALABSORPTION AND INTESTINAL FAILURE

Impairment in the ability of the gastrointestinal tract to transport nutrients into the portal circulation is known as *malabsorption* and is attributable to a range of conditions that may be transient or lifelong (e.g. viral gastroenteritis, celiac disease, inflammatory bowel disease). *Intestinal failure* is a life-limiting chronic condition in which the functional gut mass is insufficient to meet nutritional and fluid requirements to sustain growth and hydration. The most common form of intestinal failure is short bowel syndrome resulting from surgical intestinal resection for necrotizing enterocolitis.

ETIOLOGY

Malabsorption

- Inflammatory/immune-mediated (infection, celiac, IBD, IPEX/IPEX-like)
- Inadequate surface area (surgical resection, celiac)
- Fat malabsorption (pancreatic exocrine insufficiency, e.g. cystic fibrosis, Schwachman–Diamond syndrome; chronic liver disease)
- Bile acid defects (ileal resection, chronic liver disease)
- Congenital diarrheas and enteropathies (microvillous inclusion disease, tufting enteropathy, congenital lactase deficiency, DGAT1 deficiency)
- Disorders of lipoprotein metabolism (abetalipoproteinemia, hypobetalipoproteinemia, chylomicron retention disease)

Intestinal failure:

Above etiologies of malabsorption may lead to intestinal failure. The most common are:

- Surgical short-bowel syndrome (originating from, for example, necrotizing enterocolitis, gastroschisis, malrotation with midgut volvulus, intestinal atresia)
- Dysmotility (e.g., chronic intestinal pseudo-obstruction)
- Congenital diarrheas and enteropathies (e.g., microvillous inclusion disease, tufting enteropathy, congenital lactase deficiency, DGAT1 deficiency)

CLINICAL MANIFESTATIONS

- Diarrhea is defined by stool output of >10 mL/kg/day or >200 g/day in older children; stool output of >20 mL/kg/day is common in intestinal failure.
- Diarrhea for longer than 14 days requires diagnostic evaluation.
- Weight loss or failure to gain weight, diarrhea, abdominal distention, anemia, edema, and osteopenia are all indicative of malabsorption.
- In addition to insufficient macronutrient uptake (carbohydrates, proteins, fats), micronutrient deficiencies may develop depending on the region of the gastrointestinal tract affected (e.g., vitamin B_{12}—terminal ileum, iron—stomach, vitamins A/D/E/K—pancreas/liver)

DIAGNOSTICS

- Workup for suspected malabsorption should focus on both underlying etiology and processes that are amenable to treatment.
- Infectious stool studies (PCR-based, where available): stool culture, ova and parasites, *Giardia lamblia, C. difficile*
- Blood tests: Hemoglobin/MCV (micronutrient deficiencies, gastrointestinal loss), albumin (nutritional status), C-reactive protein/sedimentation rate (inflammation), total IgA and tissue transglutaminase IgA (celiac disease), electrolyte panel (acidosis, renal function), serum aminotransferases/bilirubin (liver disease)
- Micronutrients: 25-hydroxyvitamin D, vitamin A, vitamin E, INR (vitamin K), iron/TIBC/ferritin, vitamin B_{12}/folate and methylmalonic acid/homocysteine, copper, zinc, thiamine
- Stool tests: stool-reducing substances (carbohydrate loss), stool A1AT (protein loss), 72-hour fecal fat (fat loss), fecal calprotectin (intestinal inflammation), fecal pancreatic elastase (pancreatic exocrine function)
- Upper endoscopy/colonoscopy with intestinal biopsy: specifically to evaluate suspected chronic conditions of lumen (IBD, celiac disease, congenital enteropathy)

MANAGEMENT

- Ensure adequate nutrition, which may include parenteral nutrition via central access.
- Address underlying disease process (e.g., for celiac disease, omit gluten from diet; for IBD, target immune system).
- Promote intestinal absorption: micronutrient supplementation, modification of enteral feeding composition (fat/protein/carbohydrate), and site of delivery in gastrointestinal tract.
- For intestinal failure, the following therapies may be employed:

    Medical: H_2-blockers/PPIs (reduce hyperacidity from resection), loperamide (slow transit to increase time for absorption), bile-acid sequestrant (reduce bile acid diarrhea in TI resection), antibiotics (intestinal dysbiosis or small intestinal bacterial overgrowth, also central venous catheter–associated line infections), ursodeoxycholic acid (cholestasis)

    Surgical: LILT or Bianchi procedure or STEP to increase absorptive capacity of remaining bowel; small intestine or multivisceral transplantation for intestinal failure–associated liver disease, inadequate central vascular access, recurrent central venous catheter–associated bloodstream infections.

MOTILITY DISORDERS

The impaired movement of contents through the gastrointestinal tract is known as a motility problem. Motility disorders may result from diseases that affect the innervation of the gastrointestinal tract (e.g., gastroparesis, Hirschsprung disease), congenital malformations (esophageal atresia, anorectal malformation), or systemic illnesses causing secondary effects (ileus). Common conditions such as GERD and constipation are also considered motility disorders because of the abnormal movement that is inherent to their pathophysiology.

ETIOLOGY

Innervation:
- Achalasia
- Gastroparesis
- Chronic Intestinal Pseudo-obstruction
- Hirschsprung disease

Congenital malformation:
- Esophageal atresia/tracheoesophageal fistula
- Anorectal malformation
- Gastroschisis
- Congenital diaphragmatic hernia

Systemic illness/effect:
- Neuromuscular disease (scleroderma, muscular dystrophy)
- Metabolic/endocrine disease (thyroid, mitochondrial)
- Postsurgical
- Medications

CLINICAL MANIFESTATIONS

- Region of gastrointestinal tract affected relevant to symptoms: vomiting, bloating, abdominal pain, limited oral intake, difficulty with defecation
- Variable onset of presentation, depending on underlying etiology
- Intolerance of baseline feeding is common in transient motility problems from acute systemic illness (e.g., postinfectious ileus, postinfectious gastroparesis)
- Accompanying urinary retention in CIPO

DIAGNOSTICS

- Exclude obstruction: abdominal plain radiograph, upper gastrointestinal series with small-bowel follow-through, CT/MRI
- Assess for modifiable etiologies: medications (e.g., opiates, anticholinergics), electrolyte disturbance (e.g., hypomagnesemia), hypothyroid (free T_4/TSH), CNS (e.g., increased ICP, encephalopathy), renal (e.g., uremia), psychological (e.g., anxiety)
- Evaluate transit: Esophagography (limited but for esophageal clearance; achalasia), multichannel intraluminal impedance (acidic and nonacidic reflux; GERD), gastric emptying study (nuclear scintigraphy–radiolabeled meal, 4-hour test, gastroparesis)
- Interrogate underlying innervation: Esophageal manometry (achalasia, rumination), antroduodenal manometry (pseudo-obstruction—distinguish neuropathic from myopathic), colonic manometry, anorectal manometry (Hirschsprung disease, internal anal sphincter achalasia)
- Rectal suction biopsy and barium enema remain important diagnostic tools to evaluate for Hirschsprung disease.

MANAGEMENT

- Treat underlying causes, if modifiable.
- Goals of therapy are to ensure optimal nutrition, facilitate defecation, and minimize debilitating symptoms.
- Use feeding strategy to maximize absorption: nasogastric/gastric feeding if esophageal impairment, postpyloric feeding (nasojejunal/gastrojejunal) if medically refractory gastroparesis, parenteral nutrition if inadequate absorption via jejunal route.
- Gastroparesis: diet (low in fat, frequent small-volume meals), medication (erythromycin, metoclopramide), therapeutic endoscopy (pyloric botulin toxin injection)
- Pseudo-obstruction/ileus: amoxicillin–clavulanic acid for small-bowel motility, antibiotic therapy (rifaximin, metronidazole) for intestinal dysbiosis/small intestinal bacterial overgrowth
- Hirschsprung disease: colectomy with pull-through surgery

LIVER, GALLBLADDER AND PANCREAS

ALPHA$_1$-ANTITRYPSIN DEFICIENCY

An autosomal recessive disorder associated with chronic liver disease and premature pulmonary emphysema that is caused by a deficiency of the serine protease inhibitor, A1AT.

EPIDEMIOLOGY

- Most common inherited cause of liver disease in children
- Affects 1 in 2000 live births of White children in the United States

PATHOPHYSIOLOGY

- A1AT is predominantly produced in hepatocytes, is released into the bloodstream, and functions in the lung to inhibit cleavage of connective-tissue proteins.
- Genetic mutation of A1AT leads to protein misfolding. Resultant protein cannot be released from the endoplasmic reticulum of hepatocytes, leading to hepatotoxicity.
- Absence of A1AT or abnormal function allows uninhibited cleavage of connective tissue by elastase, leading to lung injury.

CLINICAL MANIFESTATIONS

- May present at any age from infancy to adulthood
- Variable presentation: Some allele variants cause both liver and lung disease, while others cause only lung disease
- Liver disease (neonate to adult): Prolonged conjugated hyperbilirubinemia in neonate, small for gestational age, acholic stools, elevated transaminases, severe bleeding episode (vitamin K deficiency from liver disease), severe liver failure, hepatomegaly, portal hypertension, varices, chronic hepatitis, cirrhosis, hepatocellular carcinoma
- Lung disease (adult): Emphysema
- On physical exam: Jaundice, hepatomegaly, splenomegaly, ascites, excoriations from pruritus

DIAGNOSTICS

- Serum A1AT level: Normal is 150–350 mg/dL; may be misleading because it is an acute-phase reactant and could be falsely elevated in a proinflammatory state. Further, a normal serum level does not equate to normal protein function.
- PI typing: Defines alleles present, which indicates a normal (MM genotype) or mutant (ZZ genotype) A1AT protein. Other genotypes exist, leading to variable phenotypes.
- Liver biopsy: Necessity for diagnosis is controversial

MANAGEMENT

- Supportive care for liver dysfunction
- Counsel against cigarette smoking.
- Protein replacement therapy (recombinant or purified): Only for established emphysema; does not help liver disease
- Surgical options: Orthotopic liver transplantation, portacaval or splenorenal shunt, lung transplantation

AUTOIMMUNE HEPATITIS

A chronic inflammatory liver disease of unknown etiology characterized by elevated serum aminotransferases, hypergammaglobulinemia, autoantibodies, histologic

findings of a portal tract mononuclear infiltrate and interface hepatitis between the portal tract and the lobule, and clinical response to immunosuppressive therapy. There are two primary types of AIH:

- Type I: Presence of ANA and anti-SMA
- Type II: Presence of LKM antibody; more common in pediatrics
- SLA antibody can be found in either type and is associated with more aggressive disease; LC1 antibody may be found in type II.

EPIDEMIOLOGY

- Relatively uncommon; may present at any age
- Female predominance (4:1)
- About 20% of patients have at least one other autoimmune disorder: Associations observed with autoimmune thyroiditis, nephrotic syndrome, type I diabetes mellitus, Behçet disease, vitiligo, IBD, aplastic anemia, and Addison's disease

PATHOPHYSIOLOGY

- Likely autoimmune process in genetically susceptible persons
- Associated with certain HLA haplotypes (A1, B8, DR3, DR4)
- May overlap with autoimmune sclerosing cholangitis

CLINICAL MANIFESTATIONS

- Extremely variable from asymptomatic to liver failure; may be acute or insidious and progressive
- An acute hepatitis syndrome is the most common presentation, characterized by fatigue, malaise, nausea, anorexia, upper abdominal discomfort, arthralgia, myalgia, oligomenorrhea, skin rashes, mild pruritus, jaundice, dark urine, and pale stools.
- Physical exam should evaluate for signs of chronic liver disease: Jaundice, cutaneous stigmata of liver disease, ascites, hepatomegaly, splenomegaly, rash, altered mental status

DIAGNOSTICS

- ALT, AST levels are increased. ALP and GGT levels are normal or increased.
- INR/PT, *albumin:* To evaluate synthetic liver function
- Quantitative immunoglobulin levels (high IgG, normal IgA)
- ANA, anti-SMA, and anti-LKM-1 for initial diagnostic evaluation. Additional antibodies may be indicated: F-actin antibodies, anti-SLA, anti-LC1, p-ANCA; rarely patients with AIH are negative for traditional antibodies (seronegative autoimmune hepatitis).
  - ✓ During evaluation alternative causes should be pursued: Infection (antibody titers to hepatitis A, B, or C; EBV; CMV), celiac disease (total IgA, TTG-IgA), Wilson disease (ceruloplasmin, 24-hour urinary copper), and myositis (creatine phosphokinase) as source of enzyme elevation (CKP)
- Liver biopsy: Required to confirm diagnosis and rule out other causes of chronic hepatitis. "Interface hepatitis" is the hallmark of AIH on biopsy. Treatment may be initiated without a biopsy in the setting of acute liver failure and coagulopathy when risks of biopsy outweigh benefits.
  - ✓ The overall diagnosis is based on clinical, laboratory, and histologic findings. A scoring system for diagnosis likelihood is provided in the American Association for the Study of Liver Diseases practice guidelines on the diagnosis and management of autoimmune hepatitis.

MANAGEMENT

- Prednisone 2 mg/kg/day (maximum, 60 mg/day); gradually decrease dose over 6–8 weeks to the minimal dose required to maintain normal ALT/AST.
- Azathioprine (0.5 mg/kg/day [maximum, 2 mg/kg/day]): Add if steroid alone not leading to improvement
- Initial relapse after achieving remission is often treated by returning to the initial prednisone dose with addition of azathioprine for long-term maintenance therapy.
- Discontinuation of therapy is considered in a subset of patients who have been treated for more than 3 years, have normal ALT/AST for 2 consecutive years, and demonstrate histologic remission on liver biopsy; discontinuation of therapy just before or during puberty may be associated with higher rates of relapse; many patients require lifelong immunosuppressive therapy.
- Liver transplantation for initial presentation with severe liver failure or progressive disease unresponsive to medical therapy

BILIARY ATRESIA

A disease of unknown etiology in which there is progressive destruction of the extrahepatic biliary tree with variable involvement of the intrahepatic biliary system

EPIDEMIOLOGY

- Incidence: 1 in 10,000–20,000
- Slight female predominance
- 10–25% of cases associated with other congenital anomalies (see "Clinical Manifestations")

PATHOPHYSIOLOGY

- Natural history is complete obliteration of bile ducts leading to biliary cirrhosis and liver failure.
- Most cases affect the entire extrahepatic biliary tree.
- 10% of cases affect only the distal biliary tree.
- Untreated extrahepatic disease: Life expectancy is 11 months.

CLINICAL MANIFESTATIONS

- Usually normal at birth
- Conjugated hyperbilirubinemia most commonly presents around 2–6 weeks of age. Approximately 10–35% will be jaundiced at birth, with the bile ductular injury occurring in the prenatal period.
- Associated anomalies: Polysplenia, abdominal heterotaxy, intestinal malrotation, cardiovascular malformations, and anomalies of hepatic arteries/portal vein
- On physical exam: Jaundice/greenish hue to skin, hepatomegaly, splenomegaly, dark urine, acholic stools, ascites, edema

DIAGNOSTICS

- Bilirubin (total, conjugated, and unconjugated): Conjugated fraction greater than 2 mg/dL or greater than 20% of total bilirubin
- ALT/AST two to three times normal; GGT/ALP markedly elevated; PT/PTT elevated; albumin low owing to synthetic liver dysfunction
- Platelets/leukocyte count: Thrombocytopenia/neutropenia common if there is hypersplenism

- Abdominal ultrasound: May not be diagnostic but important to rule out choledochal cyst and to detect polysplenia or heterotaxy. Absence of the gallbladder raises suspicion for biliary atresia.
- HIDA scan (iminodiacetic-based acid labeled with 99m-technetium): Normally after injection, this lipid-soluble, albumin-bound substance is found in the liver and followed by excretion into the small bowel. In biliary atresia, there is normal uptake by liver, but excretion occurs into the urinary tract because of an absent/obstructed biliary tree.
- Liver biopsy: Typically shows bile-duct proliferation with cholestasis and fibrosis, characteristic of biliary obstruction
- Surgical cholangiography: Gold standard to demonstrate lack of excretion from biliary tree to intestinal lumen; performed intraoperatively immediately prior to Kasai procedure.

MANAGEMENT

Hepatoportoenterostomy (Kasai procedure)

- Anastomosis of intrahepatic biliary tract directly to bowel at the portal plate
- 80% eventually require liver transplantation even if done early
- 70–80% success of palliation if done before 60 days of age; only 20–30% success if done after 90 days of age
- High morbidity and mortality
- Complications include cholangitis, portal hypertension/varices, malnutrition/fat-soluble vitamin deficiency

Liver Transplantation

- Indicated for extrahepatic biliary atresia when diagnosis is delayed past time window for Kasai procedure
- Indicated after Kasai procedure if hepatic insufficiency, portal hypertension with recurrent variceal bleeding, irreversible failure to thrive, recurrent cholangitis, persistent cholestasis, hepatopulmonary syndrome

GALLBLADDER DISEASE

DEFINITIONS

- Cholelithiasis: Gallstones
- Choledocholithiasis: Stones in CBD
- Cholecystitis: Infected or inflamed gallbladder
- Calculous cholecystitis: Infected or inflamed gallbladder that contains stones
- Acalculous cholecystitis: Infected or inflamed gallbladder that does not contain stones

EPIDEMIOLOGY

- Cholelithiasis and cholecystitis are uncommon in children and are often secondary to a predisposing condition.
- More than 50% of cholecystitis in children is acalculous.
- Biliary symptoms develop in only 20% of patients with gallstones.

ETIOLOGY

- Conditions that predispose to cholelithiasis in children: Prematurity, congenital anomaly of biliary tract, hemolytic disorders (e.g., sickle cell disease), ileal resection or disease, obesity, pregnancy, cystic fibrosis, chronic furosemide use, TPN, long-term ceftriaxone

PATHOPHYSIOLOGY
Cholelithiasis

- Due to alteration in relative proportions of bile components
- Cholesterol gallstones due to bile supersaturated with cholesterol
- Pigment gallstones: Black pigment stones due to bile supersaturated with unconjugated bilirubin that forms complexes with free ionized calcium. Brown pigment stones involve biliary stasis and bacterial infection.

Choledocholithiasis

- Primary: Stones formed in CBD
- Secondary: Stone migrates from gallbladder and lodges in CBD
- Causes obstructive cholestasis; may lead to pancreatitis, cholangitis

Cholecystitis

- Calculous: Obstruction of cystic duct by stone leads to acute inflammatory response of gallbladder mucosa; secondary bacterial infection may occur.
- Acalculous: Biliary stasis (e.g., postsurgery, TPN, infectious illness) causes acute symptoms whereas functional disorders (e.g., biliary dyskinesia) cause chronic symptoms.

CLINICAL MANIFESTATIONS

- Cholelithiasis: 80% asymptomatic; biliary colic with RUQ pain
- Choledocholithiasis: Biliary colic, obstructive jaundice, cholangitis, pancreatitis
- Calculous cholecystitis: Acute presentation involves abdominal pain (RUQ or diffuse), low-grade fever, nausea, vomiting, anorexia. Chronic presentation often includes history of biliary colic or history of acute cholecystitis episode that resolved. Symptoms may be minimal.
- Acalculous cholecystitis: Acute presentation similar to acute calculous cholecystitis. Chronic presentation involves recurrent biliary type pain
- Patient may appear ill, with abdominal tenderness, rebound, guarding, palpable gallbladder, jaundice, and/or splenomegaly.
- Murphy's sign: On palpation of RUQ, pain worsens with inspiration, which leads to cessation of breathing; indicative of gallbladder pathology.

DIAGNOSTICS

- Bilirubin, aminotransferases, ALP: May be elevated or normal
- Leukocytosis: Variable
- Amylase/lipase: May be elevated
- Abdominal x-ray: May show calcified stones
- Ultrasound: Best to detect cholelithiasis, choledocholithiasis, and acute cholecystitis
- HIDA scan: No filling of gallbladder in acute cholecystitis; delayed filling in chronic cholecystitis (delayed ejection fraction with CCK or pain with CCK stimulation suggests either chronic cholecystitis or biliary dyskinesia).
- MR cholangiopancreatography: MRI of the biliary duct system. Improved resolution compared to ultrasound; may identify stones or other anomalies of the ducts missed on previous ultrasound.
- ERCP: Endoscopic cholangiography, advantage of being diagnostic and therapeutic for CBD obstruction due to stones

MANAGEMENT
Cholelithiasis

- Observation in asymptomatic patients

Choledocholithiasis

- ERCP with or without sphincterotomy and biliary stent
- Elective cholecystectomy
- Surgical correction of anatomic abnormality of biliary tree, such as choledochal cyst

Acute Cholecystitis

- Rehydration, analgesia, antibiotics, observation (usually resolves spontaneously in 2–3 days)
- Typical antibiotic regimens: Ampicillin–sulbactam; ampicillin–sulbactam plus gentamicin; third-generation cephalosporin plus metronidazole; ticarcillin–clavulanate; piperacillin–tazobactam; imipenem (if life-threatening)
- Elective cholecystectomy after resolution of acute illness (early or up to 2–3 months later) in uncomplicated cases
- Emergent cholecystectomy is indicated if complicated by necrosis, perforation, or empyema.

Chronic Cholecystitis

- Cholecystectomy for chronic calculous cholecystitis (in general)
- For biliary dyskinesia, cholecystectomy has variable results, with many children continuing to experience pain in the postoperative period.

PANCREATITIS

DEFINITIONS

Acute pancreatitis: An acute inflammatory process of the pancreas characterized by two of the following three characteristics: acute abdominal pain, elevated pancreatic enzymes at least three times the upper limit of normal, and radiologic evidence of pancreatic inflammation.

Acute recurrent pancreatitis: At least two episodes of acute pancreatitis with resolution of pain and pancreatic enzymes between episodes.

Chronic pancreatitis: A condition of recurring or persisting abdominal pain, pancreatic inflammation, and progressive destruction of the pancreas that often leads to pancreatic insufficiency or failure

EPIDEMIOLOGY

- All ages; male = female incidence
- Heritable forms of pancreatitis are the most common forms of chronic pancreatitis in children (cationic trypsinogen, *SPINK1, CFTR* gene mutations)

ETIOLOGY

Acute Pancreatitis

- Systemic disease: Infections; inflammatory/vascular (Henoch–Schönlein purpura, hemolytic–uremic syndrome, Kawasaki disease, IBD, collagen vascular); sepsis/shock; transplantation
- Mechanical/structural: Trauma (blunt injury, child abuse, post-ERCP); anatomic (annular pancreas, pancreas divisum, choledochal cyst, stricture); obstruction (stones, tumor)
- Metabolic/toxic: Hyperlipidemia, hypercalcemia, cystic fibrosis, severe malnutrition, refeeding, renal disease, organic acidemia, drugs/toxins
- Idiopathic: Up to 25% of cases

Chronic Pancreatitis

- Obstructive: Congenital anomaly (choledochal cyst), ductal fibrosis or stricture, tumor, pseudocyst, sphincter of Oddi dysfunction, trauma, idiopathic fibrosing pancreatitis, autoimmune pancreatitis, sclerosing cholangitis
- Calcific: Heritable pancreatitis (cationic trypsinogen deficiency, *SPINK1* and *CFTR* mutations), hypercalcemia, hyperlipidemia, juvenile tropical pancreatitis
- Idiopathic

PATHOPHYSIOLOGY

- Acute pancreatitis: Inappropriate activation of enzymes within pancreatic parenchyma leads to inflammation and tissue destruction resulting in necrosis of peripancreatic fat, interstitial edema, and cytokine release
  - ✓ Complications include hypocalcemia, hyperglycemia, gastrointestinal hemorrhage, severe necrosis, pseudocyst rupture, abscess, acute tubular necrosis, gastritis, duodenitis, and pleural effusion.
- Chronic pancreatitis: Fibrotic parenchymal disease resulting from obstructive or calcific processes; exact mechanisms unknown.
  - ✓ Complications include pancreatic exocrine and endocrine insufficiency or failure
- Hereditary pancreatitis (e.g., cationic trypsinogen deficiency): Autosomal dominant form of calcific chronic pancreatitis due to mutations of cationic trypsinogen, resulting in recurrent bouts of acute pancreatitis
- Autoimmune pancreatitis: Associated with increased IgG levels (particularly IgG4), presence of autoantibodies, diffuse enlargement of pancreas, narrowing of main pancreatic duct, and lymphocytic infiltration of the pancreas with fibrotic changes

CLINICAL MANIFESTATIONS

- Acute pancreatitis: Severe abdominal pain of acute onset; with or without epigastric location; nausea, vomiting, anorexia. Clinical course is highly variable.
  - ✓ Most commonly is a self-limited process resolving over a period of 5–8 days on average in previously healthy children.
  - ✓ A minority of patients may develop SIRS with hypotension, renal failure, pulmonary edema or pleural effusions, hemorrhage, and shock
- Chronic pancreatitis: Recurring or persistent abdominal pain or painless; some patients have recurrent episodes of acute pancreatitis; pain diminishes as pancreas burns out (may take 10–20 years)
  - ✓ Other manifestations include pancreatic exocrine or endocrine insufficiency (end-stage), steatorrhea, excessive appetite, growth failure, obstructive jaundice.

DIAGNOSTICS

- Amylase: Level increases early; lasts 3–5 days
- Lipase: More specific than amylase; typically elevated longer
- In chronic pancreatitis, enzyme levels may not be increased
- C-reactive protein: Peaks at 36–48 hours
- Markers of severe disease: Hyperglycemia, hypocalcemia, hypoxemia, hypoproteinemia, high BUN, high white blood cells, low hematocrit
- Imaging not necessary in majority of cases of isolated acute pancreatitis, but may consider:
- Abdominal x-ray: To exclude other causes of abdominal pain
- Chest x-ray: To evaluate for pleural effusion
- Ultrasound: To assess pancreatic inflammation, calcification, ductular dilatation, stones, pseudocyst

- CT: If ultrasound is technically unsatisfactory (sensitivity >90% if necrosis involves >30% of pancreas). Consider CT-guided fine-needle aspiration if diagnosis of necrosis/infection uncertain.
- MRCP: To noninvasively visualize biliary and pancreatic ducts, especially if recurrent pancreatitis and to assess for anatomic anomalies

MANAGEMENT

- Supportive care, bed rest
- Nothing by mouth and nasogastric decompression if vomiting
- Fluid and electrolyte replacement. May need aggressive fluid resuscitation, requiring 1.5–2 × maintenance intravenous fluids in early phases of disease
- Early nutrition with enteral feedings
- TPN reserved for patients who cannot safely tolerate enteral feedings
- Monitor acid–base status, electrolytes, renal function.
- Analgesia: Ibuprofen, tramadol, narcotics
- Adjuncts in chronic pancreatic pain: Amitriptyline, nortriptyline, gabapentin (Neurontin)
- Antibiotics: For severe systemic illness or pancreatic necrosis (imipenem, ticarcillin–clavulanate, piperacillin–tazobactam, or ciprofloxacin plus metronidazole)
- Repeat ultrasound or an alternative imaging study may be useful for patients not improving as expected to evaluate for pseudocyst, abscess, necrosis, or hemorrhage.
- Attempt to identify underlying cause to help prevent recurrence
- ERCP both diagnostic and therapeutic to relieve stones, strictures, or other anatomic anomalies. Risk of worsening pancreatitis.
- Surgical management of complications such as symptomatic pseudocyst, abscess, necrosis, hemorrhage. Surgical correction of structural lesions is performed after acute illness resolves.
- Once symptoms resolve and patient is able to tolerate oral feedings, maintain on low-fat diet until complete recovery or indefinitely in chronic cases; consider pancreatic enzymes

WILSON DISEASE

Autosomal recessive disease of copper metabolism that involves defective biliary copper excretion, which leads to abnormal copper accumulation in the liver, CNS, eyes, and kidneys

EPIDEMIOLOGY

- Prevalence: 1:30,000

PATHOPHYSIOLOGY

- Wilson disease gene on chromosome 13 encodes a transmembrane copper-transporting ATPase protein (ATPase 7B). Mutations result in an abnormal transporter protein, which prevents normal export of copper from hepatocytes.
- Copper accumulates first in the liver and then spills over to other tissue.

CLINICAL MANIFESTATIONS

- Frequently presents in childhood but rarely before age 5 years
- Classic triad: Hepatic disease, neurologic disease, Kayser–Fleischer rings (brown-yellow ring around the corneoscleral junction resulting from copper deposits)
- In children, hepatic effects precede neurologic effects and typically present in the second decade of life

- Liver: Acute hepatitis, chronic active hepatitis, cirrhosis, fulminant hepatic failure (especially in pubertal females)
- CNS: Basal ganglia involvement leads to dystonia, incoordination, tremor, fine motor skill difficulty, rigidity, dysarthria, and gait disturbances. Psychiatric manifestations include depression, aggressive behaviors, impulsivity, compulsivity, poor school performance, psychosis
- Ophthalmologic: Kayser–Fleischer rings, sunflower cataracts (cataract related to copper deposits described as brown-green deposits in anterior and posterior lens capsule)
- Other: Hemolytic anemia, proximal renal tubular dysfunction, bone demineralization, osteoporosis, pathologic fractures, cardiac dysrhythmias, cholelithiasis

DIAGNOSTICS

- Laboratory tests: Ceruloplasmin level less than 20 mg/dL; serum copper low or high; 24-hour urine copper greater than 100 mcg/day; CBC (hemolysis); LFTs (hepatitis, cholestasis)
- Liver biopsy: Gold standard; quantitation of hepatic copper, typical findings of steatosis, inflammation, with or without fibrosis
- Head CT: Ventricular dilatation, brain atrophy, basal ganglia abnormalities
- Head MRI: More sensitive than CT for specific changes

MANAGEMENT

- D-penicillamine (20 mg/kg/day divided four times a day, maximum 1 g/day; start with reduced dose): Copper chelator used as initial treatment in hepatic disease. Give 1 hour before or 2 hours after meals. Supplement with vitamin B$_6$.
- Trientine: A copper chelator and alternative to D-penicillamine. Typical dose in range of 20 mg/kg/day in two to three divided doses rounded to nearest 250 mg.
- Zinc: Antagonist of copper absorption used as adjunctive therapy or alternative maintenance therapy after chelation. Typical dose is 150 mg/day in larger children and adults, and 75 mg/day in smaller children. Daily dose is divided two to three times per day.
- Ammonium tetrathiomolybdate: Still experimental
- Diet: Restrict dietary sources of copper: animal liver and kidney, shellfish, chocolate, dried beans, peas, unprocessed wheat
- Liver transplantation: For severe disease with fulminant hepatic failure or worsening disease unresponsive to medical therapy
- Screening of asymptomatic relatives of patients with Wilson disease

Elizabeth J. Bhoj, MD, PhD
Tara L. Wenger, MD, PhD

GENETIC APPROACH TO EVALUATION OF COMMON PROBLEMS

AN INFANT WITH DYSMORPHIC FEATURES OF MULTIPLE ANOMALIES

Major anomalies are structural defects that require surgery or ongoing medical care (e.g., cleft palate, cardiac defects, hypospadias). Minor anomalies are unusual morphologic features that are of no serious medical or cosmetic consequence to the patient (e.g., single palmar crease, low-set ears, clinodactyly).

EPIDEMIOLOGY

- Major anomalies are detected in 3% of newborns, but up to 7% of children will have a defect identified by the age of 5 years.
- Minor anomalies are found in 15% of children.
- Only 1% of children have three or more minor anomalies, 90% of whom also have at least one major anomaly.
- A child with multiple minor anomalies should be evaluated for the presence of a major anomaly.

IMPACT

- Birth defects are the second leading cause of death in the first month of life (second only to prematurity).

ETIOLOGY

- Chromosome rearrangements: 5–10%
- Single-gene defects: 10–15%
- Environmental (nongenetic) factors: 10%
- Polygenic/multifactorial causes: 35–40%
- Unknown: 30%

DIAGNOSTIC CONSIDERATIONS

- Age of parents:
  - ✓ Advanced maternal age is associated with increased rate of trisomy 21, and other chromosomal disorders (**Table 11-1**)
  - ✓ Advanced paternal age is associated with increased rate of de novo autosomal dominant single-gene disorders.
- Multiple pregnancy losses:
  - ✓ Can indicate a balanced translocation or X-linked disorder that is lethal in males
  - ✓ If available, genetic testing from these fetuses should be reviewed.
- Assisted reproductive technology:
  - ✓ Rate of birth defects is higher in infants conceived using assisted reproductive technology (8.3%) and is highest in infants conceived via intracytoplasmic sperm injection (9.9%).
  - ✓ Preimplantation genetic testing during in vitro fertilization does not rule out mosaic disorders or types of genetic disorders that were not evaluated.

TABLE 11-1	Incidence at Live Birth for Chromosomal Abnormalities	
Maternal Age at Delivery (Years)	**Trisomy 21**	**All Chromosomal Anomalies**
20	1/1667	1/526
25	1/1200	1/476
30	1/952	1/385
35	1/378	1/192
40	1/106	1/66
45	1/30	1/21

Reproduced with permission from Heffner LJ: Advanced maternal age—how old is too old? *N Engl J Med* 2004 Nov 4;351(19):1927-1929.

✓ Higher risk of growth restriction and/or placental dysfunction when the mother is not genetically related to the infant (e.g., egg donor, embryo donor, surrogate gestation)

✓ Ovarian hyperstimulation (e.g., clomiphene [Clomid], in vitro fertilization) increases the risk of methylation defects (e.g. Beckwith-Wiedemann syndrome is 18 times more likely in an infant conceived via in vitro fertilization)

✓ Records should be reviewed to determine what types of carrier screening and preimplantation genetic testing and/or screening were completed

- Family history:

✓ Identification of family members with similar birth defects, pregnancy losses, infertility, and whether the child resembles his or her family members

✓ Ethnicity should be elicited to determine the rarity of physical features (e.g., synophrys [hypertrophy and fusion of the eyebrows] is common in children of Middle Eastern descent, epicanthal folds are common in children of Asian descent) and to identify genetic conditions prevalent in certain ethnic groups.

✓ Presence of consanguinity increases likelihood of autosomal recessive disorder in offspring.

✓ Maternal immunization status prior to pregnancy and titers if possible, with special attention to viruses that are associated with birth defects if primary exposure occurs during pregnancy (e.g. measles, rubella, varicella).

- Medication/drug exposure during pregnancy:

✓ Many medications (e.g., anticonvulsants, warfarin, retinoic acid) and other substances (e.g., alcohol) are associated with an increased rate of birth defects.

- Travel history before and during pregnancy:

✓ Travel to Zika virus—endemic regions should be elicited for the mother as well as her sexual partners in the months prior to and during the pregnancy.

- Maternal medical conditions during pregnancy:

✓ Risk due to medical condition itself (e.g., maternal diabetes associated with an increased risk of many birth defects including cardiac defects, duplicated great toe) or because of exposure to teratogenic medications (e.g., anticonvulsants, warfarin, retinoic acid)

- Genetic screening or diagnostic testing during pregnancy:

✓ Results of genetic screening (offered to all women) and diagnostic genetic testing (often done following abnormal screening or identification of anomalies) may not be recorded in the infant's chart, and these records should be requested.

✓ Prenatal karyotypes are often limited to Fluorescence in situ hybridization (FISH) for 13, 18, 21 and sex chromosomes. Request actual report to determine if full karyotype or limited karyotype was done, as both may be listed as "normal karyotype" in infant's chart.

✓ Non-invasive prenatal screening (NIPS) has variable sensitivity and specificity for different genetic disorders, and confirmatory diagnostic testing before or after birth is required (Table 11-2).

TABLE 11-2	Types of clinical genetic testing				
Test	**Use**	**Detects**	**Cost**	**Turnaround Time**	**Special Considerations**
NIPS	Pregnancy screening	Chromosomal disorders, microdeletions	+	+	Variable sensitivity/specificity. Confirmatory testing required.
PGS	Pre-implantation testing in IVF	Chromosomal disorders, microdeletions	+++	+/+++ (if PGD added)	Panels vary by lab, targeted testing can be added (PGD)
FISH	Detects specific chromosome segments	Disorders of copy number (e.g., microdeletions), rearrangements	+	+	Need to know exact region of interest
Karyotype	Suspected chromosomal disorder	Large chromosomal abnormalities	+	+	Prenatal karyotypes may be limited to FISH of chromosomes 13, 18, 21, X, Y
SNP array	Detection of microdeletions/ duplications	Microdeletions/duplications, some uniparental disomy, loss of heterozygosity	++	+++	First-line testing for most undiagnosed patients
Targeted Sanger testing	Detection of variants in a small number of genes	Sequence variants in specific genes	+/+++	++	Often used for familial testing of known disorder
Targeted NGS panel testing	Detection of variants in multiple specific genes	Sequence variants in multiple genes	++/+++	+++	First-line for genetic disorders with multiple causative genes
MLPA	Copy number analysis in specific region	Specific microdeletions and microduplications	+	+	Need to know exact region of interest

			Cost	Turnaround Time	Comments
Exome Sequence	Sequence analysis of (*Continued*) ~20,000 genes	Sequence variants in most genes, as long as good coverage. Mitochondrial genetic testing can be added.	+++	++++	Not used for detection of copy number variants, trinucleotide repeat disorders, methylation defects. Detects cause of abnormalities in ~1/3 of patients
Genome Sequence	Sequence analysis of most regions of genome, also usually involves copy number analysis	Sequence variants that would be detected in exome sequencing in addition to intronic and other regions	++++	++++	Increasing clinical availability
Methylation Analysis	Determination of methylation status of imprinted genes	Aberrant gene methylation	++	++	Usually only targeted testing for specific genes

Note: Testing can be for multiple tissues, including amniocentesis or chorionic villus sampling

FISH = fluorescence in situ hybridization; IVF = in vitro fertilization; MLPA = multiplex ligation-dependent probe amplification; NIPS = noninvasive prenatal screening; NGS = next-generation sequencing; PGD = preimplantation genetic diagnosis; PGS = preimplantation genetic screening; SNP = single-nucleotide polymorphism

For Cost: + = least costly; +++ = most costly. For Turnaround Time: + = quicker turnaround time; +++ = longer turnaround time

✓ If NIPS was attempted during pregnancy and the lab reported that the test was unable to be performed, it may indicate an abnormality (e.g., long stretches of homozygosity, which could increase the likelihood of a recessive or imprinting disorder).

✓ Children with congenital heart disease may have also undergone FISH for 22q11.2 deletion syndrome, which may not identify cases with duplications or smaller nested deletions or duplications, which cause a similar spectrum of defects

- Pregnancy complications:
  ✓ Some birth defects may be caused by pregnancy complications (e.g., maternal diabetes resulting in cardiac defects, oligohydramnios resulting in deformations), while some pregnancy complications may be the result of carrying an affected fetus (e.g., polyhydramnios in 22q11.2 deletion syndrome, HELLP syndrome with fetus affected by long-chain fatty acid dehydrogenase deficiency)

- Medical state of infant:
  ✓ Consider Apgar score, resuscitation, and continued support.
  ✓ Determine whether appropriate exams and imaging have been done to identify other structural defects (e.g., echocardiography, ophthalmologic exam, renal ultrasonography, skeletal films)
  ✓ For critically ill infants with suspected genetic disease: consider obtaining blood for DNA extraction prior to performing ECMO or cardiopulmonary bypass, before administering whole blood, or for any critically ill infant in whom a genetic disease is suspected but not yet identified.

PHYSICAL EXAM

- Length, weight, and head circumference percentile should be corrected for gestational age, even within the "term" window and also compared to one another.
- Careful identification of most severe features (e.g., tetralogy of Fallot) along with most unusual features (e.g., epibulbar dermoids on eye exam) can help to narrow differential diagnosis.
- Systematic head-to-toe approach by body part (e.g., skull, hair, eyes, eyebrows, nose, ears) with focus on structure (e.g., ear placement, ear formation, presence of ear pits/folds) rather than on functional organ system (e.g., cardiac exam, respiratory exam, neurologic exam) is crucial for identification of minor anomalies.
- Unusual features or abnormal measurements should be compared to those of family members (e.g., measure parental head circumferences, look at photographs of siblings)

Mimickers of Genetic Diseases

Some recognizable syndromes are not known to be associated with an identifiable genetic cause and typically have a low recurrence risk. As there is no specific test for these conditions, the workup in these cases primarily involves excluding other genetic causes.

- Decreased fetal movement (including fetal akinesia sequence):
  ✓ Decreased fetal movement from a primary neurologic or neuromuscular cause can be associated with breech position, high arched or cleft palate, micrognathia, long fingers, abnormal skull shape, myopathic facies, and abnormal creases
- VACTERL association:
  ✓ Children may have two or more of the following defects: Vertebral anomalies (V), anal atresia (A), cardiovascular anomalies (C), tracheoesophageal fistula (TE), renal or radial ray defects (R), and limb anomalies (L).

✓ Children with VACTERL have favorable cognitive outcomes and low recurrence risk.

✓ Workup includes search for potential comorbid conditions (e.g., echocardiography, spine imaging, limb films, renal ultrasonography) and exclusion of other genetic conditions that may mimic VACTERL (e.g., genomewide microarray testing to rule out aneuploidy, chromosome breakage studies to rule out Fanconi anemia in patients with involvement of radial ray).

• Amniotic band syndrome:
  ✓ Disruption of developing embryo or fetus by strands from amnion
  ✓ Characterized by limb or digit amputations (with normal-appearing limb or digit up to the point where it is missing), hemangiomas, cleft lip and/or cleft palate
  ✓ Nongenetic; low risk of recurrence

• Diabetic embryopathy: Maternal diabetes is associated with increased rate of common birth defects as well as rare malformations, including duplicated hallux. Congenital heart disease, such as transposition of the great arteries, ventricular septal defect, and atrial septal defects are often found, as well as caudal regression, situs inversus, ureter duplex, renal agenesis, and anencephaly.
  ✓ May be associated with macrosomia or growth restriction
  ✓ As maternal diabetes is common, genetic workup should not be limited because of the presence of maternal diabetes. Diagnostic workup is focused on excluding other causes of specific malformations (e.g., microarray testing for congenital heart disease, sequencing of *GLI3* for duplicated hallux)

• Möebius sequence:
  ✓ Möebius sequence is caused by palsy of the sixth and seventh cranial nerves and is characterized by inturned eyes and limited facial movement, giving an unusual facial appearance.
  ✓ Möebius sequence has been linked to prenatal vascular insults.

• Goldenhar syndrome/craniofacial microsomia:
  ✓ Usually limited to underdevelopment of one or both sides of face and ear (including anotia in some), ear tags, lateral facial clefts, epibulbar dermoids, hearing loss
  ✓ Can include malformations of multiple organ systems (e.g., severe cardiac or skeletal anomalies)
  ✓ If suspected, cervical-spine anomalies should be ruled out prior to neck hyperextension (e.g., procedures requiring intubation.)
  ✓ Risk of recurrence is low.

DIAGNOSTIC WORKUP

• First-line genetic testing will depend on level of suspicion for a specific syndrome.
• Karyotype should be done for patients with suspected trisomies.
• Specific gene sequencing should be done for suspected single-gene disorders
• If a diagnosis is not clear from the initial exam, genomewide microarray testing should be done to rule out aneuploidy.
• Exome or genome sequencing may be considered for cases in which diagnosis remains elusive despite standard testing.
• Metabolic workup should be considered, especially for patients with electrolyte abnormalities, involvement of multiple systems, or unexplained worsening of medical course.
• Additional medical workup (e.g., ophthalmologic exam, echocardiography, spine imaging) may help to identify comorbid conditions and narrow genetic differential diagnosis.

GROWTH DISTURBANCES

More than 1300 distinct genetic entities are associated with poor growth; one fourth have a prenatal onset. In addition, prenatal-onset growth disturbances can occur because of placental dysfunction, infections and drug exposures during pregnancy. Most genetic syndromes associated with prenatal-onset growth disturbances have additional features, such as structural abnormalities, dysmorphic features, or developmental delay. When a genetic cause of poor or excessive growth is suspected, focused history taking and physical exam will help narrow the differential diagnosis. There are fewer genetic causes of overgrowth, but careful evaluation remains important for accurate categorization.

DIAGNOSTIC CONSIDERATIONS

- Prenatal versus postnatal onset: Birth weight, length, and head circumference should be plotted by gestational age at birth, including among term infants (37–42 weeks).
- Degree of similarity to family member growth patterns: Pedigree should be reviewed for recognizable inheritance pattern or size very different than relatives.
- Proportionate versus disproportionate: Includes comparison of height, weight, and head circumference percentiles as well as individual body segment abnormalities (e.g., shortened long bones in skeletal dysplasia)
- Symmetric versus asymmetric: Should include comparison of limb length and girth to one another (left vs. right) as well as obvious organomegaly (e.g., macroglossia) or differences in facial symmetry
- Determine whether growth abnormality followed change in feeding patterns: Assess for feeding difficulties or excessive eating. The presence of feeding difficulties does not preclude a genetic cause for poor growth, as some syndromes are associated with extreme feeding difficulties.
- Presence of dysmorphic features, birth defects, or intellectual disability: When present, these features are helpful in syndrome identification.

Notable syndromes in which altered growth may be a major presenting feature:
Poor growth:
- Prenatal onset: Russell–Silver syndrome (normal head circumference but short stature and low birth weight), skeletal dysplasias, chromosomal aberrations, microdeletion syndromes (e.g., Williams syndrome, 22q11.2 deletion syndrome)
- Postnatal onset: Any syndrome with poor feeding or increased energy expenditure as a prominent feature

Overgrowth:
- Prenatal onset: Sotos syndrome, Weaver syndrome, Beckwith–Wiedemann syndrome, maternal diabetes
- Postnatal onset: Marfan syndrome

Mixed growth pattern:
- Prader–Willi syndrome: Weight gain is initially poor owing to feeding difficulties; then excessive weight gain occurs because of insatiable appetite. Very small hands and feet and short stature are usually present, sometimes requiring administration of growth hormone. Infants will also have profound hypotonia.

Asymmetric growth:
- Can be due to underdevelopment of one side, or overgrowth of the other. Identification of an abnormality on one side can be helpful in subtle cases (e.g., ear tags on smaller side of face in Goldenhar syndrome).

- Underdevelopment of one or both sides of face: Goldenhar syndrome, craniofacial microsomia
- Overgrowth (asymmetry) of face or limbs: Beckwith–Wiedemann syndrome, neurofibromatosis type I, Proteus syndrome, mosaicism (especially segmental)

DIAGNOSTIC EVALUATION

- Karyotype, genomewide microarray or specific gene testing may be indicated based on suspicion for individual syndromes.
- Consider skeletal survey if skeletal dysplasia is suspected.
- Additional medical workup including referral to endocrinology or gastroenterology may be necessary to rule out nongenetic etiologies while awaiting results of testing.
- Must be distinguished from other causes of facial asymmetry due to distortion, including positional plagiocephaly and craniosynostosis.
- Consider other etiologies when a focal region becomes larger (e.g., plexiform neurofibroma) or loss of tissue on one half of face (e.g., Parry–Romberg hemifacial atrophy).

HYPERTROPHIC CARDIOMYOPATHY

Increased wall thickness of the left ventricle without chamber expansion, in the absence of abnormal ventricular load (i.e., not due to hypertension, structural heart disease, or valve disease), with associated diastolic dysfunction

EPIDEMIOLOGY

- Adult prevalence estimates of 1 in 500 adults have been reported; however, good pediatric data are lacking.
- Estimated incidence in adults and children is reported to be between 0.24 and 0.47 per 100,000 per year.

GENETIC ETIOLOGIES

- Nonsyndromic: Isolated cardiac sarcomeric gene mutations are present in at least 50% of cases where syndromic and metabolic etiologies have been excluded.
- Common sites of sarcomeric gene mutations include the myosin light and heavy chains, troponins, and titin.
- Usually inherited or de novo dominant mutations
- No dysmorphic features on exam
- Syndromic: Approximately 10% of cases are associated with a malformation syndrome.
- Mutations in the RAS-MAPK pathway (Noonan, LEOPARD, and Costello syndromes):
- Owing to mutations in the members of the RAS-mitogen activated protein kinase pathway, most commonly *PTPN11*.
- Physical features can include short stature, epicanthal folds, ptosis, hypertelorism, low posterior hairline, webbed neck, and shield chest.
- LEOPARD is characterized by lentigines (L), ECG abnormalities (E), ocular hypertelorism and obstructive cardiomyopathy (O), pulmonic stenosis (P), abnormalities of genitalia (A), retardation of growth (R), and deafness (D)
- Costello syndrome, due to mutations in *HRAS*, is associated with increased risk of malignancy and intellectual disability.
- Pompe syndrome (glycogen storage disease type II):
  ✓ Due to decreased enzyme activity of acid alpha-glucosidase.
  ✓ In addition to cardiomegaly and hypertrophic cardiomyopathy, there is often hypotonia, feeding difficulties, failure to thrive, and hearing loss
  ✓ Enzyme-replacement therapy is available.

OTHER ETIOLOGIES

- Inborn errors of metabolism: Glycogen storage diseases, fatty acid oxidation defects, lysosomal storage diseases, mitochondrial disease
- Neuromuscular disorders: Friedreich's ataxia, myotonic dystrophy
- Dilated cardiomyopathy: Enlarged chamber volumes with normal or thinned walls and associated systolic dysfunction

EPIDEMIOLOGY

- Annual incidence in children younger than 18 is 0.57 case per 100,000.
- Higher in boys than in girls (0.66 vs. 0.47 case per 100,000)
- Higher in African Americans than Caucasian children (0.98 vs. 0.46 per 100,000)
- Higher in infants (<1 year) than in children (4.40 vs. 0.34 case per 100,000)

GENETIC ETIOLOGIES

Nonsyndromic: Up to 40% of dilated cardiomyopathy presents as inherited isolated cardiac disease.
- Autosomal dominant:
  ✓ Extremely variable penetrance
  ✓ Most mutations are confined to individual families.
  ✓ A significant portion of nonfamilial cases are also found to have mutations.
  ✓ Unlike hypertrophic cardiomyopathy, mutations affect proteins with a variety of functions, including sarcomeric, cytoskeleton, nuclear envelope, sarcolemma, calcium handling, RNA splicing, and trafficking proteins.
- Arrhythmia associated:
  ✓ A minority of patients may have conduction disease or supraventricular arrhythmias that may precede the diagnosis of dilated cardiomyopathy
  ✓ Usually due to mutations in the genes encoding the nuclear envelope proteins lamin A/C or emerin, or the *SCN5A*-encoded cardiac sodium channel
- Syndromic: The vast majority of patients have isolated cardiac disease; however, a few extracardiac phenotypes are known.
- Dystrophinopathies:
  ✓ Dilated cardiomyopathy can occur in Duchenne and Becker muscular dystrophies owing to mutations in *DMD* gene.
  ✓ In Duchenne muscular dystrophy, patients present with delayed milestones and progressive proximal weakness in early childhood; however, the cardiomyopathy usually presents after age 18.
  ✓ In Becker muscular dystrophy, presentation and cardiomyopathy occur later in life.
- Barth syndrome (3-methylglutaconic aciduria type 2):
  ✓ Due to mutations in *TAZ*, which lead to infant-onset dilated cardiomyopathy, skeletal myopathy, and neutropenia.
- Sensorineural hearing loss:
  ✓ Can occur in association with dilated cardiomyopathy in patients with *EYA4* mutations
  ✓ Initial workup: Physical exam (with particular attention to motor exam and hearing), family history (including sudden cardiac death, arrhythmias), chest x-ray, echocardiography, ECG, metabolic evaluation, genomewide microarray, targeted gene sequencing

STRUCTURAL CONGENITAL HEART DISEASE

EPIDEMIOLOGY

- CHD is the most common major congenital anomaly.

- In North America estimated prevalence is 8.1 per 1000 live births.
- Unlike in the past, now more than 75% of patients with CHD survive the first year, and the population of adult CHD patients is growing at a rate of almost 5% per year.

NONGENETIC ETIOLOGIES

- Causes include maternal exposures such as alcohol or antiepileptic medications, environmental exposures such as pesticides, and congenital infections such as rubella.

GENETIC ETIOLOGIES

Syndromic due to aneuploidy:
- Trisomy 21 (Down syndrome)
  ✓ 40–50% of patients have CHD.
  ✓ AV canal lesions are the prototypic finding.
  ✓ Associated features include distinctive facial features, intellectual disability, hearing loss, thyroid disease, and short stature.
- Trisomy 13 (Patau syndrome)
  ✓ 80–100% of patients have CHD.
  ✓ A wide variety of cardiac lesions can be present.
  ✓ Associated features include very low survival rates, microphthalmia, polydactyly, and poor growth.
- Trisomy 18 (Edwards syndrome)
  ✓ 80–100% of patients have CHD.
  ✓ A wide variety of cardiac lesions can be present.
  ✓ Associated features include very low survival rates, rocker bottom feet, clenched fists, distinctive facies, and poor growth.
- Monosomy X (Turner syndrome)
  ✓ 20–50% of patients have CHD.
  ✓ Coarctation of the aorta is the prototypic lesion.
  ✓ Associated features include short stature, webbed neck, wide-spaced nipples, and infertility.

Syndromic due to copy number variants (deletions or insertions):
- 22q11.2 deletion syndrome (formerly known as DiGeorge or velocardiofacial syndrome):
  ✓ 70–80% of patients have CHD, which is the major cause of mortality in 22q11.2 deletion syndrome.
  ✓ Lesions include tetralogy of Fallot, aortic-arch abnormalities, and ventricular septal defects. Cardiac defects linked to deletion of *TBX1*,
  ✓ Associated features include underdevelopment of the thymus and parathyroid glands, cleft lip and/or palate, short stature, feeding difficulties, immunodeficiency, learning difficulties, and psychiatric disorders.
- Williams syndrome (7q11.23 deletion):
  ✓ Up to 80–100% of patients have CHD.
  ✓ Common lesions include supravalvar aortic stenosis, pulmonary artery stenosis, and valve abnormalities.
  ✓ CHD due to deletion of *ELN*.
  ✓ Associated features include distinctive facies, intellectual disability, feeding difficulties, hypercalcemia, outgoing personality, and anxiety.

Syndromic due to point mutations:
- Noonan and Costello syndromes: See full description in "Cardiomyopathy," genetic etiologies.
  ✓ Both syndromes can have associated pulmonic stenosis and atrial or ventricular septal defects.

- Alagille syndrome (due to JAG1 or NOTCH2 mutations):
  ✓ >90% of patients have CHD.
  ✓ Common findings include peripheral pulmonary hypoplasia, pulmonic stenosis, and tetralogy of Fallot.
  ✓ Associated features include cholestasis with a paucity of bile ducts, eye abnormalities, and distinctive facies.
- CHARGE syndrome (due to CHD7 mutations):
  ✓ 85% of patients have CHD.
  ✓ Common lesions include pulmonic stenosis, atrial septal defects, and tetralogy of Fallot
  ✓ Associated features include eye coloboma (C), heart defect (H), choanal atresia (A), retarded growth and development (R), genital hypoplasia (G), and ear and hearing abnormalities (E)

Nonsyndromic genetic etiologies:
- Copy-number variants
  ✓ About 10–15% of patients with isolated, sporadic CHD may have a rare copy-number variant.
- Point mutations
  ✓ Isolated CHD can be due to mutations in transcription factors and signaling molecules involved in the patterning and development of the embryonic heart. To date, there have been dozens of genes identified, and this list is rapidly expanding.
  ✓ Initial workup: Physical exam, family history, chest x-ray, echocardiography, ECG, genomewide microarray, targeted gene sequencing

HYPOTONIA

Decreased tone in any muscle or muscle group, can be divided into central hypotonia, which affects the core trunk muscles, axial hypotonia, which affects the limbs, and specific muscle group hypotonia, such as facial hypotonia. It may be very mild and noticed only on close testing, or so profound that respiration, swallowing, and reflexes are affected.

DIFFERENTIAL DIAGNOSIS

Hypotonia in an infant can be due to primary genetic cause (e.g., trisomy 21, Prader–Willi syndrome), neurologic abnormality (e.g., lissencephaly, hypoxic–ischemic encephalopathy, myotonic dystrophy, spinal muscular atrophy), metabolic disease (e.g., Zellweger syndrome, Pompe disease, congenital disorder of glycosylation), or other medical issue (e.g., prematurity, sepsis, botulism).

DIAGNOSTIC CONSIDERATIONS

The search for a genetic cause of hypotonia, especially in a neonate, should consider the following:
- Major malformations: The presence of major malformations in an infant with hypotonia makes a genetic cause more likely (e.g., CHD more likely in hypotonia due to trisomy 21 than in hypotonia due to neuromuscular disease).
- Minor dysmorphic features: Minor dysmorphia that result from decreased fetal movement (e.g., high arched palate, long fingers, breech presentation with abnormal skull shape, abnormal creases) should be distinguished from minor dysmorphia unrelated to fetal movement (e.g., coarse facies, epicanthus)
- Prader–Willi syndrome should be considered in any infant with hypotonia and feeding difficulty. Many children with Prader–Willi syndrome will be fair as compared with their family members and have very small hands and feet (less than the third percentile).

DIAGNOSTIC TESTING

- Genomewide microarray testing should be done to rule out aneuploidy
- SNP microarray testing is preferred because it can assess loss of heterozygosity in cases where Prader–Willi syndrome is suspected.
- Additional testing for Prader–Willi syndrome (methylation studies) may be indicated.
- Karyotype should be done when trisomy 21 is suspected. Additional sequencing for suspected single-gene disorders can be done.
- Additional nongenetic workup may include neuromuscular evaluation, electromyography, brain MRI to assess structural defects, and metabolic testing (e.g., transferrin isoelectric focusing to test for congenital disorders of glycosylation, 7-dehydrocholesterol to test for Smith–Lemli–Opitz syndrome, very-long-chain fatty acids to test for peroxisomal disorders)

PIERRE ROBIN SEQUENCE

Microretrognathia and airway obstruction due to glossoptosis, with or without U-shaped cleft palate. There are notable genetic and nongenetic etiologies. Microretrognathia can be due to a primary effect of a genetic variant on mandibular development, or as a secondary cause of restricted movement of the fetal chin and tongue. This restricted movement can be due to hypotonia or mechanical constraint of the chin. Though Pierre Robin sequence can be diagnosed by physical examination, a thorough history, physical examination, and genetic testing are needed to determine the etiology.

DIFFERENTIAL DIAGNOSIS

- Stickler syndrome, 22q11.2 deletion syndrome, auriculocondylar syndrome, Treacher Collins syndrome, other syndromic and nonsyndromic causes

DIAGNOSTIC CONSIDERATIONS

- Stickler syndrome is the most common genetic cause of Pierre Robin sequence, and it is often inherited from an affected parent. Ophthalmologic examination can be helpful to establish the diagnosis, prior to the return of genetic testing results.

DIAGNOSTIC TESTING

- Many patients will receive testing for Stickler syndrome in addition to microarray testing.
- A variety of microdeletion syndromes and single-gene disorders have been associated with Pierre Robin sequence, so physical examination and history are needed to guide the sequence of genetic testing.

NOTABLE SYNDROMES LIKELY TO BE ENCOUNTERED IN AN INPATIENT SETTING

22q11.2 DELETION SYNDROME

Formerly known as DiGeorge syndrome and velocardiofacial syndrome 2 2q11.2 DS is the most common contiguous gene deletion syndrome. Most cases affect the same approximately 3-Mb region encompassing about 45 genes.

EPIDEMIOLOGY

- Prevalence: 1 in 4000 births, males and females affected equally

ETIOLOGY

- Approximately 90% of cases of 22q11.2 DS are de novo, with 10% inherited from a parent.
- There is a 50% chance of an affected parent passing the deletion to each offspring.

CLINICAL CHARACTERISTICS

- Cardiovascular malformations: Most common defects include tetralogy of Fallot, ventriculoseptal defect, interrupted aortic arch, truncus arteriosus, and vascular ring.
- Immune: Immunodeficiencies including T-cell lymphopenia, delayed IgG production, and thymic hypoplasia/aplasia
- Palate: Palatal defects including velopharyngeal insufficiency, cleft palate
- Endocrine: Endocrinologic abnormalities, including hypocalcemia
- Neurodevelopmental: Mild-to-moderate developmental delay, autism spectrum disorder (20%), psychosis (25%), and ADHD (50%)

DIAGNOSIS

- Genomewide microarray testing or multiplex ligation-dependent probe amplification is the preferred diagnostic method for 22q11.2 DS.
- The classic 22q11.2 deletion can be identified using FISH, but this technique may not identify patients with duplications or cases with atypical nested deletions.

BECKWITH–WIEDEMANN SYNDROME

Disorder of imprinting that leads to somatic overgrowth and tumor predisposition, often diagnosed by the classic triad of symmetric or asymmetric gigantism, exomphalos, and macroglossia

EPIDEMIOLOGY

- Prevalence: 1 in 14,000, with equal numbers of males and females
- No predominance in any ethnic group
- Increased risk with assisted reproduction (including in vitro fertilization and ovulation stimulating drugs)
- About 85% sporadic, 15% familial

ETIOLOGY

- There are multiple causes of BWS, all leading to aberrant methylation at 11p15.5.
- Sporadic loss of methylation at imprinting center (IC) 2 is the cause in about 50% of cases, with gain of methylation at IC1 accounting for 5% of cases.
- 20% of cases are the result of paternal uniparental disomy of chromosome 11p15.5.
- Another 5% are secondary to spontaneous and 40% to inherited *CDKN1C* mutations. Rarer causes include de novo and maternally derived translocations and inversions and paternally derived duplications.

CLINICAL CHARACTERISTICS

- Growth: Height and weight are above the normal range early in life but final adult heights are normal (i.e., near the 50th percentile); head circumference typically remains in the 50th percentile. Hemihypertrophy can be prominent.

- Macroglossia: May cause secondary feeding difficulties, speech problems, and obstructive sleep apnea
- Malignancy: Children with BWS are at greatly increased risk (5–10%) of hepatoblastoma and Wilms tumor, usually occurring in the first decade of life. The absolute risk of different types of malignancies and recurrence risk vary greatly depending on molecular subtype.
- Hypoglycemia: Elevated risk of hypoglycemia and hyperinsulinism
- Other major anomalies: Abdominal-wall defects, organomegaly, renal anomalies, and cardiac malformations can also occur
- Minor anomalies: Common facial features include anterior earlobe creases, posterior helical pits, small midface with large mandible, facial nevus flammeus, infraorbital creases, and macroglossia; these become less striking in adulthood.
- Development: Normal in most cases

DIAGNOSIS

- Molecular testing is diagnostic in some cases, with slightly greater yield when an affected tissue is sampled (e.g., skin fibroblasts from the side with hypertrophy). Methylation-sensitive multiplex-ligation probe analysis, or sequencing of multiple methylation sensitive areas affected, is the standard test.
- Genomewide testing: SNP rather than CGH array should be performed because SNP array can identify some cases due to uniparental disomy.

NOONAN SYNDROME

Genetic syndrome due to a defect in the RAS-MAPK pathway characterized by distinctive facial features, congenital heart anomalies, and short stature

EPIDEMIOLOGY

- Estimated prevalence: 1 in 1000 to 1 in 2500.

ETIOLOGY

Mutations in genes encoding RAS-MAPK pathway proteins (most commonly PTPN11) lead to overactivation of several different growth factor, cytokine, and hormone cell-signaling pathways.

CLINICAL CHARACTERISTICS

- Facial features: Hypertelorism, epicanthal folds, ptosis, downslanting palpebral fissures, short broad nose, webbed neck
- Growth: Normal birth weight and length followed by short stature, feeding difficulties, failure to thrive, delayed puberty
- Cardiac: Pulmonic stenosis, hypertrophic cardiomyopathy, atrial septal defects, etc.; 25% of patients die of heart failure in the first year.
- Hematologic: Coagulation defects, thrombocytopenia, myeloproliferative disorder
- Other: Hearing loss, cryptorchidism, male infertility, lymphatic abnormalities, chest deformities, widely spaced nipples, acid reflux, variable cognitive impairment

DIAGNOSIS

- Sequencing of genes in the RAS-MAPK pathway known to cause Noonan syndrome

PRADER–WILLI SYNDROME

Imprinting defect due to lack of expression from paternally derived chromosome 15q11.2-q13 resulting in profound hypotonia, neonatal feeding difficulties with later hyperphagia and obesity, and developmental delay

EPIDEMIOLOGY

• Prevalence: 1 in 10,000 to 1 in 30,000

ETIOLOGY

• Lack of expression of paternal genes from chromosome 15q11.2-q13, either from deletion of the region of paternally chromosome 15 (70%), maternal uniparental disomy 15 (25%), or imprinting defect (<5%)

CLINICAL CHARACTERISTICS

• Hypotonia: Neonatal hypotonia, which may be profound
• Feeding difficulty in infancy: Poor sucking and difficulty eating, often with failure to thrive as an infant
• Hyperphagia: After infancy period, hyperphagia predominates, with resultant obesity
• Endocrine: Short stature, pubertal delay, and small genitalia
• Sleep: Sleep apnea
• Neurodevelopment: Developmental delay, increased rate of autism spectrum disorder, skin picking, speech articulation defects
• Minor dysmorphic features: Characteristic facial features of almond-shaped eyes, narrow bifrontal diameter, narrow nasal bridge, and down-turned mouth with thin upper lip; small hands and feet

DIAGNOSIS

• Genetic testing should evaluate different mechanisms that can result in the phenotype, including methylation-sensitive PCR of 15q11.2-q13, SNP genomewide microarray to assess for microdeletion or maternal uniparental disomy, sequencing of imprinting center for defects

TRISOMY 21

Also known as "Down syndrome," a genetic condition caused by an additional copy of chromosome 21, characterized by hypotonia, CHD, and intellectual disability

EPIDEMIOLOGY

• Prevalence: 1 in 660 newborns; risk increases with increasing maternal age (see Table 11-1).

ETIOLOGY

• Caused by an additional copy of chromosome 21, by nondisjunction (94% with full trisomy 21, 2.4% with mosaic trisomy 21) or Robertsonian translocation (3.3%)
• Risk of recurrence low in nondysjunction (approximately 1%), high in Robertsonian translocation carriers

CLINICAL CHARACTERISTICS

Principle features in the neonate: Evaluation of a neonate for trisomy 21 should include systematic evaluation, rather than just relying on facial features. This is particularly important

right after birth, when facial features may be distorted. Features seen in most neonates with trisomy 21 include:

- Hypotonia (80%)
- Poor Moro reflex (85%)
- Hyperflexibility of the joints (80%)
- Excess skin on the back of the neck (80%)
- Flat facial profile (90%)
- Slanted palpebral fissures (80%)
- Anomalous auricles (60%)
- Dysplasia of pelvis (70%)
- Dysplasia of midphalynx of fifth finger (60%)
- Single transverse palmar crease (45%)

At least four features are found in 100%, and at least six features in 89% of neonates with trisomy 21.

- Congenital heart disease: Cardiac defect in 40% (most often endocardial cushion defect)
- Gastrointestinal tract abnormalities: Hirschsprung disease, duodenal atresia, tracheo-esophageal fistula, omphalocele, pyloric stenosis, annular pancreas, imperforate anus.
- Endocrine: Hypothyroidism
- Hematologic: Leukemia
- Skeletal: Atlantoaxial instability, hip dysplasia, avascular necrosis or slipped capital femoral epiphyses.
- Neurodevelopmental: Developmental delay, hearing loss

DIAGNOSIS

- Standard karyotype
- Accurate identification can often be made shortly after birth by physical characteristics, but standard karyotype should be done to confirm diagnosis and determine mode of inheritance for determination of recurrence risk

WILLIAMS SYNDROME

Second most common contiguous gene deletion syndrome, characterized by supravalvar aortic stenosis, hypercalcemia, feeding difficulties, outgoing personality, anxiety, and developmental delay.

EPIDEMIOLOGY

- Prevalence: 1 in 10,000

ETIOLOGY

- About 98% of patients have a classic 1.5- to 1.8-Mb deletion on chromosome 7q11.23, encompassing 26–28 genes.
- 2% have a smaller deletion with a milder phenotype.

CLINICAL CHARACTERISTICS

- Cardiac disease: Most commonly supravalvular aortic stenosis
- Growth: Failure to thrive in infancy with poor growth, should use Williams syndrome-specific growth charts
- Endocrine: Hypercalcemia
- Musculoskeletal: Joint laxity early in life; stiffness and joint contractures may develop.

- Neurodevelopment: Profound intellectual disability is common, with relatively preserved language, outgoing personality, and anxiety.
- Facial features: Delicate facial features with a low nasal bridge, described as "elfin facies"

DIAGNOSIS

- Genomewide microarray testing or multiplex ligation-dependent probe amplification is preferred for diagnosis, as FISH may miss children with atypical, nested deletions and duplications.

12 Hematology*

Esther Berko, MD, PhD
Kandace Gollomp, MD

ANEMIA

RED BLOOD CELL INDICES

- Hematocrit (HCT): Volume percentage of RBCs in blood. See **Table 12-1** for age-related normal levels
- Mean corpuscular volume (MCV): Average RBC volume
- Mean corpuscular hemoglobin (MCH): Average quantity of hemoglobin per RBC
- Mean corpuscular hemoglobin concentration (MCHC): Grams of hemoglobin per 100 mL of packed RBCs (amount of hemoglobin per unit volume)
- Red cell distribution width (RDW): Index of the variation in RBC size
- Reticulocyte count: Percentage of young RBCs in the plasma

DIFFERENTIAL DIAGNOSIS BASED ON MCV

Microcytic Anemia

- Iron deficiency, thalassemia, anemia of inflammation, lead poisoning, sideroblastic anemia, copper deficiency
- Iron deficiency versus thalassemia trait: RBC count and RDW are often normal in thalassemia trait; in iron deficiency, low RBC count and elevated RDW; Mentzer index (MCV/RBC) serves as a useful screen (<13 suggests thalassemia trait, >13 suggests iron deficiency).

Normocytic Anemia

- In normocytic anemia, assess the reticulocyte count. The reticulocyte index accurately reflects erythropoiesis by adjusting for the degree of anemia.
- Reticulocyte index (RI) = % Reticulocyte × Patient HCT/Normal HCT
- RI is greater than 3% in compensated bleeding or hemolysis and less than 2% in anemia owing to decreased RBC production; 1% is normal marrow activity without anemia.
- Reticulocytes low:
  ✓ Indicates hypoproductive process
  ✓ Pure RBC dysplasia (Diamond–Blackfan anemia)
  ✓ Transient erythroblastopenia of childhood
  ✓ Aplastic crisis (e.g., secondary to parvovirus B19 infection)
  ✓ Renal disease; acute bleeding (without compensation)
  ✓ Marrow infiltration (e.g., leukemia, solid tumor, hemophagocytosis, or myelofibrosis)

---

*The views expressed in this presentation are those of the authors and do not necessarily reflect the official policy or position of the Department of the Navy, Department of Defense, or the U.S. government.

†I am a military service member. This work was prepared as part of my official duties. Title 17, USC, §105 provides that "Copyright protection under this title is not available for any work of the U.S. Government." Title 17, USC, §101 defines a US Government work as a work prepared by a military service member or employee of the US Government as part of that person's official duties.

TABLE 12-1	Normal Hemoglobin, Hematocrit, and Mean Corpuscular Volume Values by Age		
Age	Hemoglobin (g/dL)*	Hematocrit (%)*	MCV (Mean −2 SD)
Newborn	16.8 (13.7–20.1)	55 (45–65)	108 (98)
2 weeks	16.5 (13.0–20.0)	50 (42–66)	105 (86)
3 months	12.0 (9.5–14.5)	36 (31–41)	91 (74)
6 months–2 years	12.0 (10.5–14.0)	37 (33–42)	78 (70)
7–12 years	13.0 (11.0–16.0)	38 (34–40)	86 (77)
Women (adult)	14.0 (12.0–16.0)	42 (37–47)	90 (80)
Men (adult)	16.0 (14.0–18.0)	47 (42–52)	90 (80)

*Mean values with ranges in parentheses.
MCV = mean corpuscular volume.
Note: These data have been compiled from several sources.

✓ Marrow aplasia (aplastic anemia)
✓ Hormone deficiencies (e.g., hypothyroidism or growth hormone deficiency)
✓ Anemia of inflammation
- Reticulocytes high:
  ✓ Chronic blood loss with compensatory erythropoiesis
  ✓ Extrinsic hemolysis: Antibody-mediated hemolysis (e.g., auto- or drug-induced), DIC, HUS, TTP, prosthetic heart valve, vitamin E deficiency, Wilson disease, liver disease, renal disease, burns
  ✓ Intrinsic hemolysis: Membrane disorders (e.g., hereditary spherocytosis), enzyme deficiencies (e.g., G6PD), hemoglobin disorders (e.g., sickle cell disease)

Macrocytic Anemia

- Folic acid deficiency, vitamin B_{12} deficiency, normal newborn (MCV, 100–125), trisomy 21, medications (e.g., valproate, trimethoprim–sulfamethoxazole, hydroxyurea, azathioprine), bone marrow failure (e.g., Fanconi anemia), dyserythropoietic anemia, hypothyroidism, liver disease, inborn errors of metabolism (e.g., orotic aciduria, Lesch–Nyhan syndrome)
- To evaluate for nutritional deficiencies causing macrocytic anemia, consider obtaining RBC or serum folate, MMA, and homocysteine:
  ✓ B_{12} is a cofactor in the metabolism of MMA and homocysteine, and both are therefore elevated in vitamin B_{12} deficiency.

IRON DEFICIENCY ANEMIA

Microcytic anemia with a decreased reticulocyte count and increased RDW due to a deficiency of iron

ETIOLOGY

- Inadequate oral intake: Malnutrition, dietary restriction, or excessive/exclusive cow's milk intake typically in toddlers. The most common cause in children ages 1–3 years is dietary.
- Inadequate iron absorption: Loss or dysfunction of absorptive enterocytes (celiac disease, inflammatory bowel disease, bowel resection, or rare genetic defects in intestinal iron uptake)

- Excessive blood loss: Gastrointestinal blood loss (Meckel diverticulum, gastritis, ulcer, vascular malformation, varices, inflammatory bowel disease, tumor (rare in children), parasitic infection, cow's milk–induced enteropathy), hematuria, menstrual blood loss, other excessive bleeding (epistaxis), idiopathic pulmonary hemosiderosis
- Increased iron demand: Neonatal growth, adolescent growth, pregnancy

PATHOPHYSIOLOGY

- Iron is required for heme synthesis as well as for other systemic enzymes (i.e., cytochromes).

CLINICAL PRESENTATION

- Mild or moderate iron deficiency may have few overt symptoms
- Progressive pallor, irritability, difficulty sleeping, shortness of breath, headaches, fatigue, pica (including pagophagia [ice chewing])
- In toddlers, a history of drinking greater than 24 ounces of cow's milk a day or transition to cow's milk before 12 months is common.

DIAGNOSTICS

- CBC with reticulocyte count. MCV and reticulocyte count will be low. Thrombocytosis or thrombocytopenia may also occur.
- Smear: hypochromic microcytic RBC with pencil forms
- Iron studies: High TIBC, low transferrin, and low ferritin (first value to recover with iron supplementation). Of note, ferritin is an acute-phase reactant and can be elevated in inflammatory conditions. The plasma iron level indicates recent intake and does not accurately reflect iron stores.

MANAGEMENT

- Iron deficiency is always secondary to an underlying cause. It is imperative that the etiology is determined in concert with iron replacement.
- Oral iron: 4–6 mg/kg/day of elemental iron in two to three divided doses. Best absorption occurs with intake of high ascorbic acid foods like orange juice; do not administer with milk.
- Continue iron for 8–12 weeks after the Hb has normalized (total of 3–4 months of replacement)
- For toddlers with excessive mild intake make dietary changes: Limit milk intake (≤8 ounces per day); only offer milk once the child has eaten a meal, stop using the bottle (if appropriate), increase intake of iron-rich foods.
- Response to therapy: Reticulocyte count will start to increase in 2–3 days, increase in Hb in 1 week, normalization in Hb within 4–6 weeks, normalization of RDW after 3 months of therapy.
- Consider IV iron in patients with poor enteral absorption (i.e., inflammatory bowel disease) or inability to tolerate oral iron supplementation

THALASSEMIAS

The thalassemias encompass a group of inherited disorders of hemoglobin synthesis that involve decreased or defective synthesis of one or more globin chains. Thalassemias are named after the affected globin chain, with α- and β-thalassemia being the most common and clinically important types. Imbalances of globin chains can lead to impaired erythropoiesis and increased hemolysis, resulting in a hypoproductive microcytic anemia.

β-Thalassemia is usually the result of point mutations that lead to impaired β-globulin production. The notation β^+ indicates decreased production, while β^0 indicates absent

production. The clinical phenotype depends on the combination of the normal (β) or abnormal (β^+ or β^0) alleles. The terms β-thalassemia intermedia and β-thalassemia major are clinical designations based on the severity of anemia and the need for transfusions.

- β-Thalassemia trait (β^+/β or β^0/β): Heterozygous condition (one copy), causes a mild reduction in β-chain synthesis with a resultant mild microcytic anemia
- β-Thalassemia intermedia (β^+/β^+ or β^0/β^+): Homozygous condition that results in markedly reduced β-chain synthesis and moderate anemia that will occasionally require transfusion
- β-Thalassemia major (β^0/β^0 or β^0/β^+): Homozygous condition with no detectable to severely reduced β-chain production resulting in a severe microcytic hypochromic anemia that requires lifelong RBC transfusions (a.k.a. Cooley anemia)

α-Thalassemia is usually due to large deletions that result in impaired α-globulin production. There are two α-globin genes on each chromosome and, therefore, four different forms of inherited conditions.

- Silent carrier: Loss of one α gene ($-\alpha/\alpha\alpha$), with minimal effect on hemoglobin production
- α-thalassemia trait: can occur in two configurations, trans ($-\alpha/-\alpha$) or cis ($--/\alpha\alpha$). Trans deletions are common in patients of african descent.
- HbH (β4) disease: Deficient in three α genes ($-\alpha/--$), with tetrameric β-chain production (HbH) that results in a microcytic hemolytic anemia with variable severity
- Hydrops fetalis: Deficient in all four α genes ($--/--$); not compatible with life; in utero, the fetus develops hydrops fetalis.

CLINICAL MANIFESTATIONS

- α- and β-thalassemia trait: Mild microcytic anemia, asymptomatic
- HbH: Moderate hemolytic anemia, jaundice, hepatosplenomegaly, gallstones, occasional need for transfusions during illness
- β-Thalassemia intermedia: Moderate hemolytic anemia (Hb >7 g/dL), splenomegaly, intermittent transfusion requirement
- Beta-thalassemia major: Massive hepatosplenomegaly, growth retardation, bony deformities including frontal bossing and maxillary prominence from extramedullary hematopoiesis (all preventable with aggressive transfusion therapy)
- If iron overload from chronic transfusions is not adequately treated with chelation therapy, patients can develop cirrhosis, endocrine abnormalities, cardiac dysfunction, and skin hyperpigmentation

DIAGNOSTICS

- Hematologic parameters vary depending on severity of condition
- α-Thalassemia trait: Mild microcytic anemia, normal levels of HbA, HbA$_2$, and HbF; +Hb Barts (γ-chain tetramer) on newborn screen
- β-Thalassemia trait: Mild microcytic anemia. HbA$_2$ level 3.5–8%; HbF level 1–5%, but significant variability depending on type of mutation. May not be detected on newborn screen.
- HbH: Moderate hypochromic, microcytic anemia (Hb 7–10 g/dL); Variation in RBC shape and size on peripheral-blood smear and other findings of chronic hemolysis, reticulocytosis, HbH (β_4) on electrophoresis. Newborn screen >25% Hb Barts
- β-Thalassemia intermedia (β^+/β^+ or β^0/β^+): Clinical designation based on having a moderate microcytic anemia, Hb > 7 g/dL, that only necessitates intermittent transfusion with normal growth
- β-Thalassemia major (β^0/β^0 or β^0/β^+): Clinical designation with a resultant severe anemia (Hb 3–7 g/dL); reticulocytosis; HbF 30–100%; HbA$_2$ 2–7%; MCV 50–60 fL. The newborn screen will demonstrate only HbF in patients without any β-hemoglobin chain production.

MANAGEMENT

- No intervention for α- or β-thalassemia trait
- Folic acid supplementation for those with HbH
- Chronic transfusion therapy for β-thalassemia major may be required as early as 2 months, but necessary by 2 years; 10–15 mL/kg of packed RBCs required every 3–4 weeks; goal pretransfusion hemoglobin 9.0–10 g/dL
- Chelation therapy for chronically transfused patients with iron overload; oral/SC/IV chelators available and necessary 5–7 days per week
- In patients receiving chronic transfusion, ferritin levels should be monitored to screen for iron overload, but annual MRI should be used to more accurately assess cardiac and liver iron concentrations and guide chelation therapy.
- Stem cell transplantation is currently the only curative therapy for thalassemia.

HEMOLYTIC ANEMIA

Disorders in which RBCs are destroyed because of intrinsic RBC defects or immune-mediated destruction. These anemias are characterized by an elevated reticulocyte count with high unconjugated bilirubin and elevated LDH.

G6PD DEFICIENCY

Deficiency in the major enzyme in the hexose monophosphate shunt; results in a decrease in the oxidative protective mechanism of the RBC. An oxidative stress may cause RBC hemolysis.

EPIDEMIOLOGY

- X-linked inheritance; most common enzyme deficiency, affects more than 500 million people worldwide (African, Mediterranean, and Asian origins)
- African American (10–15% affected) variant is less severe than Mediterranean variant

CLINICAL MANIFESTATIONS

- Neonatal jaundice (further discussed in "Management" section)
- For milder forms patients are clinically and hematologically normal until they have an "oxidative challenge." Severe forms can have a baseline hemolytic anemia.
- 6–24 hours after exposure to oxidative agent: Dark urine, jaundice, pallor, tachycardia, nausea, abdominal pain
- 24–48 hours: Low-grade fever, irritability, listlessness, splenomegaly, and hepatomegaly

DIAGNOSTICS

- G6PD quantitation: The G6PD concentration is highest in young RBCs, so the presence of reticulocytosis can lead to overestimation of true G6PD level.
- Can be confirmed genetically. Many newborn screens already genetically test for the five most common mutations.

During Hemolytic Episode:

- Normocytic, normochromic anemia with reticulocytosis
- Smear: Anisocytosis (reflected by increased RDW), spherocytosis, blister cells, Heinz bodies on supravital staining with methyl violet (precipitates of denatured hemoglobin)
- Elevated unconjugated bilirubin
- Urine dipstick positive bilirubin
- Direct antiglobulin test (DAT) negative (excludes autoimmune hemolysis)

MANAGEMENT

- Avoid oxidative stressors including sulfonamides, fava beans, mothballs containing naphthalene, or certain antimalarial agents (primaquine, pamaquine, chloroquine)
- Most episodes of acute hemolysis are self-limited with hemoglobin returning to normal within 3–6 weeks
- If hemoglobin greater than 7 mg/dL and clinically stable and no hemoglobinuria, observe closely for 24–48 hours. If hemoglobin less than 7 mg/dL or between 7 and 9 mg/dL with continued brisk hemolysis (persistent hemoglobinuria), consider packed RBC transfusion (see Transfusion Medicine section)
- Management of neonatal jaundice associated with G6PD deficiency similar to approach for other causes of neonatal jaundice. Initiate prompt phototherapy per neonatal guidelines. Infants with the more severe type may require exchange transfusion to prevent kernicterus (more common in Mediterranean and Asian variants)

HEREDITARY SPHEROCYTOSIS (HS)

Disorder of the RBC membrane resulting in a decreased membrane surface area to intracellular volume ratio

EPIDEMIOLOGY

- Most common in people of northern European heritage
- 75% inherited (two-thirds as autosomal dominant) and 25% new mutations

PATHOPHYSIOLOGY

- Defect or deficiency of red-cell skeletal proteins (ankyrin, spectrin)
- Decreased deformability of the RBCs due to membrane loss results in sequestration in the spleen and depletion of membrane lipid results in spherocytes and premature destruction of RBCs

CLINICAL MANIFESTATIONS

- Anemia: Mild to severe; patients may have hyperhemolytic periods and are susceptible to an aplastic crisis from parvovirus infection.
- Jaundice, splenomegaly, gallstones
- 50% of HS patients present in the newborn period with jaundice.

DIAGNOSTICS

- Normocytic hemolytic anemia with increased reticulocyte count, high RDW, and MCHC
- Smear: Spherocytes, anisocytosis, polychromasia
- HS-EMA (eosin-5′-maleimide) binding assay: A flow cytometry assay with improved sensitivity and specificity over the osmotic fragility test for detecting hereditary spherocytosis

MANAGEMENT

- Daily folic acid supplementation
- Splenectomy: For severe cases (i.e., failure to thrive or recurrent transfusions). This stops red-cell destruction in the spleen and lengthens the red-cell lifespan. If possible, delay splenectomy until the patient is 5 years of age or older to decrease risk of infection.
- Transfusion support if needed

SICKLE CELL DISEASE

Sickle cell disease (SCD) is a group of inherited hemoglobinopathies secondary to the production of abnormal hemoglobin complicated with an associated hemolytic anemia and vaso-occlusion. Normal adult hemoglobin (HbA) is composed of four polypeptide globulin chains ($2\alpha2\beta$). Sickle cell disease results from a genetic mutation in both β-globulin genes, with at least one mutation resulting in HbS. Homozygous SS is the most common form of SCD and is the most severe. Additional forms of SCD include compound heterozygous states in which HbS is combined with either another abnormal hemoglobin or a β-thalassemia mutation (e.g., HbC, HbE, beta-plus (β^+) thalassemia, or beta-zero (β^0) thalassemia).

EPIDEMIOLOGY

- Sickle cell trait, present in up to 8% of African Americans, is the heterozygous state where one gene produces normal beta globin and the other produces HbS resulting in a primarily asymptomatic carrier.
- SCD occurs in approximately 1 in 365 African American infants and is thought to affect 100,000 individuals in the United States.

PATHOPHYSIOLOGY

- Point mutations in the beta-globin gene yield hemoglobin that is prone to polymerization, causing red cells to "sickle" taking on an elongated, rigid shape.
- Sickle cells obstruct the microvasculature and cause microinfarcts that lead to endothelial injury, painful vaso-occlusive episodes, and end-organ damage to the spleen, bones, kidneys, lungs, and brain.

CLINICAL COMPLICATIONS AND MANAGEMENT

Painful episodes:

- Definition: Vaso-occlusive event resulting in an acute onset of severe pain commonly in the back, chest and extremities; can result in swelling of the hands and feet in infants (dactylitis).
- Management: Patients may be treated as outpatients with oral medications (antiinflammatory drug with or without an oral opioid) and hydration; severe pain not responsive to oral pain medications requires hospitalization, appropriate pain control includes a combination of an antiinflammatory agent such as ibuprofen or ketorolac (IV) with an opioid, and IV hydration.

Fever:

- Definition: Temperature >38.5°C. Patients with SCD are more susceptible to bacterial infections because of functional asplenia. They are at highest risk for sepsis from encapsulated organisms, such as *Streptococcus pneumoniae*, *Neisseria meningitidis*, and *Salmonella*.
- Management: All patients with SCD and fever need to be urgently evaluated with a physical examination, blood culture, CBC with differential and a reticulocyte count; consider a urine culture, chest x-ray (dependent on age and symptoms); administration of antibiotics (ceftriaxone or high-dose ampicillin) with observation.
- To prevent bacterial infections, children with SCD should be vaccinated (pneumococcal conjugate vaccine [PCV13] and the 23-valent pneumococcal polysaccharide vaccine, as well as meningococcal vaccination) and take prophylactic penicillin.

Splenic sequestration:

- Definition: Intrasplenic trapping of RBCs and platelets
- Clinical manifestations: A decrease in hemoglobin and often platelets with an acute enlargement of the spleen that can lead to life-threatening anemia; in SCD-SS approximately 30% will have an episode by 5 years of age; often associated with acute viral/bacterial illnesses; in milder forms of SCD, such as SCD-SC or SCD-Sβ^+-thalassemia, splenic sequestration can occur at an older age. Patients with SCD-SS treated with hydroxyurea from a young age may have delayed splenic auto-infarction and may develop splenic sequestration at older ages.
- Management: Follow the hemoglobin and spleen size closely. Administration of fluids may be helpful in clinically stable patients with a mild decrease in hemoglobin. If splenomegaly and anemia result in hypoxia, tachypnea, or significant tachycardia, then transfuse with RBCs (5–10 mL/kg), then reassess. RBC transfusion causes remobilization of sequestered blood, resulting in a higher posttransfusion hemoglobin than expected from the transfused blood alone.

Acute chest syndrome:

- Definition/clinical manifestations: Clinical diagnosis based on the findings of fever, respiratory symptoms, and a new pulmonary infiltrate on chest x-ray (radiologic findings can lag behind the clinical symptoms). Causes include bacterial infection (*Mycoplasma pneumoniae*, *Chlamydia pneumoniae*, *Staphylococcus aureus*, *S. pneumoniae*, or *Haemophilus influenzae*), viral infection, fat emboli, in situ vaso-occlusion, pulmonary edema, or thromboembolism.
- Management: Antibiotics—ampicillin or a third-generation cephalosporin (cefotaxime or ceftriaxone), a macrolide (erythromycin, azithromycin, or clarithromycin), and oxygen if hypoxic; pain control; incentive spirometry; RBC transfusion (simple or exchange) for respiratory or hemodynamic instability. May require intensive care monitoring.

Aplastic crisis:

- Definition: Marked anemia with reticulocytopenia, frequently secondary to parvovirus infection, that causes a maturation arrest of RBC production in the bone marrow for 1–2 weeks. Patients with SCD are dependent on their high reticulocyte count to maintain their hemoglobin secondary to their shortened RBC lifespan (10–20 days in SCD-SS vs. 120 days in patients without hemolysis).
- Clinical manifestations: Increased fatigue, pallor, fever. Reticulocytopenia begins approximately 5 days after exposure and continues for 7–10 days.
- Management: Packed RBC transfusion may be necessary if the patient is symptomatic

Stroke:

- Children with SCD-SS and Sβ^0-thalassemia have a 10% risk of stroke by 20 years of age. The predominant etiology is a large-vessel vasculopathy with proliferative intimal hyperplasia.
- Clinical manifestations: Hemiparesis, facial droop, aphasia, generalized symptoms such as mental status changes, stupor, or seizures
- Management:
  ✓ Head MRI or CT Scan (if MRI is not available);
  ✓ Immediately obtain a CBC with reticulocyte count, hemoglobin electrophoresis to assess HbS percentage, and type and screen.
  ✓ Principle treatment is exchange transfusion to decrease percent HbS.
  ✓ Long term: Placed on a chronic RBC transfusion protocol to minimize the risk for further strokes.

- Stroke prevention is possible through routine transcranial Doppler imaging, which measures the velocity of cerebral blood flow and detects those children who are at an increased risk for a first stroke.
- Children with persistently elevated transcranial Doppler measurements are placed on a chronic RBC transfusion protocol to prevent stroke. After an appropriate period of transfusions, some of these patients can be transitioned to hydroxyurea.

DIAGNOSTIC TESTS

- Often diagnosed on newborn screen and family history
- Hemoglobin electrophoresis will show presence of S or C hemoglobin; should be confirmed genetically with sequencing of B globin genes.

PREVENTIVE MANAGEMENT

- Penicillin prophylaxis for coverage of encapsulated organisms due to functional asplenia
- Folic acid supplementation to support increased rate of erythropoiesis
- Hydroxyurea therapy increases hemoglobin levels by increasing hemoglobin F production. When adherent, patients develop a rise in MCV. Leads to decreased frequency of pain crises and may help prevent the development of vasculopathy. Recommended for all patients with SCD-SS older than 9 months.

AUTOIMMINUE HEMOLYTIC ANEMIA (AIHA)

Formation of autoantibodies to components of RBC surface antigens that leads to hemolysis

EPIDEMIOLOGY

- The incidence is approximately 1 in 100,000 to 3 in 100,000 persons per year.
- Peak incidence in childhood in the first 4 years of life, most commonly due to warm AIHA.

ETIOLOGY

- In neonates, occurs due to passive transfer of maternal antibodies
- Often secondary to an underlying virus (e.g. *Mycoplasma,* Epstein–Barr virus, cytomegalovirus, hepatitis, HIV) or bacterial infection (e.g., *Streptococcus,* typhoid, *Escherichia coli*)
- Drug-induced: Antimalarials, antipyretic, sulfonamides, penicillin, ceftriaxone, rifampin
- Can be associated with hematologic malignancy (leukemia, lymphoma) and some solid tumors
- Autoimmune disorders: Lupus, mixed connective tissue disorder, rheumatoid arthritis, common variable immune deficiency, Evan's syndrome, autoimmune lymphoproliferative disorder (ALPS)
- May occur following hematopoietic stem-cell transplantation or solid-organ transplant due to alloimmunity or the effects of immunosuppression

PATHOPHYSIOLOGY

- Warm autoantibodies (~80% of cases): IgG antibodies with maximal activity at 37°C bind to RBC antigens, leading them to be cleared extravascularly by splenic macrophages.
- Cold autoantibodies or cold agglutinin disease (~7–25% of cases): IgM antibodies with maximal activity in vitro at 0–30°C bind to RBC antigens leading to complement-fixation that induces intravascular hemolysis. Commonly associated with *Mycoplasma* infection.
- Paroxysmal cold hemoglobinuria (PCH): IgG directed against the RBC P-antigen (Donath–Landsteiner antibody) fixes complement at cooler areas (i.e., extremities) leading to intravascular hemolysis when coated RBCs return to warmer areas of the body

CLINICAL MANIFESTATIONS

- Patients may develop fatigue, pallor, and jaundice, as well as dark urine
- Exam findings include hepatosplenomegaly, tachycardia, systolic flow murmur, orthostasis.

DIAGNOSTIC TESTS

- Labs are typical of hemolytic process: falling hemoglobin, elevated reticulocyte count, elevated LDH, hyperbilirubinemia, increased AST
- Urinalysis will show large blood but few RBCs, indicating hemoglobinuria
- Positive DAT (direct Coomb's test) is diagnostic:
  - ✓ Warm AIHA: IgG detected on RBC surface with or without complement (C3)
  - ✓ Cold AIHA and PCH: C3 detected on RBC surface

MANAGEMENT

- MEDICAL EMERGENCY: As hemoglobin falls rapidly, patients may become hemodynamically unstable. Must initiate treatment promptly.
- RBC transfusion: Although fully cross-matched blood may not be possible, transfusions should be given to patients with life-threatening anemia or rapid hemolysis. Clinicians should communicate with the transfusion service to coordinate.
- Immunosuppression:
  - ✓ Corticosteroids: Treat severe cases with IV methylprednisolone 1–4 mg/kg/day divided every 6–8 hours. Transition to oral prednisone 1–2 mg/kg/day divided over 2–3 days, maintained for 2–3 weeks until hemoglobin stabilizes, followed by gradual taper.
  - ✓ Second-line treatments: Used in patients who cannot tolerate steroids or experience relapse with weaning. Include rituximab, mycophenolate mofetil, sirolimus, and splenectomy.

TRANSIENT ERYTHROBLASTOPENIA OF CHILDHOOD

An acquired, self-limited anemia in a previously healthy child characterized by bone marrow erythroblastopenia, which can be severe

ETIOLOGY

- Unknown; often preceded by viral illness (can be 1–2 months prior to presentation)

EPIDEMIOLOGY

- Age at onset: 6 months–4 years (80% are >1 year at diagnosis)

CLINICAL MANIFESTATIONS

- Gradually progressive pallor in an otherwise healthy child
- No organomegaly, ecchymosis, petechiae, or jaundice
- Spontaneous recovery within 1–2 months

DIAGNOSTICS

- Diagnosis of exclusion
- Hb level: 3–8 g/dL (normocytic and normochromic)
- Low reticulocyte count
- White blood cell and platelet counts typically normal
- Neutropenia (ANC <1000/mm^3) in 10% of cases
- Bone marrow: Decreased RBC precursors (not required for diagnosis)

MANAGEMENT

- Transfusions for symptomatic anemia (see "Transfusion Medicine" section)
- Recovery typically occurs within 1–2 months but in rare cases may take as long as 12 months
- Neutropenia
  - ✓ Decreased ANC. For Caucasian and Asian children, neutropenia is defined as ANC <1500 cells/µL for those over 1 year and <1000 cells/µL for children under 1 year.
  - ✓ 5% of children of African descent have benign ethnic neutropenia with a baseline ANC <1500 cells/µL. This finding does not lead to an increased risk of infection.
  - ✓ For all patients, severe neutropenia is defined as an ANC <500 cells/µL

DIFFERENTIAL DIAGNOSIS

- Benign ethnic neutropenia, viral suppression, AIN, SCN, cyclic neutropenia, neonatal immune neutropenia (can be either alloimmune or autoimmune), medication effect, hypothyroidism, nutritional deficiency (vitamin B_{12}, folate, copper), bone marrow failure syndromes, glycogen storage disease 1b, immunodeficiency syndromes, hematologic malignancy

COMMON CAUSES

- Autoimmune neutropenia:
  - ✓ Epidemiology: AIN is the most common chronic neutropenia of childhood. It typically presents in the first 2 years of life, occurring in approximately 1 in 6300 children. Neutropenia in children older than 5 is more likely to be due to secondary causes such as autoimmune conditions.
  - ✓ Pathophysiology: The development of autoantibodies directed against neutrophil surface antigens leads to their clearance primarily by splenic macrophages. During infection, many patients release a high number of neutrophils from the marrow that overwhelm their antineutrophil antibodies, causing a transient rise in the ANC.
  - ✓ Diagnosis: Physical exam is usually unremarkable, without dysmorphic features, growth retardation, or organomegaly. History may include recurrent oral ulcerations, frequent episodes of otitis media, or upper respiratory infections, but children with AIN rarely develop severe bacterial infections. Antineutrophil antibody testing can confirm the diagnosis, but the test is limited by low sensitivity. A bone marrow biopsy is not required for patients with a typical presentation.
  - ✓ Management: AIN typically has a benign course, with spontaneous resolution in >95% of patients. Conservative management is sufficient for most patients. G-CSF can be used to raise the ANC in the rare child who develops a serious bacterial infection. It may also be used prior to surgery to minimize infection risk by temporarily raising the ANC.
- Severe congenital neutropenia (SCN): Also known as Kostmann syndrome, this is a heterogeneous group of conditions that lead to persistent severe neutropenia (ANC <500), with an increased risk of life-threatening bacterial infections; 20–30% of these patients develop myelodysplastic syndromes or leukemia.
  - ✓ Pathophysiology: Genetic mutations in genes such as *ELANE* and *HAX1* cause a maturational arrest that leads to reduced production of neutrophils.
  - ✓ Diagnosis: Physical exam may show dysmorphic features and growth failure, history may include deep-tissue infections, pneumonias, and sepsis. A bone marrow biopsy will likely reveal a neutrophil maturational arrest at the promyelocyte phase. Genetic testing can identify the causative mutation in most cases.
  - ✓ Management: Treatment varies depending on the underlying cause. Some patients will respond to G-CSF; others will require a hematopoietic-cell transplantation as curative therapy.

- Cyclic neutropenia: A rare autosomal dominant disorder that causes patients to develop recurrent 3- to 5-day periods of severe neutropenia regularly over 3-week intervals
  - ✓ Pathophysiology: 80% of cases occur due to mutations in the neutrophil elastase gene (*ELANE*), leading to cyclic episodes of accelerated myeloid cell death.
  - ✓ Diagnosis: Patients usually present with recurrent episodes of severe neutropenia that may be associated with oral ulcers, fevers, lymphadenopathy and bacterial infections. Serial blood counts (two to three times a week over 6 weeks) is the gold standard for diagnosis. Genetic testing for *ELANE* mutations is also valuable.
  - ✓ Management: Most patients are treated conservatively, but those with recurrent infections or recurrent painful oral ulcerations can be treated with G-CSF.

THROMBOCYTOPENIA

DIFFERENTIAL DIAGNOSIS

INCREASED PLATELET DESTRUCTION

- Immune thrombocytopenia purpura (ITP), DIC, neonatal alloimmune thrombocytopenia, HUS, artificial heart valves or grafts, uremia, Kasabach–Merritt syndrome (see Chapter 6), TTP, other immune-mediated thrombocytopenias (human immunodeficiency virus [HIV], systemic lupus erythematosus), sepsis
- Medication-induced: Aspirin, nitrofurantoin, heparin, sympathetic blockers, clofibrate, nonsteroidal antiinflammatory drugs (NSAIDs), sulfonamides, penicillin, quinidine, quinine, digoxin, procainamide, methyldopa, phenytoin, valproic acid, barbiturates, gold, cimetidine, ranitidine

DECREASED PLATELET PRODUCTION

- Hereditary thrombocytopenias: Thrombocytopenia-absent radii syndrome, congenital amegakaryocytic thrombocytopenia, Wiskott–Aldrich syndrome, Fanconi anemia, trisomy 13, trisomy 18, inherited giant platelet disorders, DiGeorge syndrome
- Marrow infiltration: Acute lymphocytic leukemia, histiocytosis, lymphomas, neuroblastoma, storage diseases, marrow failure, aplastic anemia
- Medications: Thiazide diuretics, chemotherapeutic agents, alcoholism, estrogen, furosemide, trimethoprim–sulfamethoxazole
- Infection-induced: Cytomegalovirus, Epstein–Barr virus, varicella, rubella, rubeola, mumps, parvovirus B19, tuberculosis, typhoid

PLATELET SEQUESTRATION

- Splenomegaly, hypothermia, burns

OTHER

- Pseudothrombocytopenia—platelet clumping induced by ethylenediaminetetraacetic acid (EDTA). Clumping can be identified on peripheral-blood smear. Thrombocytopenia should resolve when blood is collected in citrated tubes.

IMMUNE THROMBOCYTOPENIA

DEFINITION

- An autoimmune disorder characterized by thrombocytopenia and associated mucocutaneous bleeding.
- Chronic ITP is defined as platelet counts of <100,000/μL that persist for more than 12 months after presentation.

EPIDEMIOLOGY

- Frequency: 1.9–6.4 cases per 100,000 children per year
- Peak age: 5 years; range, 2–6 years; males affected more frequently during young childhood, females affected more commonly in older childhood and adolescence
- About 80% resolve within 6 months.

PATHOPHYSIOLOGY

- Autoantibodies (IgG) to multiple membrane glycoproteins on the surface of platelets and megakaryocytes
- Autoantibody-coated platelets are cleared by opsonization and phagocytosis primarily in the spleen, but also throughout the reticuloendothelial system

CLINICAL MANIFESTATIONS

- Sudden onset of widespread bruising, petechiae and/or purpura, typically days or weeks after a viral illness. Some patients develop mucosal bleeding symptoms, including epistaxis, wet purpura, and gastrointestinal bleeding
- Intracranial hemorrhage is rare; incidence is 0.1–0.5%.

DIAGNOSIS

- History and physical examination
- CBC with isolated severe thrombocytopenia. Immature platelet fraction should be elevated as the marrow tries to compensate for increased peripheral destruction of platelets.
- Peripheral-blood smear with normal red and white cell morphology and few observed platelets. Those that are seen may be enlarged.
- Bone marrow aspiration may be helpful in atypical cases. It is not routinely recommended for the diagnosis of ITP.
- ITP is a diagnosis of exclusion. Other causes of thrombocytopenia need to be considered (see "Differential Diagnosis" section in section on "Thrombocytopenia").

MANAGEMENT

- There is little evidence that treatment changes the long-term outcome. Cases of no to mild bleeding (skin bleeding only) may be managed with observation only, regardless of the platelet count. Treatment should be considered in patients with significant bleeding symptoms (e.g., mucosal, gastrointestinal, menstrual). The goal of treatment is to obtain adequate hemostasis.
- First-line therapy:
  ✓ Intravenous immunoglobulin: Is thought to work by saturating Fc receptors on cells in the MPS, preventing platelet clearance. Treat with 1 g/kg/day for 1–2 days; improves platelet count in 75% of patients within 48 hours (usually does not increase until 24 hours after first dose given); premedicate with acetaminophen and diphenhydramine to decrease side effects (flu-like symptoms and headache are common; aseptic meningitis occurs rarely).
  ✓ Anti-D (WinRho): Binds to RBC surface in RhoD-positive patients; opsonized RBCs saturate cells in the MPS and prevent phagocytosis of platelets. Administer 50–75 mcg/kg; generally tolerated well; side effects include extravascular hemolysis (mean decreased hemoglobin of 1–2 g/dL); rare intravascular hemolysis or DIC. Should not be given to patients with anemia, evidence of bleeding, autoimmune hemolysis, or signs of infection.
  ✓ Corticosteroids: Multiple dosing strategies are reported. The most common is 1 mg/kg/day (maximum, 60–80 mg) of prednisone for 2–4 weeks followed by a taper. Briefer higher dosing regimens have also been found to be effective, as has treatment with dexamethasone

- Second-line therapy:
  - ✓ Splenectomy: The spleen is the major site of platelet phagocytosis and autoantibody production, and 80% of patients have improvement in platelet counts after surgery. However, splenectomy leads to increased risk of infection, thrombosis, and pulmonary hypertension. In children, surgery should be deferred for 12 months after diagnosis and should be used only in patients with refractory bleeding symptoms.
  - ✓ Rituximab: Anti-CD20 antibody that leads to temporary clearance of mature B lymphocytes. 60% of patients respond to treatment. It can induce prolonged hypogammaglobulinemia, and baseline immunoglobulin levels should be obtained
  - ✓ TPO-RAs: Mimic the effect of the cytokine, TPO, which stimulates megakaryocytes to produce platelets. Eltrombopag and Romiplostim are now both FDA-approved for use in children and are effective in the majority of patients
- Other agents: MMF, azathioprine, cyclophosphamide, cyclosporine, sirolimus, vincristine, danazol, dapsone

BLEEDING DISORDERS

COAGULATION STUDIES

Activated partial thromboplastin time (aPTT): Measures the intrinsic clotting system, which includes factors V, VIII, IX, X, XI, XII, fibrinogen, prothrombin, and the other contact factors

Prothrombin time (PT): Measures the extrinsic clotting system which includes factor V, VII, X, fibrinogen, and prothrombin (standardized with the international normalized ratio [INR])

Thrombin time: Measures the final step of the coagulation cascade with the conversion of fibrinogen to fibrin

Bleeding time (Rarely used because of its low sensitivity.): Evaluates platelet plug formation Differential diagnosis for abnormal PT and/or PTT: Usually due to insufficient sample volume, as the laboratory test is dependent on the ratio of blood to preservative in the collection tube. When real, abnormal coagulation values can result from factor-specific deficiencies (like hemophilia), nutritional deficiencies (vitamin K), organ dysfunction (liver disease) or systemic illness (DIC). Clinical history and relevant factor levels can help with diagnosis, as detailed in the **Table 12-2**. Factors II, VII, IX, and X are vitamin K–dependent. All factors other than VIII are synthesized in the liver. Factor VII has the shortest half-life of all factors.

HEMOPHILIA

Bleeding disorder affecting primarily males that results from an inherited deficiency of either factor VIII (hemophilia A) or IX (hemophilia B)

TABLE 12-2	Factor Levels with Different Causes of Abnormal Coagulation		
	Vitamin K Deficiency	**Liver Disease**	**Disseminated Intravascular Coagulation**
Factor V	Normal	Decreased	Decreased
Factor VII	Decreased	Decreased	Decreased
Factor VIII	Normal	Normal	Decreased
Factor X	Decreased	Decreased	Decreased

EPIDEMIOLOGY

- Hemophilia A: 1 in 5000 live male births (85%)
- Hemophilia B: 1 in 30,000 live male births (15%)
- Both are X-linked recessive; 30% spontaneous mutation rate

PATHOPHYSIOLOGY

- Factors VIII and IX participate in the activation of factor X.
- Factor Xa converts prothrombin to thrombin, which can then cleave fibrinogen to fibrin, leading to clot formation.
- Deficiency of either factor VIII or IX results in impaired clot formation.

CLINICAL MANIFESTATIONS

- Hemophilia A and B are clinically indistinguishable
- Three major classifications (bleeding related to amount of residual factor clotting activity present): Less than 1% = severe; 1–5% = moderate; >5–40% = mild
- Most common cause of morbidity is bleeding into joints (hemarthrosis), especially the knees, elbows, shoulders, ankles, and hips.
- Life-threatening bleeding episodes may occur in the CNS or in the pharynx or retropharynx
- Other bleeding sites include the urinary tract (with or without trauma), muscle bleeding, or excessive delayed postoperative bleeding. Postcircumcision bleeding is often the initial presentation in patients without a family history of hemophilia.

DIAGNOSTICS

- Prolonged PTT, normal PT, normal bleeding time
- Factor VIII or IX activity: Decreased (factor IX levels are low in normal newborns making diagnosis difficult in the newborn period)
- Carrier testing and prenatal diagnosis are available. Delivery by either vaginal or cesarean section is appropriate, but avoid using instruments (e.g., vacuum or forceps) .

MANAGEMENT

- Replace the missing factor; in the past these factors were derived from pooled plasma, now there are recombinant factor products.
- Prophylaxis is indicated in patients who have had significant bleeding.
- Factor replacement therapy: Determined by the type and severity of the bleed. Hemostatic levels are 35–40%. For life-threatening or major bleeding or head trauma, replace 100%. The initial half-life of factor VIII concentrate is 6–8 hours, with a subsequent half-life of 8–12 hours. The initial half-life of factor IX concentrate is 4–6 hours, with a subsequent half-life of 18–24 hours. Factors with extended half-lives are now available with prolonged half-lives ranging from 14 to 19 hours for factor VIII and 80 to 100 hours for factor IX
- Dose of factor VIII (units) = % desired rise in plasma factor VIII × body weight (kg) × 0.5 (may vary per patient)
- Dose of factor IX (units) = % desired rise in plasma factor IX × body weight (kg) × 1.4 (may vary depending on product or patient)
- DDAVP: For mild hemophilia A only; patients should have a DDAVP trial prior to using therapeutically. DDAVP causes the release of stored endogenously produced factor VIII and von Willebrand factor
- Recombinant factor VIIa: Directly activates the intrinsic pathway; can be used in patients with inhibitors

- Emicizumab: monoclonal antibody that binds to factor IX and X, mimicking the effect of factor VIII. Can be used as a bypass agent in patients with inhibitors.
- Aminocaproic or tranexamic acid: Antifibrinolytic medications, useful for mucosal bleeding; see formulary for dosing.
- Avoid medicines that negatively affect platelet function (e.g., aspirin, NSAIDs).
- Complications: Chronic joint destruction, causing pain and limiting mobility; transfusion-transmitted diseases (not reported from recombinant products); inhibitor (neutralizing antibody) formation to factor VIII or factor IX

VITAMIN K DEFICIENCY

Vitamin K is a fat-soluble vitamin found in green, leafy vegetables, pork, soybeans, and liver. Vitamin K is required for the posttranslational carboxylation of specific coagulation factors (factors II, VII, IX, and X and proteins C and S).

PATHOPHYSIOLOGY

- Infants not supplemented with vitamin K after delivery may develop hemorrhagic disease of the newborn (peak incidence at 2–5 days of life); infants born to mothers who were taking anticonvulsants, phenobarbital, and phenytoin are at higher risk.
- Insufficient dietary intake
- Altered gut colonization: Vomiting, diarrhea, malabsorption (celiac disease, cystic fibrosis, biliary atresia, gastrointestinal tract obstruction), antibiotic use
- Hepatocelluar disease
- Drugs: Warfarin

DIAGNOSTICS

- PT and PTT are prolonged.
- Low vitamin K–dependent factors (factors II, VII, IX, and X proteins C and S)

MANAGEMENT

- Vitamin K may be given orally, SC, IM, or IV; see formulary for dosing; risk of anaphylaxis with IV administration.
- Infants should be treated with vitamin K shortly after birth to prevent hemorrhagic disease of the newborn.

VON WILLEBRAND DISEASE

Most common inherited bleeding disorder; caused by an abnormality of von Willebrand factor (vWF)

- Type 1: 70–80% of cases; decreased vWF levels (normal structure)
- Type 2A: Decreased high-molecular-weight multimers; more severe than type 1
- Type 2B: Increased binding of vWF to normal platelets resulting in a mild thrombocytopenia and a decrease in high-molecular-weight multimers
- Type 2N: Defect of the vWF factor VIII binding region; low factor VIII levels; mild hemophilia phenotype
- Type 2M: Functional defect of vWF poor binding to platelets; normal multimers
- Type 3: Homozygous deficiency; vWF levels are undetectable with resultant low factor VIII levels because of increased clearance; severe disease; presents like hemophilia A.

EPIDEMIOLOGY

- About 1% of the population
- Autosomal dominant inheritance is most common (type 1).
- Acquired vWF deficiency may be due to neoplasms (e.g., Wilms tumor), autoimmune disorders (e.g., hypothyroidism or systemic lupus erythematosus), myeloproliferative disorders, lymphoproliferative disorders, or cardiac defects resulting in high shear stress (i.e., aortic stenosis).

PATHOPHYSIOLOGY

- vWF is a large glycoprotein synthesized in megakaryocytes and endothelial cells
- vWF has two roles in hemostasis: (1) It allows platelets to adhere to damaged endothelium. (2) It serves as a carrier protein for factor VIII.
- DDAVP can induce the release of stored vWF from endothelial cells.

CLINICAL MANIFESTATIONS

- Mucocutaneous bleeding: Easy bruising, recurrent epistaxis, menorrhagia
- Postsurgical or traumatic bleeding

DIAGNOSTICS

Levels of vWF can fluctuate. Normal study results do not necessarily exclude vWD. When the diagnosis is strongly suspected, patients may require up to three sets of laboratory studies before excluding the diagnosis.

- Bleeding time (no longer performed): Often prolonged (but can be normal)
- PTT: Can be prolonged if factor VIII is decreased (can be normal)
- vWF antigen level: Measures the total vWF plasma concentration
- vWF activity (ristocetin cofactor): Decreased in all types, except it can be normal in type 2N. (Ristocetin is an antibiotic that stimulates platelet aggregation in the presence of vWF.)
- Factor VIII activity: Normal to decreased
- vWF multimers: Helps distinguish type of von Willebrand disease (vWD)

MANAGEMENT

- DDAVP: Causes endothelial release of stored vWF with a twofold to fivefold increase in plasma levels; most helpful for patients with type 1 vWD; side effects include hyponatremia, facial flushing, and headache; available in IV or intranasal formulations; see formulary for dosing. Not recommended in type 2B because it can worsen thrombocytopenia.
- Plasma-derived vWF concentrates (Humate P, Alphanate)

Dosed in ristocetin units:

1 ristocetin U/kg = About 2% increase in vWF antigen

No. of ristocetin units = (weight in kg) × (% desired) × 0.5

- Cryoprecipitate: Use only if concentrates are not available; not treated with detergent for viruses, but lower donor exposure than with FFP.
- Aminocaproic acid or tranexamic acid: Antifibrinolytic therapy; helpful in oral bleeding and menorrhagia respectively, see formulary for dosing. Can be taken orally.

THROMBOSIS

Complete or partial occlusion of deep veins or arteries

EPIDEMIOLOGY

- Incidence of venous thromboembolism in children is 58 in 10,000 hospital admissions.
- Usually occurs in children with acquired and/or congenital risk factors for thrombosis
- Congenital risk factors: Antithrombin deficiency, protein C deficiency, protein S deficiency, factor V Leiden (activated protein C resistance), prothrombin mutation, elevated lipoprotein(a), hyperhomocysteinemia, dysfibrinogenemia, heparin cofactor II deficiency
- Acquired risk factors: CVC (most common), antiphospholipid antibody syndrome, cancer, congenital heart disease, trauma, surgery, infection, severe dehydration, prematurity, pregnancy, nephrotic syndrome, inflammatory bowel disease, cystic fibrosis, SCD, medications (e.g., estrogen or L-asparaginase)

PATHOPHYSIOLOGY

- Related to endothelial damage, venous stasis, or hypercoagulability and usually in combination

CLINICAL MANIFESTATIONS

- Extremity DVT: Extremity pain, swelling, and discoloration. Consider this diagnosis in patients with a current or recent CVC in the affected extremity.
- Superior vena cava syndrome: Swelling and plethora of the head and neck, and distended neck veins; caused by a large thrombus obstructing the superior vena cava (also associated with compression of SVC by malignancy)
- Pulmonary embolism: Shortness of breath, pleuritic chest pain, cough, hemoptysis, fever and in the case of massive PE, hypotension and right heart failure
- Cerebral sinovenous thrombosis: Neonates often present with seizures, whereas older children often complain of headache, vomiting, seizures, and focal signs. They may also have papilledema and abducens nerve palsy.
- Renal-vein thrombosis: Hematuria, abdominal mass, thrombocytopenia
- Arterial thrombosis: Cold, pale, blue extremity with poor or absent pulses

DIAGNOSTICS

- Laboratory studies: See **Box 12-1.**
- Doppler ultrasound: Best for lower-extremity DVT, decreased sensitivity for upper-extremity DVT

BOX 12-1 RECOMMENDED LABORATORY EVALUATION FOR A NON–LINE-ASSOCIATED OR UNPROVOKED THROMBOSIS

Complete blood cell count
Prothrombin time
Activated partial thromboplastin time
Antithrombin activity
Protein C activity
Protein S activity
Factor V Leiden mutation
Prothrombin mutation
Homocysteine
Lipoprotein(a)
Anticardiolipin antibody (IgG, IgM)
Anti-beta-2 glycoprotein antibody (IgG, IgM)
Dilute Russell viper venom time (or alternative test for a lupus anticoagulant)

- Venography: Helpful for upper-extremity DVT if ultrasound is negative and clinical suspicion is high; requires contrast
- Spiral CT (ventilation-perfusion scan used previously): To evaluate for PE
- Magnetic resonance venography of brain: Best test for sinovenous thrombosis (can be missed on CT)
- CT or MR angiogram/venogram: Helpful for proximal thrombosis or to confirm questionable findings on ultrasound

MANAGEMENT

- Anticoagulation: Patients with symptomatic DVT should receive anticoagulation with unfractionated heparin or LMWH. Unfractionated heparin can be immediately reversed and should be used in patients who may require urgent procedures, are at high risk for bleeding, or have renal failure. Maintaining a therapeutic effect is often easier with LMWH. Length of therapy is dependent on cause of underlying thrombosis.

MEDICATIONS FOR ANTICOAGULATION

HEPARIN

- Mechanism of action: Complexes with natural anticoagulant antithrombin and accelerates activity; limits the expansion of thrombi by preventing fibrin formation; causes prolongation of aPTT (Table 12-3)
- Dosage form: Parenteral
- Dose:
  ✓ Initial bolus: 50–75 U/kg
  ✓ Infusion: younger than 1 year, 28 U/kg/hr; older than 1 year, 20 U/kg/hr
- Monitoring: Therapeutic aPTT is 60–85 seconds. Check first aPTT 4 hours after the loading dose and adjust according to Table 12-3. A therapeutic heparin anti-Xa level is 0.3–0.7 U/mL.
- Antidote: Protamine sulfate
- Side effects:
  ✓ Bleeding
  ✓ Osteoporosis with long-term use

TABLE 12-3	Unfractionated Heparin Dose Adjustment Based on Activated Partial Thromboplastin Time	
aPTT	**Dose Adjustment**	**Time to Repeat aPTT**
<50	50 U/kg bolus	4 hours after rate change
	↑ Infusion rate by 10%	
50–59	↑ Infusion rate by 10%	4 hours after rate change
60–85	Keep rate the same	Next day
86–95	↓ Infusion rate by 10%	4 hours after rate change
96–120	Hold infusion for 30 minutes	4 hours after rate change
	↓ Infusion rate by 10%	
>120	Hold infusion for 60 minutes	4 hours after rate change
	↓ Infusion rate by 15%	

Adapted with permission from Michelson AD, Bovill E, Andrew M. Antithrombotic therapy in children. *Chest.* 1995 Oct;108(4 suppl):506S–522S.

TABLE 12-4	Enoxaparin Dosing	
	Enoxaparin Treatment	**Enoxaparin Prophylaxis**
<2 months	1.5 mg/kg every 12 hours	0.75 mg/kg every 12 hours
>2 months	1 mg/kg every 12 hours	0.5 mg/kg every 12 hours

✓ Heparin-induced thrombocytopenia (HIT): Incidence is not clearly defined in pediatric patients with a reported range of 0–2.3%. Higher-risk pediatric groups include patients undergoing cardiopulmonary bypass. HIT is characterized by symptoms appearing 5–10 days after heparin exposure, with a 50% fall in the platelet count (rarely the platelet count is less than 20,000/mm^3), and there can be venous or arterial thrombosis. Treatment includes the removal of all heparin treatment, including avoidance of LMWH. Anticoagulation should be initiated with a nonheparin anticoagulant such as a direct thrombin inhibitor (i.e., argatroban or bivalirudin)

LOW-MOLECULAR-WEIGHT HEPARIN

- Mechanism of action: Accelerates antithrombin but inhibits factor Xa more than thrombin; long half-life, good bioavailability; monitor with anti-factor Xa levels
- Dosage form: Subcutaneous
- Dosing (enoxaparin) (**Table 12-4**)
- Monitoring: Therapeutic enoxaparin anti–factor Xa level is 0.5–1 U/mL. Check anti–factor Xa level 4–6 hours after the second dose, and adjust as needed.
- Antidote: Protamine causes partial reversal.
- Side effects: Bleeding; HIT
- Use with caution in patients with renal insufficiency and avoid in renal failure

WARFARIN (COUMADIN)

- Mechanism of action: Inhibits vitamin K epoxide reductase, the vitamin K regenerative enzyme; decreases the plasma concentration of vitamin K–dependent factors II, VII, IX, and X along with proteins C and S; causes prolongation of PT
- Dosage form: Oral only (no intravenous formulations)
- Dosing: Start while patient is at therapeutic levels on heparin or LMWH; initially reduces protein C (shortest half-life) before other factors, so initially there is a prothrombotic effect. Prolongation of PT/INR begins at 24–48 hours but takes 5–7 days for full anticoagulant effect. See formulary for dosing.
- Monitoring: Use the INR; therapeutic range depends on clinical scenario. For patients with DVT, therapeutic INR is 2–3.
- Antidote: Vitamin K, four-factor prothrombin complex concentrate (Kcentra)
- Side effects: Bleeding; warfarin-related skin necrosis (result of starting warfarin without adequate anticoagulant coverage)
- Efficacy is affected by dietary intake/absorption of vitamin K as well as significant interactions with other medications. Therefore, patients on warfarin should be monitored closely during illness, significant changes in the diet, or with changes in medication

DIRECT ORAL ANTICOAGULANTS

This is a new class of anticoagulants that are highly effective in adults and are currently being studied in children, including rivaroxaban, apixaban, edoxaban, and dabigatran

- Mechanism of action: Direct Xa or thrombin inhibitors

- Dosing: Varies by agent. Administered orally and usually taken once or twice daily
- Monitoring: Not routinely monitored. DOACs interfere with coagulation assays, which cannot be used to assess their effect.
- Side effects: Typically very well tolerated. Bleeding can occur and can be reversed with direct antidotes.

THROMBOLYTIC THERAPY

Necessary for life- or limb-threatening thrombosis and should be considered in patients with large PE with hemodynamic instability, renal artery or vein thrombosis with compromised end-organ perfusion, or massive iliofemoral thrombosis. Options for therapy include recombinant tPA as either local or systemic therapy.

- Mechanism of action: Activates plasminogen to plasmin, which then degrades the fibrin clot
- Dosing for systemic therapy: tPA (wide variation)
  - ✓ Low dose: 0.03–0.06 mg/kg/hr; duration depends on dose and clinical response; can be used for a relatively prolonged duration 48–86 hours.
  - ✓ High dose: 0.1–0.6 mg/kg/hr; reassess after 6 hours consider another 6 hours if clot not resolved
- Dosing for catheter directed tPA: 0.5–2 mg/hr
- Monitoring: CBC, PT, PTT, fibrinogen, and D-dimer should be checked prior to the initiation of thrombolytic therapy and every 4–8 hours while on the infusion. An elevated D-dimer and a drop in fibrinogen are indicative of a lytic state. To minimize the risk of bleeding, it is important to maintain the fibrinogen >100 mg/dL and the platelet count >75,000/mm³.
- Antidote: None; if bleeding, stop the drug (short half-life)
- Side effect: Bleeding
- Precautions: No IM injections; no urinary catheterization, rectal temperatures, or arterial puncture; patient should be in intensive care unit.
- Contraindications: CNS ischemia/trauma/hemorrhage/surgery within 30 days, CNS pathology (e.g., neoplasm), seizures (within 48 hours), severe bleeding, surgery, or invasive procedure within 7–14 days, uncontrolled coagulopathy, inability to maintain a platelet count >75,000/mm³ or fibrinogen >100 mg/dL, uncontrolled hypertension, serum creatinine >2 mg/dL, prematurity (gestation age <32 weeks)

TRANSFUSION MEDICINE

CRYOPRECIPITATE TRANSFUSION

PRODUCT

- Contains fibrinogen, factor VIII, vWF, and factor XIII
- One unit volume will vary, maximum is 15 mL; >150 mg/unit fibrinogen and >80 IU/unit factor VIII, vWF, and factor XIII

INDICATION

- Bleeding associated with hypofibrinogenemia
- Bleeding in patients with factor VIII deficiency or vWF if factor products are not available

DOSAGE

- Rule of thumb: 1–2 units/10 kg (will result in a 60–100 mg/dL rise in fibrinogen)

FRESH-FROZEN PLASMA TRANSFUSION

PRODUCT

- Contains all of the clotting factors
- FFP about 220 mL/unit; contains approximately 1 unit/mL of all coagulation factors

INDICATION

- To correct a factor deficiency in a patient with coagulopathy and bleeding or perioperatively (DIC, vitamin K deficiency, liver disease, congenital factor deficiency, warfarin overdose)

DOSE

- 10–15 mL/kg, provides an approximate 10–15% factor correction with ideal recovery
- Can follow response by measuring PT/PTT and/or monitoring clinical bleeding

PLATELET TRANSFUSION

PRODUCT

- Whole-blood–derived versus single-donor apheresis platelets (single-donor product decreases the risk of antiplatelet antibodies and is preferable for patients who require multiple platelet transfusions)
- Whole-blood–derived platelets: About 50 mL/unit
- Apheresis platelets: 250–300 mL, equivalent to 6 units of whole-blood–derived platelets

INDICATION

- Thrombocytopenic patient who is bleeding, critically ill, or requires surgical intervention. Most procedures can be done if platelet count is maintained at >50,000/mm^3.
- Given to prevent bleeding in patients with hypoproductive bone marrow (e.g., chemotherapy, aplastic anemia) when platelet count less is than 10–20,000/mm^3
- Patients with platelet-function defects who require surgical procedures or have active bleeding uncontrolled with local measures

DOSE

Whole-blood–derived platelets:

- Children less than 10 kg: 5–10 mL/kg (increases platelet count by 50,000/mm^3–100,000/mm^3)
- Patients greater than 10 kg: 1 platelet unit/10 kg will increase by about 50,000/mm^3 (maximum volume, 15 mL/kg)

Apheresis platelets:

- <35 kg: 10 mL/kg
- >35 kg: 1 unit/patient (with a maximum volume 15 cc/kg)
- Platelets are stored at room temperature so there is a higher risk of bacterial contamination

RED BLOOD CELL TRANSFUSION

PRODUCT

- Packed red blood cells (PRBCs); 180–350 mL/unit (**Table 12-5**)
- Patient should be typed and cross-matched prior to transfusion, but can use O-negative or O-positive blood in emergent situation (O-negative is preferable, especially in females).
- Hematocrit varies depending on the preservative solution: 55–65% in adenine–saline units to 70–75% in citrate–phosphate–dextrose-adenine units.

TABLE 12-5	Risk of Virus Transmission with Red Blood Cell Transfusion in the United States
Virus	**Risk of Transmission**
HIV1/HIV2	1 in 2,135,000
Hepatitis C	1 in 1,935,000
Hepatitis B	1 in 205,000
HTLV	1 in 2,993,000

Data from Dodd RY, Notari EP, Stramer SL: Current prevalence and incidence of infectious disease markers and estimated window-period risk in the American Red Cross blood donor population, *Transfusion*. 2002 Aug;42(8):975–979.

TABLE 12-6	Risk of Adverse Transfusion Reactions
Hazard	**Risk per Unit**
Allergic transfusion reaction	1:50 to 1:100
Febrile transfusion reaction	1:100
Sepsis (bacterial contamination)	1:400 to 1:12,500
Anaphylaxis	1:20,000 to 1:50,000
Acute hemolysis (ABO mismatch)	1:6000 to 1:33,000
Death	1:500,000
Transfusion-related acute lung injury	1:5000

Data from AuBuchon JP, Kruskall MS. Transfusion safety: realigning efforts with risks, *Transfusion* 1997 Nov-Dec;37(11–12):1211–1216.

- Leukocyte-reduced product greatly reduces risk of cytomegalovirus transmission and febrile transfusion reactions.
- Washed PRBCs: Used for patients with IgA deficiency or a history of severe allergic transfusion reactions
- Irradiated PRBCs: Prevents transfusion associated graft versus host disease, which is important for neonates, young infants, and immunocompromised patients

INDICATION

- Treatment of symptomatic anemia (e.g., tachycardia, hypotension, hypoxia) or acute blood loss greater than 15%

DOSE

- Rule of thumb: 5 ml/kg of PRBCs increases hemoglobin 1 g/dL
- In patients who weigh more than 70 kg, 1 unit of PRBCs increases hemoglobin by 1 g/dL.
- For severe anemia in a hemodynamically compensated child, transfuse small volume, slowly (over approximately 4 hours) because of the risk of precipitating heart failure; initial PRBC transfusion volume estimated as: (1 ml/kg of PRBCs) × (current hemoglobin).

TRANSFUSION COMPLICATIONS

Multiple reactions—Hemolytic, nonhemolytic, allergic, infectious (see Table 12-6), circulatory overload, transfusion related acute lung injury, hypothermia, rarely electrolyte

abnormalities in the setting of massive transfusion protocols (hypoglycemia or hypocalcemia or hyperkalemia). Descriptions of more common reactions are given below.

HEMOLYTIC TRANSFUSION REACTION

- Acute: Rapid destruction of red cells; usually due to blood-type incompatibility (**Table 12-6**). Can result in fever, chills, hypotension shock, DIC, and renal failure; high mortality rate. If suspected, stop transfusion and institute supportive measures (fluids, pressors). Evaluation: Check for clinical errors, confirm patient blood type, screen for antibodies, repeat DAT on posttransfusion serum, culture donor blood for bacteria
- Delayed: 3–10 days after transfusion, usually in patients who had previous transfusion as a result of an antibody that was present, but undetectable at the time of the transfusion. May result in fever, fatigue, jaundice, and dark urine. Additional evaluation would include urine for hemoglobin, CBC and reticulocyte count, and markers of hemolysis.

FEBRILE NONHEMOLYTIC TRANSFUSION REACTION

- Temperature increase of at least 1°C in association with transfusion, with or without chills; usually due to antibody to donor white blood cells or plasma proteins; uncommon with leuko-reduced products. Stop transfusion and evaluate (see previous section). Consider premedication with acetaminophen.

ALLERGIC TRANSFUSION REACTION

- Reaction to donor plasma proteins; ranges from minor urticaria to anaphylaxis. Stop transfusion and treat with antihistamines (epinephrine and steroids if respiratory compromise).

13 Human Immunodeficiency Virus Infection

Fabian Engelbertz, MD
Eimear Kitt, MD
Andrew P. Steenhoff, MBBCh, DCH
Richard Rutstein, MD

HUMAN IMMUNODEFICIENCY VIRUS INFECTION

Human Immunodeficiency virus (HIV) may lead to acquired immunodeficiency syndrome (AIDS). Progression to AIDS is associated with opportunistic infections, cancers, and death. Advances in antiretroviral treatments (ARTs) have transformed HIV infection into a chronic illness with near normal life expectancy for those with access and adherence to lifelong therapy. See Table 13-1 for currently approved antiretroviral drugs.

EPIDEMIOLOGY IN THE UNITED STATES

- Mother-to-child transmission (MTCT): In the United States, advances in HIV testing, combination ART (cART) use in pregnant HIV-infected women consisting of a minimum of three drugs from at least two different classes of antiretroviral agents, and postexposure prophylaxis of HIV-exposed infants have reduced MTCT to less than 1%. In 2017 in the United States, 73 infants were perinatally infected with HIV.
- Pediatric infection: There are about 2200 children under the age of 13 years with HIV infection in the United States. While this number has been decreasing, there is now a growing number of foreign-born HIV-infected children living in the United States.
- Adolescent and young adult infection:
  ✓ Perinatally acquired infection: With marked improvement in the safety and efficacy of antiviral therapies, perinatally infected children usually into adulthood. However, most HIV-infected young adults have non–perinatally acquired HIV.
  ✓ Non–perinatally acquired infection: The Centers for Disease Control and Prevention (CDC) classifies modes of transmission as: male-to-male sexual contact (men who have sex with men [MSM]); injection drug use (IDU); MSM and IDU; heterosexual contact; or other. The incidence of HIV infection has remained stable or decreased, with MSM still representing the largest risk group. African Americans and Hispanics remain disproportionately affected by HIV.
    - 44% of adolescents and young adults who tested positive for HIV were previously unaware of their diagnosis.

DIFFERENTIAL DIAGNOSIS

- Infancy and childhood:
  ✓ Congenital immunodeficiencies; congenital infections; infections, such as *Mycobacterium tuberculosis*; malignancies; malnutrition; or other causes of failure to thrive, such as inflammatory bowel disease, celiac disease, or cystic fibrosis
- Adolescents and young adults:
  ✓ Acute infection: Any viral syndrome such as influenza, mononucleosis (EBV, CMV); primary HSV; bacterial or viral meningitis; arbovirus or rickettsial infections; gastrointestinal infections; malignancy; rheumatologic disease and primary or secondary syphilis

TABLE 13-1	FDA-Approved and Still Marketed Antiretroviral Medications (July 2019)*
Nucleoside/Nucleotide Reverse Transcriptase Inhibitors (NRTIs)	**Multiclass Combination Formulations**
Abacavir	Abacavir/lamivudine/dolutegravir
Emtricitabine	Emtricitabine/tenofovir/bictegravir
Lamivudine	Emtricitabine/tenofovir/efavirenz
Tenofovir alafenamide	Emtricitabine/tenofovir/rilpivirine
Tenofovir disoproxil fumarate	Emtricitabine/tenofovir/darunavir/cobicistat
Zidovudine	Emtricitabine/tenofovir/elvitegravir/cobicistat
Combination NRTIs	Lamivudine/tenofovir/doravirine
Abacavir/lamivudine	Lamivudine/tenofovir/efavirenz
Tenofovir alafenamide/emtricitabine	Rilpivirine/dolutegravir
Tenofovir disoproxil fumarate/emtricitabine	**Protease Inhibitors (PI)**
Tenofovir disoproxil fumarate/lamivudine	Atazanavir
Zidovudine/lamivudine	Darunavir
Zidovudine/lamivudine/abacavir	Atazanavir/cobicistat
Nonnucleoside Reverse Transcriptase Inhibitors (NNRTIs)	Darunavir/cobicistat
Doravirine	Lopinavir/ritonavir
Efavirenz	**Integrase Strand Transfer Inhibitors (INSTI)**
Etravirine	Bictegravir
Nevirapine	Dolutegravir
Rilpivirine	Elvitegravir
Entry and Fusion Inhibitors	Raltegravir
Ibalizumab	
Maraviroc	

*Not all agents are approved for pediatric use.

✓ Advanced infection: Differential diagnosis will vary depending on presentation, some examples are the following:
  ▪ Infectious: Pneumonia (bacterial, viral, fungal, parasitic); meningitis (bacterial, viral, fungal); sepsis, chronic fatigue syndrome; syphilis, tuberculosis, chronic vaginal candidal infection
  ▪ Wasting: Malignancy, anorexia nervosa, inflammatory bowel disease, celiac disease, or cystic fibrosis
  ▪ Malignancy: Burkitt lymphoma, Kaposi sarcoma, cervical dysplasia or cancer

PATHOPHYSIOLOGY

• Most consequences result from the steady decline of CD4+ T lymphocytes over a period of years with additional immune dysfunction caused by B-cell dysregulation.
• Perinatally acquired infection:
  ✓ Intrauterine: Virus crosses the placenta to infect an unborn infant. Providing cART to HIV-infected pregnant women reduces the viral load and reduces the chance of intrauterine infection.

✓ Intrapartum: Passage through the birth canal exposes the infant to the virus from genital secretions and blood. This poses the highest risk of perinatally acquired HIV infection among non-breastfed HIV-exposed infants. Having therapeutic levels of antiretroviral drugs in the infant's system is analogous to preexposure prophylaxis. Postexposure prophylaxis is provided to protect the infant from the possibility of acquisition of HIV during delivery.

✓ Breastfeeding: An additional 10–20% of mother-to-child HIV transmission may occur through breastfeeding. HIV-infected women in the United States are advised to avoid breastfeeding because there is ready access to infant formulas.

• Non–perinatally acquired infection: The virus is introduced into the bloodstream directly (e.g., through intravenous drug use) or from transmucosal exposure (e.g., sexual exposure).

CLINICAL MANIFESTATIONS

Clinical manifestations vary by age at time of presentation.

• Infancy (<12 months of age):
  ✓ HIV-infected infants have a high risk of pneumonia due to *Pneumocystis jirovecii* during the first 6 months of life.
  ✓ 30–80% will present with some abnormal physical finding by 1 year of age, mainly lymphadenopathy, hepatosplenomegaly (though generally mild), recurrent oral thrush and failure to thrive

• Childhood (≥12 months of age to adolescence):
  ✓ Later presentations during childhood include recurrent pneumonia, invasive bacterial infections, developmental delay or regression in development, lymphocytic interstitial pneumonia, HIV-related renal disease and HIV-related cardiomyopathy.

• Adolescents and young adults:
  ✓ Acute HIV infection: Consider acute HIV infection in any sexually active adolescent or young adult with fever of unknown origin or strep-negative exudative pharyngitis (especially with a rash) or in association with a newly diagnosed sexually transmitted infection, particularly syphilis.
  ✓ Asymptomatic HIV Infection: Due to the long duration of asymptomatic latency, infected persons may have no symptoms and may not be aware of their HIV infection
  ✓ Advanced HIV infection: Varied clinical manifestations include pneumonia (recurrent bacterial, *P. jirovecii*, *M. tuberculosis*); meningitis (toxoplasmosis, cryptococcal); fever of unknown origin (e.g., disseminated *Mycobacterium avium–intercellulare* (dMAI), CMV, HSV, lymphoma); candidiasis (oropharyngeal, vaginal, or esophageal); diarrheal illness (e.g., *Microsporidium, Cryptosporidium, Isospora,* CMV, dMAI), malignancy (e.g., Burkitt lymphoma, cervical cancer, Kaposi sarcoma), renal failure (from HIV nephropathy) and cardiomyopathy.

DIAGNOSTICS

• Initial testing (except for young infants): send fourth- or fifth generation HIV antigen/antibody combination immunoassays that detect HIV1/2 antibodies as well as HIV1 p24 antigen (https://stacks.cdc.gov/view/cdc/50872).
• MTCT:
  ✓ Women whose HIV status is unknown or undocumented should have a rapid HIV test during delivery.
  ✓ Nearly all exposed infants will test positive for HIV antibody because of the passage of maternal immunoglobulin G (IgG) antibodies across the placenta. These antibodies may remain in the infant until age 18–24 months.

✓ Quantitative HIV RNA plasma PCR assays (viral load) or qualitative HIV DNA (same sensitivities as RNA viral load testing), are used to confirm the presence or absence of HIV transmission from HIV-infected mothers.
- Diagnostic testing in infants with perinatal HIV exposure:
  ✓ Testing at birth in high-risk infants is recommended
  ✓ PCR testing should be performed at:
    - 14–21 days of life
    - 1–2 months of life
    - 4–6 months of life
  ✓ If any PCR test is positive, a second test should be performed as soon as possible on a separate specimen.
  ✓ Confirmation of negative HIV status in non-breastfed infants: Two negative PCR-based tests, one obtained at ≥1 month of age and one obtained at ≥4 months of age, or two negative HIV antibody tests from separate specimens obtained at ≥6 months of age
  ✓ Weaker evidence (grade BIII) supports HIV-negative status if HIV-negative by antibody testing at 12–18 months of age
- Suspected acute HIV infection in children and adolescents:
  ✓ Because of the lag in the development of HIV antibodies, HIV antibody testing can provide false negative results (based on the assay, antibody testing may not be positive until 3–12 weeks after infection). The fourth- and fifth-generation HIV antigen/antibody combination assay will become positive earlier after infection (around 10–14 days after infection) because of the early identification of p24 antigenemia.
  ✓ Quantitative HIV RNA testing should also be done whenever acute HIV is considered: ≥10,000 copies/mL are diagnostic of acute HIV infection with a sensitivity of close to 100%; specificity = 98%; will be positive within about 7 days after infection.
- Latent HIV infection:
  ✓ See **Figure 13-1** for current testing algorithm; Newer FDA-approved fourth- and fifth-generation HIV antigen/antibody combination immunoassays should be used.
  ✓ The American Academy of Pediatrics, the CDC, and the U.S. Preventive Services Task Force recommend routine HIV screening and testing in all adolescents and young adults beginning at as early as age 13 years; at least annual repeat screening and testing should be performed in those with a higher risk of HIV exposure (e.g., MSM, IDU, unprotected sexual intercourse, diagnosed sexually transmitted diseases, or sexually active youth in areas with high HIV prevalence of ≥0.1%).

MANAGEMENT

- Infants and children:
  ✓ Intrapartum ART/prophylaxis:
    - All HIV-infected pregnant women should be treated with cART upon diagnosis, without respect to their viral load.
    - For pregnant women on cART and not optimally suppressed, HIV genotype testing should be considered prior to modifying cART.
    - For HIV-infected pregnant women in the United States who have never received treatment, genotyping should be done, but medications can be initiated prior to receiving the results. General recommendations are listed here, but given the rapidly developing changes in this field, refer to the most updated guidelines for added guidance available at https://aidsinfo.nih.gov/guidelines/html/3/perinatal/0.
      ▷2 Nucleoside/nucleotide reverse transcriptase inhibitors (NRTIs) should be part of any regimen. Preferred dual NRTI backbone combinations are abacavir

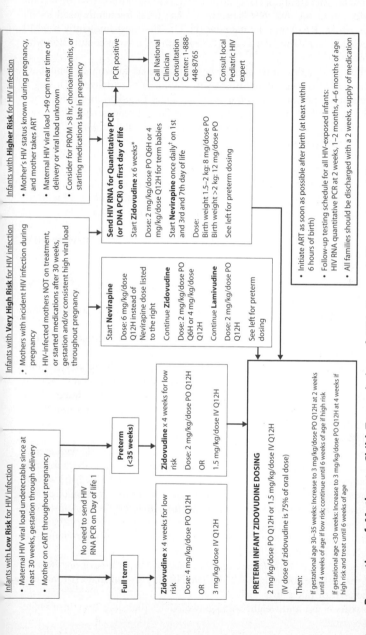

FIGURE 13-1 Prevention of Mother-to-Child Transmission of HIV. Neonatal Diagnostic and Treatment Algorithm. Children's Hospital of Philadelphia's Neonatal HIV Post-Exposure Prophylaxis Algorithm. *The decision to start an infant on treatment, dosing for nevirapine, and length of that treatment, should always be made in consultation with an HIV treatment specialist. †Some HIV treatment specialists also include lamivudine as well (2 mg/kg/dose for 4–6 weeks). ART = antiretroviral treatment; cART = combination antiretroviral treatment; cpm = copies/mL; PCR = polymerase chain reaction; PO = per os (orally); PROM = premature rupture of membranes; Q6H = every 6 hours; Q12H = every 12 hours. Data from U.S. guidelines on the Use of Antiretroviral Drugs in Pregnant Women with HIV In-fection and Interventions to Reduce Perinatal HIV Transmission, August 2019.

(abacavir)/lamivudine (3TC) and tenofovir disoproxil fumarate (TDF)/emtricitabine (FTC) or TDF/3TC. Abacavir has a high placental transfer rate.

▷ Integrase-strand transfer inhibitors (INSTIs) and protease inhibitors (PIs) are recommended in addition to the dual NRTI backbone. The most frequently used INSTI agents are raltegravir (RAL) and dolutegravir (DTG). The most frequently used PI agents are atazanavir (ATV) and darunavir (DRV), both are used in conjunction with ritonavir or cobicstat.

- Continuous infusion of zidovudine should be administered to women who have HIV RNA levels >1000 copies/mL (or unknown viral load) near delivery. Dosing is 2 mg/kg IV over first hour followed by continuous infusion of 1 mg/kg/hr until delivery.
- If the HIV RNA viral load is >1000 copies/mL near time of delivery, a scheduled cesarean section should take place at 38 weeks' gestation. For women with HIV RNA viral load <1000 copies/mL, vaginal delivery is acceptable.
- The infant should receive oral zidovudine as soon as possible after birth. High-risk infants (those born to HIV-infected women who started therapy late in gestation, who have not received cART during pregnancy, or who have a detectable viral load before labor or during delivery) should receive combination therapy consisting of zidovudine, nevirapine, and possibly lamivudine (see algorithm in **Figure 13-2** for dosing and length of treatment).
- Breastfeeding is not recommended for infants born in the United States to HIV-infected women.

• HIV-infected children
  ✓ HIV-infected infants and children should be treated with cART regardless of CD4 count or percentage or viral load.
  ✓ In children <5 years old, the CD4 percentage is generally preferred to stage immune status due to age-related variability in absolute CD4 counts.
  ✓ Immunologic monitoring including CD4 count, percentage, and viral load should be performed every 3–4 months.
  ✓ Age-specific case definitions for HIV infections based on CD4+T-lymphocyte counts and percentages are available through the CDC's Morbidity and Mortality Weekly Report Revised Surveillance Case Definition for HIV Infection—United States, 2014: Recommendations and Reports (https://www.cdc.gov/mmwr/preview/mmwrhtml/rr6303a1.htm?s_cid=rr6303a1_e).
  ✓ Initiation of cART in children who have never received it:
    - Treatment should generally include two NRTIs, plus either a nonnucleoside reverse transcriptase inhibitor (NNRTI), an INSTI or a boosted PI. Refer to the guidelines for most up-to-date recommendations (https://aidsinfo.nih.gov/guidelines/html/2/pediatric-arv/0).
    - HIV genotyping for viral resistance should be performed prior to initiation of cART.
    - Initial recommended regimens vary by age. Refer to guidelines for the most up-to-date recommendations (https://aidsinfo.nih.gov/guidelines/html/2/pediatric-arv/0).
      ▷ Children from birth to <14 days of age: Zidovudine plus NRTI (emtricitabine or lamivudine), NNRTI (nevirapine), or INSTI (raltegravir)
      ▷ Children ≥14 days and <3 years of age: two NRTIs plus lopinavir/ritonavir or raltegravir
      ▷ Children ≥3 years of age and weight <25 kg: two NRTIs plus atazanavir/ritonavir or darunavir/ritonavir or raltegravir
      ▷ Children ≥3 years of age and weight >25 kg: two NRTIs plus dolutegravir or elvitegravir and cobicistat
• Adolescents and young adults
  ✓ cART is recommended for all HIV-infected individuals to reduce disease progression and likelihood of transmission to others.

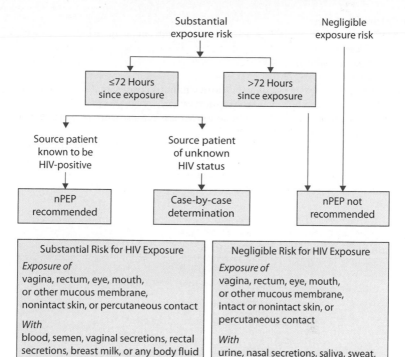

FIGURE 13-2 Algorithm for evaluation and treatment of possible nonoccupational HIV exposures. nPEP = nonoccupational postexposure prophylaxis. Reproduced with permission from Centers for Disease Control and Prevention. Updated Guidelines for Antiretroviral Postexposure Prophylaxis After Sexual, Injection Drug Use, or Other Nonoccupational Exposure to HIV - United States, 2016. Website: https://www. cdc.gov/hiv/pdf/programresources/cdc-hiv-npep-guidelines.pdf.

✓ HIV genotyping should occur prior to starting cART. If necessary, treatment may begin pending results and then modified if resistance to a particular drug is discovered.

✓ HLA B*5701 testing should be done in anyone for whom treatment with abacavir is being considered.

✓ An antiretroviral combination generally consists of two NRTIs in combination with a third active antiviral medication from one of three drug classes: an INSTI, a NNRTI, or a PI with a booster (ritonavir or cobicistat). Refer to guidelines for the most up-to-date recommendations (https://aidsinfo.nih.gov/guidelines/html/1/adult-and-adolescent-arv/0).

- Preferred dual NRTI backbone
  ▷ TDF or tenofovir alafenamide (TAF) + FTC or 3TC (Caution with tenofovir use in those with renal insufficiency and prior to Tanner stage 4)
  ▷ Abacavir (only for those without a positive mutation at HLA-B57*01) + 3TC

- PI-based regimen
  ▷ DRV + ritonavir + TDF + FTC (caution with tenofovir use in those with renal insufficiency)
- INSTI-based regimens
  ▷ Bictegravir (BIC) + TAF + FTC
  ▷ DTG + Abacavir + 3TC (only for those without a positive mutation at HLA-B57*01; DTG with caution during preconception or early pregnancy)
  ▷ DTG + TDF + FTC (caution with tenofovir use in those with renal insufficiency and prior to Tanner stage 4)
  ▷ RAL + TDF + FTC (only for use in those with pretreatment creatinine clearances >70 mL/min)

✓ Alternative regimens may be appropriate in some situations.
✓ Common side effects of cART medications are given in **Table 13-2**

TABLE 13-2	Common Side Effects of HIV Medicine Classes
Medication	**Common Side Effects**
NRTIs	Anemia, neutropenia (zidovudine)
	Diabetes mellitus/insulin resistance (zidovudine, didanosine)
	Hyperpigmentation (emtricitabine)
	Gastrointestinal symptoms (nausea, emesis)
	Lactic acidosis
	Myopathy (zidovudine)
	Neuropathy (didanosine)
	Pancreatitis
	Hepatotoxicity
	Dyslipidemia/lipoatrophy
	Osteoporosis (tenofovir disoproxil fumarate)
	Renal impairment (tenofovir disoproxil fumarate)
	Hypersensitivity reaction (abacavir, contraindicated if HLA-B*5701 positive)
NNRTIs	Rash
	Psychiatric effects (efavirenz)
	Abnormal dreaming
	Insomnia
	Depression
	Anxiety
	Dyslipidemia (efavirenz)
	Hepatotoxicity (efavirenz, nevirapine)
	QT interval prolongation (efavirenz, rilpivirine)
	Hypersensitivity reaction (nevirapine)
	Teratogenic (efavirenz)

(Continued)

TABLE 13-2	Common Side Effects of HIV Medicine Classes (*Continued*)
Medication	**Common Side Effects**
PIs	Gastrointestinal symptoms (nausea, diarrhea)
	Dyslipidemia
	Hyperglycemia
	Hyperbilirubinemia (atazanavir)
	Hepatotoxicity
	Nephrolithiasis
	Headache
	Rash
INSTIs	Gastrointestinal symptoms (nausea, diarrhea, flatulence)
	Elevations in amylase and liver-function tests
	Headache
	Dizziness, abnormal dreams
	Pruritus, rash
	Fatigue, muscle pain
	Possible teratogenicity (dolutegravir)
Entry and fusion inhibitors	Gastrointestinal symptoms (nausea, diarrhea, abdominal pain)
	Rash
	Dizziness
	Cough/upper respiratory tract infections (maraviroc)
	Hepatotoxicity (maraviroc)
	Pyrexia (maraviroc)

PRIMARY PROPHYLAXIS OF OPPORTUNISTIC INFECTIONS (OI)

Refer to guidelines for most up-to-date recommendations (HIV-exposed and HIV-infected children: https://aidsinfo.nih.gov/guidelines/html/5/pediatric-opportunistic-infection/0; adolescents and adults with HIV: https://aidsinfo.nih.gov/guidelines/html/1/adult-and-adolescent-arv/0)

- Cytomegalovirus (CMV)
- The primary method of preventing CMV infection is by treating with ART and recognizing the early manifestations of disease. If this is not possible, prophylaxis can be considered as outlined below.
  ✓ Children 1–5 years of age: CD4 <5% and CMV antibody positivity
  ✓ Children ≥6 years of age: CD4 count <50 cells/mm^3 and CMV antibody positivity
  ✓ Valganciclovir is the drug of choice for primary prophylaxis
- *Mycobacterium avium* complex (MAC)
  ✓ Children ≤1 year of age: <750 CD4 cells/mm^3
  ✓ Children 1–2 years of age: <500 CD4 cells/mm^3
  ✓ Children 2–5 years of age: <75 CD4 cells/mm^3
  ✓ Children ≥6 years of age: <50 CD4 cells/mm^3
  ✓ Azithromycin or clarithromycin may be used.

- Pneumocystis jiroveci pneumonia: Chemoprophylaxis is based on a combination of age and CD4 count or percentage, as follows:
  - ✓ Children 4-6 weeks to ≤1 year of age: all HIV-infected infants
  - ✓ Children 1–5 years of age: CD4 count <500 cells/mm^3 or CD4 <15%
  - ✓ Children ≥6 years of age: CD4 count <200 cells/mm^3 or CD4 <15%
  - ✓ Trimethoprim–sulfamethoxazole (TMP-SMX) is the drug of choice for primary prophylaxis
- *Toxoplasma gondii*
  - ✓ Children 1–5 years of age: CD4 <15% and IgG antibodies to toxoplasma
  - ✓ Children ≥6 years of age: CD4 count <100 cells/mm^3 and IgG antibodies to toxoplasma
  - ✓ TMP-SMX is the drug of choice for primary prophylaxis.
- Vaccine-preventable diseases:
  - ✓ Follow recommendations of the Advisory Committee on Immunization Practices (https://www.cdc.gov/vaccines/hcp/acip-recs/index.html).
  - ✓ In general, live vaccines should be avoided in HIV-infected infants with severe immunosuppression (for children ≤5 years: CD4 <15% for ≥6 months; for children ≥6 years: CD4 count ≥200 cells/mm^3).
  - ✓ Vaccines against encapsulated organisms can reduce risk of disease burden in HIV-infected children, as follows:
    - Meningococcal conjugate vaccination (MCV-4): two doses given soon after age 2 years separated by 8 weeks
    - Polysaccharide pneumococcal vaccination (PCV-23) should be given after 2 years of age and then repeated in 5 years
  - ✓ Hepatitis B vaccine:
    - Immunogenicity is reduced in children with HIV infection. Titers should be checked after the three-dose vaccine series and if <10 mIU/mL, a repeat of the three-dose vaccine series is recommended.

MANAGEMENT OF OPPORTUNISTIC INFECTIONS (OI) AND INFLAMMATORY SYNDROMES

OIs remain an important cause of morbidity and mortality. Risk factors include undiagnosed HIV infection, lack of proper prophylaxis of OI, virologic and immunologic failure while on cART, and suboptimal adherence to cART.

- **Differential Diagnosis**
  - ✓ Distinguishing between OI and infections that nonimmunocompromised individuals may also acquire can be difficult. Immune reconstitution inflammatory syndrome (IRIS), a paradoxical systemic inflammatory reaction to either an active or a latent infection, can present weeks to months after the initiation of cART. Its presentation is similar to that for an infectious illness, but it is purely inflammatory in nature.
  - ✓ A good rule of thumb is to always consider common infections that can present in any child without HIV infection, then consider the OIs, oncologic processes, and IRIS.
  - ✓ Common presentations of OIs and their differential diagnoses include
    1) Pneumonia: viral, bacterial, Pneumocystis pneumonia, fungal, tuberculosis (TB)
       → General pneumonia workup should also include lactate dehydrogenase, silver stain or pneumocystis jiroveci pneumonia PCR, TB sputum/gastric aspirate
    2) Fever: Invasive bacterial infection (osteomyelitis, subacute bacterial endocarditis), CMV, dMAI, cryptococcosis, oncologic diseases
       → Consider adding CMV PCR, dMAI blood culture, *Cryptococcus* antigen, bone marrow or lymph node biopsy to general fever workup.

3) Chronic diarrhea: dMAI, cryptosporiodiosis, isosporiasis, CMV, bacterial dysentery
   → Stool cultures, ova and parasites, dMAI blood cultures, CMV PCR from gastrointestinal tissue
✓ See complete **Table 13-3** for diagnosis and treatment of OIs.

POSTEXPOSURE PROPHYLAXIS

- *Occupational PEP:* Guidelines available from the "Updated US Public Health Service Guidelines for the Management of Occupational Exposures to Human Immunodeficiency Virus and Recommendations for Post-exposure Prophylaxis" (https://npin.cdc.gov/publication/updated-us-public-health-service-guidelines-management-occupational-exposures-human).
  ✓ Risk of HIV transmission following a percutaneous exposure is about 0.3% and 0.09% after contact with mucous membranes or nonintact skin. Higher HIV viral load in infected persons, a larger, hollow-bore needle, or an arterial source increase risk of transmission
  ✓ HIV testing of the source patient is preferred when possible
  ✓ Initiate PEP as soon as possible, preferably within hours. If the source patient is later found to be HIV-negative PEP can be discontinued.
  ✓ Baseline testing of the exposed individual should be performed:
    - HIV (rapid HIV antigen/antibody combination immunoassay)
    - Syphilis (RPR, VDRL)
    - Hepatitis B (HBsAg/HBsAb)
    - Hepatitis C (HCV antibody)
  ✓ Three drug regimens are now recommended in all exposures in which PEP is being recommended:
    - The preferred regimen is RAL 400 mg orally twice daily or 600 mg orally daily or DTG 50 mg once daily (may not be used during preconception or early pregnancy), plus TDF 300 mg + FTC 200 mg orally daily
    - Treatment duration is 4 weeks
  ✓ Follow-up should occur at 72 hours, 6 weeks, 12 weeks, and 6 months after exposure.
  ✓ Local expert guidance should be sought. PEP guidance is also available at PEPline at www.nccc.ucsf.edu/about_nccc/pepline, or by phone at 888-448-4911
- Nonoccupational postexposure prophylaxis (nPEP):
  ✓ Defined as nonoccupational exposure to blood, genital secretions, or other potentially infectious body fluids
  ✓ If prophylaxis is chosen, it should be started as soon as possible after exposure; prophylaxis started after 72 hours is unlikely to be effective and generally is not recommended.
  ✓ **Table 13-4** shows relative risk of HIV transmission per exposure type
  ✓ **Figure 13-2** shows the Center for Disease Control's algorithm for determining the need for nPEP.
  ✓ Baseline testing of the exposed individual should be performed:
    - HIV (rapid HIV antigen/antibody combination immunoassay)
    - Syphilis (RPR, VDRL)
    - Hepatitis B (HBsAb)
    - Hepatitis C (HCV antibody)
    - CBC, BMP, LFTs
    - For sexual abuse victims, consider further STI + pregnancy + toxicologic + forensic-evidence testing

TABLE 13-3 Opportunistic Infections (OIs) in HIV-Infected Infants and Children, Adolescents, and Young Adults

Etiology	Clinical Presentation	Laboratory/Radiological Findings	Preferred Treatment
Bacterial Infections			
Bartonella henselae and *Bartonella quintana*	FUO, bacillary angiomatosis, endocarditis, osteomyelitis, splenitis	CD4 count <100 cells/mm³ Elevated antibody titer to organism Histopathology or PCR	Children: Doxycycline 2–4 mg/kg orally per day for 3–4 months. Adolescents/adults: Bacillary angiomatosis, peliosis, bacteremia, and osteomyelitis: • Doxycycline 100 mg orally per day for 3 months. Endocarditis: • Doxycycline 100 mg IV every 12 hours; PLUS • Gentamicin 1 mg/kg IV every 8 hours for 2 weeks, then • Doxycycline 100 mg by mouth twice daily for 3 months.

Syphilis: The spirochete *Treponema pallidum* is the cause. While not necessarily an OI, there has been a resurgence in the United States in recent years.	• Congenital syphilis: Infants should be evaluated and treated as per CDC guidelines
	
	• HIV coinfection can alter the clinical presentation in every stage.
	
	• Primary syphilis: Painless chancre at the site of inoculation.
	
	• Secondary syphilis: Almost any rash, adenopathy, malaise, headache.
		• Dark-field microscopy, where available, can detect treponemes in primary syphilis.
		
		• Non–treponemal-specific screening tests:
		  ○ Venereal Disease Research Laboratory
		  ○ RPR
		  ○ EIAs
		
		• RPR allows for the assessment of titer levels
			Congenital syphilis (proven or highly probable; refer to CDC guidelines):
			• Aqueous penicillin G 100,000–150,000 units/kg/day, administered as 50,000 units/kg/dose IV every 12 hours during the first 7 days of life and every 8 hours thereafter, for a total of 10 days
			• Alternatively, Procaine penicillin G 50,000 units/kg/dose IM in a single dose for 10 days
			
			Primary, secondary, and early-latent syphilis:
			• Penicillin G 2.4 million units IM × 1

Syphilis: (continued)

- Latent syphilis:
  - Early: Absence of symptoms, but positive RPR and treponema-specific confirmatory assay within 12 months of a previously negative RPR
  - Late/unknown duration: Asymptomatic and + RPR and treponemal specific confirmatory assay over 12 months beyond a previously negative RPR

- Neurosyphilis:
  - Can occur at any stage of syphilis and manifest in varied clinical presentations, such as cranial-nerve dysfunction, stroke, meningitis, acute or chronic change in mental status, loss of vibration sense, and auditory or ophthalmic abnormalities. It is important to note that asymptomatic neurosyphilis may be more common in HIV-infected individuals.

- Treponemal specific confirmatory tests:
  - FTA-ABS: Generally remains positive after one episode of syphilis

Late-latent or syphilis of unknown duration:
- Penicillin G 2.4 million units IM weekly × 3 weeks

Neurosyphilis:
- Penicillin G 24 million units IV per day divided every 4 hours for 14 days

(Continued)

TABLE 13-3 Opportunistic Infections (OIs) in HIV-Infected Infants and Children, Adolescents, and Young Adults (*Continued*)

Etiology	Clinical Presentation	Laboratory/Radiological Findings	Preferred Treatment
Mycobacterial Infections			
Mycobacterium tuberculosis	Pulmonary: Cough, fever, failure to thrive, weight loss Extrapulmonary: Most common sites in children are lymph nodes or CNS. However, blood (miliary), cardiac, joint, bone, skin, kidney, eye, and abdomen can be initial sites. In adolescents/adults, common sites may involve blood (miliary), cardiac, joint, bone, skin, kidney, CNS, eye, and abdomen. Increasing immunosuppression increases likelihood of extrapulmonary presentation.	• + Mantoux PPD ≥5 mm • + Interferon-gamma release assay: Caution in those <5 years of age • Sputum sample with acid-fast bacilli • Gastric aspiration (early morning) • Tissue sampling • Chest x-ray	Children: Disseminated disease may progress quickly in infants; prompt initiation of treatment should be considered. Caution with drug–drug interactions with cART. 4 drug regimen recommended: • Ethambutol 20 mg/kg daily dose (maximum, 2.5 g) • Isoniazid 10–15 mg/kg daily dose (maximum, 300 mg) • Pyrazinamide 30–40 mg/kg daily dose (maximum, 2 g) • Rifampin 10–20 mg/kg daily dose (maximum, 600 mg) Adolescents/Adults: Caution with drug–drug interactions with cART. Four-drug regimen recommended: • Ethambutol: Weight-based dosing 20 mg/kg, for person >40–55-kg 800 mg daily, for 56–75 kg 1200 mg daily, for >76 kg 1600 mg daily • Isoniazid: 10 mg/kg (usual dose, 300 mg) daily • Pyrazinamide: Weight-based dosing 35 mg/kg, for person >40–55 kg 1000 mg daily, for 56–75 kg 1500 mg daily, for >76 kg 2000 mg daily • Rifampin: 15 mg/kg (usual dose, 600 mg) daily (Note interactions with cART!)

| *Mycobacterium avium–intracellulare* | • Pulmonary: Less common presentation in children
• Disseminated: More common in children. Rare in first year of life. Symptoms include: hectic fevers, night sweats, weight loss, abdominal pain, diarrhea, lymphadenitis
• In patients with AIDS who are not on ART, MAC disease typically is a disseminated, multiorgan infection.
• Early symptoms may be minimal and can precede detectable mycobacteremia by several weeks | • CD4 counts <50 copies/mm³ or CD4 % ≤15–25% depending on age, with the lower % for younger children
• Positive blood culture or culture from site. May use culture of normally sterile site (e.g. bone marrow)
• Perform susceptibility testing to azithromycin and clarithromycin | Two drug combination therapy for 12 months, three drugs for disseminated disease
Preferred regimen:
Children:
• Clarithromycin 7.5–15 mg/kg orally twice daily (maximum, 500 mg per dose) + Ethambutol 15–25 mg/kg once daily (maximum, 2.5 g/day)
• Severe disease add rifabutin 10–20 mg/kg once daily (maximum, 300 mg daily)
Alternative regimen:
• Azithromycin 10–12 mg/kg once daily (maximum, 500 mg daily) may be substituted for clarithromycin
Secondary prophylaxis is needed after treatment completion.
Adolescents/adults:
• Clarithromycin 500 mg orally twice daily
• Ethambutol 15 mg/kg orally daily, OR
• Azithromycin 500–600 mg + ethambutol 15 mg/kg orally daily if drug interaction or intolerance precludes the use of clarithromycin
• Severe disease add Rifabutin 300 mg once daily (dose adjustment may be needed due to drug interaction)
Duration:
• At least 12 months of therapy, can discontinue if no signs and symptoms of MAC disease and sustained (>6 months) CD4 count >100 cells/mcL in response to cART |

(Continued)

TABLE 13-3 Opportunistic Infections (OIs) in HIV-Infected Infants and Children, Adolescents, and Young Adults (*Continued*)

Etiology	Clinical Presentation	Laboratory/Radiological Findings	Preferred Treatment
Viral Infections			
CMV: End organ disease typically occurs in those with profound immunosuppression (CD4 counts <50 cell/mm³).	• Retinitis: Most common presentation; may be unilateral: floaters, central or peripheral visual loss. • Other sites: GI, liver, kidney, sinuses, or CNS Symptoms often nonspecific: Fever, weight loss, odynophagia, or profuse bloody diarrhea • Pneumonitis is very uncommon	• CMV can be isolated in cell culture from blood leukocytes, urine, or tissue • Positive blood buffy-coat culture • DNA PCR of blood, fluid, or tissue • Ophthalmoscopic exam • End-organ disease diagnosis requires tissue biopsy for diagnosis (GI, lung)	*Children:* Symptomatic congenital infection: • Ganciclovir 6 mg/kg IV every 12 hours for 6 weeks Disseminated disease and retinitis: • Ganciclovir 5–7.5 mg/kg IV every 12 hours for 14–21 days • Followed by 5 mg/kg IV per day for 5–7 days per week for chronic suppression CNS disease (also followed by chronic suppression): • Ganciclovir 5–7.5 mg/kg IV every 12 hours; PLUS • Foscarnet 60 mg/kg IV every 8 hours until symptoms improved Adolescents/Adults: CMV retinitis: *Induction therapy: For immediate sight-threatening lesions (adjacent to the optic nerve or fovea):* • Intravitreal injections of ganciclovir (2 mg) or foscarnet (2.4 mg) for 1–4 doses over a period of 7–10 days to achieve high intraocular concentration faster; PLUS *Preferred systemic induction therapy:* Valganciclovir 900 mg orally twice daily for 14–21 days *For peripheral lesions:* • Valganciclovir 900 mg orally twice daily for 14–21 days

CMV: (continued)

Chronic maintenance (secondary prophylaxis):

- Valganciclovir 900 mg orally daily

For CMV esophagitis or colitis:

- Ganciclovir 5 mg/kg IV every 12 hours; may switch to valganciclovir 900 mg orally twice daily once the patient can tolerate oral therapy

- Duration: 21–42 days or until symptoms have resolved

- Maintenance therapy is usually not necessary, but should be considered after relapses.

Histologically confirmed CMV pneumonia:

- Experience for treating CMV pneumonitis in HIV patients is limited.

- Use of IV ganciclovir or IV foscarnet is reasonable (doses same as for CMV retinitis)

CMV neurologic disease:

Note: Treatment should be initiated promptly.

- Ganciclovir 5 mg/kg IV every 12 hours + (foscarnet 90 mg/kg IV every 12 hours or 60 mg/kg IV every 8 hours) to stabilize disease and maximize response, continue until symptomatic improvement and resolution of neurologic symptoms.

The optimal duration of therapy and the role of oral valganciclovir have not been established for pulmonary or CNS CMV.

(Continued)

TABLE 13-3 Opportunistic Infections (OIs) in HIV-Infected Infants and Children, Adolescents, and Young Adults (*Continued*)

Etiology	Clinical Presentation	Laboratory/Radiological Findings	Preferred Treatment
Jackson Canyon (JC) virus: The causative agent of PML; causes demyelinating disease of the CNS. Rare in children.	Usually insidious in onset. May present with focal neurologic deficits, cognitive dysfunction, visual disturbances, paralysis, ataxia, or aphasia.	• PML is generally associated with profound immunosuppression, i.e., CD4% <15. • MRI of white matter will reveal: o Deceased signal on T1 images o Increased signal on T2 and FLAIR sequences o Presence of JC virus in CNS by PCR in conjunction with MRI findings o Brain biopsy is gold standard with specificity of 100%, but carries significant risk.	• Poor prognosis in pre-cART era. • cART has increased survival time and is the only treatment that has demonstrated benefit.
Fungal Infections			
Aspergillosis: Most common species causing infection are *A. fumingatus*, followed by *A. flavus* Rare in the post-cART era, but significantly lethal in pre-cART era.	• Invasive pulmonary aspergillosis is the most common: Fever, cough, dyspnea, pleuritic pain • Other sites: Tracheobronchitis, CNS, skin, and sinuses	• Profound immunosuppression (CD4 <15%) associated with higher risk • Blood cultures generally not helpful • Chest x-ray or CT scan for pulmonary involvement • Biopsy for fungal culture of suspected site • BAL galactomannan is very specific.	Invasive pulmonary aspergillosis: • Voriconazole 6–8 mg/kg IV every 12 hours for two doses followed by 7 mg/kg either IV or orally twice daily for 12 weeks

Candida Infections	• Oral thrush and diaper dermatitis occur in a majority of HIV-infected children; primarily caused by *C. albicans*. • Esophageal candidiasis presents with odynophagia and retrosternal pain, and children can present with nausea, vomiting, and weight loss. • Vulvovaginal candidiasis: Presents similarly to HIV-uninfected women with a white, cottage cheese–like vaginal discharge and vaginal itching. • Disseminated candidiasis: Blood infections are generally caused by non-*albicans* species of *Candida*.	Oral thrush: • Potassium hydroxide preparation of samples will show budding yeast cells. • Culture may need to be done in refractory cases or failure of treatment. Esophageal thrush: • Barium swallow will demonstrate a classic cobblestone appearance • Refractory causes may require endoscopy to rule out other causes. Vulvovaginal candidiasis: • May be made clinically • Potassium hydroxide preparation of samples will show budding yeast cells and hyphae.	Children: Oral thrush: • Uncomplicated infection: Nystatin suspension 1 ml (100,000 U) four times daily for infants and 4–6 ml (400,000–600,00 U) swish and swallow four times daily for children for 7–14 days or topical clotrimazole troche (>3 years of age) 10 mg five times daily for 7–14 days • Moderate to severe, or recurrent infection: Fluconazole 3–6 mg/kg orally once daily (maximum, 400 mg/dose) for 7–14 days. Esophageal thrush: • Fluconazole 6 mg/kg orally once daily on day 1 followed by 3–6 mg/kg orally once daily (maximum, 400 mg/dose) for 14–21 days. • Itraconazole cyclodextrin oral solution 5 mg/kg once daily for 14–21 days. Disseminated candidiasis: • Amphotericin B 0.5–1.5 mg/kg IV once daily • Treat for at least 2–3 weeks after the last positive blood culture. • Longer treatment may be needed for some sites (e.g., CNS, lung)

(*Continued*)

TABLE 13-3 Opportunistic Infections (OIs) in HIV-Infected Infants and Children, Adolescents, and Young Adults (*Continued*)

Etiology	Clinical Presentation	Laboratory/Radiological Findings	Preferred Treatment
Candida Infections (continued)		Disseminated candidiasis: • Blood cultures (1–2 days for growth and 1–2 days for speciation) • Beta-**D**-glucan assays (limited validation in children) • PCR, but can currently only identify to the *Candida* species level. • Consider ultrasound to identify liver and kidney dissemination • Ophthalmology exam to detect eye involvement.	Adolescents/adults: <u>Oral thrush:</u> • Fluconazole 100 mg orally daily for 7–14 days. <u>Esophageal thrush:</u> • Fluconazole 100 mg orally once daily for 14–21 days. • Itraconazole oral solution 200 mg once daily for 14–21 days.
Coccidioidomycosis: Caused by two species, *C. immitis* and *C. posadasii. C. immitis* is confined to California while *C. posadasii* is more widely distributed throughout the Southwest, Mexico, and Latin America.	Pulmonary: • Fever, malaise, cough and chest pain. • Hemoptysis is less common Meningitis: • Headache, change in mental status, focal deficits, vomiting often occur. Hydrocephalus is common. Disseminated disease: • Generalized lymphadenopathy • Skin nodules or ulcers • Peritonitis • Liver involvement	• Tissue histology that shows spherules containing endospores are diagnostic. • Blood cultures and CSF cultures are rarely positive. • Sputum cultures often positive. • Serologic assays, such as complement fixation assays of IgG and IgM may be helpful; however may be falsely negative in severely immunocompromised children. • Clinical symptoms are nonspecific, so consider evaluation in those with travel to endemic areas.	Children: <u>Pulmonary or disseminated nonmeningeal disease:</u> • Amphotericin B 0.5–1 mg/kg IV once daily until clinical improvement (min of several weeks). <u>Meningeal infection:</u> • Fluconazole 5–6 mg/kg IV or orally twice daily (max 800 mg/day). Adolescents/adults: <u>Mild disease (e.g., focal pneumonia):</u> • Fluconazole 400 mg orally daily <u>Severe, non-CNS infection, or disseminated disease:</u> • Liposomal amphotericin B 4–6 mg/kg IV daily until clinical improvement and then switch to an azole.

Coccidioidomycosis: (continued)			Meningeal infection: • Fluconazole 400–800 mg IV or orally daily. Chronic suppressive therapy: • Fluconazole 400 mg orally daily Children: CNS disease: Acute therapy (2-week induction) is followed by consolidation therapy. • Amphotericin B 0.7–1 mg/kg IV daily; PLUS • Flucytosine 100 mg/kg orally divided four times daily Consolidation therapy: • Fluconazole 12 mg/kg on day 1, followed by 6–12 mg/kg (maximum, 800 mg daily) either IV or orally for minimum of 8 weeks.

Cryptococcosis: Generally caused by *Cryptococcus neoformans*. Infections are rare in children, particularly in the post-cART era.	Generally occurs in profoundly immunocompromised individuals.
	Meningoencephalitis:
	• Insidious onset
	• Fever, headaches, possibly nuchal rigidity
	Disseminated cryptococcosis:
	• Cutaneous lesions that resemble molluscum contagiosum
	• Nodules
	• Ulcers
	Pulmonary:
	Rare in children, but may include fever, dry cough, x-ray with focal or diffuse infiltrates.
		• Cryptococcal antigen in serum, CSF, or other body fluid is the recommended test.
		• CSF analysis:
		  ○ High opening pressure
		  ○ India-ink stained wet mount of CSF (no longer performed in some centers)
		• Culture of blood, CSF, and sputum
			Localized diseased (not CNS):
			• Fluconazole 12 mg/kg on day 1, followed by 6–12 mg/kg (maximum, 800 mg daily) either IV or orally. Treatment duration varies
			
			Disseminated disease (no CNS):
			Amphotericin B 0.7–1 mg/kg IV daily (+/− flucytosine)

(Continued)

TABLE 13-3 Opportunistic Infections (OIs) in HIV-Infected Infants and Children, Adolescents, and Young Adults (*Continued*)

Etiology	Clinical Presentation	Laboratory/Radiological Findings	Preferred Treatment
Cryptococcosis: (continued)			Adolescents/adults: <u>CNS disease:</u> Acute therapy (2-week induction) is followed by consolidation therapy. • Liposomal amphotericin B 3–4 mg/kg IV daily; PLUS • Flucytosine 100 mg/kg orally divided 4 times daily (renal dosing needed) Consolidation therapy: For minimum of 8 weeks followed by maintenance therapy. • Fluconazole 400 mg daily either IV or orally Maintenance therapy: • Fluconazole 200 mg orally daily for at least 12 months. <u>Non-CNS, extrapulmonary, and diffuse pulmonary disease:</u> • Treat the same as meningitis, above. <u>Non-CNS with mild to moderate symptoms and focal pulmonary infiltrates:</u> • Fluconazole 400 mg orally daily for 12 months.
Histoplasmosis: Caused by inhalation of microconidia of *Histoplasma capsulatum*. Most highly endemic in the Ohio and Mississippi river valleys. It is been rare in children in both the pre- and post-ART eras.	<u>Progressive disseminated histoplasmosis:</u> Most common presentation in HIV-infected children. • Prolonged fever • Failure to thrive • Hepatosplenomegaly • Cough	• Culture is often invasive and slow to grow organism • EIA probes can detect infection in serum, sputum, and CSF • CSF can also be tested for histoplasma antigen.	Children: <u>Disseminated disease:</u> • Itraconazole oral solution. Loading dose of 2–5 mg/kg (maximum, 200 mg) orally for days 1–3, followed by 2–5 mg/kg (maximum, 200 mg) per dose twice daily for 12 months. (Urine antigen should be checked for relapse)

Histoplasmosis:
(continued)

- Lymphadenopathy
- Ulcerative cutaneous lesions
  - Fatigue
  - Weight Loss
  - Cough

CNS disease:
  - Fever
  - Headache
  - Focal deficits

GI disease:
  - Diarrhea
  - Abdominal pain
  - Weight loss

Pulmonary disease:
  - Cough
  - Fever
  - Pleuritic chest pain

Adolescents/adults:

Moderately severe to severe disseminated disease:

Induction therapy (for at least 2 weeks or until clinically improved):

- Liposomal amphotericin B 3 mg/kg IV daily

Maintenance therapy:

- Itraconazole 200 mg orally three times daily for 3 days, then 200 mg orally twice daily.

Less severe disseminated disease:

Induction and maintenance therapy:

- Itraconazole 200 mg orally thrice daily for 3 days, then 200 mg orally twice daily for at least 12 months

Meningitis:

Induction therapy (4–6 weeks):

- Liposomal amphotericin B 5 mg/kg/day IV daily

Maintenance therapy:

Itraconazole 200 mg orally twice daily for ≥1 year and until resolution of abnormal CSF findings

(Continued)

TABLE 13-3 Opportunistic Infections (OIs) in HIV-Infected Infants and Children, Adolescents, and Young Adults (*Continued*)

Etiology	Clinical Presentation	Laboratory/Radiological Findings	Preferred Treatment
Pneumocystis jiroveci pneumonia: Caused by *Pneumocystis jirovecii*. The organisms are found in lungs of humans worldwide.	Pneumonia: • Remains a common AIDS-defining illness • Highest incidence in first year of life (peak age, 3–6 months) • Fever • Cough (nonproductive) • "Quiet" tachypnea or quiet inspiratory crackles may be only respiratory finding • Dyspnea	• CD4 counts are generally <200 cells/mm³ or <15%. In infants <12 months of age, pneumocystis jiroveci pneumonia can occur at any CD4 count or percentage • Hypoxia is hallmark • LDH is nonspecific, but often elevated • Chest x-ray classically shows bilateral diffuse interstitial infiltrates described as "ground glass" in appearance, but can be normal. • Stains of sputum (obtained through induced mechanism, BAL) include silver stain, toluidine blue, and Wright stain. • Direct fluorescent antibody stains or PCR may also be used.	TMP-SMX: TMP 15–20 mg/kg/day IV or orally divided every 8 hours. • Duration of treatment is 21 days followed by suppressive therapy. • In adolescents or adults moderate or severe disease, corticosteroids may reduce morbidity and mortality In infancy, pneumocystis jiroveci pneumonia may be more rapidly progressive and has higher mortality; therefore many HIV pediatric experts recommend corticosteroids in all infants with pneumocystis jiroveci pneumonia.
Parasitic Infections			
Cryptosporidiosis/ microsporidiosis: *Cryptosporidium* spp. are ubiquitous protozoal parasites. *Microspora* spp. are intracellular spore-forming protozoa.	Cryptosporidiosis: • Nonbloody watery diarrhea • Abdominal cramping • Fever • Vomiting • Can invade biliary duct causing acalculous cholecystitis or sclerosing cholangitis	Cryptosporidiosis: • EIA preferred • Cannot be cultured Microsporidiosis: • Trichrome stain	Cryptosporidiosis: • Effective cART treatment Microsporidiosis: • Effective cART treatment • Albendazole 7.5 mg/kg (maximum, 400 mg/dose) orally twice daily may be used for disseminated, but not ocular infection for microsporidia other than *Enterocytozoon bienuesi*.

Cryptosporidiosis/
microsporidiosis:
(continued)

Microsporidiosis:
- Diarrheal illness, nonbloody
  - Hepatitis
  - Peritonitis
  - Myositis
  - Keratoconjunctivitis
  - Cholangitis

Toxoplasmosis: Caused by *Toxoplasma gondii*. Infection can occur congenitally or through exposure later in life. Even in pre-cART era, CNS toxoplasmosis was rare in children.

CNS disease:
- Focal encephalitis
- Headache
- Fever

With progression:
- Seizures
- Coma

Non-CNS presentations are rare in those with HIV/AIDS.

- CT or MRI with contrast will show ring-enhancing lesions in the gray matter of the cortex or basal ganglia. Edema is often present.
- IgG antibodies are uniformly present.
- Stereotactic CT-guided brain biopsy is the only definitive diagnostic tool.
- Detection of *T. gondii* by PCR in CSF is very specific, but has low sensitivity.

Children:

Congenital toxoplasmosis:
- Pyrimethamine: Loading dose, 2 mg/kg orally once daily for 2 days, then 1 mg/kg orally once daily for 2–6 months, then 1 mg/kg orally 3 times weekly; PLUS
- Leucovorin(folinic acid), 10 mg orally or IM with each dose of pyrimethamine; PLUS
- Sulfadiazine, 50 mg/kg orally twice daily
- Treatment duration: 12 months

Acquired toxoplasmosis, acute induction therapy (followed by chronic suppressive therapy):
- Pyrimethamine: Loading dose, 2 mg/kg (maximum, 50 mg) orally once daily for 3 days, then 1 mg/kg body weight (maximum, 25 mg) orally once daily; PLUS
- Sulfadiazine, 25–50 mg/kg (maximum, 1.0–1.5 g/dose) orally per dose four times daily; PLUS
- Leucovorin, 10–25 mg orally daily
- Followed by long-term suppressive therapy

(Continued)

261

TABLE 13-3	Opportunistic Infections (OIs) in HIV-Infected Infants and Children, Adolescents, and Young Adults (Continued)		
Etiology	**Clinical Presentation**	**Laboratory/Radiological Findings**	**Preferred Treatment**
Toxoplasmosis: (continued)			Treatment duration (followed by long-term suppressive therapy): ≥6 weeks (longer if clinical or radiologic disease is extensive or response is incomplete at 6 weeks).
			Adolescents/adults:
			Treatment of acute infection:
			• Pyrimethamine 200 mg orally once, followed by weight-based therapy:
			• If <60 kg, pyrimethamine 50 mg orally once daily + sulfadiazine 1000 mg orally every 6 hours + leucovorin 10–25 mg orally once daily
			• If ≥60 kg, pyrimethamine 75 mg orally once daily + sulfadiazine 1500 mg orally every 6 hours + leucovorin 10–25 mg orally once daily
			• Leucovorin dose can be increased to 50 mg daily or twice daily.
			Duration for acute therapy:
			• At least 6 weeks; longer duration if clinical or radiologic disease is extensive or response is incomplete at 6 weeks
			Chronic maintenance therapy:
			• Pyrimethamine 25–50 mg orally daily + sulfadiazine 2000–4000 mg orally daily (in two to four divided doses) + leucovorin 10–25 mg orally daily. This should be continued for at least 6 months after CD4 counts have exceeded 200 cells/mm³ before consideration of stopping secondary prophylaxis.

BAL = bronchoalveolar lavage; CMV = cytomegalovirus; CNS = central nervous system; CSF = cerebrospinal fluid; CT = computed tomography; EIA = enzyme-linked assay; FLAIR = fluid-attenuated inversion recovery; FTA-ABS = fluorescent treponemal antibody absorption test; FUO = fever of unknown origin; IM = intramuscularly; PPD = purified protein PML = progressive multifocal leukodystrophy; PPD = purified protein

TABLE 13-4	Estimated Per-Act Risk for Acquisition of HIV, by Exposure Route
Exposure type	**Rate for HIV acquisition per 10,000 exposures**[a]
Parenteral	
Blood transfusion	9,250
Needle sharing during injection drug use	63
Percutaneous (needlestick)	23
Sexual	
Receptive anal intercourse	138
Receptive penile-vaginal intercourse	8
Insertive anal intercourse	11
Insertive penile-vaginal intercourse	4
Receptive oral intercourse	Low
Insertive oral intercourse	Low
Other[b]	
Biting	Negligible
Spitting	Negligible
Throwing body fluids (including semen or saliva)	Negligible
Sharing sex toys	Negligible

Source: http://www.cdc.gov/hiv/policies/law/risk.html

[a]Factors that may increase the risk of HIV transmission include sexually transmitted diseases, acute and late-stage HIV infection, and high viral load. Factors that may decrease the risk include condom use, male circumcision, antiretroviral treatment, and preexposure prophylaxis. None of these factors are accounted for in the estimates presented in the table.

[b]HIV transmission through these exposure routes is technically possible but unlikely and not well documented.

Adapted with permission from Patel P, Borkowf CB, Brooks JT, et al: Estimating per-act HIV transmission risk: a systematic review, AIDS 2014 Jun 19;28(10):1509-1519.

✓ Preferred antiretroviral medication for nPEP based on age (adapted from CHOP's Suspected Sexual Abuse Clinical Pathway)
  ▪ Adults and adolescents >13 years old, weight >40 kg and Tanner stage ≥3: RAL 400 mg twice daily or 600 mg once daily (DTG 50 mg once daily may be used for male individuals as an alternative, but should be used with caution in females of child-bearing age because of possible risks during early pregnancy), plus TDF 300 mg + FTC 200 mg orally daily (replace with zidovudine + lamivudine for existing renal disease)
  ▪ Children 6–12 years old, weight >30 kg, or age >13 years and Tanner stage <3: Zidovudine 300 mg + lamivudine 150 mg orally twice daily plus RAL 400 mg orally twice daily

- Children 2–12 years old, weight <30 kg or who cannot swallow whole tablets/capsules: Lamivudine 4 mg/kg/dose + zidovudine 240 mg/m^2/dose formulation orally twice daily plus RAL chewable tablet (10–14 kg: 75 mg BID, 14–20 kg: 100 mg BID, 20–28 kg: 150 mg BID, 28–40 kg: 200 mg BID, >40 kg: 300 mg BID) or plus lopinavir/ritonavir 300 mg/m^2/dose orally twice daily
- For sexual abuse victims, consider STI prophylactic treatment + emergency contraception

Katie Kennedy, MD
Juhee Lee, MD
Soma Jyonouchi, MD

APPROACH TO PRIMARY IMMUNODEFICIENCY

Clinical Red Flags for Immunodeficiency:

- Frequent infections (respiratory, GI, or skin)
- Severe or unusual infections
- Unusual pathogen (*Pneumocystis jirovecii, Burkholderia cepacia, Serratia marcescens, Aspergillus* spp.)
- Hospitalization for a common pathogen
  - ✓ Sepsis with an encapsulated organism (*Streptococcus pneumoniae, Haemophilus influenzae*)
  - ✓ *Neisseria* spp. infection
  - ✓ EBV or CMV
- Persistence of a common pathogen that is usually cleared (*Candida* spp., HPV, molluscum)
- Recurrent fevers without a source
- Multisystem or early-onset autoimmunity

Recurrent urinary tract infections or streptococcal pharyngitis are not typically associated with immunodeficiency.

MAJOR CATEGORIES

Major categories of primary immune deficiencies reflect various parts of the immune system (**Table 14-1**).

HUMORAL IMMUNODEFICIENCIES

DIFFERENTIAL DIAGNOSIS

- Immunoglobulin loss: Nephrotic syndrome or renal failure, severe burns, intestinal lymphangiectasia, chylous loss, severe enteropathy
- Drug-induced: Antimalarial agents, captopril, carbamazepine, glucocorticoids, rituximab, phenytoin, sulfasalazine
- Malignancy: Chronic lymphocytic leukemia, thymoma, Non-Hodgkin's lymphoma, B-cell malignancy
- Prematurity
- Maturational delay (Transient Hypogammaglobulinemia of Infancy)

X-LINKED AGAMMAGLOBULINEMIA (XLA)

A defect of B-cell maturation that results in B-cell and antibody deficiencies with recurrent bacterial infections

TABLE 14-1	Features and Diagnostic Approach for Primary Immunodeficiencies		
Category	**Select Conditions**	**General Features**	**Diagnostic approach**
B-cell (antibody/ humoral) disorders	• X-linked agamma-globulinemia • Common variable immunodeficiency • Specific antibody deficiency • Transient hypogam-maglobulinemia of infancy • IgA deficiency	• Usually present after 3–6 months of age, after maternal antibodies decrease • Predisposition for infections of the upper and lower respiratory tract with encapsulated bacteria	*Quantitative measures:* • Serum immuno-globulin levels (IgG, IgA, IgM) • B-cell counts (CD19, CD20) *Functional measures:* • IgG responses to vaccinations—Pneumococcus, tetanus, and diphtheria antibody titers
T-cell and combined (T- and B-cell) disorders	• SCID • 22q11.2 deletion syndrome • Wiskott–Aldrich syndrome • Ataxia—telangiectasia • *STAT3* • *DOCK8* deficiencies	• Present at birth or in early infancy • FTT, chronic diarrhea • Prolonged and severe respiratory viral infections • Predisposition for fungal and opportunistic infections • Association with autoimmune diseases (ITP, hemolytic anemia)	*Quantitative measures:* • Absolute lymphocyte count on CBC with differential (80% of the ALC is comprised of T cells) • T cell counts (CD3, CD4, CD8) • TREC assay on SCID newborn screen *Functional measures:* • Mitogen proliferation assay
Phagocyte disorders	• Chronic granulomatous disease • Leukocyte adhesion deficiency • Severe congenital neutropenia	• Present in early childhood • Predisposition to skin infections, pneumonia, lymphadenitis, and osteomyelitis • Poor wound healing, delayed separation of the umbilical cord, and omphalitis	*Quantitative measures:* • Absolute neutrophil count on CBC with differential *Functional measures:* • Neutrophil oxidative burst (DHR assay)

(Continued)

TABLE 14-1	Features and Diagnostic Approach for Primary Immunodeficiencies (*Continued*)		
Category	**Select Conditions**	**General Features**	**Diagnostic approach**
Complement disorders	• C1–C9 deficiencies	• Extremely rare • Early complement component defects (C1, C4, C2): predisposition for lupus • C3 defects: predisposition for recurrent infections with encapsulated organisms • Terminal complement component defects (C5–C9): predisposition for recurrent meningococcal disease	• CH50 • AH50 • Individual complement levels (if CH50 or AH50 abnormal)
Immune dysregulation disorders	• IPEX syndrome • APECED	• Polyendocrinopathies • Early-onset autoimmunity • Chronic diarrhea and/or FTT (IPEX) • Candidiasis (APECED)	• *FOXP3* gene sequencing (IPEX) • Autoimmune regulator gene sequencing (APECED)

APECED = autoimmune polyendocrinopathy–candidiasis–ectodermal dystrophy; CBC = complete blood count; FTT = failure to thrive; IPEX = immunodysregulation, polyendocrinopathy, enteropathy, X-linked; TREC = T-cell receptor excision circles.

EPIDEMIOLOGY

• Approximately 1 in 100,000–200,000

ETIOLOGY

• Mutations in *Btk* (Bruton tyrosine kinase) gene

PATHOPHYSIOLOGY

• Btk is required for B-cell maturation after the pre-B stage. As a result, patients with XLA have arrest of B-cell development in the bone marrow at the pro-B to pre-B stage. Mature B cells and plasma cells do not develop, causing a deficiency of all antibody isotypes.
• Btk is also expressed in myeloid stem cells, causing some patients to present with neutropenia.

CLINICAL MANIFESTATIONS

• Bacterial respiratory-tract infections such as sinusitis, otitis, pneumonia, and bronchitis with encapsulated organisms (*S. pneumoniae*, *H. influenzae*) are very common. More invasive infections with these organisms (sepsis, meningitis, septic arthritis) can also occur
• Patients do not have difficulty with common viral respiratory infections.
  ✓ There is, however, an increased susceptibility to enterovirus infections (e.g., poliovirus, coxsackievirus, echovirus), which can cause chronic diarrhea, meningitis, or fatal disseminated infection.

- Profound neutropenia is found in 10% of XLA patients at initial presentation (usually in the setting of acute infections). The neutropenia typically resolves after the infectious episode is treated. Sepsis, especially with *Pseudomonas aeruginosa* and *Staphylococcus aureus*, can occur during episodes of neutropenia.
- Absence of tonsils on physical examination is a classic finding.

DIAGNOSTICS

- Very low levels of IgG, IgA, and IgM antibodies and absent vaccine titers in children beyond the first 6 months of life
- Typically, <1% peripheral B lymphocytes (CD19, CD20)
- Neutropenia (with ANC as low as 0) can be seen during acute infectious episodes.
- Absence of Btk protein (by flow cytometry or Western blotting) and genetic testing confirms the diagnosis

MANAGEMENT

- Lifelong IVIG or subcutaneous immunoglobulin replacement to prevent serious infectious complications. IVIG provides passive immunity against common pathogens such as tetanus, diphtheria, pneumococcus, and hepatitis B.

COMMON VARIABLE IMMUNODEFICIENCY (CVID)

A heterogeneous group of disorders characterized by decreased antibody levels and antibody function resulting in recurrent bacterial infections

EPIDEMIOLOGY

- 1 in 25,000 individuals

ETIOLOGY

- The exact genetic cause of most CVID cases remains unknown. This is likely a heterogeneous disorder with a common clinical phenotype

PATHOPHYSIOLOGY

- Defects in B-cell differentiation or B-cell costimulatory signaling result in impaired immunoglobulin production.

CLINICAL MANIFESTATIONS

- Onset can occur at any age.
- >90% of patients suffer from recurrent infections of the sinopulmonary tract (sinusitis and pneumonia).
- Autoimmune diseases are common (25% of patients) and include autoimmune hemolytic anemia and immune thrombocytopenic purpura (ITP). Other manifestations include rheumatoid arthritis, autoimmune thyroiditis, pernicious anemia, and inflammatory bowel disease. Autoimmune complications can precede the onset of infections.
- Patients are also at greater risk for developing certain malignancies, including lymphoma (incidence, 8%) and gastric carcinoma (incidence, 2%).
- Chronic infectious diarrhea (often *Giardia lamblia* or *Campylobacter jejuni*) can occur.
- Noncaseating granulomas of lungs, liver, and spleen can occur.

DIAGNOSTICS

- IgG with either IgM or IgA 2 SD below age-appropriate normal levels
- Poor antibody response to vaccine antigens 4 weeks post-vaccination

- T- and B-cell enumeration by flow cytometry
  - ✓ A CD4 lymphopenia may be present in some patients.
  - ✓ B cell numbers are typically normal but may be low in some patients.
  - ✓ Patients with low or absent switched memory B cells appear to be at greatest risk for bronchiectasis and autoimmune complications

MANAGEMENT

- Lifelong IVIG or subcutaneous immunoglobulin replacement to prevent serious infections
- Prophylactic antibiotics can be considered as adjunctive therapy in patients with recurrent infections. The type of prophylaxis should be directed at the site of infection and offending pathogens (e.g., amoxicillin 20 mg/kg/day. with a maximum of 250 mg twice daily or azithromycin 10 mg/kg/week with a maximum of 1g weekly).
- Routine or screening imaging studies are not recommended for detection of malignancy in the absence of suggestive signs or symptoms.
- Routine screening for autoimmune and infectious complications
  - ✓ CBC to monitor for autoimmune cytopenias (e.g., ITP hemolytic anemia)
  - ✓ Other testing should be guided by clinical symptoms.

TRANSIENT HYPOGAMMAGLOBULINEMIA OF INFANCY (THI)

A prolongation of the physiologic nadir of immunoglobulin production, which typically occurs between 3 and 6 months of life

EPIDEMIOLOGY

- Approximately 0.061 in 1000 live births

ETIOLOGY

- A maturational delay in endogenous IgG production

PATHOPHYSIOLOGY

- Transplacental transfer begins during the second trimester of pregnancy and peaks during the third trimester; IgG measured in the infant at birth is almost entirely maternal. Maternal IgG gradually declines and a physiologic nadir is reached around 6 months of age, when the infant's endogenous IgG production begins to develop.
- THI is a delay in endogenous IgG production leading to prolonged hypogammaglobulinemia.

CLINICAL MANIFESTATIONS

- Low IgG levels
- Normal vaccine antigen responses
- Many patients are asymptomatic and identified incidentally, but some may present with recurrent bacterial sinopulmonary infections.
- Spontaneous improvement in IgG levels usually occurs by 18 months of age, but some may not have full recovery until 5 years of age.
  - ✓ 67% normalize by 24 months of age
  - ✓ 100% normalize by 5 years of age

DIAGNOSTICS

- Low IgG levels with decreased or normal IgM and IgA levels
- Normal or low normal vaccine responses. If vaccine antibody levels are low, patients should be revaccinated and have levels rechecked 4–6 weeks later.

- Absolute T, B, and NK cells are normal.
- THI remains a diagnosis of exclusion.

MANAGEMENT

- No therapy is needed if patients are asymptomatic. Immunoglobulin levels and vaccine antibody responses should be rechecked every 6–12 months until resolution of hypogammaglobulinemia can be documented.
- Antibiotic prophylaxis (e.g., amoxicillin 20 mg/kg divided twice daily with a maximum of 250 mg twice daily) can be considered for those with recurrent sinopulmonary infections.
- IVIG is typically not indicated for THI of infancy unless patients continue to suffer from severe infections despite antibiotic prophylaxis. IVIG therapy should be stopped within 1–2 years after initiation to assess endogenous antibody levels and vaccine responses.

IgA DEFICIENCY

The most common immunodeficiency, characterized by isolated undetectable serum IgA

EPIDEMIOLOGY

- 1 in 300 Caucasians

ETIOLOGY

- A selective deficiency in IgA production secondary to a B-cell maturational defect

PATHOPHYSIOLOGY

- IgA is normally concentrated in mucosal secretions (pulmonary secretions, saliva, tears, breast milk, GI secretions); its concentration in the serum is relatively low.
- In IgA deficiency, a maturational defect in B cells leads to expression of immature IgA on the cell surface with coexpression of IgM and IgD. Development into IgA-secreting plasma cells is impaired.

CLINICAL MANIFESTATIONS

- Most patients (85%) with selective IgA deficiency are asymptomatic and do not require treatment or regular follow-up.
- A minority of patients may present with sinopulmonary infections with encapsulated bacteria.
- Autoimmune disorders (ITP, autoimmune hemolytic anemia, SLE, vitiligo), GI disorders (giardiasis, inflammatory bowel disease), and atopic diseases (asthma, allergic rhinitis, atopic dermatitis, food allergy) are also increased in patients with IgA deficiency.
- Very rarely, anaphylactic transfusion reactions to IgA containing blood products may occur.
- Selective IgA deficiency may progress to CVID. Thus, patients who are symptomatic with sinopulmonary infections should be followed longitudinally to determine whether CVID develops.

DIAGNOSTICS

- Undetectable IgA levels, with normal IgG and IgM levels
- Normal antibody responses to vaccines

MANAGEMENT

- No treatment is required for asymptomatic patients who do not suffer from increased infections

TABLE 14-2	Normal Immunoglobulin Levels for Age (mg/dL)		
	IgG	IgM	IgA
Newborn	1031±200	11±5	2±3
1–3 mo	430±119	30±11	21±13
4–6 mo	427±186	43±17	28±18
7–12 mo	661±219	54±23	37±18
13–24 mo	762±209	58±23	50±24
25–36 mo	892±183	61±19	71±37
3–5 yr	929±256	56±18	93±27
6–8 yr	923±256	65±25	124±45
9–11 yr	1124±235	79±33	131±60
12–16 yr	946±124	59±20	148±63
Adult	1159±305	99±27	200±31

Adapted with permission from Stiehm ER, Fudenberg HH. Serum levels of immune globulins in health and disease: a survey, *Pediatrics* 1966 May;37(5):715-727.

- If patient suffers from recurrent infections, prophylactic antibiotics can be considered. These should be tailored to the pathogens and sites of repeated infections (e.g., amoxicillin 20 mg/kg/day, with a maximum of 250 mg twice daily, azithromycin 10 mg/kg/week, with a maximum of 1 g weekly).
- Patients with selective IgA deficiency are not candidates for IVIG therapy (IVIG does not contain IgA).
- Normal immunoglobulin levels for age are shown in **Table 14-2**.

COMBINED IMMUNODEFICIENCIES

DIFFERENTIAL DIAGNOSIS

- Genetic syndromes: 22q11.2 deletion syndrome, CHARGE syndrome, chromosome 10p deletions
- Infections: HIV, parasites, malaria
- Inherited thrombocytopenias or autoimmune thrombocytopenia
- DNA breakage syndromes: Nijmegen breakage syndrome, Bloom syndrome

SEVERE COMBINED IMMUNODEFICIENCY (SCID)

A heterogeneous group of disorders characterized by profound T-cell dysfunction that results in severe infections and death within the first year of life without stem-cell transplantation

EPIDEMIOLOGY

- Incidence between 1 in 50,000 and 1 in 70,000 live births

ETIOLOGY

- More than 30 different genetic defects are know to cause SCID.

PATHOPHYSIOLOGY

- The unifying feature shared by all types of SCID is a complete absence of T-cell development. Some mutations allow for B-cell development to occur, but B-cell function is invariably impaired because of the absence of T cell costimulatory signaling.
  - ✓ In common gamma-chain receptor SCID, the gamma chain forms the functional signaling unit of specific receptors affecting T- and NK-cell development (B-cell development is not impaired)
  - ✓ In adenosine deaminase and purine nucleoside phosphorylase deficiency SCID, accumulation metabolites that are toxic to all types of lymphocytes results in a T–B–NK–SCID phenotype.

CLINICAL MANIFESTATIONS

- SCID patients present during early infancy with pneumonia, diarrhea, otitis, sepsis, or skin infections. Recalcitrant oral candidiasis, *P. jirovecii* lung infections, and severe viral respiratory infections are common.
- Lymphoid tissue, including the thymus, is often decreased or absent.
- Thymic tissue is typically absent on chest x-ray.
- Failure to thrive secondary to recurrent infections
- Patients can develop severe infections after receiving live virus vaccines (rotavirus, BCG, MMR, varicella)
- Graft-versus-host reactions from engrafted maternal T cells can result in severe cutaneous, gastrointestinal, and hematologic disease. Lymphadenopathy and hepatosplenomegaly can also occur.

DIAGNOSTICS

- Newborn screening for SCID is now available in most states and is based on measuring T cell receptor excision circles (TRECs), which are by-products of T-cell development. Patients with SCID typically have undetectable TREC values.
- A CBC with differential typically reveals a low absolute lymphocyte count (ALC) $<3000/mm^3$ because 80% of the ALC is comprised of T cells (however, a normal CBC does not exclude SCID).
  - ✓ A CBC with differential yielding an ALC $<1000/mm^3$ is highly concerning for SCID.
- Flow cytometry to enumerate T, B, and NK cells (T-cell numbers are markedly reduced. B- and NK-cell numbers vary depending on the type of SCID.)
- Immunoglobulin levels are markedly reduced (although IgG can be normal in young infants because of maternally transferred immunoglobulin).
- T-cell proliferation in response to mitogens usually reveals poor T-cell function.
- HIV DNA PCR to exclude HIV infection.

MANAGEMENT

- Isolation—Minimize sick contacts.
  - ✓ Contact and respiratory precautions should be instituted immediately.
  - ✓ Hospitalization is often necessary.
- TMP-SMX prophylaxis to prevent *P. jirovecii* infections
- Fluconazole prophylaxis to prevent *Candida albicans* infections
- IVIG replacement therapy
- Avoid all live-virus vaccinations (rotavirus, BCG, varicella, MMR).
- All blood products must be irradiated, CMV-negative, and leukocyte-reduced. Patients can develop graft-versus-host disease from retained leukocytes and CMV infections from blood products.

- Breastfeeding should be avoided to prevent transmission of CMV.
- HLA typing should be performed for the patient and any siblings for bone marrow transplantation. There is a 95% success rate (i.e., survival >10 years) for bone marrow transplantation performed within the first 3 months of life.

22q11.2 DELETION SYNDROME

A genetic disorder characterized by cardiac defects, hypocalcemia, developmental delay, facial dysmorphology, and variable T-cell defects

EPIDEMIOLOGY

- 1 in 3000 to 1 in 4000 live births
- In about 10% of cases, the 22q11.2 deletion is inherited from a parent; 90% of cases occur spontaneously.
- Found in 8% of children with cleft palates and in 1% of children with congenital heart disease

ETIOLOGY

- Wide array of gene deletions in the 22q region, including the *TBXI* gene

PATHOPHYSIOLOGY

- Impaired embryogenesis of the third and fourth pharyngeal arches results in thymic hypoplasia (which impairs T-cell development), parathyroid hypoplasia (which results in hypocalcemia), conotruncal heart defects, and facial dysmorphology
- DiGeorge syndrome, velocardiofacial syndrome, and similar syndromes involve deletions within the 22q region, but wide heterogeneity of the phenotype results from differing amounts of chromosomal loss.

CLINICAL MANIFESTATIONS

- Low T-cell numbers are present in 80% of patients with 22q11.2 deletion syndrome (22q11.2DS). The decrease in T-cell numbers is typically mild to moderate but T-cell function is preserved.
- A severe life-threatening form of this syndrome resulting from complete thymic aplasia (resulting in the near-total absence of T cells) occurs in approximately 1% of patients (complete DiGeorge). Patients with this condition require a thymic transplantation in order to survive.
- Patients typically have normal B-cell numbers and immunoglobulin levels.
- Tetany and seizures from hypocalcemia are present in 10–30% of neonatal patients. The hypocalcemia is typically self-limiting; most children do not require calcium supplementation beyond 1 year of age. However, it is important that calcium levels be followed over time because hypocalcemia may develop again in a patient who previously had been able to come off of calcium supplementation. Patients with complete athymia often require lifelong calcium supplementation).
- 80–90% of patients have congenital heart disease. The most common are interrupted aortic arch, right-sided aortic arch, ventricular septal defect, aberrant right subclavian and internal carotid arteries, tetralogy of Fallot, and truncus arteriosus.
- Speech delay, nonverbal learning disorders, and mild developmental delay (40–50%)
- Paranoid schizophrenia and bipolar disorder in adolescence and adulthood
- Autoimmune diseases occur in 9%. The most common are juvenile idiopathic arthritis, ITP, and autoimmune hemolytic anemia.
- Characteristic facial features: Low-set, cupped or folded ears, small mouth, short philtrum, broad nasal bridge, hooded eyelids, hypertelorism, high-arched or cleft palate, micrognathia

DIAGNOSTICS

- Fluorescence in situ hybridization (FISH) or multiplex ligation-dependent probe amplification (MPLA) assays for chromosome 22q11.2 deletions
  ✓ Patients with heart disease, characteristic facial features, and hypocalcemia should be screened immediately.
- Genomewide assay—This has become the preferred method for diagnosis because it has the ability to identify atypical deletions and other chromosomal abnormalities, such as 10p deletions, CHD7 deletions, and chromosomal duplications
- Newborn TREC screening for SCID (which is designed to detect low T cells) may also identify patients with 22q11.2DS.
- Serum calcium levels (including ionized calcium)
- Parathyroid hormone level (frequency depends on initial levels as some patients never develop hypocalcemia)
- Echocardiography, ECG, and chest x-ray to identify conotruncal or other cardiovascular abnormalities in all infants with a high degree of clinical suspicion for disease
- Flow cytometry for T- and B-cell subsets (along with CBC)
  ✓ Low T-cell numbers may result from thymic hypoplasia.
  ✓ T-cell numbers may be normal if the thymus is well developed.
- Immunoglobulin levels and antibody responses to vaccinations
  ✓ Low IgG levels and poor specific antibody responses to vaccinations occur in 5–10% of patients.

MANAGEMENT

- Live viral vaccines are generally given to patients who have a CD8 T-cell count >300 cells/mm^3 and normal specific antibody responses to non-live viral vaccine antigens.
- Thymic transplantation is indicated for patients with complete thymic aplasia resulting in complete absence of T cells and severe immunodeficiency.
- Antibody deficiency can be present in a minority of patients who may require IVIG therapy.
- Calcium supplementation, if necessary

WISKOTT–ALDRICH SYNDROME (WAS)

A combined T- and B-cell immunodeficiency associated with thrombocytopenia (with small platelets), eczema, recurrent infections, autoimmunity, and malignancy

EPIDEMIOLOGY

- 1 in 250,000 live male births
- There are case reports of heterozygotic females due to inactivation of the unaffected X-chromosome.

ETIOLOGY

- Defect in the WAS gene (Xp11.23)

PATHOPHYSIOLOGY

- WAS protein functions to enhance actin polymerization and branching, allowing cells to rearrange their actin cytoskeleton. Cytoskeletal rearrangement is vital for a number of key functions in immune cells such as endocytosis, exocytosis, chemotaxis, and formation of the immunologic synapse

CLINICAL MANIFESTATIONS

- 30% have classic triad of thrombocytopenia, eczema, and chronic sinopulmonary infections
- Recurrent otitis media, sinusitis, and pneumonia. Other infections include sepsis, meningitis, severe viral infections, and opportunistic infections (including *P. jirovecii*)
- Infants often present with petechiae and bleeding (e.g., bloody diarrhea, epistaxis, or prolonged bleeding after circumcision), especially if platelet counts are less than 10,000/mm^3
- Mild to severe eczema develops in a majority of patients with WAS. The eczema is often complicated by superinfection with bacterial and viral (e.g., HSV) pathogens.
- Malignancies develop in 13% of patients and occur during adolescence or adulthood (most commonly EBV-positive B-cell lymphoma and leukemia)
- Autoimmune disease (e.g., autoimmune cytopenia, vasculitis, colitis) occurs in 40% of patients

DIAGNOSTICS

- Thrombocytopenia (typically <70,000/mm^3) with small platelets (mean platelet volume, 3.8–5.0 fL)
- T-cell lymphopenia and reduced lymphocyte proliferation to mitogens
- Normal IgG, reduced IgM, and increased IgA and IgE levels
- Assess antibody responses to protein and polysaccharide vaccine antigens, as these can be decreased, most commonly following pneumococcal vaccination.
- Reduced WAS protein expression (by flow cytometry or Western blot). Protein expression can be normal in some patients but protein function is reduced.
- Genetic testing for mutations in the *WAS* gene can confirm the diagnosis.

MANAGEMENT

- WAS patients with antibody deficiency benefit from IVIG or subcutaneous immunoglobulin replacement therapy
- *P. jirovecii* prophylaxis with TMP-SMX
- While splenectomy may improve thrombocytopenia, the risk of fatal invasive bacterial infections increases significantly. Therefore, splenectomy is not recommended.
- Patients with severe disease who have an HLA-identical donor are good candidates for bone marrow transplantation. This therapy can cure both the immunologic and hematologic abnormalities seen in patients. Five-year survival following fully matched transplantation is 90% (survival for haploidentical transplantations is approximately 50%). Outcomes are significantly better when transplant occurs before 5 years of age.

ATAXIA–TELANGIECTASIA

Combined T- and B-cell immunodeficiency with neurocutaneous findings and a predisposition for malignancy

EPIDEMIOLOGY

- Incidence between 1 in 100,000 and 1 in 300,000; equal across races

ETIOLOGY

- Ataxia–telangiectasia, mutated (ATM), protein (gene on chromosome 11q22.3)
- Autosomal recessive inheritance

PATHOPHYSIOLOGY

- ATM protein functions to detect double-stranded DNA breaks and to initiate cell-cycle checkpoint arrest—this delay in cell-cycle progression allows for the repair of DNA damage.

CLINICAL MANIFESTATIONS

- Although walking develops normally by 1 year of life, progressive ataxia develops, and patients are generally wheelchair-bound after 10 years of age. Other neurologic abnormalities include oculomotor apraxia, dysarthria, and choreoathetosis.
- The onset of ataxia *precedes* the development of cutaneous telangiectasias, which are present by 3–5 years of age.
  ✓ Telangiectasias typically develop on the bulbar conjunctiva, ear pinna, and nose.
- Patients suffer from a high frequency of recurrent sinopulmonary infections, but opportunistic infections are rare. Aspiration pneumonia secondary to dysfunctional swallowing is common.
- There is an increased risk of malignancy in patients with ataxia–telangiectasia; approximately one-third of patients develop non-Hodgkin's lymphoma, leukemia, or solid malignancies.

DIAGNOSTICS

- Definitive diagnosis is established by identification of mutations in the *ATM* gene.
- Elevated serum alpha-fetoprotein (AFP) after 1 year of age; AFP can normally be elevated in infants.
- Brain MRI may reveal cerebellar atrophy in older children with ataxia–telangiectasia.
- B-cell abnormalities include low immunoglobulin levels and low antibody responses to vaccinations.
- T-cell abnormalities include low T-cell numbers via T-cell enumeration and reduced T-cell function via T-cell proliferation in response to mitogens.

MANAGEMENT

- IVIG or subcutaneous immunoglobulin supplementation for hypogammaglobulinemia.
- X-rays and ionizing radiation should be avoided to minimize the risk of future malignancies.

HYPER-IgE SYNDROME (*STAT3* DEFICIENCY)

A primary immunodeficiency characterized by invasive bacterial skin and lung infections, dermatitis, elevated IgE levels, and musculoskeletal abnormalities

EPIDEMIOLOGY

- Incidence unknown, but rare; equal incidence in males and females and across races

ETIOLOGY

- Autosomal dominant mutations in the *STAT3* gene

PATHOPHYSIOLOGY

- Mutations in *STAT3* impair differentiation and function of interleukin (IL)-17–secreting (Th17) cells. IL-17 secreted by Th17 cells stimulate granulopoiesis through induction of granulocyte colony-stimulating factor, recruit neutrophils to the site of infection through induction of IL-8, and stimulate production of antimicrobial peptides such as β-defensins.

CLINICAL MANIFESTATIONS

- Eczematous rash in infancy or early childhood
- Failure to shed primary teeth (60–70%), often requiring dental extraction
- Recurrent bacterial infections, including upper and lower respiratory tract infection (90%). Pneumatoceles following pneumonias are common.
  - ✓ Organisms include *S. aureus, H. influenzae, P. aeruginosa,* and *Aspergillus fumigatus.*
- Skin infections are common, including hot and cold abscesses.
- Mucocutaneous fungal infections, including thrush, esophageal candidiasis, and onychomycosis in 80% of patients.
- Pathologic fractures following minor trauma (60–70%)
- Hyperextensible joints (60%)
- Characteristic facial features: Coarse facies—wide nose, deep-set eyes, prominent chin and forehead, high-arched palate

DIAGNOSTICS

- Elevated IgE greater than 2000 IU/mL, although not a reliable biomarker
  - ✓ Elevated IgE is also commonly seen in patients with atopic disease and is not specific for *STAT3* deficiency.
- Elevated eosinophil count greater than 2 SD above normal (93% of patients)
- Dental x-rays: Delayed development and retained primary teeth
- Antibody responses to pneumococcus, diphtheria, and tetanus should be assessed, as some patients have impaired antibody responses to vaccine antigens.
- Low Th17-cell numbers
- Genetic testing to identify mutations in the *STAT3* gene can confirm the diagnosis.

MANAGEMENT

- Antistaphylococcal antibiotic prophylaxis (usually TMP-SMX at a dose of 2.5 mg/kg/day of the trimethoprim component, with 160 mg TMP/dose)
- IVIG or subcutaneous immunoglobulin for patients with impaired antibody immunity

DOCK8 DEFICIENCY

A primary immunodeficiency characterized by severe atopic disease, recurrent viral cutaneous infections, as well as invasive bacterial skin and lung infections (previously referred to as autosomal recessive hyper-IgE syndrome)

EPIDEMIOLOGY

- Incidence unknown, but rare
- Equal incidence in males and females, with a higher prevalence in consanguineous populations

ETIOLOGY

- Autosomal recessive mutations in the *DOCK8* gene

PATHOPHYSIOLOGY

- *DOCK8* functions in the regulation of *STAT3* phosphorylation. Thus, a deficiency impairs the differentiation and function of Th17 cells and subsequent recruitment of neutrophils to the site of infection via IL-8.

- Actin cytoskeleton regulation is also impaired, causing defective immune synapse formation.
- *DOCK8* assists in B-cell signaling. Mutations also cause defective antibody production and impair the formation of memory B cells.

CLINICAL MANIFESTATIONS

- Severe atopic conditions include eczema, food and environmental allergies, eosinophilic esophagitis, and allergic rhinitis.
- Cutaneous viral infections, including molluscum contagiosum, varicella–zoster, herpes simplex, and human papillomaviruses, are a hallmark of this disease.
- Frequent sinopulmonary infections are often experienced and can lead to bronchiectasis. Typical pathogens include *Staph. aureus*, *H. influenzae*, *P. aeruginosa*, and *A. fumigatus*.
- Autoimmune disease, including autoimmune hemolytic anemia, hypothyroidism, systemic lupus erythematosus, and uveitis
- Increased risk of virally driven cancers (up to 17% of patients)

DIAGNOSTICS

- Elevated IgE; IgG may also be elevated, but IgM and IgA may be low.
- Elevated eosinophil count
- Antibody responses to pneumococcus, diphtheria, and tetanus should be assessed, as some patients have impaired antibody responses to vaccine antigens.
- T-cell lymphopenia is present in a majority of patients.
- Low Th17 cell numbers
- Genetic testing to identify mutations in the *DOCK8* gene can confirm the diagnosis.

MANAGEMENT

- Antistaphylococcal antibiotic prophylaxis (usually TMP-SMX at a dose of 2.5 mg/kg/day of the trimethoprim component, with a maximum of 160 mg TMP/dose)
- IVIG for patients with impaired antibody immunity
- Stem-cell transplantation is curative.

INNATE DEFECTS

DIFFERENTIAL DIAGNOSIS

- Leukemoid reaction malignancy: Acute lymphoblastic leukemia
- SLE, specifically with complement defects

CHRONIC GRANULOMATOUS DISEASE (CGD)

A phagocyte immunodeficiency resulting from impaired activation of the neutrophil oxidative burst

EPIDEMIOLOGY

- Prevalence varies by mutation (e.g., genes for gp91, a component of the nicotinamide adenine dinucleotide phosphate [NADPH] oxidase complex, have mutations as follows: CYBB 1 in 250,000; CYBA 1 in 2,000,000)
- 65–70% X-linked inheritance; remainder autosomal recessive. X-linked CGD is typically more severe clinically than autosomal recessive CGD.

ETIOLOGY

- Mutations affecting the NADPH oxidase complex

PATHOPHYSIOLOGY

- CGD is caused by defects in the NADPH oxidase system, which consists of six proteins (two membrane-bound and four cytosolic). Upon cellular activation, the cytosolic components assemble with the membrane-bound components to form the active complex. Oxygen and NADPH+H are reduced by NADPH oxidase to produce NADP+ and superoxide radical. This stimulates an influx of potassium cations into the cell, which then activates the release of neutrophil proteases (neutrophil elastase and cathepsin G).

CLINICAL MANIFESTATIONS

- Patients present within the first few years of life with severe deep-seated infections: Pneumonia (79%), skin or visceral abscesses (68%), lymphadenitis (53%), and osteomyelitis (25%)
- Patients susceptible to bacterial and fungal organisms: *Staph. aureus*, *S. marcescens*, *B. cepacia*, *Nocardia* spp., and *A. fumigatus*
- Early-onset inflammatory bowel disease resulting in malabsorption may occur, particularly in X-linked CGD. Obstructive GI tract and urinary tract noninfectious granulomas are problematic complications.

DIAGNOSTICS

- Flow cytometry for dihydrorhodamine 123 (DHR) dye conversion to rhodamine 123 has largely replaced the less accurate nitroblue tetrazolium (NBT) test. It can be used to detect carrier status and can differentiate X-linked CGD from other forms in a majority of cases.

MANAGEMENT

- Long-term prophylaxis with TMP-SMX and itraconazole to reduce severe bacterial and fungal infections
- Interferon-gamma prophylaxis has also been shown to reduce the frequency of infectious complications.
  ✓ Side effects such as fever and flu-like symptoms limit use of this medication.
- Bone marrow transplantation (BMT) is curative and currently considered the standard of care for patients with absent neutrophil function. CGD patients with little or no reactive oxygen intermediate [ROI] production have markedly reduced long-term survival compared with patients with residual production of ROI.
- BMT should be considered as soon as possible for patients with X-linked CGD and those with autosomal recessive CGD with severe symptoms.

LEUKOCYTE ADHESION DEFICIENCY (LAD)

An autosomal recessive phagocyte immunodeficiency that results from a defect in neutrophil migration leading to recurrent bacterial infections

EPIDEMIOLOGY

- Extremely rare, with less than 400 cases of LAD type 1 reported in the United States
- LAD type 2 reported primarily in Middle East

ETIOLOGY

- LAD 1: Deficiency or defect in the common beta chain of the β_2-integrin family CD18
- LAD 2: Mutations in the gene encoding GDP-fucose transporter 1 (FUCT1)
- LAD 3: Mutations in the gene for KINDLIN3, which is a protein involved in integrin activation

PATHOPHYSIOLOGY

- Patients with LAD have normal ANCs and normal neutrophil function. However, their neutrophils are unable to adhere to the endothelium of vessels and migrate to sites of active infection or inflammation.
  - ✓ LAD 1: Defective firm adhesion of neutrophils to endothelium
  - ✓ LAD 2: Defective leukocyte rolling but intact firm adhesion
  - ✓ LAD 3: Normal integrin expression and structure but impaired integrin activation and thus binding)

CLINICAL MANIFESTATIONS

- LAD 1: This is the most common form of LAD; it is characterized by markedly elevated WBC count (50,000–100,000/mcL) even in the absence of infection, delayed separation of the umbilical cord with omphalitis, recurrent bacterial skin infections, impaired wound healing, absent pus formation, and pneumonia with staphylococcus and gram-negative bacilli. Delayed umbilical-cord separation is defined as greater than 7 weeks. Patients with severe forms of LAD 1 often die during infancy without bone marrow transplantation.
- LAD 2: This is characterized by a milder phenotype than LAD 1. Patients develop mild leukocytosis (10,000–40,000/mcL) and have reduced (but not absent) pus formation. Bacterial skin and lung infections are typically not life-threatening. Patients have severe mental, growth, and motor retardation, as well as microcephaly.
- LAD 3: The clinical phenotype is identical to that for LAD 1, with significant platelet aggregate dysfunction leading to bleeding complications such as cerebral hemorrhage, hematoma, and bloody stools.

DIAGNOSTICS

- Marked leukocytosis in the absence of infection on CBC with differential count
- Decreased or absent expression of CD18 via flow cytometry in LAD 1 (normal in LAD 2 and LAD 3)
- Absence of CD15a on leukocytes on LAD 2 (flow cytometry)
- Gene sequencing: *ITGB2* (LAD 1), *SLC35C1* (LAD 2), or *KINDLIN* 3 (LAD 3)

MANAGEMENT

- LAD 1: BMT should be considered for patients with severe forms of LAD 1. BMT has a success rate of 80% when a matched donor is available and 50% in cases of haploidentical transplants.
- LAD 2: Aggressive treatment of infections and prophylactic antibiotics. Fucose supplementation should be started as early as possible to help prevent psychomotor retardation.
- LAD 3: As with LAD 1, early intervention with BMT should be considered.

EARLY COMPLEMENT DEFECTS

A primary immunodeficiency characterized by recurrent infections and systemic lupus erythematosus (SLE), caused by a deficiency in the early components of the complement cascade. In contrast, patients with terminal complement defects (C5–C9) present with recurrent invasive meningococcal disease.

EPIDEMIOLOGY

• C2 mutation is the most common, with an incidence of 1 in 10,000.

ETIOLOGY

• Defects can occur in C1q, C1r, C1s, C4, or C2 components.

PATHOPHYSIOLOGY

• Early complement components, C1Q in particular, play a role in the clearance of apoptotic cells, which may create conditions that are more prone to the development of lupus. C3b is an opsonin that is critical for defense against encapsulated bacteria.

CLINICAL MANIFESTATIONS

• Patients can have difficulty with infections with encapsulated organisms.
• SLE is the most common presenting symptom (incidence is 90% in patients with C1q deficiency) and can present very early in life.

DIAGNOSTICS

• CH50 will invariably be low. A normal CH50 essentially rules out C1–C9 deficiencies, and measurement of individual complement proteins is not required).
• Testing for individual components if CH50 is low (C1q, C1s, C1r, C2, C4)

MANAGEMENT

• Appropriate management of lupus is imperative, as this can often be the cause of mortality.
• Vaccination for encapsulated bacteria should be given (*S. pneumoniae, H. influenzae*)
• Prompt treatment for infections with antibiotics is essential.

DISORDERS OF IMMUNE DYSREGULATION

DIFFERENTIAL DIAGNOSIS

• Infections: HIV, parasitic infection, as well as other causes of infectious diarrhea
• Early-onset inflammatory bowel disease, chronic malabsorption

IPEX (IMMUNODYSREGULATION, POLYENDOCRINOPATHY, ENTEROPATHY, X-LINKED) SYNDROME

A primary immunodeficiency characterized by profound diarrhea and autoimmune disease. This disorder has a poor prognosis, with death occurring in early childhood if untreated.

EPIDEMIOLOGY

• Rare. Fewer than 300 cases have been described.

ETIOLOGY

• X-linked mutation in the *FoxP3* gene

PATHOPHYSIOLOGY

• *FoxP3* is a transcription factor responsible for the development of T-regulatory (Treg) cells.
• Tregs suppress autoreactive T cells in the periphery.
• Dysfunctional Treg cells lead to loss of peripheral tolerance and development of multisystem autoimmune disease from infancy.

CLINICAL MANIFESTATIONS

- Clinical triad of autoimmune enteropathy, autoimmune disease and dermatitis
- Diarrhea is typically severe and watery but can appear mucous or bloody.
- Failure to thrive
- Early-onset multisystem autoimmune problems; typically, type I diabetes, autoimmune thyroiditis, and autoimmune cytopenias.
- Mild to moderate eczema and in some cases a generalized erythematous rash

DIAGNOSTICS

- Eosinophilia is a consistent finding.
- Anemia, neutropenia, and thrombocytopenia may also be present and warrant additional testing for autoimmune antibodies
- IgE is elevated, with normal IgM, IgG, and IgA levels
- Villous atrophy classically seen on small bowel biopsy.
- *FoxP3* flow cytometry and gene sequencing are diagnostic.

MANAGEMENT

- Immunosuppressive medications (such as rapamycin or cyclosporine) are used to target autoreactive T-cell activation
- Most patients require total parenteral nutrition because of malabsorption from severe enteropathy.
- Stem-cell transplantation is curative and should be initiated as soon as possible.

Kathleen Chiotos, MD
Lori Handy, MD, MSCE
Salwa Sulieman, DO
Leila Posch, MD
Jeffrey S. Gerber, MD, PhD

SYNDROMES AND COMPLEXES

BITE-WOUND INFECTIONS

Infections usually localized to the site of a bite. Rare sequelae include meningitis, brain abscess, endocarditis, and septic arthritis.

EPIDEMIOLOGY

- Infection in 10–15% of dog bites and approximately 50% of cat bites
- Greatest rate of infection after bites to the hands (28–63%)
  - ✓ Other common sites: Face/head/neck (6–16%), arm/leg (10–32%), and trunk (2–10%)

ETIOLOGY

- Usually polymicrobial; derived from oral flora of biting animal
- Cat and dog bite infections: *Pasteurella canis* (dog), *Pasteurella multocida* (cat), *Capnocytophaga* spp (dog) streptococci, *Staphylococcus aureus, Moraxella* spp., *Neisseria* spp., and anaerobes
- Human bites: *S. aureus,* viridans group Streptococci, *Streptococcus pyogenes, Eikenella corrodens, Streptococcus intermedius, Neisseria* spp., *Haemophilus* spp.
- Horse/sheep bite: *Actinobacillus* spp, *Streptococcus equisimilis*
- Marine settings/fish bite: *Halomonas venusta, Vibrio* spp, *Aeromonas hydrophila, Plesiomonas shigelloides, Pseudomonas* spp., *Mycobacterium marinum*
- Monkey bite: B virus

PATHOPHYSIOLOGY

- Infection follows direct inoculation of bacteria into tissues.
- Hematogenous dissemination may occur.

CLINICAL MANIFESTATIONS

- Note wound type (puncture, laceration, avulsion), edema, erythema, tenderness, drainage, depth of penetration, bruising, deformity, involvement of underlying structure, sensation, regional lymphadenopathy.
- Look for signs of systemic infection (e.g., fever, hypotension).
- Animal: Record type of animal, health of animal, provoked or unprovoked attack; observe for signs of rabies if applicable.
- Patient: History of asplenia (increased risk of *Capnocytophaga* spp.); immunosuppression or other illnesses; last tetanus immunization

DIAGNOSTICS

- Gram stain and culture of wound if time from injury is longer than 8 hours or if signs and symptoms of infection exist.
- Consider blood culture if fever present.
- Radiography indicated for penetrating injuries overlying bones or joints, suspected foreign body, or fracture.

MANAGEMENT

Immediate Management

- Examine for foreign body, irrigate with copious amounts of normal saline, and debride devitalized tissue.
- Suturing is controversial. Leave wound open if greater than 8 hours old or a puncture wound; primary wound closure for injuries to face and when cosmetic outcome is important
- Indications for operative exploration and debridement: Extensive tissue damage; involvement of metacarpophalangeal joint from clenched fist injury; cranial bites by large animals

Tetanus Prophylaxis

- Clean minor wounds: Administer tetanus toxoid if >10 years since last tetanus-containing vaccine dose, if vaccine history is unknown, or if fewer than three doses received.
- Puncture or severe wounds: If fewer than three doses received, administer tetanus toxoid and tetanus immunoglobulin. If patient has completed primary immunization but it has been ≥5 years since last tetanus-containing vaccine dose, administer tetanus toxoid.

Rabies Postexposure Prophylaxis

- Prophylaxis:
  - ✓ Active: Four doses of rabies vaccine on days 0, 3, 7, and 14 (five doses for immunocompromised hosts)
  - ✓ Passive: Rabies immunoglobulin (RIG) given on day 0 with the first dose of vaccine, infiltrate wound with as much as possible and give remainder IM.
- Dogs, cats, ferrets: If animal is healthy and available for 10 days of observation, prophylaxis (immunization) only if animal develops signs of rabies; if animal is suspected or determined to be rabid, administer both immunization and RIG; if unknown, consult public health officials.
- Bats, skunks, raccoons, foxes, woodchucks, and most other carnivores: Regarded as rabid unless geographic area is known to be free of rabies or proven negative via laboratory tests; patients require rabies immunization and RIG.
- Livestock, rodents, and lagomorphs: Typically not high risk, but consult local public health officials

Antibiotic Management

See **Table 15-1.**

BRONCHIOLITIS

Acute lower respiratory tract infection that causes inflammation of the bronchioles and results in distal airway obstruction and frequently accompanied by wheezing

TABLE 15-1	Antibiotic Management of Bite Wounds		
Source	Most common Organisms	Antibiotic	Comments
Dog, cat	*Pasteurella* spp, *Staphylococcus aureus*, *Streptococcus* spp., anaerobes, *Capnocytophaga* spp., *Moraxella* spp., *Corynebacterium* spp., *Neisseria* spp.	Orally: Amoxicillin–clavulanate IV: Ampicillin–sulbactam *Alternative if penicillin-allergic:* Third-generation cephalosporin or trimethoprim–sulfamethoxazole PLUS Clindamycin	• Consider MRSA coverage for severe wounds or refractory infections • 3–5 days for prophylaxis; treatment of infected wounds typically 7–10 days depending upon source control and wound severity
Human	*Streptococcus* spp., *Staph. aureus, Haemophilus* spp., *Eikenella corrodens*, other anaerobes	Orally: Amoxicillin–clavulanate IV: Ampicillin-sulbactam *Alternative if penicillin-allergic:* Third-generation cephalosporin or trimethoprim–sulfamethoxazole PLUS Clindamycin	

MRSA = methicillin-resistant *Staphylococcus aureus*.

EPIDEMIOLOGY

- Usually younger than 2 years of age
- One-third of children develop bronchiolitis in the first 2 years of life; approximately 10% of these children will be hospitalized.
- All geographic areas; winter to early spring
- Risk factors for severe illness: Age less than 3 months, gestational age less than 34 weeks, ill or toxic appearance, respiratory rate >70 breaths per minute, pulse oximetry <94%, cardiac or pulmonary disease, immunodeficiency

ETIOLOGY

- Infectious agents: Respiratory syncytial virus (RSV; 50–80% of cases); parainfluenza viruses types 1, 2, and 3; adenovirus; influenza virus; rhinovirus; coronaviruses; human metapneumovirus. Patients may have coinfections.

PATHOPHYSIOLOGY

- Necrosis of airway epithelium and ciliated lining causes mucosal inflammation. Lymphocytic infiltration of peribronchial and peribronchiolar epithelium causes edema of submucosa and adventitia.
- Impaired mucociliary clearance leads to obstruction of smaller-caliber distal airways without significant alveolar involvement, causing partial or total obstruction to airflow
- Varying degrees of obstruction lead to rapidly changing clinical signs and symptoms.
- Epithelial regeneration lags behind clinical recovery.

CLINICAL MANIFESTATIONS

- Incubation period of causal pathogens ranges from 2 to 8 days. Acute illness ranges from 3 to 7 days. Recovery is gradual over 1–3 weeks.

- Signs and symptoms: Rhinorrhea (profuse), cough, low-grade fever, lethargy, increased work of breathing, tachypnea, wheezing, cyanosis, apnea (especially in ages <3 months), and retractions (suprasternal, subcostal, intercostal, and, with severe illness, supraclavicular)
- Auscultation: Prolonged expiratory phase, wheezing, rales, rhonchi

DIAGNOSTICS

- Diagnostic testing is typically not indicated for routine bronchiolitis.
- Chest x-ray is not typically required, but if performed, it reveals hyperinflation, patchy atelectasis, peribronchial cuffing .
- Rapid viral identification from nasopharyngeal aspirate may be useful for cohorting hospitalized patients but has little impact on management; routine viral testing is not necessary.
- Consider arterial blood gas and serum electrolyte measurements if there is concern for impending respiratory failure.

MANAGEMENT

- Respiratory support:
  - ✓ Initiate supplemental oxygen in previously healthy infants only if oxygen saturation values persistently fall below 90% while awake or 88% while asleep. Discontinue oxygen if oxygen saturation is greater than 90% while feeding well with minimal respiratory distress.
  - ✓ Discontinue use of pulse oximetry or transition to intermittent pulse oximetry during the convalescent stage of illness (e.g., if oxygen saturation >90% in room air for >2–4 hours).
  - ✓ High-flow nasal cannula decreases intubation rate, respiratory rate, and ICU length of stay.
  - ✓ Mechanical ventilation should be considered for infants with signs of respiratory failure, shock, or persistent apnea.
- Pharmacologic interventions:
  - ✓ Nebulized β_2-adrenergic agonists (albuterol, levalbuterol) are *not routinely* indicated. For moderate to severely ill infants, consider trial doses with assessment of clinical response. May have more benefit in those with asthma history or in ventilated patients. Potential exists for paradoxical effects and increased airway resistance.
  - ✓ Nebulized α- or β-adrenergic agonists (racemic epinephrine) are *not routinely* indicated. In moderately ill infants, consider trial doses with assessment of clinical response.
  - ✓ Current research does not support treatment with hypertonic (3%) saline; consider for patients with prolonged hospital stay (either 1.5 mg racemic epinephrine mixed with 4 mL of 3% saline or 1–2.5 mg albuterol mixed with 4 mL 3% saline; administered every 2–8 hours).
  - ✓ Corticosteroids *not routinely* indicated; studies do *not* show consistent clinical improvement with either systemic or inhaled formulations; infants with a strong family history of asthma *and* a previous episode of wheezing might benefit from early systemic steroid administration, though data are conflicting.
  - ✓ Antivirals (ribavirin) are virtually never indicated.
- Suctioning: Lapses in suctioning for >4 hours are associated with increased length of stay.
- Chest physiotherapy has not been shown to reduce the length of disease, improve clinical scores, or reduce hospital stay.
- Infants with extreme tachypnea are at risk of aspiration; consider nothing-by-mouth status, IV hydration, and nasogastric tube for enteral feeds.
- Infection prevention and control: Viruses causing bronchiolitis are transmitted primarily by direct contact with secretions and/or fomites. Appropriate hand hygiene is paramount. Contact precautions and patient cohorting are indicated.

- Palivizumab (humanized monoclonal RSV antibody) prophylaxis:
  - ✓ Recommended during the first year of life to infants born before 29 weeks 0 days' gestation and to infants with hemodynamically significant heart or chronic lung disease of prematurity
  - ✓ The recommended dose is 15 mg/kg/dose for a maximum of 5 monthly doses during RSV season.
  - ✓ The American Academy of Pediatrics (AAP) guidelines provide additional guidance on eligibility for administration (*Pediatrics* 2014;134:e1474–e1502).
  - ✓ Palivizumab does not interfere with response to vaccines

CENTRAL-LINE ASSOCIATED BLOODSTREAM INFECTION

Bacteria or yeast cultured in the presence of a central venous catheter (CVC).

EPIDEMIOLOGY

- Most common device-associated infection in children
- Associated with increased morbidity and mortality
- Neonatal central line-associated bloodstream infections are associated with adverse neurodevelopmental outcomes.
- Risk with nontunneled is greater than with tunneled, which is greater than totally implantable catheter
  - ✓ Tunneled = Hickman, Broviac, Groshong, and Quinton catheters
  - ✓ Totally implantable = portacath, permacath (hemodialysis)
- Lower risk with silver-chelated collagen cuff, antibiotic-impregnated catheter (e.g., minocycline + rifampin, chlorhexidine + silver sulfadiazine), and chlorhexidine preparation compared to betadine preparation

ETIOLOGY

- Coagulase-negative *Staphylococcus* spp., *S. aureus*, *Enterococcus*, *Pseudomonas aeruginosa*, and other gram-negative bacilli, *Candida* spp., rapid-growing mycobacteria (e.g., *Mycobacterium chelonae*, *M. fortuitum*, *M. abscessus*)

PATHOPHYSIOLOGY

- Medical devices are portal of entry for migration of skin organisms into catheter
- Contamination of catheter hub by health care worker hands or environmental sources
- Hematogenous seeding of catheter from another focus of infection or translocated bacteria from the gastrointestinal tract

CLINICAL MANIFESTATIONS

- Fever alone
- Fever, hypotension, tachycardia, tachypnea (septic shock)
- Abscess or cellulitis at catheter-insertion site (tunnel infection)
- Complications include sepsis, bacterial endocarditis, mycotic aneurysms, disseminated candidiasis (endophthalmitis, endocarditis, or hepatosplenic or renal candidiasis)

DIAGNOSTICS

- Blood cultures from the catheter *and* periphery are preferred. The following criteria implicate CVC as source of infection:
  - ✓ *Quantitative blood cultures (rarely used):* (1) CVC culture yields a colony count at least fivefold *higher* than peripheral-blood culture; (2) 15 or more CFUs from catheter tip

by *semiquantitative* culture (colony counts directly from agar plate); or (3) 100 or more CFUs from catheter tip by *quantitative* culture
  ✓ *Differential time to positivity*: Positive result from CVC culture at least 2 hours earlier than from peripheral culture with similar culture volume. Compared to quantitative blood culture methods, differential time to positivity has sensitivity of 80–90% and specificity of 75–94%.
- Consider echocardiography if:
  ✓ Culture grows *S. aureus* or HACEK organism
  ✓ Culture positive longer than 3 days despite appropriate therapy
  ✓ New murmur develops
- Rapid-growing mycobacteria grow in conventional blood culture bottles. Isolation of MAI requires special AFB isolator blood culture tubes (check with microbiology laboratory)
- If culture grows *Candida* spp., risk of dissemination to at least one organ is about 17%, including dissemination to the eye (3%), central nervous system (12%), abdomen (8–23%), and heart (8%). Obtain ophthalmologic exam and consider imaging the brain and abdomen as well as echocardiography.

MANAGEMENT

- Follow institutional central-line associated bloodstream infection prevention practices.
  ✓ Verify device necessity.
  ✓ Review local prevention bundles, including hand hygiene, aseptic technique, standards around dressings, bathing, and access.
- Empiric antibiotic regimens may vary depending on regional antibiotic susceptibility patterns. Guiding principles include coverage for skin flora, which may include MRSA and nosocomial gram-negative organisms if patient is ill or frequently hospitalized. If the patient is already on antimicrobial therapy, empiric antibiotics should be broader than the current regimen (**Figure 15-1**).
- Fever alone in presence of a central catheter:
  ✓ Suggested resource: https://www.chop.edu/clinical-pathway/fever-non-oncology-cvc-clinical-pathway
    Authors: B. Ku, MD; M.K. Abbadessa, RN; L. Riede, RN; R. Mann, CRNP; J. Gerber, MD; M. Hayes, PharmD; T. Bales, MD; L. Copelovitch, MD; D. Friedman, MD; B. Laskin, MD; P Mazzeo, MD; L. Rand, MD; C. Witmer, MD; D. Barsky, MD; J. Lavelle, MD
  ✓ Cefepime (gram-negative should be selected on the basis of local antibiogram) with or without vancomycin, depending on host and institutional recommendations for inpatients
- Shock in presence of a central catheter:
  ✓ Vancomycin and cefepime (choice of gram-negative agent should be selected on the basis of local antibiogram); consider also source of infection and patient history of drug resistant organisms.
  ✓ Consider antifungal coverage if the patient is immunocompromised, has been on prolonged antibiotics, or is on inserted TPN
- Reasons to discontinue the central catheter: (1) Rapid clinical deterioration; (2) cellulitis or abscess at or along catheter site; (3) persistently positive blood culture results despite appropriate therapy; (4) endocarditis/septic thrombophlebitis; (5) organism is known to be difficult to clear —e.g., *Bacillus, Burkholderia, Candida, S. aureus, Stenotrophomonas,* and *Mycobacteria*
- Treatment duration is individualized according to organism, clinical course, CVC status (salvage or removal), and clearance of bacteremia.

FIGURE 15-1 Antimicrobial Spectrum of Commonly Used Antibacterial Agents. Results may vary; consult local clinical microbiology laboratory for most relevant data. S = synergy when used in combination with cell wall active agent; empty cells = no data; + = active, − = not recommended, +/− = variable activity.

	Penicillin	Ampicillin	Oxacillin	Ampicillin–sulbactam	Ticarcillor–clavulanate	Piperacillin–tazobactam	Cefazolin	Cefuroxime	Cefoxitin	Ceftriaxone	Ceftazidime	Cefepime	Imipenem	Meropenem	Doxycycline	Clindamycin	Aminoglycosides	Ciprofloxacin	Levofloxacin	Azithromycin	Tmp-smx	Vancomycin	Linezolid	Metronidazole
Gram +																								
GBS	+	+	+	+	+	+	+	+	+	+	+	+	+	+	+	+	−	+/−	+	+/−	−	+	+	−
S. pneumoniae	+	+	+	+	+	+	+	+	+	+	+	+	+	+	+	+	−	+/−	+	+/−	+	+	+	−
E. faecalis	+	+	−	+	+/−	+	−	−	−	−	−	−	+	+/−	−	−	S	+/−	+	−	−	+	+	−
E. faecium	+/−	+/−	−	+/−	+/−	+/−	−	−	−	−	−	−	+/−	−	−	−	S	−	−	−	−	+/−	+	−
Staph. aureus	−	−	+	+	+	+	+	+	+	+	−	+	+	+	+	+	+	+	+	−	+	+	+	−
MRSA	−	−	−	−	−	−	−	−	−	−	−	−	−	−	+	+	S	+/−	+/−	−	+	+	+	−
Listeria	+	+	−	+	−	−	−	−	−	−	−	−	+	+	+	−	S	+	+	+	+	+	+	−
Gram −																								
H. influenzae	−	+/−	−	+	+	+	+	+	+	+	+	+	+	+	+	−	+	+	+	+	+/−	−	−	−
N. meningitidis	+	+	−	+	+	+	−	+	+/−	+	+/−	+	+	+	+	−	−	+	+	+	+	−	+/−	−
E. coli	−	+/−	−	+	+	+	+	+	+	+	+	+	+	+	+	−	+	+	+	−	+/−	−	−	−
Klebsiella	−	−	−	+	+	+	+	+	+	+	+	+	+	+	+/−	−	+	+	+	−	+/−	−	−	−
Enterobacter	−	−	−	−	+	+	−	+/−	−	+	+	+	+	+	−	−	+	+	+	−	+	−	−	−
Serratia	−	−	−	−	+	+	−	+/−	−	+	+	+	+	+	−	−	+	+	+	−	+	−	−	−
Pseudomonas	−	−	−	−	+	+	−	−	−	−	+	+	+	+	−	−	+	+	+/−	−	−	−	−	−
Anaerobes																								
Oral anaerobes	+	+	−	+	+	+	−	−	+	−	−	−	+	+	−	+	−	−	+	−	−	−	+	+
Gut anaerobes (Bacteroides fragilis)	−	−	−	+	+	+	−	−	+	−	−	−	+	+	−	−	−	−	−	−	−	−	+/−	+

289

- General recommendations include:
  - ✓ *Candida* spp: Minimum 14 days (line removal recommended)
  - ✓ *S. aureus*: Minimum 14 days (line removal recommended)
  - ✓ Coagulase-negative staphylococci: 5–10 days if line remains in place, 3 days if line removed
  - ✓ *Enterococcus* and viridans streptococci: 7 days
  - ✓ Gram-negative organisms: 7–10 days (line removal preferred)
- Antibiotic or ethanol locks can be considered as part of salvage therapy and for CVC maintenance (prevention) for patients with recurrent CVC infection.

CELLULITIS/ABSCESS

A primary, superficial skin infection

ETIOLOGY

- Immunocompetent children: *S. pyogenes* (predominant with simple cellulitis), *S. aureus* (predominant with purulence/abscess formation). Consider *S. agalactiae* in neonates.
- Immunocompromised children: Also *Pseudomonas* spp., Enterobacteriaceae, *Cryptococcus neoformans*, anaerobes

PATHOPHYSIOLOGY

- Acute infection of the skin involving the dermis and subcutaneous tissues, most commonly following local trauma (e.g., abrasions)

CLINICAL MANIFESTATIONS

- Constitutional symptoms including fever, chills, malaise
- Skin edema, warmth, erythema, tenderness, or fluctuance
- Red, lymphangitic streaks
- Regional lymphadenopathy
- Break in skin may be found on exam.

DIAGNOSTICS

- Culture of aspirate, skin biopsy, and blood cultures collectively yield causal organism in 25% of cases; blood cultures positive in <1% of uncomplicated cellulitis and roughly 12% of complicated infections.
- Blood cultures should be performed in young patients or those who are systemically ill.
- Drain areas of fluctuance (especially in areas of high MRSA prevalence).

MANAGEMENT

- Well-appearing children can be treated as outpatients: Cephalexin or amoxicillin–clavulanate can be used for simple cellulitis and for purulent cellulitis/abscess formation in regions with low MRSA prevalence; trimethoprim–sulfamethoxazole (TMP-SMX) or clindamycin for purulent cellulitis/abscess formation in areas of high MRSA prevalence
- Consider ultrasound to identify drainage collection.
- Incision and drainage of abscesses is paramount and obviates antimicrobial therapy for simple abscesses.
- Hospitalize and initiate antibiotics for ill-appearing patients with high fever, rapid progression, or lymphangitis. Consider oxacillin, cefazolin, or clindamycin. Critically ill patients require coverage with vancomycin due to possible MRSA resistance to clindamycin. (*Refer to section on MRSA.*)
- Duration of therapy depends on clinical response and adequate drainage; typically 5 days

Age	Etiology	
	Bacteria	**Virus**
Neonate	Group B *Streptococcus*, enteric gram-negative rods, *Listeria monocytogenes*	Cytomegalovirus, herpes simplex virus
1 to 3 months	*S. pneumoniae, Chlamydia trachomatis, Bordetella pertussis*	RSV, parainfluenza viruses
3 months to 4 years	*S. pneumoniae, Haemophilus influenzae, S. aureus, Mycoplasma pneumoniae*	RSV, parainfluenza viruses, influenza, adenovirus
5 to 15 years	*S. pneumoniae, M. pneumoniae, C. pneumoniae*	Influenza

TABLE 15-2   Etiology of Community-Acquired Pneumonia by Age

COMMUNITY-ACQUIRED PNEUMONIA

Infection of lung parenchyma

EPIDEMIOLOGY/ETIOLOGY

- Viruses account for up to 35% of childhood community-acquired pneumonia (CAP), but almost 80% of CAP in children <2 years.
- The etiology of CAP by age is shown in **Table 15-2**.
- Clinically significant pleural effusions:
  - ✓ Common: *S. pneumoniae* and *S. aureus*
  - ✓ Less common: *S. pyogenes, M. tuberculosis*
- Aspiration pneumonia: Enteric gram-negative rods, oral anaerobes; frequently polymicrobial

PATHOPHYSIOLOGY

- Absent systemic or secretory immunity to an organism
- Impaired lower respiratory tract defenses
- Direct inhalation or hematogenous seeding of organism

CLINICAL MANIFESTATIONS

- Fever, cough, tachypnea (most sensitive indicator)
- Hypoxia, nasal flaring, grunting, retractions, dyspnea
- Crackles, decreased breath sounds, egophony, whispered pectoriloquy
- Wheezing suggests a viral or atypical bacterial cause
- Chest or abdominal pain, malaise

DIAGNOSTICS

Chest Radiography

- Chest x-ray findings suggest etiology but may lag behind clinical symptoms:
  - ✓ Lobar or segmental abnormality, pleural effusion: Bacterial infection
  - ✓ Bilateral, diffuse infiltrates: Viral, *M. pneumoniae, Legionella pneumophila*

✓ Hilar adenopathy: *M. tuberculosis*, endemic fungi (e.g., *Histoplasma capsulatum*, *Coccidioides immitis*), *M. pneumoniae*; Epstein–Barr virus

✓ Pneumatocele: *S. aureus*, gram-negative rods, occasionally *S. pneumoniae*

Laboratory Studies

- Blood culture:
  - ✓ Outpatient: Should *not* be routinely performed in nontoxic, fully immunized children
  - ✓ Inpatient: Should be obtained in those with presumed moderate to severe bacterial pneumonia, particularly those with complications
  - ✓ Blood cultures should be obtained in all children who have progressive symptoms and in those who fail to demonstrate clinical improvement.
  - ✓ Blood culture result positive in 10–25% with pleural effusion; 3–7% of hospitalized children with pneumonia; less than 2% of outpatients with pneumonia
- Pleural fluid:
  - ✓ Transudate: pH >7.2; LDH less than 1000 U/L; WBC count <1000/mm^3; no bacteria on Gram stain; glucose >40 mg/dL; pleural/serum LDH ratio <0.5
  - ✓ Exudate: pH l<7.1; LDH >1000 U/L; WBC count >10,000/mm^3; bacteria present on Gram stain; glucose l<40 mg/dL; pleural/serum LDH <0.5
  - ✓ Send acid-fast culture and stains if concerned about *M. tuberculosis*

Diagnosis of Specific Agents

- Viral pathogens: Nasopharyngeal aspirate PCR, antigen detection, or culture
- *M. pneumoniae* and *C. pneumoniae*: PCR (rapid, accurate); serology (time-consuming); cold agglutinins (poor sensitivity)
- Tuberculosis: Tuberculin skin test; interferon-gamma release assay (IGRA), culture and acid-fast smear of sputum, bronchoalveolar lavage, or gastric aspirates

MANAGEMENT

- Specific treatment ultimately depends on cause
- Antibiotic selection depends on clinical presentation: See **Table 15-3**.
- Possible causes of persistent fever despite antibiotics include development of effusion/empyema, viral or mycoplasma etiology, necrotizing pneumonia, or, less likely, resistant bacteria.
- Chest ultrasound is preferred imaging method to quantify and characterize pleural effusions identified on chest x-ray.
  - ✓ Small: <10 mm on lateral decubitus film or opacifies less than ¼ of hemithorax; fluid drainage not required
  - ✓ Moderate: >10 mm but opacifies less than ½ of hemithorax; drainage required if patient has respiratory compromise or if suggestive of empyema.
  - ✓ Large: Opacifies greater than ½ of hemithorax; drainage should be performed
  - ✓ If exudative/simple fluid, requires chest tube with or without fibrinolysis
  - ✓ If loculated/complex fluid, may warrant video-assisted thoracoscopy (VATS) or chest tube with fibrinolysis; open decortication not usually necessary but may be used in cases of treatment failure despite chest tube or VATS.
- Complications: Empyema, lung abscess, necrotizing pneumonia
- Suggested resource: https://www.chop.edu/clinical-pathway/pneumonia-community-acquired-clinical-pathway

Authors: J. Gerber, MD, PhD; T. Metjian, PharmD; M. Siddharth, MD; D. Davis, MD; MSCE, T. Florin, MD; J. Zorc, MD; T. Kaur, MD; T. Blinman, MD; D. Mong, MD; X. Bateman, CRNP; E. Pete Devon, MD; Ron Keren, MD, MPH; L. Bell, MD; L. Utidjian, MD; E. Moxey, RN, MPH

TABLE 15-3 Empiric Therapy for Community-Acquired Pneumonia in Children >3 Months of Age

Pneumonia Category	First-Line Therapy*	β-Lactam Allergy†	Target Pathogen(s)	Duration of Therapy/Comments
Mild (outpatient)	Amoxicillin	First-line: Clindamycin OR Second-line: Levofloxacin	S. pneumoniae	• Duration: 7 days • High-dose amoxicillin active against most S. pneumoniae • Clindamycin active against most S. pneumoniae • Levofloxacin active against virtually all S. pneumoniae, Mycoplasma pneumoniae, and L. pneumophila • Oral cephalosporins inferior to high-dose amoxicillin for S. pneumoniae • Azithromycin resistance in up to 40% of S. pneumoniae; therefore, not recommended
Moderate (inpatient)	Ampicillin	First-line: Clindamycin OR Second-line: Levofloxacin	S. pneumoniae	• Duration: 7 days, with minimum 48 hours since last fever • High-dose ampicillin active against most S. pneumoniae • Ceftriaxone for incompletely immunized patients or treatment failure‡ with outpatient amoxicillin
Complicated[3] (inpatient)	Clindamycin AND Ceftriaxone	Clindamycin AND Levofloxacin	S. pneumoniae S. pyogenes S. aureus	• Duration: 7 days from drainage or resolution of fever (if not drained) • Consult infectious diseases and surgery for pneumonia with mod–large effusion/empyema to consider alternate etiologies and evaluate for drainage
Severe/complicated (ICU)	Vancomycin AND Ceftriaxone	Vancomycin AND Levofloxacin	S. pneumoniae S. pyogenes S. aureus	• Duration: 7 days from drainage or resolution of fever (if not drained) • Consult Infectious Diseases and Surgery for pneumonia with mod–large effusion/empyema to consider alternate etiologies and evaluate for drainage

(Continued)

TABLE 15-3 Empiric Therapy for Community-Acquired Pneumonia in Children >3 Months of Age (Continued)

Pneumonia Category	First-Line Therapy*	β-Lactam Allergy†	Target Pathogen(s)	Duration of Therapy/Comments
Atypical	Azithromycin (in addition to treatment above—see comment) OR Levofloxacin		Mycoplasma pneumoniae Legionella pneumophila	• Duration for proven infections: ○ Mycoplasma pneumoniae • Azithromycin: 5 days • Levofloxacin: 10 days ○ Legionella pneumophila • Azithromycin: 5–10 days • Levofloxacin: 14–21 days • Azithromycin does not have sufficient coverage for S. pneumoniae or S. aureus and thus requires addition of standard CAP therapy • Levofloxacin typically covers S. pneumoniae and S. aureus; therefore, does NOT need additional coverage • If requires hospital admission and treatment, send Mycoplasma nasopharyngeal PCR or Legionella urine antigen to aid in diagnosis

*For typical, presumed bacterial community-acquired pneumonia.

†Defined by urticaria or anaphylaxis (type 1–mediated hypersensitivity)

‡After >48 hours of therapy with high dose amoxicillin in a patient tolerating an oral regimen

¶Includes pneumonia with moderate-large parapneumonic effusion

Note: Atypical pneumonia (characterized by nonlobar, patchy, or interstitial pattern on chest x-ray; insidious onset; low-grade fever, malaise, headache, cough; minimal auscultatory findings relative to chest x-ray) is often caused by respiratory viruses, but may be caused by atypical bacterial pathogens including *Mycoplasma pneumoniae.* Most atypical pneumonia is mild and self-limited; however, for disease requiring hospitalization, consider PCR testing for respiratory viruses and *M. pneumoniae.*

CROUP

Upper airway obstruction due to infection-induced inflammation that may involve the larynx, infraglottic tissues, and trachea (laryngotracheitis), leading to inspiratory stridor, respiratory distress, barking cough, and hoarseness

EPIDEMIOLOGY

- Usually between ages 6 months and 3 years (peak at 18 months), though can occur up until age 6
- Epidemics begin in late fall and peak in early winter

ETIOLOGY

- Common: Parainfluenza viruses (50–80% of cases)
- Less common: RSV, influenza viruses A and B, adenovirus, coxsackieviruses, and measles
- Bacterial croup (laryngotracheobronchitis and laryngotracheobronchopnemonitis) is due to secondary bacterial infection from organisms such as *S. aureus*, group A *Streptococcus*, *S. pneumoniae*, *H. influenzae*, and *Moraxella catarrhalis*
- Most common noninfectious cause of airway obstruction/stridor is foreign body.

PATHOPHYSIOLOGY

- Viral infection of the nasopharynx spreads to respiratory epithelium.
- Infection causes diffuse inflammation and edema of the trachea and vocal cords.
- Inflammation of the subglottic trachea (narrowest part of child's upper airway) leads to dramatic airflow restriction and obstruction.
- Bacterial croup is due to inflammatory cell infiltrate, ulceration, formation of pseudomembranes and microabscesses.

CLINICAL MANIFESTATIONS

- Initial rhinorrhea, pharyngitis, and low-grade fevers
- Upper airway obstruction 8–12 hours later
- Signs of obstruction include "barking" cough, hoarseness, inspiratory stridor, accessory muscle use, and hypoxia. Dysphagia is not typical.
- Fever, tachypnea, restlessness, coryza
- Children with bacterial infections are toxic.

DIAGNOSTICS

- Croup is a clinical diagnosis.
- Neck x-rays are not required but can support the initial diagnosis.
- Only 50% of cases demonstrate abnormal neck x-ray findings. Anteroposterior view: narrowed airway in subglottic area (steeple sign). Lateral view: overdistention of the hypopharynx.
- Respiratory viral PCR testing rarely changes management. However, in severe cases, or with concern for bacterial superinfection, a nasal-wash specimen or tracheal secretions can be used for direct identification of organisms.

MANAGEMENT

- Cool mist tent or vaporizer is not recommended, as it may increase patient anxiety, leading to worsening respiratory distress.
- Corticosteroids: Routinely recommended for croup regardless of severity to decrease subglottic edema. Associated with fewer admissions, fewer return visits, and shorter duration

of stay in the ED or hospital Most recommend dexamethasone (0.3 mg/kg) orally or intramuscularly for one dose) or nebulized budesonide (2–4 mg) for one dose; no current evidence to suggest that longer courses provide additional benefit.

- Nebulized racemic epinephrine (2.25%): Effective for symptomatic improvement in moderate to severe croup (stridor at rest, significant respiratory distress, hypoxemia). Adrenergic effects induce vasoconstriction leading to decreased subglottic edema. Onset occurs in less than 10 minutes. Duration of effect is less than 2 hours; requires 2- to 4-hour observation before discharge. Repeated treatments may decrease need for intubation in ill patients.
- Criteria for discharge include: No stridor at rest; normal air entry, no cyanosis, and level of consciousness. Ensure close follow-up; symptom rebound can occur once steroids wear off.
- Supplemental oxygen for hypoxemia. Use of heliox therapy (70% helium, 30% oxygen mixture) has been described for severe distress: Helium improves laminar gas flow in edematous airway and decreases the mechanical work of respiratory muscles. However, more evidence of efficacy in this setting is needed.
- Patients with superimposed bacterial laryngotracheobronchitis or laryngotracheobronchopneumonia often require endotracheal intubation and should receive antimicrobials targeting the most common organisms.

ENCEPHALITIS

Inflammation of the brain parenchyma leading to altered mental status

EPIDEMIOLOGY

- Most frequently observed in summer and early fall when enteroviruses and arboviruses are most prevalent
- Reported incidence is between 1.5 in 100,000 and 10 in 100,000. More common in children than in adults. Epidemiologic studies are difficult to perform because of lack of standard case definitions.
- Commonly associated with meningitis (meningoencephalitis)

ETIOLOGY

- Pathogen identified in less than 50% of cases
- Viruses most commonly implicated: Arboviruses (West Nile, La Crosse, St. Louis, Eastern and Western equine, Venezuelan equine, California, Powassan, and Colorado tick fever), enteroviruses, parechoviruses, herpes simplex virus (HSV) 1 and 2, human herpesvirus 6 (HHV-6) and human herpesvirus 7 (HHV-7) , varicella–zoster virus (VZV), influenza A and B, parainfluenza 1–3, mumps, measles, RSV, rotavirus, adenovirus, Epstein–Barr, rabies, Nipah virus, cytomegalovirus (CMV), parvovirus, lymphocytic choreomeningitis virus, Japanese encephalitis virus
- Bacteria: *H. influenzae*, *Neisseria meningitidis*, *S. pneumoniae*, *M. tuberculosis*, *Bartonella henselae*
- Other infections: *Mycoplasma pneumoniae*, Rocky Mountain spotted fever, *Ehrlichia*, *Cryptococcus neoformans*, *Coccidioides immitis*, *Histoplasma*, parasites including malaria, and helminths
- Postinfectious diseases: Guillain–Barré, Miller–Fisher, acute cerebellar ataxia, acute disseminated encephalomyelitis (ADEM), acute flaccid myelitis, acute necrotizing encephalopathy
- Other: Metabolic disorder, seizure disorder, toxin ingestion, mass lesion, subarachnoid hemorrhage, acute demyelinating disorder, acute confusional migraine, vasculitis, N-methyl-D-aspartate (NMDA) receptor and other autoimmune/autoinflammatory encephalitis

PATHOPHYSIOLOGY

- Most commonly occurs by hematogenous spread to the brain following viremia or bacteremia
- May occur as a result of retrograde movement through the peripheral nerves (e.g., HSV and rabies)
- Pathogenesis can include direct viral cytopathology and/or a parainfectious or postinfectious inflammatory response.

CLINICAL MANIFESTATIONS

- Common: Acute febrile illness, headache, altered mentation
- Other: Behavioral or personality changes, generalized or focal seizures, hemiparesis, ataxia, movement disorders
- Neurologic abnormalities are based on areas of the brain affected; altered level of consciousness, cranial-nerve palsies, ataxia, weakness
- If associated meningitis: Nuchal rigidity, Kernig and Brudzinski signs (see "Meningitis" section)

DIAGNOSTICS

- Clinical diagnosis is based on fever and altered mental status.
- See Table 15-4.
- Detailed vaccination, travel, and exposure history should guide additional diagnostics.
- Laboratory or imaging features may be suggestive of more unusual causes and consultation with infectious diseases expert and neurologist can guide additional testing.

TABLE 15-4	Diagnostic Approach for Encephalitis
Routine Studies	

Cerebrospinal fluid (CSF)

Opening pressure, WBC count + differential, RBC count, protein, glucose

Gram stain and bacterial culture

Herpes simplex virus PCR

Varicella–zoster virus PCR

Enterovirus PCR

Autoimmune/inflammatory CSF studies (recommend expert consultation)

Serum

Blood culture

CBC with differential

Chemistry panel

Liver-function tests

Toxicology screen

HIV antibody/antigen screen

Hold extra acute and collect convalescent serum 10–14 days later for paired antibody testing

Other

Nasopharyngeal respiratory viral PCR panel (if symptomatic)

(Continued)

TABLE 15-4	Diagnostic Approach for Encephalitis (*Continued*)

Imaging/Neurophysiology

Neuroimaging (MRI preferred to CT if available)

Chest imaging if respiratory symptoms present

EEG

Conditional Studies

Immunocompromised Patients

CSF cytomegalovirus PCR

CSF human herpesvirus 6/7 PCR

CSF HIV PCR

CSF Epstein–Barr virus PCR

CSF JC virus PCR

CSF *Toxoplasma gondii* PCR with serum serology

CSF acid-fast bacilli culture and smear

CSF fungal culture

CSF and serum West Nile virus serologies plus additional regional arboviruses

CSF and serum PCR for arboviruses

CSF Cryptococcal antigen and/or India Ink staining

Serum *Coccidioides immitis* complement fixation antibodies

Urine *Histoplasma capsulatum* antigen

Season and Exposure

Summer/Fall: Serum and CSF IgG and IgM for arboviruses specific to geographic location; serum serology of tick-borne diseases

Cat exposure: Serum Bartonella antibody, ophthalmologic evaluation

Tick exposure: Serum serology of tick-borne diseases endemic to region

Animal bite/bat exposure: Rabies testing in concert with regional health department

Sexually active/maternal concern: CSF VDRL, serum Treponemal testing

Swimming/diving in fresh water or sinus irrigation: CSF wet mount and PCR for *Naegleria fowleri*

MANAGEMENT

- If associated with meningitis suggestive of bacterial disease then begin appropriate empiric antibiotics (see "Meningitis" section) after obtaining CSF culture
- HSV encephalitis: In 0–3 months, IV acyclovir 60 mg/kg/day divided every 8 hours; 3 months to 11 years, 30–45 mg/kg/day divided every 8 hours; >12 years, 30 mg/kg/day divided every 8 hours. Acyclovir may also be indicated in VZV infections—consult with infectious diseases specialist.
- Most patients with other viral encephalitides require only supportive care. In select cases, corticosteroids and/or IV immune globulin may be considered to decrease inflammation, though further studies are need to demonstrate efficacy—consultation with neurology and infectious diseases is recommended.

- Physical, occupational, and speech therapy are important in children with severe disease and long-term complications.
- Complications: Cerebral edema, long-term neurologic dysfunction, seizure disorder, death

FEVER IN NEONATES AND YOUNG INFANTS

Temperature 38.0°C or greater in neonate (age, 0–28 days) or young infant (age. 29–56 days)

EPIDEMIOLOGY

- Serious bacterial infection (SBI) occurs in 5–15% of febrile neonates, including urinary-tract infections (UTIs) (4–10%), bloodstream infections (1–2%), pneumonia (1%), and meningitis (0.5–1%). Additional sources of infection to consider, guided by history and physical exam, include osteomyelitis, gastroenteritis, and skin/soft tissue infections. Viral infection is a common cause of fever in this age group.

ETIOLOGY

- Urinary tract infections: *Escherichia coli*, *Klebsiella*, and *Enterobacter* spp., group B *Streptococcus* (GBS), *Enterococcus*
- Bloodstream infections: GBS, *E. coli*, *Klebsiella*, and *Enterobacter* spp.; *Listeria monocytogenes*; coagulase-negative staphylococci (catheter-associated infection); *S. aureus*; enteroviruses; HSV; *S. pneumoniae*
- Pneumonia: GBS; *E. coli*, *Klebsiella*, and *Enterobacter* spp; *L. monocytogenes*; *Chlamydia trachomatis*; respiratory viruses; CMV; *S. pneumoniae*
- Meningitis: GBS; *E. coli*, *Klebsiella*, and *Enterobacter* spp; *L. monocytogenes*; enteroviruses; HSV (see "Neonatal HSV" section); *S. pneumoniae*

PATHOPHYSIOLOGY

- Degree of neonatal immune compromise is inversely related to gestational age and birth weight.
- Neonates at higher risk of systemic dissemination from any bacterial infection
- Labor and delivery expose neonates to unique pathogens.

CLINICAL MANIFESTATIONS

- Important history: Maternal fever or infection (particularly history of GBS or HSV), birth history, ill contacts, level of activity, irritability, feeding, lethargy, vomiting, bowel habits, urine output, jaundice, respiratory symptoms or distress, fever, skin lesion or rash
- Medical history should include immunization status, existing medical conditions (e.g., human immunodeficiency virus [HIV], asplenia), prematurity
- Neurologic: Bulging fontanelle, lethargy, irritability, hypotonia, hypertonia, weak suck or cry
- Respiratory: Tachypnea, grunting, nasal flaring, retractions, hypoxemia, apnea, cyanosis
- Cardiovascular: Tachycardia, bradycardia, hypotension, delayed capillary refill, diminished pulses
- Gastrointestinal: Abdominal tenderness, distended or firm abdomen, diminished bowel sounds, periumbilical ecchymoses or erythema, discharge from umbilical stump
- Skin: Jaundice, mottled skin, petechiae
- Skeletal: Focal bone tenderness, decreased activity of one limb (asymmetric movement)

DIAGNOSTICS AND MANAGEMENT

- Specific protocols may vary by hospital.
- The Pediatric Emergency Care Applied Research Network prediction rule:
  ✓ Recommends lumbar puncture (LP) if any of the following are present: Urinalysis positive, absolute neutrophil count >4090/mm³, or procalcitonin >1.7 ng/mL (high sensitivity [97.7%] and negative predictive value [99.6%]) (Kuppermann N, et al. A clinical prediction rule to identify febrile infants 60 days and younger at low risk for serious bacterial infections. *JAMA Pediatr* 2019;173:342–351.)
- The Philadelphia protocol is described subsequently:
- All infants 28 days old or younger undergo complete evaluation because of inability to rely on physical exam. All ill-appearing infants 0–56 days of age should also receive complete evaluation: Complete blood count (CBC) with differential; blood culture; urinalysis with Gram stain and cell count; urine culture; CSF cell count, glucose, protein and culture; chest x-ray (if respiratory signs)
- Hospitalize all neonates (ages 0–28 days) to administer empiric intravenous antibiotic therapy until either an organism is identified or all culture results are negative for 48 hours or longer: Ampicillin + gentamicin OR ampicillin + ceftazidime (or cefepime), using meningitis dosing. Add acyclovir for neonates ages 0–21 days (see "Neonatal HSV" section). Consider discharge at 24–36 hours for well-appearing neonates and infants with reassuring CSF studies and all negative cultures. Diagnosis of UTI in neonates does not obviate lumbar puncture, as coexisting meningitis may occur.
- In young infants (age 29–56 days), the Philadelphia protocol identifies those at low risk for bacterial disease who may not require a complete evaluation or empiric antibiotic therapy. Criteria to identify low-risk infants (29–56 days) are:
  ✓ Exam: Well appearance and normal exam
  ✓ Full term (≥37 weeks' gestation), no significant medical history
  ✓ CBC: ≥5000 and ≤15,000 WBC/mm³; band-to-neutrophil ratio <0.2
  ✓ Spun urinalysis: <10 WBC per high-power field; no bacteria on Gram stain
  ✓ CSF (if performed): <8 WBC/mm³; no bacteria on Gram stain
  ✓ Chest x-ray (if performed): No evidence of infiltrate
- If *all* blood and urine results meet low-risk criteria and the infant appears well, CSF does not need to be obtained. For low-risk infants 29–56 days old for whom follow-up within 24 hours by a physician can be ensured, consider outpatient management without antibiotics. If any results are abnormal or patient appears ill, obtain CSF and admit to the hospital and treat empirically with intravenous antibiotics (may use ceftriaxone alone). If culture results are negative after 48 hours and suspicion for SBI no longer exists, then discharge. If any culture result is positive, alter therapy appropriately.
- Infants 29–60 days who test positive for RSV and have clinical symptoms consistent with bronchiolitis are at lower risk for an SBI than those who test negative, although a clinically important rate of UTIs has been documented (requiring evaluation of blood and urine). Lumbar puncture and empiric antibiotic therapy may be deferred in some cases.
- Consider viral PCR testing for enterovirus, parechovirus, and HSV from the serum and CSF when testing is readily available, particularly with CSF pleocytosis.

FEVER OF UNKNOWN ORIGIN

Fever (documented temperature 38.3°C or greater) for 14 days or longer with cause not apparent after physical exam and initial screening laboratory tests

EPIDEMIOLOGY

- Infection (28–52%), collagen vascular disease (6–20%), malignancy (3–16%)
- Resolution of fever without diagnosis in 20–40%

DIFFERENTIAL DIAGNOSIS

- See **Table 15-5**.

PATIENT HISTORY/DIAGNOSTIC CONSIDERATIONS

- Constitutional: Time of fever onset and measured temperature, method used to take temperature, weight loss, night sweats, chills, anorexia
- History: Travel, animal exposure, exposure to unpasteurized dairy products, tick bite, blood transfusion, trauma, fractures or puncture wounds, congenital or acquired heart disease, immunodeficiency, foreign-body ingestion, CVC, medications
- Family stressor (Munchausen by proxy, pseudofevers)
- Perform repeated and thorough physical exams searching for findings that suggest specific cause.

TABLE 15-5	Differential Diagnosis of Fever of Unknown Origin		
Common Infectious Causes	**Less Common Infectious Causes**	**Rare Infectious Causes**	**Noninfectious Causes**
Systemic viral syndrome	Tuberculosis	Q fever	Collagen vascular diseases
Respiratory tract infection	Cat-scratch disease	Brucellosis	Juvenile rheumatoid arthritis
Osteomyelitis	Infectious mononucleosis	Tularemia	Systemic lupus erythematosus
Urinary-tract infection	Lyme disease	Leptospirosis	Dermatomyositis
CNS infection	Rickettsial diseases	Intraabdominal abscess	Scleroderma
Enteritis	Malaria	Toxoplasmosis	Vasculitis
	Periodontal abscess	Syphilis	Malignancy
	Endocarditis	Endemic fungi (e.g., histoplasmosis)	Kawasaki syndrome
	HIV	Psittacosis	Inflammatory bowel disease
	Viral hepatitis	Chronic meningococcemia	Munchausen syndrome by proxy
	Acute rheumatic fever		Factitious fever
			Periodic fever syndrome
			Central fever
			Dysautonomia
			Hyperthyroidism
			Drug fever

MANAGEMENT

Initial Studies (Select Tests Based on History and Exam)

- Blood:
  - ✓ Blood culture, CBC, C-reactive protein (CRP), erythrocyte sedimentation rate (ESR), hepatic-function panel
  - ✓ Serology for HIV, EBV, CMV, cat-scratch disease, Lyme disease, and streptococcal enzyme titers (anti-streptolysin O, anti-DNase B)
  - ✓ Antinuclear antibodies
- Urine: Urinalysis and culture
- Stool: Hemoccult testing, culture or PCR (bacterial/viral), ova and parasite exam
- Radiologic: Chest radiograph
- Miscellaneous: Tuberculin skin test/IGRA, throat culture

Additional Studies to Consider

- Blood:
  - ✓ Repeat blood culture
  - ✓ Serology for toxoplasmosis; hepatitis A, B, and C; tularemia; brucellosis; leptospirosis; Rocky Mountain spotted fever; ehrlichiosis; and Q fever
- Stool: *Clostridiodes difficile* toxins A and B
- Radiologic: Radiographs of involved bones if tenderness or edema on exam, sinus CT, gastrointestinal barium study with small -follow-through (if symptoms suggest inflammatory bowel disease), abdominal ultrasound, MRI of pelvis, spine, or specific extremity, echocardiography
- Miscellaneous: Ophthalmologic exam, bone marrow biopsy (if abnormal CBC or suspected malignancy), lumbar puncture, evaluation for immune deficiency

GASTROENTERITIS

Infection of the gastrointestinal tract associated with vomiting and diarrhea (more than three episodes of loose or watery stools per day)

EPIDEMIOLOGY

- Infectious cases due to viruses (75–90%), bacteria (10–20%), or parasites (up to 5%)

ETIOLOGY

- See **Table 15-6**

PATHOPHYSIOLOGY

- Osmotic/malabsorptive: Intestinal epithelial damage leads to malabsorption and osmotic diarrhea (e.g., *Giardia*)
- Inflammatory: Exudation of mucus, blood, and protein into the luminal space exacerbates water and electrolyte loss (e.g., *Shigella*, Shiga-toxin–producing [STEC])
- Secretory/toxigenic: Toxin release results in active secretion of water into the luminal space (e.g., cholera toxin, rotavirus)

CLINICAL MANIFESTATIONS

- See **Table 15-6.**

TABLE 15-6 Clinical Features of Common Gastrointestinal Pathogens

Pathogen	Clinical Manifestations	Epidemiologic Clues	Diagnosis	Management
Viral				
Rotavirus	Generally begins with vomiting followed by watery diarrhea, associated with high fevers in one-third of cases	Children <5, peaks in cooler months	Antigen detection via EIA, PCR	Supportive once infected; prevention by universal rotavirus vaccination
Norovirus	Sudden onset of vomiting, watery diarrhea, abdominal pain, and fever	Outbreaks in day care centers, cruise ships; most common cause of foodborne disease outbreaks	PCR; stool antigen tests have lower sensitivity and specificity	Supportive
Sapovirus, adenovirus (40 or 41), and astrovirus	Milder illness than norovirus or rotavirus characterized by watery diarrhea, less commonly associated with vomiting or fever	Primarily in children <4	PCR for sapovirus and astrovirus; EIA for adenovirus	Supportive
Bacterial				
Bacillus cereus	Nausea, abdominal cramps, can be predominantly vomiting (preformed toxin ingestion) or predominantly diarrhea (spore ingestion)	Foodborne; preformed toxin most commonly in fried rice, spores in contaminated meat or vegetables; vomiting onset in 0.5–6 hours, diarrhea onset in 6–15 hours	Organism or toxin can be detected in *food or recovery from stool of 2 or more ill people*	Supportive
Campylobacter jejuni	Bloody diarrhea with severe abdominal pain, fever, occasionally bacteremia; immune-mediated manifestations including Guillain–Barré syndrome, Miller–Fisher syndrome, and reactive arthritis can occur following infection	Ingestion of improperly cooked poultry, unpasteurized milk, untreated water; exposure to young animals (i.e., new pets); travel to dairy farms; occasionally person-person transmission	Culture using selective media (preferred); commercially available EIA and PCR	Generally supportive, but azithromycin × 3 days or erythromycin × 5 days can shorten duration of illness and organism shedding when given early in illness

(Continued)

TABLE 15-6 Clinical Features of Common Gastrointestinal Pathogens (*Continued*)

Pathogen	Clinical Manifestations	Epidemiologic Clues	Diagnosis	Management
Clostridioides difficile	See section on *C. difficile*			
Escherichia coli				
• Shiga-toxin–producing (STEC)	Hemorrhagic colitis with bloody diarrhea appearing 3–4 days after onset of symptoms, may cause HUS (O157:H7)	Undercooked beef, contaminated greens, unpasteurized milk, petting zoos, person–person	Culture on sorbitol containing selective media, EIA for Shiga toxin production; monitor CBC, BUN, and creatinine for development of HUS	Supportive; antibiotic therapy in patients with STEC is associated with increased risk of developing HUS in some studies but no increased risk or benefit found on meta-analysis of trials. Most experts recommend no antibiotic treatment.
• Enteropathogenic	Watery diarrhea	Exclusively in children <2 and in resource-limited countries	Clinical/epidemiological; cultures cannot distinguish from normal flora	Supportive
• Enterotoxigenic	Watery diarrhea, abdominal cramping; "traveler's diarrhea"	Resource-limited settings (and travelers to these settings, "traveler's diarrhea")	Clinical/epidemiological or PCR; cultures cannot distinguish from normal flora	Azithromycin or ciprofloxacin × 3 days may reduce duration of diarrhea
• Enteroinvasive	Fever, watery or bloody diarrhea	All age groups, occasionally food borne	Clinical/epidemiological; cultures cannot distinguish from normal flora	Supportive
• Enteroaggregative	Mild watery diarrhea, may be chronic	All age groups	Clinical/epidemiological; cultures cannot distinguish from normal flora	Supportive

	Clinical Features	Epidemiology/Transmission	Diagnosis	Treatment
Nontyphoid *Salmonella*	Diarrhea, abdominal cramps, and fever; can be complicated by bacteremia, osteomyelitis, brain abscesses, and meningitis	Undercooked poultry or beef, dairy products, contaminated water, contact with reptiles or amphibians; most common in children <4	Stool culture; FDA-cleared PCR assay available, but limited clinical experience and stool culture is still required for serotyping and susceptibility testing	Treatment of gastroenteritis is only indicated for those at high risk of invasive disease: Children <3 months, chronic GI disease, HIV, or other immunocompromising condition. An initial dose of ceftriaxone should be given, followed by oral azithromycin, or amoxicillin or TMP-SMX for susceptible strains.
Salmonella typhi	Initially fever, malaise, myalgias, abdominal pain, constipation or bloody diarrhea, then hepatosplenomegaly and rose spots by the second week of illness; associated with bacteremia and sometimes meningitis	Humans are the only hosts; most common in resource-limited settings and travelers to those settings.	Blood culture, bile culture, or bone marrow aspirate; stool cultures are often negative.	Empiric treatment with ceftriaxone or azithromycin with definitive therapy determined based on sensitivities. Drug, route, and duration depend on susceptibilities, clinical response, site of infection, and host, but generally should be continued for at least 7 days, with up to 14 days considered for patients treated with amoxicillin or TMP-SMX. Fluoroquinolones may be alternatives, depending on local prevalence of resistance. Corticosteroids may be beneficial in children with severe enteric fever (delirium, coma, shock).

(Continued)

TABLE 15-6 Clinical Features of Common Gastrointestinal Pathogens *(Continued)*

Pathogen	Clinical Manifestations	Epidemiologic Clues	Diagnosis	Management
Shigella	Varies from watery stools without constitutional symptoms to bloody stools associated with high fever, abdominal pain, and tenesmus; can be complicated by pseudomembranous colitis, toxic megacolon, and HUS (Shiga-toxin producing *S. dysenteriae*). Generalized seizures and postinfectious reactive arthritis have been associated	Low inoculum required for infection, often associated with childcare outbreaks	Stool culture preferred, PCR available but may lack specificity	Indicated for severe illness, dysentery, or underlying immunosuppressive conditions. Ampicillin (not amoxicillin) or TMP-SMX can be given for susceptible strains for 5 days; otherwise azithromycin × 3 days, ceftriaxone × 2–5 days, or fluoroquinolone × 3 days pending susceptibility testing
Vibrio cholerae	Painless, watery diarrhea leading to significant electrolyte imbalances	More common in the developing world; most cases in the United States are associated with consuming raw or undercooked shellfish	Stool cultures; must request selective media. Serologic testing also available but require acute and convalescent serums	Indicated for moderate to severe illness. Single dose doxycycline or azithromycin; erythromycin, ciprofloxacin, or tetracycline for 3 days. Choice of drug should be made based on local susceptibility patterns or susceptibility testing.
Yersinia enterocolitica	Fever, abdominal pain, and bloody diarrhea in young children; pseudo-appendicitis syndrome resulting from mesenteric adenitis with fever, abdominal pain, and tenderness and leukocytosis in older children; may cause bacteremia or distant foci of infection uncommonly.	Principal reservoir is swine; infection results from contaminated and incompletely cooked pork, unpasteurized milk, well water, chitterlings, and tofu. Uncommon in the United States.	Stool culture (must request selective media); PCR	Indicated only for neonates or immunocompromised hosts with gastrointestinal infection and all patients with extraintestinal foci or septicemia; parenteral third-generation cephalosporins, TMP-SMX, aminoglycosides, fluoroquinolones, tetracycline, doxycycline, and chloramphenicol are generally active.

	Clinical features	Epidemiology	Diagnosis	Treatment
Yersinia pseudo-tuberculosis	Fever, rash, diarrhea, and pseudo-appendicitis; extraintestinal manifestations include sterile pleural and joint effusions and erythema nodosum; mimics Kawasaki disease.	Reservoirs include ungulates, rodents, rabbits, and birds; outbreaks linked to contaminated fresh fruit	Stool culture (must request selective media); PCR	Same as *Yersinia enterocolitica*
Parasites				
Cryptosporidiosis	Frequent, watery diarrhea occasionally associated with fever, fatigue, abdominal pain, vomiting, and anorexia. Immunocompromised patients may have chronic diarrhea associated with weight loss and malnutrition.	Contaminated drinking and recreational water, more common in the summer. Livestock and petting zoos. Daycare outbreaks due to person–person transmission.	Direct immunofluorescent antibody, EIA, and rapid immune chromatographic tests available. Can detect oocysts on stool ova and parasite testing, but requires special specimen preparation and staining.	No specific therapy for immunocompetent hosts. HIV-positive or otherwise immunocompromised hosts, nitazoxanide (preferred). Alternatives include paromomycin with or without azithromycin.
Cyclosporiasis	Watery diarrhea with anorexia, nausea, vomiting, abdominal pain, fatigue, and weight loss. Symptoms can be relapsing.	Endemic in resource-limited settings, linked to imported fresh produce and recent travel.	Stool examination for ova and parasites, may need repeated examinations.	TMP-SMX × 7–10 days, longer in immunocompromised patients

(Continued)

TABLE 15-6	Clinical Features of Common Gastrointestinal Pathogens (*Continued*)			
Pathogen	**Clinical Manifestations**	**Epidemiologic Clues**	**Diagnosis**	**Management**
Giardia lamblia	Acute illness with watery diarrhea or more chronic illness with foul smelling stools, flatulence, and anorexia. May also have protracted course with associated anorexia, flatulence, and abdominal distention resulting in failure to thrive. Postinfectious lactose intolerance occurs in 20–40%	Daycare outbreaks, camping trips, outbreaks from contaminated water supplies.	Stool EIA or DFA testing preferred; stool examination for ova and parasites, may need repeated examinations.	Supportive for self-limited infections; otherwise metronidazole (5–10 days), tinidazole (single dose), nitazoxanide (3 days).
Entamoeba histolytica	Spectrum of disease from asymptomatic excretion of cysts to mild, noninvasive disease to intestinal amebiasis (most common) characterized by gradual onset of bloody diarrhea, lower abdominal pain, tenesmus, and weight loss; complications include toxic megacolon, fulminant colitis, and bowel perforation. Extraintestinal manifestations include most commonly liver abscesses.	Resource-limited countries	Stool ova and parasite examination; serologic testing	For asymptomatic cyst excretion: Iodoquinol, paromomycin, diloxanideFor intestinal amebiasis or extra-intestinal disease: Metronidazole or tinidazole, followed by iodoquinol or paromomycin. Percutaneous or surgical aspiration of liver abscesses may be necessary.

BUN = blood urea nitrogen; DFA = direct florescent antigen; EIA = enzyme immunoassay; HUS = hemolytic–uremic syndrome.

DIAGNOSTICS

- See **Table 15-6**.
- CBC may show excessive band forms (*Shigella*) or evidence of hemolysis (in STEC strains of *E. coli* and *Shigella*)
- Serum electrolytes not routinely indicated unless there are signs of severe dehydration or as part of evaluation for hemolytic–uremic syndrome (HUS)
- Fecal occult blood and WBC testing rarely affect clinical management.
- Stool cultures are generally low yield and should be reserved for cases of dysentery, suspected STEC, recent foreign travel, immunocompromised hosts with fevers, or when a diagnosis is needed for public health reasons. Stool cultures and ova and parasite testing are particularly low yield in patients hospitalized for >3 days and are not recommended in this population.

MANAGEMENT

- See **Table 15-5** for indications for antibiotic therapy.
- Oral rehydration is the preferred therapy in cases of mild-to-moderate dehydration, given its low failure rate (3.6%), shorter length of hospitalization, decreased costs, and fewer complications. Small but frequent oral challenges can be given with assessment of response
- Consider a single dose of ondansetron, which enhances success of oral rehydration therapy and decreases need for admission and IV hydration by approximately 50%.
- Severe dehydration can be life-threatening. Isotonic IV fluids (0.9% saline or lactated Ringer's) are recommended. IV boluses (20 mL/kg) can be given initially for resuscitation and transitioned to maintenance/replacement fluids and, ultimately, oral rehydration solutions (see, Chapter 9 on Fluids and Electrolytes)

INFECTIOUS MONONUCLEOSIS

Clinical syndrome characterized by fever, pharyngitis, lymphadenopathy, hepatosplenomegaly, and malaise. Infectious mononucleosis is classically caused by Epstein–Barr virus (EBV), but infections caused by CMV, *T. gondii*, adenovirus, or acute HIV infection can have a similar presentation.

EPIDEMIOLOGY

- Spread by close personal contact usually via saliva, but can also be transmitted through blood products, organ transplantation, and sexual contact.
- Incubation period is 30–50 days.
- Virus can be excreted in oral secretions for more than 6 months following infection and is viable in saliva for several hours outside the body.
- Often causes asymptomatic infection in early childhood.
- Approximately 90% of U.S. adults have been infected

PATHOPHYSIOLOGY

- EBV infects oropharyngeal lymphoid tissue B cells, which disseminate to involve the entire lymphoreticular system.
- Following infection, the virus remains latent within memory B cells and can later reactivate at times of immune suppression.

CLINICAL MANIFESTATIONS

- EBV can cause a wide spectrum of diseases, including asymptomatic infection (most common presentation in young children), infectious mononucleosis (most commonly in adolescents), and lymphoproliferative disease in immunocompromised hosts.
- A 3- to 5-day prodrome of malaise, fatigue, headache, and low-grade fevers may precede clinical infection.
- Classic presentation includes triad of high fever, exudative pharyngitis, and generalized lymphadenopathy, most commonly involving the cervical chain.
- Other common findings include severe fatigue, malaise, splenomegaly (more common with EBV than with CMV), hepatomegaly (10–35%), generalized maculopapular or morbilliform rash (can be triggered by amoxicillin or ampicillin use), and abdominal pain (especially in young children).
- Rare findings and complications include splenic rupture, pneumonia, myocarditis, pancreatitis, mesenteric adenitis, myositis, acute renal failure, glomerulonephritis, Guillain–Barré syndrome, meningoencephalitis, transverse myelitis, peripheral neuritis, optic neuritis, and hemophagocytic lymphohistiocytosis.
- Rash
  ✓ Can be pruritic or maculopapular and is typically generalized.
  ✓ Previously thought to occur in 80–100% of patients exposed to antibiotics, but recent data demonstrate the rash occurs in approximately 30%, most commonly with β-lactams. Rash occurs in 3–23% of patients without antibiotic exposure.
  ✓ May occur 5–10 days after the antibiotic exposure.
  ✓ Rechallenge with a β-lactam does not cause rash.
- Fever can occasionally persist for over 2 weeks.

DIAGNOSTICS

- Laboratory findings:
  ✓ Hematologic abnormalities include lymphocyte-predominant leukocytosis with >10% atypical lymphocytes, mild thrombocytopenia (platelet count *rarely* <100,000/mm^3), and hemolytic anemia (<1% of cases)
  ✓ Mild elevation of hepatic transaminases (50–65% of patients)
- Heterophile antibody tests (including mononucleosis spot (Monospot) test):
  ✓ Detects IgM, which appears over the first 2 weeks of illness
  ✓ False negative results may occur in children younger than 4 years of age (up to 50% with EBV will have a false negative result on Monospot testing).
  ✓ False positive results may also occur with leukemia, lymphoma, systemic lupus erythematosus, and serum sickness.
  ✓ Most useful for rapid diagnosis in older children, where testing is 85% sensitive and over 90% specific by the second week of illness. Becomes undetectable over 3–6 months.
- Specific EBV serologies are reliable in all ages, including with negative heterophile antibody tests.
  ✓ Acute infection: Elevated viral capsid antigen (VCA) IgM and IgG; EBV nuclear antigen (EBNA) IgG negative
  ✓ Recent infection: VCA IgM negative (disappears 4–8 weeks after infection); VCA IgG positive; EBNA negative
  ✓ Past infection: VCA IgM negative; VCA IgG and EBNA positive (appears 1–6 months after infection)
  ✓ *Note:* Early antigen assays are unreliable, so they are not useful for diagnosis.
- EBV PCR is most useful in evaluation of immunocompromised patients with suspected EBV infection; unclear role in immunocompetent host

MANAGEMENT

- Supportive care for fever and pharyngitis
- Corticosteroids reserved for patients with impending airway obstruction, which is rare (e.g., prednisone 1 mg/kg/day for 7 days followed by a taper). Steroids may also be considered for myocarditis, massive splenomegaly, hemolytic anemia, or hemophagocytic lymphohistiocytosis with expert consultation.
- Acyclovir, ganciclovir, and foscarnet demonstrate in vitro activity against EBV but have not been shown to improve clinical outcomes in previously healthy children.
- Vigorous activity and contact sports should be avoided for at least 21 days after the onset of symptoms, with return to contact sports after 4–6 weeks if asymptomatic and there is no splenomegaly
- Reduction of immunosuppressive therapy for patients with EBV-associated posttransplantation lymphoproliferative disorders

LYMPHADENITIS AND LYMPHADENOPATHY

Lymphadenopathy is defined as enlargement (>10 mm in sites other than inguinal or >15 mm in the inguinal region) of a single lymph node (isolated), a contiguous group of lymph nodes (regional), or noncontiguous groups of lymph nodes (generalized). Lymphadenitis is inflammation within a lymph node or group of lymph nodes, usually the result of infection. The condition may be acute, subacute, or chronic.

ETIOLOGY

- Depends on location and clinical presentation
- Bacterial (usually involving cervical chain):
  - ✓ Commonly due to group A beta-hemolytic streptococci or *S. aureus*
  - ✓ Less commonly due to anaerobes (dental source), cat-scratch disease, and nontuberculous mycobacteria
  - ✓ Rarely tularemia, brucellosis, leptospirosis, syphilis, or diphtheria
- Parasitic: Toxoplasmosis, leishmaniasis
- Fungal: Histoplasmosis, coccidioidomycosis, blastomycosis, cryptococcosis
- Viral: EBV, CMV, adenovirus, HIV, rubella, measles, mumps, HSV, VZV, HHV-6, HHV-7, hepatitis B, parvovirus B19, dengue
- Other: Oncologic process; Kikuchi–Fujimoto disease (a typically benign, self-limited condition characterized by painful cervical lymphadenopathy and necrosis noted on pathology); Rosai–Dorfman disease (benign histiocytic proliferation leading to lymphadenopathy, most commonly of the cervical chain)

PATHOPHYSIOLOGY

- Pyogenic lymphadenitis: Organisms enter lymph nodes and cause proliferation of lymphoid cells in response to antigenic stimuli; can cause microabscesses and suppuration; may also occur secondary to lymphatic drainage of a localized infected site
- Generalized lymphadenopathy: Organisms may enter lymphatics after hematogenous spread from a systemic infection and cause more generalized proliferation of lymphoid tissue

CLINICAL MANIFESTATIONS

- Most important to distinguish lymphadenitis from lymphadenopathy and define whether there is local or generalized involvement
- Lymphadenitis: Localized involvement; affected nodes are tender with overlying warmth or erythema. Fluctuance suggests abscess formation.

311

- Torticollis (cervical node involvement); dysphagia, drooling, and dyspnea (retropharyngeal node); cough, stridor, dyspnea (mediastinal node); abdominal pain (mesenteric adenitis); limp (inguinal node)
- Concern for malignancy if very rapid increase in node size; confluent and matted shape; firm rubbery consistency; lack of tenderness; fixation to surrounding soft tissue structures
- Overlying violaceous discoloration of skin with draining sinus is characteristic of mycobacterial adenitis, but can occasionally occur with *S. aureus*
- Specific sites:
  - ✓ Preauricular: Adenovirus, tularemia, *B. henselae* (causes Parinaud oculoglandular syndrome; see "Cat-Scratch Disease" section)
  - ✓ Postauricular: Scalp infections, HHV-6, HHV-7, rubella, parvovirus B19
  - ✓ Occipital: Tinea capitis (kerion), scalp infection (cellulitis), or superinfection of eczema or seborrheic dermatitis, rubella, toxoplasma
  - ✓ Supraclavicular: Left-sided "Virchow's node" associated with abdominal source (consider malignancy); right-sided associated with thoracic source (e.g., histoplasmosis, tuberculosis)
  - ✓ Axillary: Cat-scratch disease, bacille Calmette–Guérin (BCG) vaccination
  - ✓ Inguinal: Sexually transmitted infections including chancroid and lymphogranuloma venereum, *Yersinia pestis*
  - ✓ Generalized: CMV, EBV, toxoplasmosis, HIV, syphilis, endemic mycoses, noninfectious autoimmune or oncologic processes

DIAGNOSTICS

- Radiologic evaluation not necessary in most mild-to-moderate cases of lymphadenitis and rarely in cases of lymphadenopathy.
- Ultrasonography preferred to identify drainable abscesses complicating lymphadenitis; CT scan rarely necessary.
- Consider needle aspiration or incisional drainage of lymph node with lymphadenitis if poor response to IV antibiotics or fluctuance or evidence of extension into neck on radiologic studies. Send specimen for bacterial Gram stain and culture, mycobacterial culture and acid-fast smear, and surgical pathology. Fungal culture may be helpful in certain clinical scenarios.
- Consider need for excisional biopsy of lymph node in the setting of lymphadenopathy if supraclavicular node, massively enlarged lymph node (>4 cm), presence of systemic symptoms (e.g., >10% weight loss, night sweats, persistent fevers), or abnormalities detected on initial CBC.
- Depending on clinical situation, consider CBC (especially for generalized lymphadenopathy or massively enlarged lymph nodes [>4 cm]), ESR, CRP, cat-scratch serology, or PCR of nodal aspirate, purified protein derivative (PPD) (5–10 mm may be seen with nontuberculous mycobacteria; usually >15 mm with tuberculosis) and viral serologies or PCRs for CMV and EBV.

MANAGEMENT

- Empiric antibiotics for suspected bacterial adenitis:
  - ✓ Oral: Clindamycin (if suspected MRSA and/or anaerobic infection), amoxicillin–clavulanate, cephalexin
  - ✓ IV: Clindamycin (if suspected MRSA and/or anaerobic infection), ampicillin–sulbactam, cefazolin; rarely require vancomycin
  - ✓ If not improving on above therapy, consider repeat imaging to identify a drainable collection and/or biopsy
  - ✓ Average duration of therapy is 10 days, though may be shorter with adequate excision/drainage

- Special situations (also see "Cat-Scratch Disease" section)
  - ✓ Nontuberculous mycobacteria: Standard therapy requires surgical resection of all visibly affected nodes; incisional drainage not recommended since it may lead to a draining sinus tract. Medical management alone with clarithromycin, ethambutol, or rifampin is seldom successful.
  - ✓ *M. tuberculosis:* Isoniazid, rifampin, and pyrazinamide + ethambutol or streptomycin and infectious diseases consultation to evaluate for extent of disease

MASTOIDITIS

Acute mastoiditis: Mastoid air cell infection resulting from an extension of acute otitis media (OM)
Chronic mastoiditis: Low-grade but persistent mastoid air-cell infection resulting from chronic suppurative OM or, less commonly, inadequately treated acute mastoiditis

ETIOLOGY

- Acute mastoiditis:
  - ✓ Common: *S. pneumoniae, S. pyogenes, S. aureus*
  - ✓ Less common: *H. influenzae, Pseudomonas aeruginosa,* other enteric gram-negative bacilli, anaerobes, *M. tuberculosis*
- Chronic mastoiditis: *P. aeruginosa, S. aureus, S. pneumoniae*

PATHOPHYSIOLOGY

- Mastoid is a series of interconnected air cells located on posterior process of temporal bone, which is connected to the middle ear by a thin channel.
- Purulent material from middle ear under pressure invades mastoid air cells and can cause destruction of the bony septa within the mastoid (coalescent mastoiditis) or abscess formation
- Complications arise due to extension of infection into adjacent structures:
  - ✓ Anterior: Facial-nerve palsy, labyrinthitis due to invasion of the auditory canal, jugular vein, internal carotid
  - ✓ Posterior: Occipital osteomyelitis
  - ✓ Medial: Petrositis, intracranial complications including meningitis, subdural empyema, epidural abscess, or sinus venous thrombosis
    - Petrositis may manifest as Gradenigo syndrome, the triad of pain behind the eye, ear discharge, and abducens nerve palsy.
  - ✓ Inferior: Abscess of deep neck musculature
  - ✓ Lateral: Subperiosteal abscess within the lateral cortex of the mastoid, posterior to the pinna

CLINICAL MANIFESTATIONS

- Acute mastoiditis:
  - ✓ Fever, ear pain, tinnitus, postauricular swelling, tenderness, and erythema
  - ✓ Tympanic membrane often bulging, immobile, and opaque, or has ruptured with otorrhea present, but lack of these findings does not exclude mastoiditis
  - ✓ May have a history of recent OM (days–weeks)
  - ✓ Pinna deviated outward and downward (infant) or upward (older child)
- Chronic mastoiditis:
  - ✓ Persistent posterior auricular swelling, history of recurrent OM or effusion, chronic otorrhea, hearing loss, and ear pain

DIAGNOSTICS

- Usually clinical
- Culture from tympanocentesis or drainage procedure useful to guide therapy
- Associated lab findings can include elevated peripheral WBC count, ESR, and CRP.
- Temporal bone CT with IV contrast is imaging method of choice; destruction of bony septa, mastoid air-cell coalescence, or rim-enhancing fluid collections all suggest mastoiditis, whereas fluid-filled air cells are often seen in uncomplicated OM
- Head CT with contrast (or MRI) may reveal associated intracranial complications

MANAGEMENT

Medical

- Acute: Ampicillin–sulbactam (if no intracranial complication) or ceftriaxone with or without vancomycin; if history of recurrent otitis media, consider anti-pseudomonal antibiotic
- May switch to oral antibiotics once patient improves (amoxicillin–clavulanate; levofloxacin; or clindamycin) for a total duration of 2–4 weeks
- Chronic: Topical therapy with ofloxacin otic solution, aural irrigation; if topical therapy fails, consider systemic therapy with an anti-pseudomonal beta-lactam with or without vancomycin, with ultimate choice of antibiotic guided by microbiologic culture results
- Modify antibiotics based on culture results.

Surgical

- Ear, nose, and throat consultation: Myringotomy with or without placement of tympanostomy tubes
- Mastoidectomy if no improvement within 48 hours of myringotomy or subperiosteal abscess, facial-nerve palsy, or intracranial extension

Follow-up

- Audiology exam

MENINGITIS

Inflammation of the meninges, which manifests as increased WBCs in the CSF

EPIDEMIOLOGY

- Viral meningitis most common during late summer and early fall during enteroviral season
- Neonatal bacterial meningitis occurs in 80 cases per 100,000 live births with GBS accounting for the majority of infections
- Incidence of bacterial meningitis is 6.9 in 100,000 in children 2–23 months of age and <0.5 in 100,000 in children 2–17 years of age.

ETIOLOGY

- Bacteria
  - ✓ Neonates (0–1 month): GBS, *E. coli*, *S. pneumoniae*, enteric gram-negative bacilli, *L. monocytogenes*
  - ✓ Infants (1 month–1 year): *S. pneumoniae*, GBS, *N. meningitidis*, *H. influenzae*
  - ✓ Children older than 1 year: *S. pneumoniae*, *N. meningitidis*, *H. influenzae*. Incidence of *S. pneumoniae* is increasing, but studies are under way to track serotype replacement since introduction of pneumococcal 13-valent vaccine
  - ✓ Other bacterial causes: *Borrelia burgdorferi*, *M. tuberculosis*, *Treponema pallidum*

- Viruses: Enteroviruses, HSV 1 and 2, VZV, adenovirus, parainfluenza, mumps, measles, influenza A and B, lymphocytic choriomeningitis virus, arboviruses, HIV
- Fungi: *Blastomyces dermatitidis*, *Coccidioides immitis*, *Cryptococcus neoformans*, *Candida* species, *Histoplasma capsulatum*

PATHOPHYSIOLOGY

- Bacteria and viruses enter the bloodstream through mucosal surfaces. After entry into the blood, the organism invades the meninges and replicates, inducing an inflammatory response.

CLINICAL MANIFESTATIONS

- Neonates and infants: Fever, lethargy, poor feeding, and/or irritability. On exam: bulging fontanelle, nuchal rigidity, inconsolable irritability. In neonates, fever alone should prompt an evaluation for meningitis
- Toddlers and children: Fever, severe headache, chills, photophobia, neck stiffness, seizures, and vomiting. On exam: nuchal rigidity, photophobia, presence of Kernig and/or Brudzinski signs
- Kernig sign: While legs are flexed 90 degrees at the hip, extension of the lower legs cannot be accomplished beyond 135 degrees
- Brudzinski sign: Passive neck flexion elicits involuntary hip flexion
- Complications: Circulatory collapse, focal neurologic findings (paralysis, facial nerve palsy, visual field defects, hearing loss), seizures, hydrocephalus, brain abscess, subdural effusions, syndrome of inappropriate diuretic hormone release, death

DIAGNOSTICS

- Laboratory studies: Blood culture, CBC with differential, chemistry panel, liver function tests (especially if HSV is suspected)
- The Bacterial Meningitis Score can be used to predict children at very low risk of bacterial meningitis (see **Table 15-7**); when all five predictors are absent, outpatient management can be considered if the patient appears well and has scheduled clinical follow-up (negative predictive value >99% for absence of bacterial meningitis if all five predictors are absent)
- CSF studies (**Table 15-8**): Cell count with differential, protein, glucose, Gram stain and culture, enterovirus PCR during summer and fall, HSV PCR if consistent with clinical picture
- Radiology:
  ✓ CT scan if evidence of increased intracranial pressure or focal neurologic exam to identify masses, infarcts, and cerebral edema that may put patient at risk for cerebral herniation during lumbar puncture or to aid with prognosis
  ✓ Imaging also indicated for *Citrobacter* and *Cronobacter* infections due to high rate of abscess formation

TABLE 15-7	Bacterial Meningitis Score
Bacterial Meningitis Score Predictors Criteria[*]	
CSF Gram stain	Positive result
CSF ANC	$\geq$1000 cells/mm^3
CSF protein	$\geq$80 mg/dL
Peripheral-blood ANC	$\geq$10,000 cells/mm^3
Seizure	Onset at or prior to time of presentation

[*]Bacterial meningitis is unlikely if none of these five predictors are present.
ANC = absolute neutrophil count; CSF = cerebrospinal fluid.

TABLE 15-8	Typical Cerebrospinal Fluid Profiles			
	WBC (cells/mm³)	WBC Differential	Protein (mg/dL)	Glucose (mg/dL)
Normal neonate (0–28 days)	0–19		<115	2/3 of serum
Normal infant (29–56 days)	0–9		<89	2/3 of serum
Normal children/ adolescents	0–10		5–40	2/3 of serum
Viral meningitis	<1000	Lymphocyte predominant*	Normal or <100	2/3 of serum
Bacterial meningitis	>1000	Neutrophil predominant	>100–150	<40
Lyme meningitis	<500	Lymphocyte predominant	<100	2/3 of serum
Tuberculous meningitis	<300	Lymphocyte predominant	>200–300	<40

*Neutrophil predominance can be seen in early viral meningitis.

MANAGEMENT

- Empiric therapy in patients with suspected bacterial meningitis: Suggested resource: http://www.chop.edu/pathways.
  - ✓ Neonate (0–1 month): Ampicillin and cefepime or meropenem IV, dosed for CNS penetration. Begin acyclovir in infants <21 days of age and those who appear ill or with other stigmata of HSV disease while awaiting HSV testing results
  - ✓ All other children: Vancomycin IV and ceftriaxone, dosed for CNS penetration
- If CSF culture results remain negative for 48 hours, the antibiotics can be discontinued. However, if antibiotics are administered prior to lumbar puncture and CSF profile is abnormal, an empiric treatment course of antibiotics should be considered, which can be done in consultation with an infectious diseases specialist.
- Duration of therapy varies by organism and patient course. Typically: *N. meningitidis*, 5–7 days; *S. pneumoniae*, 10 days; GBS, 14 days
- Audiology exam indicated during follow-up

NEONATAL CONJUNCTIVITIS

Conjunctivitis (inflammation or infection of the outer membrane of the eyeball or inner portion of eyelid) occurring in infants less than 4 weeks of age

EPIDEMIOLOGY

- *C. trachomatis, Neisseria gonorrhoeae,* and HSV are the most common pathogens. Frequency related to rates of maternal genital infection; however, the incidence of nonsexually transmitted bacterial pathogens is increasing.
- *C. trachomatis* acquisition in 50% of infants born vaginally to infected mothers; after acquisition, risk of conjunctivitis is 25–50%.

ETIOLOGY

- Infectious (common): *C. trachomatis, N. gonorrhoeae,* herpes simplex virus (see "Neonatal Herpes Simplex Virus Infection"). Other organisms include *S. aureus, S. pneumoniae, groups A and B streptococci, H. influenzae* (nontypable), *P. aeruginosa* (hospitalized preterm infants)
- Chemical: Silver nitrate, erythromycin, foreign body

PATHOPHYSIOLOGY

- Modes of acquisition
  - ✓ Premature rupture of membranes
  - ✓ Transplacental hematogenous seeding
  - ✓ Direct contact with maternal genital secretions
  - ✓ Direct contact or aerosolization from caregiver's after birth
- Incubation: *N. gonorrhoeae,* 2–7 days; *C. trachomatis,* 5–14 days
- Risk factors:
  - ✓ Maternal history of untreated GC or *C. trachomatis*
  - ✓ Baby born without topical eye prophylaxis (such as a home birth), suspect *N. gonorrhoeae*

CLINICAL MANIFESTATIONS

- Conjunctival injection, edema of eyelids, chemosis (swelling)
- Eye discharge may be serosanguineous or purulent
- *C. trachomatis* pneumonia develops in 11–20% of exposed infants at 3–12 weeks of age (afebrile, nasal congestion, diffuse infiltrates, rales).
- *N. gonorrhoeae* may rapidly progress to corneal ulceration and perforation, resulting in blindness.
- *P. aeruginosa* may cause systemic infection.

DIAGNOSTICS

- Culture and Gram stain of the discharge; *N. gonorrhoeae* appears as intracellular gram-negative diplococci on Gram stain
- *C. trachomatis* can be identified by nucleic-acid amplification test (NAAT) on conjunctival or nasopharyngeal (pneumonia) swab.

MANAGEMENT

- Prevention: Perinatal ocular prophylaxis with topical 0.5% erythromycin, 1% silver nitrate, or 1% tetracycline ointment reduces risk of conjunctivitis; all active against *N. gonorrhoeae,* but do not prevent transmission of *C. trachomatis.*
- *C. trachomatis* (conjunctivitis or pneumonia)
  - ✓ Oral erythromycin for 14 days (50 mg/kg/day in four doses) has 80% efficacy. Alternative regimens include oral azithromycin (3 days) or sulfonamides.
  - ✓ Newborns born to untreated mothers with chlamydia require close observation (without treatment) because the efficacy of prophylactic oral erythromycin is unknown.
- *N. gonorrhoeae*
  - ✓ Hospitalization, consider evaluation (blood and CSF cultures) to exclude disseminated infection
  - ✓ Ceftriaxone: 25–50 mg/kg single dose IV or IM (maximum, 125 mg) for infected infants and for those born to an infected, untreated mother; ceftazidime if hyperbilirubinemia present
  - ✓ Saline eye irrigations initially every hour and then every 2–3 hours until resolution of discharge

OSTEOMYELITIS

Inflammation of bone, usually secondary to bacterial infection

EPIDEMIOLOGY

- 50% of cases occur in children <5 years of age
- Boys affected more often than girls (except in first year of life)

ETIOLOGY

- *S. aureus* is most common; MRSA should be considered depending on local epidemiology
- Other organisms: *S. pneumoniae* (less common due to widespread vaccination); *S. pyogenes*; *Kingella kingae* (6–36 months of age); enteric gram-negative rods and GBS (neonates); *N. gonorrhoeae* (adolescents); coagulase-negative staphylococci (prosthetic material-related); anaerobes (complicated sinusitis, superinfection of fracture site); *Salmonella* (sickle hemoglobinopathies); *P. aeruginosa* (puncture wound through sneaker)

PATHOPHYSIOLOGY

- Hematogenous spread (most common) or extension of contiguous skin/muscle structure infection
- In neonates, infection often extends to joint space via transphyseal capillaries, which recede by 18 months of age.

CLINICAL MANIFESTATIONS

- Most frequently occurs in long bones (in order of decreasing frequency): Femur, tibia, hands and feet, humerus, pelvis, fibula
- 75% of cases have single bone involvement
- Fever, occasionally anorexia, malaise, vomiting, irritability
- Pain and reluctance to use affected extremity ("pseudo-paralysis")
- Focal swelling, point tenderness, warmth, and erythema (usually over metaphysis)
- Tenderness out of proportion to soft-tissue findings
- Range of motion intact, limited only by pain/muscle spasm
- Neurologic deficits in vertebral osteomyelitis
- In neonates, the entire limb may have swelling, edema, and discoloration.

DIAGNOSTICS

- Leukocytosis (often but not always)
- CRP: Elevated in more than 95% (may be normal in chronic osteomyelitis)
- ESR: Elevated in 90%
- Blood culture results: Positive in 35–50%
- Bone aspirate: Culture of bone, blood, and/or joint fluid positive in 50–80%
- Plain radiographs: Low sensitivity for diagnosing early osteomyelitis; 10–20 days after onset, may detect lytic lesions, periosteal elevation, and new bone formation (7–10 days in neonates)
- MRI: Imaging method of choice, with best sensitivity (92–100%)
  - ✓ Differentiates cellulitis from osteomyelitis
  - ✓ Use of contrast allows for better differentiation of bone and soft tissue edema caused by osteomyelitis.
- Radionuclide bone scanning: Useful if MRI not available and in early diagnosis (sensitivity 80–100%)
  - ✓ Helpful if multiple sites suspected or poorly localizable pain

MANAGEMENT

Medical

- Empiric therapy: Oxacillin, cefazolin, or clindamycin (if high prevalence of MRSA). If patient is severely ill, consider vancomycin.
- CRP typically begins to decline 2–3 days after initiation of antibiotics (normal within 7–10 days). ESR begins to decline approximately 5–7 days after initiation of antibiotics (normal within 3–4 weeks).
- Early transition to oral therapy, often prior to discharge, is the preferred strategy. Treatment failure rates between children treated with early conversion to oral therapy are not different from those treated with prolonged courses of intravenous antibiotics.
- Oral therapy with either a targeted agent or empiric cephalexin (100 mg/kg/day divided every 6–8 hours; maximum, 4 g/day) or clindamycin (30–40 mg/kg/day divided every 8 hours; maximum, 600 mg/dose) may be considered. Discuss with infectious diseases specialist.
- Duration of therapy: Based on resolution of fever, pain, erythema, and/or swelling, minimum 4 weeks of therapy (typical duration, 4–6 weeks)

Surgical

- Considerations for surgery: Subperiosteal abscess; bacteremia persisting beyond 48–72 hours of treatment; continued fever, pain, swelling after 72 hours of therapy; development of sinus tract

OTITIS MEDIA

Classification of otitis media (inflammation of mucosal lining of middle ear):
   Acute otitis media (AOM): Purulent fluid in the middle ear with acute signs and symptoms of local or systemic illness
   Otitis media with effusion (OME): Asymptomatic middle ear effusion
   Chronic suppurative otitis media (CSOM): Purulent drainage through perforated tympanic membrane for more than 6 weeks

EPIDEMIOLOGY

- 90% of children have at least one episode of AOM by 2 years of age; incidence peaks between 6 and 18 months of age

ETIOLOGY

- AOM: *S. pneumoniae* (35–48%); nontypable *H. influenzae* (20–29%); *M. catarrhalis* (12–23%)
   ✓ Less common pathogens include group A *Streptococcus* and *S. aureus*.
   ✓ After initiation of pneumococcal vaccine (PCV) 7 in 2000 and PCV13 in 2010, non-vaccine serotypes of *S. pneumoniae* and nontypable *H. influenzae* have emerged as the predominant bacterial pathogens.
- Viral pathogens responsible for 10–40% of middle ear effusions in AOM, including RSV, parainfluenza, influenza, and adenovirus
- CSOM is usually polymicrobial: *Pseudomonas* spp.; *S. aureus*

PATHOPHYSIOLOGY

- AOM: Transient (e.g., upper respiratory tract infection) or chronic eustachian-tube dysfunction causes negative middle ear pressure.
- Middle ear fluid accumulates, with subsequent bacterial superinfection.

CLINICAL MANIFESTATIONS

- Abrupt onset of fever and ear pain (holding, tugging, rubbing of the ear in a nonverbal child)
- Middle ear effusion: Bulging tympanic membrane, impaired membrane mobility by pneumatic otoscopy, or air–fluid level behind membrane
- Middle ear inflammation: Tympanic membrane with red or yellow color; otalgia

DIAGNOSTICS

- Diagnosis made by physical exam with pneumatic otoscopy
- Tympanocentesis considered for: Relief of severe pain; confirmation of pathogens in neonates, in immunocompromised patients, or after failed antibiotic therapy; part of treatment for acute mastoiditis
- Tympanometry confirms middle ear effusion when pneumatic otoscopy cannot be performed.

MANAGEMENT

Based on the AAP Guideline for the Diagnosis and Management of AOM

Initial Management of Acute Otitis Media

- Pain control: Acetaminophen or ibuprofen; in children >5 years, consider topical benzocaine (e.g., Auralgan, Americaine otic)
- For ages 6 months–2 years:
  - ✓ Otorrhea or bilateral AOM—Treat with antibiotics
  - ✓ Unilateral or bilateral AOM with severe symptoms (toxic-appearing child, persistent otalgia >48 hours, fever >39°C, or uncertain follow-up)—treat with antibiotics
  - ✓ Unilateral AOM without otorrhea—Consider initial observation without antibiotics if nonsevere illness or uncertain diagnosis and then treat if no improvement within 48–72 hours. *If observation option exercised, must ensure mechanism for communication with physician, reevaluation, and obtaining medication if necessary.*
- For ages >2 years:
  - ✓ Same as above except consider initial observation of patients with bilateral AOM without otorrhea

Antibiotic Options for Acute Otitis Media

- First-line for nonsevere symptoms (if decision made to treat and/or the patient has not received amoxicillin in the past 30 days): High-dose amoxicillin, 80–90 mg/kg/day in two divided doses
  - ✓ Alternative agents for penicillin allergy: Cefdinir, cefuroxime, cefpodoxime, azithromycin, clarithromycin, or clindamycin
- First-line for severe symptoms (or the patient has received amoxicillin in the past 30 days): Amoxicillin–clavulanate using 90 mg/kg/day of amoxicillin component with 6.4 mg/kg/day of clavulanate in two divided doses
  - ✓ Alternative agent for penicillin allergy: Ceftriaxone (1–3 days)
- Clinically defined treatment failure (no improvement within 48–72 hours): Amoxicillin–clavulanate using 90 mg/kg/day of amoxicillin component (if previously on amoxicillin); otherwise use ceftriaxone (3 days) or clindamycin with or without tympanocentesis
- Duration of therapy: 5–7 days if child >6 years of age and with mild-to-moderate symptoms; 7 days if child 2–6 years of age with uncomplicated AOM; 10 days in child <2 years of age or with underlying medical conditions, recurrent AOM, or tympanic membrane perforation

Additional Considerations

- Persistence of middle ear effusion after AOM: 60–70% at 2 weeks, 40% at 1 month, and 10–25% at 3 months
- Recurrent AOM (three episodes in 6 months or four episodes in 1 year, with one episode in the preceding 6 months): Prophylactic antibiotics not indicated
- Indications for tympanostomy tubes: Chronic OME and associated conductive hearing loss greater than 15 dB or tympanic membrane retraction with ossicular erosion or cholesteatoma formation
- OME:
  - ✓ First 3 months: Observe
  - ✓ After 3 months (chronic): Tympanostomy tubes if bilateral effusions and hearing loss >15 dB. Antibiotics and corticosteroids not indicated because effusion rapidly reaccumulates upon cessation.
- CSOM: 7–14 days of ototopical antibiotics (ciprofloxacin, ofloxacin, neomycin, polymyxin B)
  - ✓ Consider oral agents as for AOM.
- Complications: Middle ear (e.g., conductive hearing loss, cholesteatoma); temporal bone (e.g., mastoiditis, petrositis; see "Mastoiditis" section); inner ear (e.g., labyrinthitis); intracranial (e.g., subdural abscess, lateral sinus thrombosis, meningitis)

PERIORBITAL/PRESEPTAL AND ORBITAL CELLULITIS

Periorbital or preseptal cellulitis: Infections anterior to orbital septum
Orbital cellulitis: Infections posterior to the orbital septum

EPIDEMIOLOGY

- Preseptal cellulitis: Usually in children under 5 years of age
- Orbital cellulitis: Mean age, 12 years; more common in boys

ETIOLOGY

Preseptal Cellulitis

- Infection after local trauma: *S. aureus*, *S. pyogenes*
- Hematogenous seeding: Usually *S. pneumoniae* (since introduction of *H. influenzae* type B vaccine)
- Soft-tissue swelling in periorbital area due to compression of ophthalmic veins secondary to sinusitis (not true cellulitis): *S. pneumoniae*, *M. catarrhalis*, nontypable *H. influenzae*

Orbital Cellulitis

- Usually extension of sinusitis into orbit
- Often polymicrobial; most commonly *S. pneumoniae*, *S. pyogenes*, *S. aureus*, and anaerobic bacteria of the upper respiratory tract

CLINICAL MANIFESTATIONS

- Fever
- Eyelid edema and erythema (>95% unilateral)

Preseptal Cellulitis

- Evidence of local trauma
- Normal visual acuity, pupillary responses, intraocular pressure, and extraocular movements
- No pain with eye movement

Orbital Cellulitis

- Proptosis
- Impaired or painful extraocular eye movements
- Loss of visual acuity or pupillary responses

DIAGNOSTICS

- Obtain CBC and blood culture for suspected or confirmed orbital cellulitis, periorbital cellulitis with fever, or toxic appearance.
- Perform a lumbar puncture if signs or symptoms of meningitis are present.
- CT scanning of orbits and sinuses is recommended if orbital involvement is confirmed by exam orbital involvement is suspected or cannot be excluded by exam, or disease progresses despite parenteral antibiotic treatment.

MANAGEMENT

Preseptal Cellulitis

- Oral antibiotics if mild infection and child nontoxic
  - ✓ First-line: Amoxicillin–clavulanate; consider clindamycin in areas of high MRSA prevalence
- IV antibiotics if child appears ill or oral treatment failed
  - ✓ First-line: Ampicillin–sulbactam; consider clindamycin or vancomycin in areas of high MRSA prevalence
- Alternative: Clindamycin, ceftriaxone, vancomycin
- Total duration: 10 days; may be completed orally if clinical improvement is documented

Orbital Cellulitis

- Requires IV antibiotics initially:
  - ✓ First-line: Ampicillin–sulbactam. Consider adding vancomycin for severe, sight-threatening infections.
  - ✓ Alternative: Clindamycin, vancomycin, ceftriaxone
  - ✓ Total duration, approximately 14 days, depending on clinical improvement and surgical drainage (if necessary); may be completed orally if clinical improvement is documented
- If no clinical improvement is noted in 36–48 hours or if symptoms progress: Repeat CT scan and consider surgical drainage.
- Surgical drainage for large, well-defined abscess on initial or repeat CT scan; complete ophthalmoplegia; significant visual impairment

RETROPHARYNGEAL AND PERITONSILLAR ABSCESS

Peritonsillar abscess: Purulent collection in the tonsillar fossa
Retropharyngeal abscess: Deep neck abscess involving the potential space between the posterior pharyngeal wall and the alar division of the deep cervical fascia

EPIDEMIOLOGY

Peritonsillar Abscess

- Typically occurs in older children/adolescents (mean age, 11 years) as a complication of streptococcal pharyngitis; 15% complicate EBV infection
  - ✓ Increasing incidence likely due to community-acquired MRSA

Retropharyngeal Abscess

- Typically occurs in young children (<5 years) and complicates pharyngitis. In older children and adolescents, it often complicates penetrating injury to the posterior pharynx.
- Prior upper respiratory infection in 50% of patients

ETIOLOGY

Peritonsillar Abscess

- Common: S. pyogenes
- Less common: *S. aureus*, anaerobes (*Fusobacterium, Peptostreptococcus, Bacteroides* spp.), *H. influenzae*

Retropharyngeal Abscess (Usually Polymicrobial)

- Common: *S. pyogenes, S. aureus*, viridans group streptococci
- Less common: Oral anaerobes (*Fusobacterium, Peptostreptococcus, Bacteroides* spp.), *Eikenella corrodens, H. influenzae, S. pneumoniae*

PATHOPHYSIOLOGY

Peritonsillar abscess

- Begins with pharyngitis or cellulitis and progresses to abscess

Retropharyngeal Abscess

- Retropharyngeal space:
  - ✓ Limited posteriorly by the alar division of deep cervical fascia and anteriorly by the posterior pharyngeal wall
  - ✓ Divided by a midline raphe into two lateral compartments with each half containing lymph nodes
- Infection of the nasopharynx spreads to retropharyngeal space by lymphatic routes; lymph node inflammation followed by necrosis leads to abscess
- Retropharyngeal abscess is unlikely in older children owing to regression of lymph nodes
- Complications: Extension to carotid sheath (carotid artery, internal jugular vein, vagus nerve) or posteriorly (atlantoaxial dislocation); spontaneous rupture may cause aspiration, asphyxiation, empyema, or mediastinitis

CLINICAL MANIFESTATIONS

Peritonsillar Abscess

- Adolescent with fever, sore throat, unilateral pain, drooling, dysphagia, and "hot potato" (muffled) voice
- Trismus in two thirds of patients
- Oropharynx: Displacement of uvula away from affected side, palpable peritonsillar fluctuance, with or without tonsillar exudate
- Ipsilateral cervical adenopathy

Retropharyngeal Abscess

- Fever, decreased oral intake, sore throat
- Drooling, dysphagia, odynophagia
- Neck stiffness or pain with neck extension
- Torticollis, trismus, stridor, and dyspnea less common (<5%)

DIAGNOSTICS

- Leukocytosis with neutrophil predominance (CBC not routinely recommended)
- Rapid streptococcal antigen test by throat swab
- Lateral neck x-ray in retropharyngeal abscess: Retropharyngeal space wider than one-half of the C2 vertebrae or greater than 7 mm (false negative rate, 14%)
- Neck CT with contrast: In peritonsillar abscess, assesses extent of infection; in suspected retropharyngeal abscess, distinguishes cellulitis from abscess (false negative rate, 10%)

MANAGEMENT

Guideline Management

Suggested resource: https://www.chop.edu/clinical-pathway/neck-infection-clinical-pathway
   Authors: R. Abaya, MD; M. Joffe, MD; L. Vella, MD; M. Dunn, MD; S. MacFarland, MD; M. Rizzi, MD; K. Shekdar, MD; R. Bellah, MD; J. Lavelle, MD

Peritonsillar Abscess

- Incision and drainage with 18-gauge needle confirms diagnosis and provides immediate relief
- Empiric therapy: Ampicillin–sulbactam/amoxicillin–clavulanate or clindamycin
- Duration of therapy: 7–10 days

Retropharyngeal Abscess

- Emergency: Secure airway (if necessary); obtain IV access; order nothing by mouth (NPO)
- Early detection (no mature abscess) may obviate surgery.
- Most cases of mature abscess require surgical drainage.
   - ✓ Transoral approach limits exposure of vessels; used to drain abscesses medial to great vessels.
   - ✓ Transcervical (i.e., external) approach limits aspiration risk; used to drain abscesses lateral to great vessels or if there is a large lateral component.
- Antibiotics: Ampicillin–sulbactam.
- Alternative: ceftriaxone + clindamycin. Use IV antibiotics initially and switch to oral antibiotics when symptoms have improved to complete 10- to 14-day course. Longer courses may be necessary for undrained collections.

SEPSIS

Historically, sepsis has been defined as systemic inflammatory response syndrome (SIRS) in response to a suspected or documented infection with or without organ system dysfunction (severe sepsis) or cardiovascular dysfunction unresponsive to fluid resuscitation (septic shock). However, these categories are expected to change in the near future because of the lack of adequate sensitivity, specificity, and clinical utility; therefore it is perhaps best to define sepsis as a syndrome of systemic inflammation, immune dysregulation, and end-organ dysfunction in response to infection.

ETIOLOGY/EPIDEMIOLOGY

- Neonatal: GBS, enteric gram-negative bacilli, less commonly *L. monocytogenes*; *S. aureus*, *Candida* spp., coagulase-negative *Staphylococcus*, other gram-negative species in hospitalized neonates, especially those with CVCs

- Community-acquired, nonimmunocompromised host: *S. pneumoniae, N. meningitidis, S. pyogenes*, enteric gram-negatives, *S. aureus*, rickettsial disease
- Immunocompromised host: Enteric gram-negative species, *S. aureus*, coagulase-negative *Staphylococcus*, viridans group *Streptococcus*, *Candida* spp.
- CVC: See "Catheter-Related Bloodstream Infection" section.
- As many as 50–75% of children with sepsis will have no confirmed cause
- **Figure 15-2** shows the laboratory classification of commonly isolated bacteria.

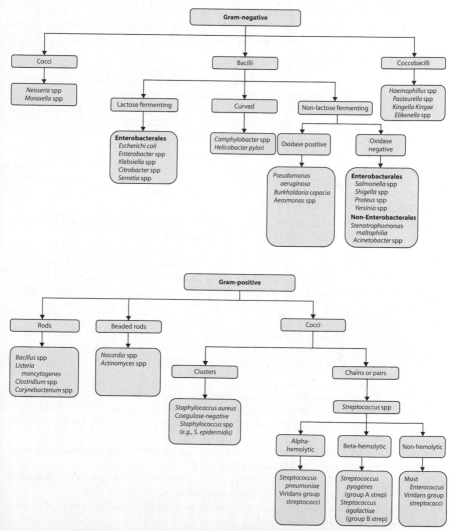

FIGURE 15-2 **Laboratory Features of Common Organisms.**

PATHOPHYSIOLOGY

- Activation of the immune response by a pathogen leads to leukocyte mobilization, upregulation of proinflammatory cytokines, complement activation, and activation of coagulation
- These processes lead to capillary and endothelial injury, vasodilation, microvascular thromboses and subsequent cardiac and other end-organ dysfunction.

CLINICAL MANIFESTATIONS

- All children presenting with signs of infection should be evaluated for signs/symptoms of organ dysfunction, including tachycardia (particularly that which persists following fever control), tachypnea, abnormal pulses (diminished or bounding), abnormal capillary refill (<1 second or >3 seconds), hypotension (late finding), diminished urine output, altered mental status (including irritability, lethargy, confusion), purpura or petechiae.
- Criteria for SIRS are as follows:
  - ✓ Temperature >38.5°C or <36°C
  - ✓ Tachycardia >2 standard deviations above normal for age or for children less than 1 year of age, bradycardia defined as a mean heart rate <10th percentile for age.
  - ✓ Tachypnea >2 standard deviations above normal for age or need for mechanical ventilation
  - ✓ Leukocytosis or leukopenia for age, or >10% bands

DIAGNOSTICS

- CBC, electrolytes, renal- and liver-function tests, dextrose stick, prothrombin time (PT), partial thromboplastin time (PTT), and fibrinogen can help evaluate for organ-system dysfunction.
- Lactate and mixed/central venous oxyhemoglobin saturation (if patient has a CVC) can be helpful in assessing adequacy of perfusion and response to therapy.
- Type and screen
- Cultures of all potential sources of infection *before* antibiotics (if doing so does not significantly delay antibiotic administration); blood culture should be obtained in all cases of sepsis (prefer cultures from both peripheral blood and central line, if present), as well as urine culture, CSF Gram stain and culture, respiratory Gram stain and culture, and wound Gram stain and culture of any identifiable soft-tissue abscesses, as clinically indicated
- Consider viral testing for HSV and/or enterovirus from serum, as well as influenza, adenovirus, and/or RSV from respiratory secretions
- Chest x-ray, imaging of possible foci of infection as clinically indicated

MANAGEMENT

- Institutions should have a resuscitation "bundle" to facilitate rapid stabilization of patients with severe sepsis or septic shock; salient elements of the resuscitation bundle are highlighted below.
- Patients with septic shock should receive 100% supplemental oxygen to optimize blood oxygen content and may require endotracheal intubation.
- Establish IV or intraosseus access (preferably at least two access points in severely ill patients) within 5 minutes after identification of severe sepsis/septic shock.
- Rapidly administer a 20 mL/kg bolus and repeated as needed within 30 minutes after identification of severe sepsis/septic shock.
- If patient's condition is not responsive to 60 mL/kg fluid resuscitation, initiate inotrope infusion via peripheral or central line within 60 minutes after identification of severe sepsis/septic shock.

- Administer broad-spectrum antibiotics within 60 minutes after identification of severe sepsis/septic shock. The recommendations below should be modified as necessary based on local susceptibility patterns, history of antibiotic resistant organisms, and suspected source of infection:
  - ✓ Neonate: Ampicillin and ceftazidime or cefepime with or without acyclovir; recommendation for ceftazidime or cefepime reflects the fact that cefotaxime is no longer being manufactured.
  - ✓ Infants and children, community acquired: Vancomycin and ceftriaxone; consider addition of a second gram-negative agent (aminoglycoside or ciprofloxacin) depending on local susceptibilities, history of antibiotic-resistant infection, or if patient in shock
  - ✓ Immunocompromised, hospitalized, or CVC: Vancomycin and an antipseudomonal beta-lactam; consider addition of a second gram-negative agent (aminoglycoside or ciprofloxacin) depending on local susceptibilities, or history of antibiotic resistant infection
  - ✓ Intraabdominal source: Add coverage for anaerobic organisms, which could include addition of metronidazole to the above regimens, or use of piperacillin–tazobactam or meropenem alone
  - ✓ Toxin-mediated process: Add clindamycin
  - ✓ Suspected rickettsial illness (Rocky Mountain spotted fever, ehrlichiosis): Add doxycycline
  - ✓ High risk for fungal infection (risk factors include neutropenia, prior broad-spectrum antibiotics, TPN-dependent): Consider adding echinocandin (caspofungin, micafungin)
  - ✓ If type I hypersensitivity to penicillin or cephalosporin: Aztreonam or fluoroquinolone in place of cephalosporins
- Source control as soon as feasible (drain soft-tissue abscesses, debride necrotic tissues, remove infected CVC)

SEPTIC ARTHRITIS

Microbial invasion of the joint space

EPIDEMIOLOGY

- Peak incidence in children <3 years of age

ETIOLOGY

- Most common across all age groups: S. aureus
- Neonates: S. aureus, GBS enteric gram-negative rods, N. gonorrhoeae
- School age: S. aureus, K. kingae, S. pyogenes, S. pneumoniae, H. influenzae
- Older children: S. aureus, S. pyogenes, N. gonorrhoeae
- Less common causes: N. meningitidis, Pseudomonas spp., Candida spp., Brucella spp., tuberculous and nontuberculous mycobacteria, B. burgdorferi (Lyme disease—seen in endemic areas)

PATHOPHYSIOLOGY

- Mechanism: Hematogenous dissemination; contiguous extension (10–16% of cases); direct inoculation
- Risk factors: Joint instrumentation, diabetes, immunodeficiency, skin or soft-tissue infection, hemoglobinopathy, IV drug use

CLINICAL MANIFESTATIONS

- Fever, malaise, poor appetite, irritability (infants)
- Frequency of joint involvement (in order of decreasing frequency): Knee, hip, ankle, elbow, shoulder, other
- Acute onset of severe joint pain, decreased mobility, refusal to walk
- Joint swelling, erythema, warmth, exquisite tenderness, decreased range of motion
- Septic hip preferentially held flexed and externally rotated
- 90% of cases are monoarticular
- Dermatitis–arthritis syndrome, sexually transmitted infections (*N. gonorrhoeae*)
- History of erythema migrans rash, significant swelling, minimal pain (Lyme disease)

DIAGNOSTICS

- CBC: 70% with elevated WBC
- CRP: Elevated at presentation in 95%
  - ✓ CRP >2 mg/dL has been shown to be the strongest independent risk factor.
- ESR: Elevated at presentation in 90%
- Blood culture results: Positive in 40% (pathogen-dependent)
- Joint fluid aspiration for cell count (**Table 15-9**)
- Joint fluid culture results: Positive in 50–60%; yield increased if joint fluid inoculated directly into blood culture bottle (for detection of *K. kingae*)
- If Lyme disease exposure: Lyme serology with or without Lyme joint fluid PCR (useful in antibiotic-refractory disease)
- Joint radiography: Important to exclude other causes of joint pain; not diagnostic for septic arthritis but may reveal distortion of fat-pad swelling, soft-tissue swelling, joint-space widening, and focal source of osteomyelitis
- Ultrasonography: Preferred initial study to identify excess joint space fluid
- MRI: Highly sensitive in early detection of joint fluid; detects involvement of adjacent bone or soft tissue

MANAGEMENT (THIS IS A MEDICAL EMERGENCY)

Guideline Management

Suggested resource: https://www.chop.edu/clinical-pathway/septic-arthritis-suspected-clinical-pathway

Authors: P. Aronson, MD, J. Posner, MD, S. Dooley, RN, S. Coffin, MD, C. Jacobstein, MD, J. Lavelle, MD

Surgical

- Hip or shoulder: Prompt surgical drainage, joint space irrigation

TABLE 15-9	Typical Synovial Fluid Findings	
Diagnosis	**Typical WBC per mm³**	**Neutrophil %**
Normal	<150	<25%
Bacterial arthritis	>50,000	>90%
Lyme arthritis	40,000–80,000*	<25%
Reactive arthritis	<15,000	<25%

*Range, 200–140,000.

- Knee, ankle, or wrist: Needle aspiration; consider joint space irrigation if unable to perform adequate drainage with aspiration.
- Open surgical drainage of joints other than hip and shoulder usually not required.

Medical

- Empiric antibiotic therapy
  ✓ Neonate: Intravenous oxacillin (or clindamycin or vancomycin if MRSA common) plus gentamicin (or ceftazidime)
  ✓ Older children: IV cefazolin–oxacillin, clindamycin, or vancomycin, depending on incidence of MRSA
  ✓ Consider both oxacillin and vancomycin if hip or shoulder involved and high rates of MRSA.
  ✓ Add ceftriaxone if risk factors for gram-negative rods.
  ✓ Consider *K. kingae* as a cause in preschool-aged children and those with poor response to clindamycin.
  ✓ Consider doxycycline if concern for Lyme disease.
  ✓ Specific antibiotic therapy based on culture results
- Oral versus intravenous antibiotics
  ✓ Oral therapy can be substituted for IV therapy after infection is adequately controlled, if an oral antibiotic appropriately covers the organism, and follow-up is ensured.
  ✓ For severe infections involving any joint space (especially the hip or shoulder): IV therapy may need to be extended.
- Duration:
  ✓ Three to 4 weeks for *S. aureus* or enteric gram-negative rods
  ✓ In general, 2–3 weeks is sufficient for most other organisms (must be individualized based on patient's course)
- Response to therapy: ESR peaks at end of first week and normalizes at 3–4 weeks. CRP peaks by day 2–3, and normalizes by day 7–9.

SINUSITIS

Inflammation of paranasal sinuses secondary to allergic, bacterial, fungal, or viral etiology
- Bacterial sinusitis is classified clinically by the duration and severity of symptoms:
  ✓ Acute bacterial sinusitis: Symptoms for <30 days
  ✓ Subacute sinusitis: Symptoms for 30–90 days
  ✓ Chronic sinusitis: Symptoms for >90 days

EPIDEMIOLOGY

- Complicates 5–10% of upper respiratory infections
- Peak prevalence in winter

ETIOLOGY

- Acute and subacute bacterial sinusitis:
  ✓ *S. pneumoniae*; *H. influenzae*; *M. catarrhalis*
  ✓ Less commonly: Group A *Streptococcus*, viridans group streptococci, anaerobes
- Chronic sinusitis:
  ✓ Aerobic bacteria found in acute sinusitis, *S. aureus*, anaerobes

PATHOPHYSIOLOGY

- Ciliary dysfunction and increased secretions lead to sinus obstruction.
- Contamination of usually sterile sinuses with nasopharyngeal bacteria
- Recurrent bacterial sinusitis should prompt investigation for underlying predisposition (e.g., allergic rhinitis, cystic fibrosis, dysmotile cilia, HIV).

CLINICAL MANIFESTATIONS

- Acute sinusitis:
  - ✓ Persistent illness: Nasal discharge of any quality, daytime cough, or both, lasting more than 10 days without improvement
  - ✓ Worsening course: Worsening or new onset of nasal discharge, daytime cough, or fever after initial improvement
  - ✓ Severe onset: Concurrent fever (temperature of 102.2°C or greater) with purulent nasal discharge and/or facial pain for at least 3 consecutive days
- Chronic sinusitis: Respiratory symptoms for longer than 90 days; nasal discharge of any quality; headache; fever uncommon
- On physical exam: Periorbital edema; mucopurulent discharge from nose or posterior pharynx; erythematous or boggy and pale nasal mucosa; tenderness to palpation and/or percussion over paranasal sinuses; malodorous breath

Complications

- Orbital complications: Orbital abscess, orbital cellulitis, optic neuritis
- Intracranial complications: Epidural or subdural empyema, cavernous or sagittal sinus thrombosis, meningitis, brain abscess, osteomyelitis (frontal bone: Pott's puffy tumor); require neurosurgical and infectious diseases consultation

DIAGNOSTICS

- Diagnosis usually based on clinical findings
- Confirmatory imaging not indicated in cases of uncomplicated sinusitis
- Imaging indicated if complicated sinusitis, numerous recurrences, protracted or unresponsive course, or anticipated surgical drainage
  - ✓ Contrast-enhanced CT better than MRI to assess suspected suppurative complications

MANAGEMENT

Medical

- Persistent illness: Either prescribe antibiotic therapy OR offer additional observation for 3 days.
- Worsening course or severe onset: Antibiotic therapy indicated
- First-line therapy: Amoxicillin or amoxicillin–clavulanate
  - ✓ High-dose amoxicillin (90 mg/kg/day) should be used in areas of high prevalence of penicillin-resistant S. pneumoniae (>10%).
  - ✓ High-dose amoxicillin with clavulanate should be used in children who attend day care, are <2 years of age, or who have had antibiotic exposure within the last 4 weeks.
- Consider alternative agent if allergy to penicillin, failure to improve on amoxicillin or amoxicillin–clavulanate after 3 days, moderate to severe illness, or protracted symptoms (>30 days)
- Alternative agents: Ceftriaxone, cefdinir, cefuroxime, cefpodoxime, levofloxacin
  - ✓ The following agents are not recommended as empiric therapy owing to high rates of resistance: Macrolides, TMP-SMX

- Duration:
  - ✓ Acute and subacute sinusitis: 10 days
  - ✓ Chronic sinusitis: 3 weeks (can be longer in complicated cases)
- Empiric therapy for complicated sinusitis (e.g., subdural extension): Vancomycin + third-generation cephalosporin + metronidazole

Sinus Aspiration

- Indications: Failure to respond to multiple course of antibiotics, severe facial pain, orbital or intracranial complications, or evaluation of an immunocompromised host

TOXIC SHOCK SYNDROME

An acute streptococcal or staphylococcal exotoxin-mediated infection resulting in fever, diffuse erythroderma, hypotension, and impairment of three or more organ systems

EPIDEMIOLOGY

- 90% of cases in 1980s occurred as a result of superabsorbent tampon use. Now <50% of cases are associated with tampon use. Other associations include foreign-body placement, primary *S. aureus* infection, postoperative wound infection, and mucous membrane or skin disruption
- *S. pyogenes*–associated toxic shock syndrome (TSS) is associated with varicella infection, diabetes mellitus, and HIV infection.

ETIOLOGY

- *S. aureus* strains producing one or more of the following exotoxins: TSS type 1, enterotoxin A, B, C, or D
- *S. pyogenes* strains producing streptococcal pyrogenic exotoxins A, B, or C, mitogenic factor, or streptococcal superantigen

PATHOPHYSIOLOGY

- TSS type 1 and other exotoxins act as superantigens, causing massive cytokine release.
- Exotoxins cause perivascular infiltrates, decreased peripheral resistance, and interstitial edema, resulting in intravascular volume depletion, hypotension, and shock.
- Activation of the coagulation cascade and thrombolytic enzymes induce microangiopathic hemolytic anemia and disseminated intravascular coagulation (DIC)

CLINICAL MANIFESTATIONS

- Fever, rash, hypotension, arthritis with multiorgan involvement and clinical illness out of proportion to degree of local infection
- Acute respiratory distress syndrome
- Diffuse erythroderma (sunburn) or blanching macular erythema that desquamates 1–2 weeks later
- Soft-tissue necrosis (necrotizing fasciitis, myositis)

DIAGNOSTICS

- Renal impairment: Elevated creatinine
- Coagulopathy: Platelets $< 100,000/mm^3$ or signs of DIC
- Liver dysfunction: Elevated alanine aminotransferase, aspartate aminotransferase, or total bilirubin
- Blood, throat, and CSF cultures are usually negative; blood cultures may be positive in *S. aureus*-related TSS.

- Diagnosis of staphylococcal TSS requires: Fever >38.9°C, diffuse macular erythrodermic rash (with subsequent desquamation), hypotension, and multisystem organ involvement (>3 organ systems)
- Diagnosis of streptococcal TSS requires: Isolation of S. *pyogenes* from a sterile or nonsterile site, hypotension, and multisystem organ involvement (>2 organ systems)

MANAGEMENT

- Anticipate shock and multisystem organ failure.
- Remove or drain any loculated source of infection.
- Empiric IV antibiotics: Beta-lactamase resistant antistaphylococcal antibiotic (e.g., oxacillin, vancomycin) plus a protein-synthesis inhibitor (clindamycin), which provides a mechanism of bacterial growth inhibition not dependent on replication (to address stationary phase S. *aureus*/S. *pyogenes*) and suppression of toxin production. Consider adding coverage against gram-negative bacteria until diagnosis is more certain.
  - ✓ For S. *pyogenes*, switch to penicillin + clindamycin.
  - ✓ For methicillin-sensitive S. *aureus*, continue with an appropriate beta-lactam antibiotic (based on susceptibility testing) and clindamycin.
  - ✓ For MRSA, continue with vancomycin and clindamycin.
  - ✓ Total antibiotic course of 10–14 days may include high-dose oral therapy when the patient is no longer critically ill.
- IVIG may be considered as adjunctive therapy for patients with an inaccessible focus of infection or those with continued deterioration following fluid and vasopressor support (one dose of 400 mg/kg); however, its effectiveness for treatment of TSS has not been established in randomized clinical trials.

URINARY-TRACT INFECTION

Infection of lower (cystitis) or upper (pyelonephritis) urinary tract

EPIDEMIOLOGY

- About 7% prevalence in young febrile children without a source
- Age and gender influence prevalence:
  - ✓ Incidence (in order of decreasing frequency): Neonates, infants, school-aged
  - ✓ Neonates: Boys affected more often than girls; uncircumcised boys at higher risk
  - ✓ Age older than 1 year: Girls affected more often than boys

ETIOLOGY

- E. *coli* (80% of urinary-tract infections [UTIs])
- Other organisms include *Klebsiella*, *Enterococcus* spp., *Proteus* spp. (boys >1 year), P. *aeruginosa*, *Staphylococcus saprophyticus* (female adolescents), GBS (neonates), S. *aureus* (suggests hematogenous seeding from additional site of infection—e.g., osteomyelitis, endocarditis, renal abscess)

PATHOPHYSIOLOGY

- Host factors: Inability to empty bladder completely (e.g., neurogenic bladder, posterior urethral valves, indwelling catheter); vesicoureteral reflux (20–30% of children with UTI)

CLINICAL MANIFESTATIONS

- Neonates and infants: Fever or temperature instability, poor feeding, vomiting, jaundice, decreased activity
- Children 2–5 years of age: Fever, abdominal pain, bedwetting or incontinence in previously toilet-trained child, foul-smelling urine
- Children older than 5 years: Fever, vomiting, abdominal pain, dysuria, frequency, urgency, bedwetting or incontinence in previously toilet-trained child, suprapubic or costovertebral angle tenderness
- Risk factors (general): History of UTI, renal disease, undiagnosed febrile episodes, sexual activity, genitourinary trauma
- Risk factors for girls: White race, age <12 months, temperature >39°C, fever >2 days, absence of other source of infection
  ✓ No more than one risk factor present: <1% probability of UTI; no more than two risk factors present: <2% probability of UTI
- Risk factors for boys: Nonblack race, temperature >39°C, fever >24 hours, absence of another source of infection
  ✓ No more than two risk factors present and uncircumcised: <1% probability of UTI; no more than three risk factors present and circumcised: <2% probability of UTI

DIAGNOSTICS

Laboratory Screening

- Urinalysis (on centrifuged urine):
  ✓ With positive leukocyte esterase, positive nitrites, or five or more WBCs per high-power field, sensitivity of 99.8% and specificity of 70%. Thus, urinalysis is a useful screening test but cannot replace culture for diagnosis.

Laboratory Confirmation

- Midstream clean catch method preferred in toilet-trained children (Table 15-10).
- Straight catherization recommended in children unable to provide clean catch specimen
- Suprapubic aspiration unsuccessful in 10% of attempts
- Urine bag specimens are *not* appropriate for culture
- To establish the diagnosis of UTI, urinalysis must show pyuria and/or bacteriuria AND >50,000 CFU/mL on urine culture; bacteriuria in the absence of pyuria should raise suspicion for asymptomatic bacteriuria or contaminated culture

TABLE 15-10	Interpretation of Urine Culture Results	
Method	**Probable**	**Possible**
Suprapubic	≥100 CFU/mL	Any growth
	One pathogen	One pathogen
Catheterization	≥50,000 CFU/mL	≥10,000 CFU/mL
	One pathogen	One pathogen
Clean catch	≥100,000 CFU/mL	≥50,000 CFU/mL
	One pathogen	One pathogen
	One culture	Two cultures

CFU = colony-forming unit.

MANAGEMENT

Guideline management

Suggested resource: https://www.chop.edu/clinical-pathway/urinary-tract-infection-uti-febrile-clinical-pathway

Authors: K. Shaw, MD, N. Plachter, CRNP, J. Lavelle, MD, T. Kolon, MD, M. Carr, MD, R. Keren, MD, R. Patel, MD, M. Dunne, MD, J. Kim, MD, J. Gerber, MD, M. Pradhan, MD, K. Ota, MD, C. Jacobstein MD, K. McGowan, PhD, T. Metjian, PharmD, M. Blackstone, MD

Medical

- Febrile UTI or suspected pyelonephritis outpatient therapy:
  - ✓ Oral therapy acceptable for uncomplicated pyelonephritis
  - ✓ Children must be older than 1 month of age, well-hydrated, and tolerating oral medications; 7–10 days of treatment. Empiric therapy (oral): Cephalexin, cefdinir, cefixime, TMP-SMX (depending on local resistance rates). Children <1 month may also be candidates for oral therapy, depending on response to initial intravenous therapy.
- Febrile UTI or suspected pyelonephritis inpatient therapy:
  - ✓ Hospitalization and initial IV therapy for those with moderate dehydration, ill appearance, significant emesis, underlying urologic abnormalities, poor compliance, and failure of outpatient therapy
  - ✓ Seven to 10 days of treatment. Empiric therapy (IV): Ampicillin + gentamicin, ceftriaxone, ciprofloxacin; may switch to oral therapy when patient clinically improved.
- No benefit to routine repeat urine cultures after initiation of therapy. Consider repeat cultures if fever or symptoms persist >72 hours.
- Consider antimicrobial prophylaxis for children with severe (grade V) vesicoureteral reflux (VUR)

Imaging

- Ultrasound of urinary tract identifies: Hydronephrosis, dilatation of distal ureters, hypertrophy of bladder wall, presence of ureteroceles
  - ✓ Recommended by AAP for: All children <2 years of age with first UTI or if clinical improvement is slower than anticipated with appropriate treatment
- Voiding cystourethrography (VCUG) identifies: VUR, posterior urethral valves, bladder abnormalities
  - ✓ VCUG should not be performed routinely after the first febrile UTI. Recommended by AAP for children with renal ultrasounds suggestive of VUR or >1 documented UTI.

SPECIFIC PATHOGENS

BARTONELLA SPECIES (CAT-SCRATCH DISEASE)

A subacute, self-limited regional lymphadenitis syndrome caused by cutaneous inoculation with *Bartonella henselae* (a fastidious pleomorphic gram-negative rod) through cat scratches or bites. Rarer causes include *Afipia felis* and *Bartonella clarridgeiae*.

EPIDEMIOLOGY

- Broad geographic distribution; peaks in fall and early winter
- Cats are the natural reservoir, with anywhere from 13 to 90% seroprevalence

- 90% of patients have a history of recent contact with healthy cats, especially cats younger than 1 year of age or cats with fleas.
- The most common cause of chronic, unilateral regional lymphadenitis in U.S. children

CLINICAL MANIFESTATIONS

- Primary cutaneous inoculation lesion (papules at site of inoculation) often precedes lymphadenopathy by 1–2 weeks.
- Unilateral subacute tender lymphadenopathy in axillary, cervical, submandibular, periauricular, supraclavicular, epitrochlear, femoral, or inguinal locations; 1–5 cm in size, up to 30% suppurate. Incubation time from cat scratch to appearance of lymphadenopathy is 5–50 days (median, 12).
- Constitutional symptoms in up to 30% of patients (fever, malaise, fatigue)
- Parinaud's oculoglandular syndrome: Conjunctival granuloma with ipsilateral preauricular lymphadenitis
- Encephalopathy may develop 1–6 weeks after primary disease and is associated with seizures and rarely coma with recovery in several weeks. Head CT is typically normal. CSF shows slight mononuclear pleocytosis. EEG is abnormal.
- Fever: Up to 5% of cases of fever of unknown origin
- Granulomatous hepatitis or splenitis
- Rare manifestations: Osteomyelitis, endocarditis, thrombocytopenic purpura, bacillary angiomatosis in immunocompromised hosts (HIV)

DIAGNOSTICS

- Serology by indirect fluorescence assay: IgG titers <1:64 = no current infection; >1:64 but <1:256 = possible infection, repeat in 10–14 days; >1:256 = current or recent infection
- PCR (blood, CSF, or tissue biopsy specimens): Useful to diagnose rare *B. henselae* manifestations
- Histopathology: Warthin–Starry silver stain may demonstrate pleomorphic bacilli in chains (not routinely necessary)
- Culture: Difficult to isolate organism from tissue or blood
- CT scan: May reveal multiple hypodense liver or spleen lesions

MANAGEMENT

- Routine antibiotic use for cat-scratch adenitis is controversial because spontaneous resolution typically occurs within 1–4 months. Azithromycin, clarithromycin, rifampin, or ciprofloxacin may hasten initial decrease in lymph node volume.
- Consider needle aspiration of painful suppurative nodes for symptomatic relief. Surgical excision is not typically required.
- No controlled trials of therapy exist for less common sites of infection (e.g., hepatosplenic cat-scratch disease, osteomyelitis, bacillary angiomatosis). Consider parenteral gentamicin or azithromycin. Transition to oral therapy with symptomatic improvement. Duration of therapy is unclear.

CLOSTRIDIOIDES DIFFICILE INFECTION

***Clostridioides difficile* is an anaerobic spore-forming bacterium that causes diarrhea and colitis.**

EPIDEMIOLOGY

- Up to 50% of infants and 1–3% of adults are asymptomatic carriers; up to 20% of recently hospitalized patients are asymptomatic carriers.
- Predisposing factors: Hospitalization, prolonged antibiotics, abdominal surgery, inflammatory bowel disease, immunodeficiency.

PATHOPHYSIOLOGY

- Disturbance of normal colonic flora, usually as a result of antibiotic exposure, allows *C. difficile* to flourish.
- Spores produce toxins (A and B) that cause mucosal damage.
- North American pulsed-field gel electrophoresis type 1 strain (NAP1) is especially virulent due to increased toxin production and has been associated with hospital outbreaks.

CLINICAL MANIFESTATIONS

- Spectrum of mild diarrhea to severe pseudomembranous colitis to toxic megacolon
- Fever and crampy abdominal pain may accompany foul-smelling, watery stools
- Pseudomembranous colitis characterized by diarrhea with blood or mucous, abdominal pain, fever, and systemic toxicity
- Toxic megacolon, intestinal perforation, and death are more common in neutropenic patients or in patients with inflammatory bowel disease.

DIAGNOSTICS

- Stool studies:
  - ✓ *C. difficile* toxins A and B by enzyme immunoassay (relatively low sensitivity, moderate specificity)
  - ✓ NAAT to detect toxin genes (high sensitivity and moderate specificity)
  - ✓ Two-step testing: Enzyme immunoassay for glutamine dehydrogenase (highly sensitive) with confirmatory toxin testing by NAAT or toxin immunoassay (to increase specificity); this approach is recommended if the clinical laboratory accepts all stool specimens for testing (including formed stools).
  - ✓ Test of cure *not* recommended.
  - ✓ Testing should *not* be performed in patients with formed stools.
  - ✓ Testing should *not* be performed in infants <1 year of age and should not be routinely performed in children ≤2 years of age unless other causes of infectious diarrhea have been excluded owing to the prevalence of asymptomatic colonization in these age groups.
- CBC: Leukocytosis, possibly anemia if stool is bloody
- Consider endoscopy when diagnosis is unclear; findings include classic pseudomembrane with a white or yellow plaque along hyperemic and inflamed colonic mucosa. Mucosa may be friable and erythematous without pseudomembrane.

MANAGEMENT

Initial Medical Management

- Discontinue offending antibiotics when possible.
- Treat any dehydration and anemia.
- Surgical consultation if toxic megacolon is present
- Mild-to-moderate infection: Either metronidazole orally/IV (orally preferred) 30 mg/kg/day (maximum, 2 g/day) divided four times daily for 10 days or oral vancomycin 40 mg/kg/day (maximum, 125 mg/day) divided four times daily for 10 days
- Severe disease (leukocytosis, leukopenia, worsening renal function): oral vancomycin 40 mg/kg/day (maximum, 2 g/day) divided four times daily for 10 days (IV not effective)

- Severe and complicated disease (ICU patient, pseudomembranous colitis, hypotension or shock): oral vancomycin 40 mg/kg/day divided four times daily for 10 days (maximum, 2 g/day) PLUS metronidazole 30 mg/kg/day IV divided every 6 hours
- In patients in whom oral therapy cannot reach the colon, add vancomycin 500 mg/100 mL normal saline and administer by enema every 8 hours until symptoms improve.

Management of Relapse

- Up to 20% relapse within 4 weeks of stopping therapy because of reinfection, persistent spores, chronic antibiotics, or a predisposing underlying disease.
- Initial relapse: Repeat metronidazole or vancomycin course.
- Second relapse: Vancomycin
- Fidaxomicin, a nonabsorbed macrolide antibiotic approved for treatment of C. difficile is associated with a lower rate of recurrence than with oral vancomycin.

Management of Chronic Relapsing C. difficile

- Prolonged oral vancomycin in a tapered or pulsed regimen; vancomycin followed by rifaximin or nitazoxanide; fecal transplantation has been effective in adults, but pediatric data are limited. Investigational therapies include human monoclonal antibodies against toxin A and B, probiotics, and immune globulin therapy.

HEPATITIS A

Hepatitis A virus (HAV) is the predominant form of viral hepatitis and is typically an acute, self-limited illness.

EPIDEMIOLOGY

- Fecal–oral transmission; rarely bloodborne, foodborne, or waterborne
- Since introduction of HAV vaccine in 1995, decrease in both sporadic cases and outbreaks
- Patients are most infectious in the 1–2 weeks prior to onset of symptoms, and risk of transmission subsequently decreases, becoming minimal within 1 week after symptom onset.

PATHOPHYSIOLOGY

- Viral shedding in stool approximately 3 weeks before onset of symptoms
- HAV replicates in hepatocytes and is released into the bloodstream, causing viremia.

CLINICAL MANIFESTATIONS

- Spectrum of disease varies greatly, ranging from asymptomatic infection to fulminant hepatitis; risk of symptomatic disease increases with age, with only 30% of infants and children under 6 experiencing clinical symptoms.
- Fever, malaise, nausea, emesis, anorexia, abdominal pain, and diarrhea during prodrome
- Jaundice, dark urine, acholic stool, and hepatomegaly are more common in older children and adults, occurring in 40–70% of infections in this age group.

DIAGNOSTICS

- Elevation of alanine aminotransferase (ALT), aspartate aminotransferase (AST), gamma glutamyl transferase, bilirubin, and alkaline phosphatase; ALT and AST elevation most prominent, peaking on days 3–10 of illness.
- Anti-HAV IgM and total anti-HAV antibody detected by immunoassay.

- Anti-HAV IgM detectable 5–10 days before onset of symptoms and suggests acute infection, whereas total anti-HAV could reflect past infection or immunization; positive anti-HAV IgM is detectable in up to 20% of vaccine recipients within 2 weeks a vaccination.

MANAGEMENT

- Supportive: No specific antiviral therapy is available.
- Prevention: Routine hepatitis A vaccination, preexposure and postexposure vaccination, and preexposure and postexposure IVIG in certain circumstances, including in children <12 months of age traveling to regions where hepatitis A is endemic.

HEPATITIS B

Hepatitis B virus (HBV) causes both acute and chronic liver disease, including cirrhosis and hepatocellular carcinoma.

EPIDEMIOLOGY

- Transmitted by perinatal, percutaneous, and sexual exposures as well as by close person–person contact, including household contacts of people with chronic hepatitis B infection
- Breastfeeding does not increase the risk of transmission, and babies who have received hepatitis B vaccination and hepatitis B immunoglobulin (HBIG) can safely breastfeed.
- Risk of vertical transmission without postexposure prophylaxis: 70–90% if mother is HBsAg -and HBeAg-positive; 5–20% if mother is HBsAg-positive but HBeAg-negative.

PATHOPHYSIOLOGY

- Cytotoxic T cells attack HBV-infected hepatocytes, causing inflammation and necrosis.
- Extrahepatic manifestations (e.g., rash, arthritis) are thought to be immune-mediated.

CLINICAL MANIFESTATIONS

- Severity of acute illness increases with age and ranges from asymptomatic seroconversion (most common in perinatal acquisition) to acute hepatitis with jaundice (occurs in 5–15% of children ages 1–5 and 33–50% of older children and adults) to fulminant fatal hepatitis (can occur at any age but is uncommon [<1%]).
- Risk of chronic infection is inversely related to the age at infection; chronic infection occurs in 90% of infants infected perinatally, 25–50% of children infected at age 1–5, and 5–10% of older children and adults.
- Incubation period ranges from 50 to 160 days, with an average of 90 days.
- Acute infection: 1–2 weeks of malaise and anorexia followed by nausea, vomiting, abdominal pain, jaundice, hepatomegaly, and splenomegaly
- Chronic infection (defined as presence of HBsAg in serum >6 months after acute infection): Often asymptomatic but can progress to cirrhosis and hepatocellular carcinoma years after infection and can be associated with extrahepatic manifestations
- Extrahepatic manifestations include arthritis, arthralgias, rash (urticarial, macular, papular acrodermatitis [Gianotti–Crosti syndrome]), membranous nephropathy, membranoproliferative glomerulonephritis, and polyarteritis nodosa

DIAGNOSTICS

- See **Table 15-11**.
- In perinatally exposed infants, testing for HBsAb and HBsAg should be done at 9–12 months of age to avoid detection of maternal antibody or HBIG and at least 4 weeks after

TABLE 15-11	Serology during Four Stages of Hepatitis B Virus Infection			
Test	**Acute Disease**	**Window Phase**	**Complete Recovery**	**Chronic Carrier**
HBsAg	Positive	Negative	Negative	Positive
HBsAb	Negative	Negative	Positive	Negative
HBcAb	Positive (IgM)	Positive (IgM)	Positive (IgG)	Positive (IgG)

HBcAb = hepatitis B core antibody; HBsAb = hepatitis B surface antibody; HBsAg = hepatitis B surface antigen; Ig = immunoglobulin.

the final dose of hepatitis B vaccine; IgM anti-HBc is unreliable for diagnosis of perinatal infection.

- HBeAg is a marker of viral replication and infectivity.
- HBV DNA PCR test is useful to follow response to therapy.

MANAGEMENT

Prevention

- Universal immunization of infants, children, adolescents, and high-risk adults
- Mother with positive HBsAg: Administer HBIG 0.5 mL IM and first dose of recombinant HBV vaccine (at different sites) within 12 hours after birth. This combination prevents perinatal transmission in 95% of exposed infants.
- Mother with unknown HBV status: Administer first HBV vaccine to infant within 12 hours after birth regardless of weight and gestational age and test mother immediately.
  ✓ If infant is <2000 g, administer HBIG within first 12 hours of life if HBV status is still unknown.
  ✓ If infant is term and >2000 g, can await mother's HBsAg testing and administer HBIG to infant as soon as possible but within 7 days

Medical

- Acute HBV infection: No specific therapy
- Chronic HBV infection: Treatment initiation based on ongoing HBV viral replication for >6 months, elevated ALT levels >6 months, age, liver biopsy findings, comorbidities, and family history. FDA-approved therapies for children include interferon alfa-2b, lamivudine, and entecavir; adefovir and tenofovir have also been approved for children >12 years, and telbivudine is approved for children >16 years.
- Children with chronic HBV infection should be screened periodically for sequelae such as hepatocellular carcinoma with laboratory testing and hepatic ultrasound, but definitive recommendations on frequency and indications for these tests are not yet available.
  ✓ Hepatitis B e antigen and hepatitis B e antibody, live- function tests, HBV DNA, presence of coinfection with HIV or other hepatitis viruses, and alpha-fetoprotein (AFP) should be evaluated at the time of chronic hepatitis B diagnosis.
  ✓ If ALT or AFP levels are elevated, or the patient has elevated HBV DNA (>2000 IU/mL), consultation with a pediatric liver specialist is recommended to determine the appropriate interval for lab follow-up as well as ultrasound imaging.
  ✓ Patients with a family history of hepatocellular carcinoma or cirrhosis should also be referred to a pediatric liver specialist.

HEPATITIS C

Hepatitis C virus (HCV) causes acute and chronic liver disease, which can lead to cirrhosis and hepatocellular carcinoma.

EPIDEMIOLOGY

- Transmitted through blood and blood-product transfusions, IV drug use, accidental needlestick injuries, sexual contact, and vertically from mother to infant
- Estimated 5–6% vertical transmission rate among patients who are HCV RNA–positive at the time of delivery, with higher rates observed in cases of HIV coinfection, fetal monitoring, prolonged rupture of membranes, and higher viremia.
- Not transmitted through breast milk; however, if nipples are cracked and bleeding, breast milk should be pumped and discarded until these symptoms have resolved.
- Incubation period: 6–7 weeks (range, 2 weeks to 6 months)

PATHOPHYSIOLOGY

- Hepatocyte death due to immune attack by cytotoxic T cells on infected hepatocytes

CLINICAL MANIFESTATIONS

- Acute symptomatic HCV infection develops in only 20% of cases, symptoms include anorexia, nausea, jaundice, dark urine, and right upper quadrant abdominal pain.
- Chronic infection: Develops in approximately 80% of perinatally infected children and less commonly in children infected postnatally
- Less than 5% go on to develop cirrhosis.
- Fulminant hepatic failure is exceedingly rare.

DIAGNOSTICS

- Anti-HCV IgG appears 8–10 weeks after infection, but can be delayed up to 6 months. Serologic testing is 97% sensitive and 99% specific, but it does not distinguish between acute and chronic infection, and no IgM assay is currently available.
- HCV RNA appears within 1–2 weeks of infection and indicates current infection. Most useful in screening perinatally exposed infants, to identify anti-HCV positive individuals with current infection, to diagnose early infection, and to monitor response to therapy. A single negative test is not conclusive because viral RNA may be only intermittently detectable.
- For neonates born to HCV-positive mothers, can either test for anti-HCV IgG after 18 months of age or by HCV PCR as early as 1–2 months of age if earlier diagnosis is desired, if there is concern about maintaining contact with the perinatally exposed infant, or if antiviral therapy were to become available in this age group.

MANAGEMENT

- Children with HCV infections should be referred to a liver specialist for close monitoring and potential therapy.
- Acute infection: Adult studies suggest that treatment in the acute phase may lead to higher sustained virologic response than treatment in the chronic phase; pediatric studies are in progress.
- Chronic infection: Several oral direct-acting antiviral drugs have been approved for adult and pediatric patients in recent years. Because treatment recommendations are rapidly

evolving, the following website should be consulted for updated guidelines: www.hcvguide-lines.org.

- If a direct acting antiviral drug is available for the patients age group, treatment is recommended, regardless of disease severity.

LYME DISEASE

Tick-borne illness caused by the spirochete *B. burgdorferi*

EPIDEMIOLOGY

- Geographic regions: Northeast, upper Midwest, West Coast
- In endemic areas: Incidence of 20–100 cases in 100,000
- Seasonal occurrence: April–October
- Incidence highest among children 5–14 years old

ETIOLOGY

- *B. burgdorferi* is transmitted by the bite of infected tick vectors: *Ixodes pacificus* (West Coast) and *Ixodes scapularis* (East Coast and Midwest)

PATHOPHYSIOLOGY

- Initial infection site: Skin
- Tick must stay attached >36 hours for transmission.
- Once disseminated into bloodstream, *B. burgdorferi* adheres to multiple cell types and persists in tissue unless treated.
- Cytokines amplify inflammatory response and cause local tissue damage

CLINICAL MANIFESTATIONS

- Three stages: Early localized, early disseminated, and late disseminated disease
- Early localized (3–32 days after bite): Erythema migrans (erythematous annular lesion with central clearing, usually >5 cm); fever, malaise, headache, myalgias, and arthralgias
- Early disseminated (3–10 weeks after tick bite): Multiple erythema migrans lesions, cranial-nerve palsies (especially VII, usually last 2–8 weeks and then resolves), fatigue, myalgia, headache, occasionally meningitis or carditis (atrioventricular block)
- Late disseminated disease (months to years after tick bite): Monoarticular arthritis of a large joint (knee in >90%); central nervous system (CNS) involvement (chronic demyelinating encephalitis, polyneuritis, memory problems) is rare in children.
- Jarisch–Herxheimer reaction: Transient fever, headache, myalgias after therapy is started

DIAGNOSTICS

- Two-test approach: enzyme immunoassay (EIA) (sensitive but not specific) and, if EIA is positive, Western blot (necessary to confirm infection)
- Positive test: 2 out of 3 IgM bands, 5 out of 10 IgG bands
- IgM peaks at 3–6 weeks; IgG peaks weeks to months after the bite
- Antibodies to *B. burgdorferi* often not detectable in patients with early localized erythema migrans rash, so at this stage can empirically treat without testing
- False positive EIA tests may be secondary to other spirochetal infections (syphilis, leptospirosis), systemic lupus erythematosus, EBV, varicella

- Lumbar puncture to confirm lymphocytic meningitis of early disseminated disease; typically reveals 10–150 WBC/mm^3 and less than 10% segmented neutrophils, elevated protein, normal glucose. PCR has poor sensitivity in CNS.
- ECG: Detect heart block in patients with disseminated Lyme
- Joint aspiration: WBC typically 25,000–80,000/mm^3 (but range from 200 to 140,000/mm^3) and positive Lyme PCR of joint fluid
- No proven utility of blood PCR or urine PCR or antigen tests

MANAGEMENT

- Early localized: 14–21 days of doxycycline in all age groups
- Early disseminated: 21 days of oral doxycycline; cefuroxime (preferred) or erythromycin may be used in young children with penicillin allergy
- Carditis with severe or symptomatic AV block: ceftriaxone 14–21 days
- Late disseminated: 21–28 days of oral doxycycline. If arthritis is unresponsive after 2 months or there is a recurrence, consider a second course of oral therapy (4 weeks) or initiate IV therapy (2–4 weeks).
- Arthritis unresponsive to oral therapy: IV ceftriaxone for 28 days

MALARIA

Intraerythrocytic parasitic infection caused by *Plasmodium* species (*Plasmodium vivax*, *Plasmodium ovale*, *Plasmodium malariae*, *Plasmodium knowlesi*, and *Plasmodium falciparum*)

EPIDEMIOLOGY

- Endemic throughout tropical areas; view countries with malaria risk at Centers for Disease Control and Prevention (CDC) website (www.cdc.gov/travel).
- Almost all cases diagnosed in the United States are acquired abroad in malaria-endemic areas; symptoms can develop as soon as 7 days after exposure to as late as several months after exposure.

PATHOPHYSIOLOGY

- Transmission is primarily through the bite of an infected *Anopheles* species mosquito. Uncommon modes of transmission include transplacental and bloodborne (e.g., transfusion, needlestick)
- Sporozoites from mosquito infect hepatocytes, differentiate to merozoites, and infect RBCs.
- Periodic RBC lysis releases merozoites to infect other RBCs.
- *P. vivax* and *P. ovale* have a dormant hepatic phase that can cause late relapse if not properly treated

CLINICAL MANIFESTATIONS

- Characteristic high fever that may have a cyclical pattern (every 48–72 hours, depending on species) or may occur daily, especially with *P. falciparum*
- Chills, headache, sweats, malaise, myalgias, nausea, vomiting, diarrhea, arthralgias, abdominal or back pain
- Pallor, jaundice, hepatosplenomegaly, anemia, and thrombocytopenia
- Symptoms are generally most severe in those who have not previously been exposed, in young children, immunocompromised hosts, and pregnant women.
- *P. falciparum* may lead to severe disease including:
  ✓ Cerebral malaria: Altered mentation, seizures, increased intracranial pressure, and progression to coma and death

✓ Severe hemolysis ("black water fever"), acute tubular necrosis, adrenal insufficiency, hypoglycemia, shock, respiratory failure, metabolic acidosis
- *P. vivax* and *P. ovale:*
  ✓ Relapse due to latent intrahepatic stage as long as 3–5 years after infection
  ✓ Hypersplenism, which may lead to splenic rupture
- *P. malariae:*
  ✓ Nephrotic syndrome, chronic asymptomatic parasitemia
- *P. knowlesi:*
  ✓ Found in southeast Asia and can cause severe disease and death due to hyperparasitemia

DIAGNOSTICS

- Giemsa-stained thick and thin peripheral-blood smears, which detect organisms (thick) and allow determination of species and percent parasitemia (thin)
- Multiple smears (every 12 hours) over 48–72 hours may be necessary if the first is negative and clinical suspicion is high, or to monitor response to therapy
  ✓ Parasitemia >2% suggests *P. falciparum.*
- Rapid antigen test is most sensitive for *P. falciparum* (90–95%), but significantly less sensitive for remaining species, so should always be accompanied by thick and thin blood smears
- Other findings: Anemia, leukopenia, thrombocytopenia, hypoglycemia, proteinuria, hematuria, elevated hepatic transaminases, acidosis, and indirect bilirubin (hemolysis)

MANAGEMENT

- Treatment regimen depends on:
  ✓ Infecting species: *P. falciparum and P. knowlesi* cause more rapidly progressive infections than other species and require rapid initiation of treatment. *P. vivax* and *P. ovale* require additional therapy (primaquine phosphate) to eradicate dormant hypnozoites in the liver
  ✓ Likelihood of chloroquine resistance: Depends on (1) the region of the world where infection was acquired and (2) whether or not chemoprophylaxis was taken (consider resistance of infecting *Plasmodium* species to chemoprophylactic regimen)
  ✓ Presence of severe illness: Parasitemia greater than 5%, signs of cerebral malaria or other end-organ involvement (renal failure, acute respiratory distress syndrome), shock, hemoglobin <7, acidosis, or hypoglycemia requires parenteral therapy with quinine, quinidine, or artesunate (investigational new drug); exchange transfusion is no longer recommended as part of management for severe malaria.
- If disease is uncomplicated, outpatient therapy is often reasonable, but consider admission for suspected or confirmed *P. falciparum* because of the potential for rapid clinical deterioration, particularly in nonimmune hosts.
- Supportive care includes monitoring for hypoglycemia, anemia, fluid and electrolyte disturbances, and renal failure.
- Parasitemia should decrease over first 48–72 hours to 25% of initial parasitemia.
- Refer to 2018 Redbook, CDC website (www.cdc.gov/malaria/resources/pdf/treatment-table_2018.pdf), or CDC malaria hotline (770-488-7788) for specific drug regimens based on patient age, severity of illness, region where infection was acquired, and clinical response.
- Travelers to malaria-endemic regions should receive chemoprophylaxis and should use bed nets, mosquito repellents, and protective clothing to minimize their contact with the *Anopheles* mosquito. Providers should consult the CDC Yellow Book (https://wwwnc.cdc.gov/travel/page/yellowbook-home) for recommendations on need for prophylaxis as well as specific regimens based on destination.

STAPHYLOCOCCUS AUREUS

S. aureus, a gram-positive coccus, is the most commonly isolated human bacterial pathogen and causes both superficial and invasive infections. MRSA isolates are resistant to all available penicillins and other β-lactam antimicrobial drugs.

EPIDEMIOLOGY

- Both methicillin-sensitive *S. aureus* (MSSA) and MRSA are major causes of hospital-acquired infections.
- MRSA has emerged as a significant cause of community-acquired infection (CA-MRSA) in both children and adults; most commonly as cutaneous abscesses but also as severe, invasive infections (e.g., pneumonia, bone/joint infections)
- Hospital-acquired MRSA infections are decreasing with better infection-control practices, but the incidence of CA-MRSA infection remains significant in many regions.

PATHOPHYSIOLOGY

- *S. aureus* infections are due to direct tissue invasion causing inflammation, hematogenous dissemination, or toxin release leading to tissue necrosis.
- MRSA strains almost universally carry the *mecA* gene, which affords β-lactam resistance.
- CA-MRSA both colonizes more body sites and displays a higher attack rate (colonization leading to infection) than MSSA.
- Transmission is via direct contact.

CLINICAL MANIFESTATIONS

- Skin and soft-tissue infections: Impetigo, abscess, cellulitis, wound infection, ocular infection, pyomyositis
- Bone/joint infections: Osteomyelitis, pyogenic arthritis, diskitis
- Respiratory tract infections: Pneumonia, lung abscess
- Cardiovascular infections: Bacteremia/sepsis, endocarditis, pericarditis, thrombophlebitis
- CNS infections: Meningitis, brain abscesses, spinal epidural abscess
- Device-related infections: Central line-associated bloodstream infections, CSF shunt infections

DIAGNOSTICS

- Culture the organism whenever possible from the infected site (e.g., blood, abscess fluid, bone, synovial fluid, CSF) for identification and antibiotic sensitivities.

MANAGEMENT

- Minor infections such as impetigo or superinfected skin lesions: Mupirocin 2% topical ointment
- For cutaneous abscesses, incision and drainage is the primary treatment. Systemic antibiotics are often not necessary after complete drainage of simple, superficial abscesses.
- Empiric oral coverage for skin/soft-tissue infection includes clindamycin, TMP-SMX, doxycycline (if ≥8 years of age), or linezolid.
- Hospitalized patients who appear ill or have severe suspected MRSA infection should receive empiric broad-spectrum antibiotics including vancomycin while awaiting culture data. Stable patients without bacteremia or intravascular infection can be treated with clindamycin, as long as local resistance rates are <10%
- *S. aureus* bacteremia without a clear focus of infection should prompt evaluation for an occult source (e.g., bone, deep muscle involvement, thrombus, endovascular source)

- Obtain echocardiogram for children with underlying heart disease, persistent bacteremia despite adequate antimicrobial therapy, or clinical signs/symptoms concerning for endocarditis.
- Consult with an infectious diseases specialist for invasive infections such as bacteremia, infective endocarditis, device-related infections, or CNS infections

NEONATAL HERPES SIMPLEX VIRUS INFECTION

Three main manifestations of neonatal HSV are:
- **Localized skin, eye, mouth (SEM) involvement (45% of cases)**
- **CNS involvement with or without SEM disease (30% of cases)**
- **Disseminated disease involving multiple organs with or without CNS involvement (25% of cases)**
- **Other TORCH infections are discussed in Neonatology chapter (Chapter 18)**

EPIDEMIOLOGY

- Incidence of 1 in 2000 to 1 in 3000 live births
- Perinatal transmission rate is higher with maternal primary genital HSV infection (25–60%) than with recurrent infection (0–5%); however, more than 75% of infants with HSV are born to women who have no history or clinical findings of HSV infection.
- Disseminated and SEM disease generally present between 7 and 14 days of life; CNS disease generally presents between 14 and 21 days of life.
- Additional risk factors for transmission include prolonged rupture of membranes, use of scalp electrodes, and vaginal delivery.

CLINICAL MANIFESTATIONS

- SEM disease: Vesicular rash in 80%; remaining patients have infection limited to the eyes and/or oral mucosa.
- Disseminated disease: Sepsis-like syndrome, hypoxia, respiratory or hepatic failure, and DIC; 60–70% have associated encephalitis and 60–80% have vesicular rash, though the rash may be a late finding.
- CNS disease:
  ✓ Temperature instability, seizures, and irritability; 60–70% have associated vesicular rash
  ✓ CSF findings show mononuclear-cell pleocytosis, normal or low glucose concentration, and mildly elevated protein; CSF findings may be normal early in the course of illness.
- Though vesicular rash and seizures are most suggestive, symptoms are generally nonspecific, and HSV disease should be considered for all cases of suspected neonatal sepsis.

DIFFERENTIAL DIAGNOSIS

- Noninfectious etiologies: Erythema toxicum, miliaria, neonatal lupus, Langerhans-cell histiocytosis, epidermolysis bullosa
- Infectious etiologies: *S. aureus*, *P. aeruginosa*, GBS, CMV, *Treponema pallidum*, varicella

DIAGNOSTICS

- In addition to routine evaluation for neonatal sepsis, obtain:
  ✓ HSV PCR (gold standard) or culture from CSF; PCR may be falsely negative early in the course of illness and should be repeated during the first week if HSV disease is strongly suspected. HSV PCR is reliable up to 7 days after initiation of acyclovir.
  ✓ HSV culture (if available) or PCR of conjunctiva, mouth, nasopharynx, and anus; any positive test after 12–24 hours of life is diagnostic of disease rather than intrapartum exposure.

✓ HSV culture or PCR from any skin vesicle
✓ HSV PCR from whole blood; blood PCR can be positive with any of the three clinical syndromes, so should not be used alone for diagnosis.
✓ Serum ALT
- Direct fluorescent antibody (DFA) staining of vesicle scraping is rapid but less sensitive than culture or PCR.
- Patients with proven HSV and possible CNS involvement should receive electroencephalography (EEG) and MRI of head during the acute period; all patients with HSV should have an ophthalmology evaluation.

MANAGEMENT

- High-dose IV acyclovir (60 mg/kg/day divided every 8 hours): 21 days for CNS or disseminated disease and 14 days for SEM disease
  ✓ A CSF HSV PCR should be repeated before completion of therapy for CNS disease. If the HSV PCR remains positive, treatment with acyclovir should be extended and weekly CSF HSV PCRs performed until negative, at which point parenteral acyclovir can be stopped.
  ✓ Suppressive therapy with oral acyclovir for 6 months after IV treatment of neonatal HSV improves neurodevelopmental outcomes and prevents cutaneous recurrences; dose is 300 mg/m²/dose three times daily
- Side effects of acyclovir: Neutropenia, renal failure
- Prognosis:
  ✓ SEM: Mortality and neurologic impairment rare, but increases with >3 recurrent episodes of skin lesions within the first 6 months of life
  ✓ CNS infection: Low risk of death in adequately treated children; >60% of survivors have neurologic impairment
  ✓ Disseminated infection: High risk of death despite treatment (approximately 30%); <20% of survivors have neurologic impairment

PERTUSSIS

Respiratory disease caused by *Bordetella pertussis*, a fastidious gram-negative rod

EPIDEMIOLOGY

- Occurs year-round, peaking late summer through fall
- Increasing in frequency among all age groups likely because of both increasing detection of cases and waning immunity from less immunogenic acellular pertussis vaccine; among young infants, lack of maternal tetanus, diphtheria, pertussis (Tdap) vaccination during pregnancy also contributes to increasing prevalence .
- Highly transmissible through respiratory droplets and direct or indirect contact with nasal secretions
- Neither natural infection nor vaccination leads to permanent immunity.

PATHOPHYSIOLOGY

- Pertussis toxin is responsible for local epithelial damage, leading to peribronchial inflammation and necrotizing bronchopneumonia

CLINICAL MANIFESTATIONS

- Incubation period is generally 7–10 days but can range from 5 to 21 days.

- Three stages of the disease usually observed, though may be variable in young infants, vaccinated children, and adults:
  - ✓ Catarrhal (1–2 weeks): Rhinorrhea, low-grade fevers, sneezing; most infectious stage
  - ✓ Paroxysmal (2–6 weeks): Paroxysmal coughing after which the child may become flushed or cyanotic or have posttussive emesis. "Whoop" occurs during sudden forceful inspiration. Infants may present with apnea or cyanosis and often lack the characteristic cough or whoop.
  - ✓ Convalescent: Chronic cough can persist for weeks to months.
- In infants <6 months of age, can be complicated by apnea in two-thirds of patients, superinfection with other bacterial pneumonia, seizures, encephalopathy, pulmonary hypertension, and death (particularly in infants <2 months)

DIAGNOSTICS

- Clinical case defined as cough lasting at least 2 weeks with one of the following: Paroxysms of coughing, inspiratory whoop, or posttussive vomiting without other apparent cause, or apnea in infants <1 year of age
- Confirmed case defined as *B. pertussis* isolated in culture, detected by PCR, or with an epidemiologic link to laboratory confirmed case
- Leukocytosis with total WBC >15,000/mm^3 with absolute lymphocytosis, particularly in infants and young children
- Chest x-ray: Perihilar infiltrates, "shaggy right heart border"
- Culture remains gold standard but is insensitive owing to the fastidious nature of *B. pertussis* and is often falsely negative in previously immunized individuals, after initiation of antibiotic therapy, or after 2 weeks of illness
- PCR of nasopharyngeal swab specimen is the preferred test at many institutions (high sensitivity and specificity) and likely provides accurate results for the first 4 weeks of illness; however, no standardized, FDA-approved assay is available.
- Serologic testing is useful in adults and adolescents who present late in the course of illness when other diagnostic tests are likely to be negative.
- Direct immunofluorescence is not recommended owing to low sensitivity.

MANAGEMENT

Prevention

- Immunization with diphtheria, tetanus, pertussis (DTaP) or TdaP vaccination according to vaccine schedule

Treatment

- Therapy can curb symptoms if started in the catarrhal stage, but will not improve the course of disease or symptoms if started later; however, antibiotic therapy is still recommended to decrease transmission.
- Azithromycin, erythromycin, and clarithromycin are first-line agents for both treatment and prophylaxis; azithromycin is recommended specifically for infants <1 month of age because of the risk of infantile hypertrophic pyloric stenosis.
- Chemoprophylaxis regardless of immunization status for close contacts, including household and child care contacts, with erythromycin, clarithromycin, or azithromycin is recommended, as is pertussis vaccination with age-appropriate vaccine. Prophylaxis should be initiated within 21 days of exposure, but could be considered beyond this time frame in high-risk contacts (i.e., young infants, pregnant women).
- TMP-SMX is an alternative for macrolide allergic patients >2 months of age.

- Respiratory isolation for hospitalized patients until patient is no longer contagious (5 days of treatment; if no therapy is given, until 3 weeks after cough onset). Routine hospitalization to complete treatment is not warranted.
- Consider hospitalization of young infants at risk for apnea.

RICKETTSIAL DISEASES

Tick-borne illnesses caused by obligate intracellular pathogens that share similar clinical and epidemiologic features and treatment: Includes ehrlichiosis, anaplasmosis, Q fever, rickettsialpox, Rocky Mountain spotted fever (RMSF), and endemic typhus. RMSF, ehrlichiosis, and anaplasmosis are the most common and are discussed subsequently.

- RMSF is caused by *Rickettsia rickettsii*
- Ehrlichiosis manifests as human monocytic ehrlichiosis (HME; *Ehrlichia chaffeensis*)
- Anaplasmosis manifests as human granulocytic anaplasmosis (HGA; *Anaplasma phagocytophilum*)

EPIDEMIOLOGY

- RMSF and HME are most prevalent in southeastern, south central, and northern Rocky Mountain states. HGA occurs predominantly in the Northeast and upper Midwest.
- Highest prevalence in late spring, summer, and early fall
- Transmission:
  ✓ RMSF: Dog tick (*Dermacentor variabilis*), Wood tick (*Dermacentor andersonii*), and Lone Star tick (*A. americanum*)
  ✓ HME: Animal reservoir for *A. americanum* is the white tail deer
  ✓ HGA: *Ixodes scapularis*; animal reservoir is the white-footed mouse.
- Incubation period: 2–14 days for RMSF (median, 7); 7–14 days for HME and HGA (median, 10)

PATHOPHYSIOLOGY

- After inoculation, rickettsia multiply in small-vessel endothelium, leading to focal areas of small-vessel inflammation, thrombus, and capillary leak

CLINICAL MANIFESTATIONS

- Early phases: Fever, headache, rash, malaise, myalgia, nausea, vomiting, abdominal pain
- RMSF rash: Typically begins on ankles and wrists spreading both centrally to the trunk (within hours) and to the palms and soles; initially blanching, erythematous, and macular but becomes petechial and then hemorrhagic; develops between third and fifth day of illness, but 10% of patients never develop rash
- Rash in 30–50% of HME; rash in less than 10% of HGA; rash can be macular, maculopapular, or petechial with variable distribution
- Other organ systems may be involved:
  ✓ Gastrointestinal: Diarrhea, hepatomegaly, splenomegaly, jaundice
  ✓ Renal: Renal failure, acute tubular necrosis
  ✓ Cardiac: Congestive heart failure, arrhythmias, shock
  ✓ Neurologic: Meningitis, encephalopathy, seizures, ataxia, aphasia, cranial-nerve palsies
  ✓ Pulmonary and generalized edema, signs of capillary leak
- Duration of illness typically 1–2 weeks; 2–3% mortality

DIAGNOSTICS

- Thrombocytopenia, anemia, and leukopenia; PT and PTT prolongation; elevated bilirubin, ALT, AST, blood urea nitrogen, and creatinine; low fibrinogen, albumin, and sodium
  ✓ Leukopenia, anemia, and hepatitis are more frequent in ehrlichiosis than in RMSF.
  ✓ WBC and platelets reach a nadir at 5–7 days of illness and then recover.
- CSF pleocytosis and elevated protein in one-third of patients
- Rickettsia-specific serology: Positive titers usually occur 6–10 days into illness. Fourfold increase in titer by indirect fluorescent antibody or EIA between acute and convalescent sera (2–3 weeks later) confirms diagnosis.
- *R. rickettsii* (RMSF) can be identified by direct antibody staining of a rash biopsy specimen.
- In HGA and HME, 50% have intraleukocytoplasmic inclusions (morulae) in neutrophils (HGA) and monocytes (HME) on buffy-coat or peripheral-blood smear.
- PCR of blood for HME and HGA are available at commercial laboratories and show promise for early diagnosis of disease.

MANAGEMENT

- Provide supportive management as indicated. Anticipate complications such as hypotension, thrombocytopenia, DIC, hypoalbuminemia, and hyponatremia.
- Recommended antibiotic is doxycycline. Alternative for RMSF is chloramphenicol, but this may have severe side effects and should only be used in rare situations. Alternative for HME and HGA is rifampin (not first line).
- Continue therapy until patient is afebrile for at least 3 days; usual course is 7–10 days for RMSF and 7–14 days for HME and HGA.
- Because delay of antibiotic treatment >5 days after onset of symptoms (and prior to detection of antibodies) is associated with greater mortality, treat suspected cases empirically.
- Expect clinical improvement in 24–36 hours and defervescence in 48–72 hours after initiation of therapy. Mildly ill patients can be treated as outpatients. Hospitalization is recommended for severely ill patients with systemic complications.

TUBERCULOSIS

Caused by *M. tuberculosis*, an acid-fast bacillus
  Latent tuberculosis infection (LTBI): Patient has positive tuberculin skin test (TST) or IGRA, no physical exam findings, and a chest x-ray that is either negative or reveals only calcifications or granulomas in lung, lymph nodes, or both.
  Tuberculosis (TB) disease: Infection in which symptoms, signs, and/or radiographic findings are apparent.

EPIDEMIOLOGY

- Increased risk of infection in certain populations: Low income; urban; non-white racial groups; foreign born; residence in jails, nursing homes, or homeless shelters; injection drug use; HIV infection; emigration from developing country
- Public health officials should be notified of all active cases of TB early in therapy

PATHOPHYSIOLOGY

- Transmission is person to person, usually via airborne droplets, but can occur by direct contact with infected body fluids.
- Children rarely infect others because they have sparse bacilli in endobronchial secretions and diminished force of cough.
- Adolescents are potentially infectious.

CLINICAL MANIFESTATIONS

Intrathoracic Disease (Includes Primary Infection and Reactivation)

- Most infected children have positive TST and no symptoms
- Hilar adenopathy, focal infiltrate, and pleural effusion are common.
- Extensive pulmonary infiltrates and cavitation are rare.
- Symptoms of primary infection and reactivation may include nonproductive cough, hemoptysis, chest pain, dyspnea, fever, night sweats, anorexia, failure to thrive, and weight loss.

Miliary Tuberculosis

- Bacteremia leads to disease in two or more organ systems. TST is nonreactive in 30%.
- Usually early complication of primary pulmonary tuberculosis in infants
- Initially malaise, anorexia, weight loss, fever
- Progresses to high fever, respiratory distress, hypoxia, and symptoms of other organ system involvement (e.g., hepatomegaly, splenomegaly, diffuse adenopathy)

Central Nervous System Disease

- Most common in ages 6 months to 4 years
- Usually occurs 2–6 months after initial infection
- Clinical manifestations vary widely. Symptoms may be mild (e.g., fever, mild but persistent headache) or severe (e.g., cranial nerve abnormalities, seizures, and decorticate posturing).

Other Manifestations

- Pericarditis, lymphadenitis, bone or joint infections, abdominal infection (peritonitis, mesenteric adenitis), cutaneous lesions

DIAGNOSTICS

TST: Use for Children at Risk of Infection

- Mantoux test containing 5 tuberculin units of PPD administered intradermally
- Delayed hypersensitivity reaction to TST peaks at 48–72 hours.
- Nonreactive TST does not exclude infection or disease.
- Time from infection to development of positive TST is 2–12 weeks.
- Special situations warranting TST include radiographic or clinical findings suggesting TB; presence of vertebral osteomyelitis or pericarditis, prior to initiation of immunosuppressive therapy, contacts of people with confirmed or suspected contagious tuberculosis, and immigration from a country with endemic infection or travel to countries with endemic infection, with contact with indigenous people.

Definition of Positive TST Based on Diameter of Induration

- Induration >5 mm in diameter: (1) Contact with infectious cases; (2) abnormal chest x-ray; (3) clinical evidence of tuberculosis disease; (4) HIV infection or other immunosuppressive conditions or therapy (e.g., corticosteroids, chemotherapy)
- Induration >10 mm in diameter: (1) Children at risk of disseminated disease (age <4 years or compromising conditions such as diabetes mellitus, chronic renal failure, and malnutrition); (2) birth in or travel to country with high TB prevalence; (3) frequently exposed to adults with TB risk factors
- Induration >15 mm in diameter: Children 4 years of age or older without risk factors
- A negative TST does not exclude LTBI or TB disease.

Immunologic Testing: IGRA

- IGRAs can be used in children 2 years of age or older; IGRA preferred in children who have received BCG vaccine.
- Sensitivity of IGRAs in children is expected to be comparable to TST; specificity is high and helps distinguish tuberculosis from BCG vaccine and most pathogenic nontuberculous mycobacteria.

Laboratory Diagnosis

- Acid-fast smear and culture are most important tests for definitive diagnosis, but organism may take 2–10 weeks to grow.
  - ✓ Early-morning gastric aspirates (three specimens on consecutive days) are best for diagnosis of pulmonary TB in young children (positive in <50% of children with pulmonary TB).
  - ✓ Cultures from sputum (in older children), CSF, pleural fluid, urine, or bone marrow biopsy specimen as indicated
  - ✓ Identification of a culture-positive source case (e.g., household member) supports the child's presumptive diagnosis and can be used for drug susceptibility testing.
- Chest x-ray to distinguish LTBI from TB disease
- Head CT: In TB meningitis, detects basilar meningitis, increased intracranial pressure, and tuberculomas

MANAGEMENT

- Exposure to contagious household contact with TB disease, after active TB is ruled out
  - ✓ Initiate treatment for LTBI even if TST is negative for children who are <5 years of age or are immunocompromised, repeat TST in 8–10 weeks. If still negative then discontinue therapy; if TST becomes positive, continue LTBI therapy.
- LTBI
  - ✓ Therapy prevents most cases of progression to TB disease.
  - ✓ Multiple options exist for treatment regimens including isoniazid (INH) for 9 months, INH and Rifapentine once weekly for 12 weeks, or rifampin for 4 months; consider 12 months of therapy for immunocompromised patients.
  - ✓ If contact has INH-resistant TB, use rifampin.
- Pulmonary TB
  - ✓ Consult infectious diseases and the local health departments.
  - ✓ Treatment: INH + rifampin + pyrazinamide for 2 months followed by INH + rifampin for 4 months. If drug resistance suspected, add either ethambutol or streptomycin to the three-drug regimen until susceptibility results are available. Supplement pyridoxine with INH for: milk- or meat-deficient diets, HIV-infected children, breast-feeding infants, and pregnant females.
  - ✓ For hilar adenopathy without other pulmonary disease, some experts recommend INH + rifampin for 6 months.
- Extrapulmonary TB (including meningitis and miliary TB): Treat in consultation with a tuberculosis or infectious diseases expert.
  - ✓ INH + rifampin + pyrazinamide + a fourth agent such as ethionamide or an aminoglycoside for 2 months followed by INH + rifampin for 10 months. Corticosteroids (e.g., dexamethasone or prednisone) for 4–6 weeks in patients with TB meningitis with appropriate tapering; consider for TB pericarditis and pleural effusion to hasten fluid absorption.

VARICELLA–ZOSTER INFECTIONS

Primary infection with VZV causes varicella (chickenpox). Reactivation of latent VZV causes herpes zoster (shingles).

EPIDEMIOLOGY

Varicella

- Transmission by airborne route to 90% of unimmunized household contacts
- Transmission to 12–33% during less sustained exposures
- Introduction of varicella vaccine has led to dramatic decrease in disease, though breakthrough disease can occur.

Herpes Zoster

- Rare in immunocompetent children <10 years of age
- Primary VZV infection acquired in utero or during first year of life is associated with increased risk of herpes zoster.

PATHOPHYSIOLOGY

Varicella

- Mucosal inoculation by respiratory droplets or by direct lesion contact
- Transmission to susceptible contacts exposed 24–48 hours before the appearance of skin lesions

Herpes Zoster

- Latent VZV infection in dorsal-root ganglion
- Transmission by direct contact with lesions: VZV is present in skin lesions but is not released into respiratory secretions in immunocompetent host.

CLINICAL MANIFESTATIONS

Varicella

- Incubation period of 10–21 days after exposure to rash
- Prodrome 24–48 hours before rash appears (fever, malaise, anorexia, headache)
- Generalized pruritic rash begins on scalp, face, or trunk and eventually involves the extremities (less intensely). Initial erythematous macules progress to clear fluid-filled vesicles with a surrounding erythematous irregular margin ("dew drops on a rose petal"). Lesions in multiple stages present on the same area of the body, especially on mucous membranes of the oropharynx, conjunctivae, and vagina.
- In 24–48 hours, lesions begin crusting.
- New lesions continue to appear for 1–7 days.
- Breakthrough varicella seen in patients with history of vaccination: maculopapular rash, typically approximately 50 lesions, afebrile, less pruritic

Herpes Zoster

- Vesicular lesions in dermatomal distribution of sensory nerve. Usually one to three dermatomal segments involved
- Discrete vesicles on erythematous base appear first and then enlarge and coalesce.
- Rash often preceded by pain, pruritis, or hyperesthesia.

Complications

- Complications of varicella: Secondary bacterial infections with *S. aureus* or *S. pyogenes* (e.g., cellulitis, necrotizing fasciitis, pneumonia), meningoencephalitis, Reye syndrome, hepatitis, nephritis, postinfectious cerebellitis
- Complications of primary varicella in high-risk populations:
  - ✓ Fetus/newborn: Congenital varicella syndrome if varicella is acquired in first 20 weeks of gestation; neonatal varicella if varicella develops in mother from 5 days before to 2 days after delivery; 30% fatality if untreated
  - ✓ Immunocompromised (lymphoproliferative malignancies, solid tumors, and solid organ transplantation): Visceral dissemination, viremia, and severe, progressive varicella
- Complications of herpes zoster:
  - ✓ Depends on distribution of involved nerve. Potential complications include conjunctivitis, keratitis, uveitis, iridocyclitis, and facial palsies.
  - ✓ Immunocompromised patients with localized skin lesions can transmit virus via aerosolized route and are at risk of visceral dissemination.

DIAGNOSTICS

- Laboratory studies are not routinely indicated, but a specific diagnosis of VZV guides treatment in immunocompromised children; can be utilized to identify breakthrough varicella.
- PCR of body fluid/tissue; viral culture if PCR not available
- Rapid diagnosis: DFA test performed on epithelial cells scraped from the base of lesions is more rapid and sensitive than culture.
- VZV IgG is detectable within 3 days after onset and persists for life after primary infection.
- Obtain liver-function test and chest x-ray in immunocompromised patients.

MANAGEMENT

Varicella

- Varicella vaccination ideally within 72 hours but up to 5 days after exposure may prevent or significantly modify disease (administer if no contraindications to varicella vaccination).
- Indications for intravenous acyclovir include immunocompromise such as malignancy, bone marrow or organ transplant, high-dose steroid therapy, HIV infection, and congenital T-lymphocyte deficiency; neonatal varicella; and varicella-associated pneumonia or encephalitis.
  - ✓ Duration: 7 days or until no new lesions have appeared
- Consider oral acyclovir for infection in the following situations: Chronic cutaneous disorders, cystic fibrosis or other pulmonary disorders, diabetes mellitus, disorders requiring chronic salicylate therapy or intermittent corticosteroid therapy, children >12 years
  - ✓ Oral administration within 24 hours after initial lesions appear
- Valacyclovir was licensed in 2008 for varicella infection in children 2 to <18 years of age, which has improved bioavailability as compared to treatment with oral acyclovir.
- Contact Infection Prevention and Control to ensure appropriate institutional isolation procedures are followed, including an airborne infection isolation room.

Herpes Zoster

- Acyclovir or valacyclovir reduce pain and duration of new lesion formation if initiated within 72 hours after infection onset and is recommended for patients at high risk for disseminated disease.
- Dose: Same as that for primary infection for total of 7 days or for 2 days after last new lesion

Passive Antibody Prophylaxis with Varicella–Zoster Immunoglobulin after Varicella Exposure

- Recommended for immunocompromised children with no history of VZV, pregnant women with no history of or antibodies to VZV, infants born to mothers whose varicella began within 5 days before or 2 days after delivery, premature infants l<28 weeks old with no maternal history of varicella, or premature infants <1000 g or hospitalized regardless of maternal immunity
- Ideally administer within 48 hours of exposure but acceptable if administered within 10 days after exposure
- Dose: 1 vial (125 U)/10 kg of body weight (maximum, 5 vials) IM
- If VZV immunoglobulin is unavailable, consider preemptive acyclovir or valacyclovir or IV immunoglobulin in high-risk patients.

Haley Newman, MD
Rebecca Tenney-Soeiro, MD, MSEd

GENERAL PRINICPLES

The term *medically complex* encompasses a diagnostically heterogeneous group of chronic conditions affecting multiple organ systems. Children with medical complexity often have greater dependence on technology and are at higher risk of infection, malnutrition, and medical errors. They require multispecialty care that is coordinated among providers and families.

RESPIRATORY CONCERNS

CLINICAL MANIFESTATIONS

- Signs and symptoms of respiratory distress include tachypnea, wheezing, hypoxia, and increased work of breathing.
- Fever may also be present with respiratory concerns.
- Poor tolerance of feeds.

DIFFERENTIAL DIAGNOSIS

- Broad differential includes infection (both viral and bacterial), difficulty with oral secretions, pain, obstruction from the upper or lower airway, asthma, neuromuscular weakness, and aspiration.

ASPIRATION

EPIDEMIOLOGY

- Common among the medically complex population, and especially prevalent in those with neurologic impairment.

PATHOPHYSIOLOGY

- Commonly due to inhalation of infectious or noninfectious oral secretions or gastric contents.

ASPIRATION PNEUMONITIS

PATHOPHYSIOLOGY

- Occurs after the acute inhalation of gastric contents into the lungs, resulting in an intense inflammatory reaction; bacteria are not often involved.

MANAGEMENT

- Many patients require ICU level of care for increased respiratory clearance and respiratory support including noninvasive ventilation and intubation.
- Can be difficult to distinguish pneumonitis from aspiration pneumonia and often antibiotics are given empirically.

ASPIRATION PNEUMONIA

ETIOLOGY

- Occurs after inhalation of nasopharyngeal and oropharyngeal contents containing normal upper respiratory tract bacteria into the lower airways.
- Organisms are usually oral anaerobes

MANAGEMENT

- Empiric treatment with amoxicillin–clavulanic acid (or ampicillin–clavulanic acid if IV required) or clindamycin

ASPIRATION FROM ABOVE

EPIDEMIOLOGY

- Increased drooling, or sialorrhea, is common in the medically complex population.

ETIOLOGY

- Increased secretion of saliva is *rarely* the underlying cause.
- Often oromotor dysfunction, lack of laryngeal sensation, and dysphagia leading to pooling of secretions.
- Oromotor dysfunction can also lead to aspiration of orally ingested foods and liquids.
- Aspiration of thin liquids is most common; this can lead to both aspiration pneumonitis and aspiration pneumonia.
- Aspiration of oral feeds can worsen over time, as oromotor dysfunction often declines, especially in neuromuscular diseases.
- Leads to ongoing pulmonary issues as well as malnutrition requiring enteral tube feeding.

DIAGNOSTICS

- Speech therapists may evaluate a child's swallowing safety at the bedside by performing a clinical assessment.
- More formal studies include videofluoroscopy or fiberoptic endoscopic evaluation of swallowing.
- A salivagram can be helpful in identifying aspiration of saliva only.

MANAGEMENT

- Suctioning to manage secretions
- Speech therapy for those who have the potential to improve oral motor skills and awareness of sensation of the lips, mouth, and oropharynx

Medical

- Glycopyrrolate can be provided enterally and has the benefit of a quick onset of action and relatively quick end of therapeutic benefit. The most common side effect is a thickening of secretions, which may lead to mucous plugging. Often decreasing the dose can be beneficial in decreasing the side effects.
- A scopolamine patch may be helpful if a patient has failed a glycopyrrolate trial, but it is not recommended in small children owing to standardized dosing of the patches.

Surgical

- Surgical therapies are usually used only in those for whom medical management has failed.
- The submandibular and parotid glands may be injected with botulinum toxin. It can take up to 2 weeks to see an effect, but the effect usually lasts for 6–9 months.
- Other surgical therapies include salivary-duct ligation or duct removal.

ASPIRATION FROM BELOW

EPIDEMIOLOGY

- Gastroesophageal reflux disease is very common in children with medical complexity.

PATHOPHYSIOLOGY

- Gastric aspirate may reflux into the oropharynx or lungs, causing irritation of the throat, chronic cough, pain with swallowing, and lung inflammation.
- Uncontrolled reflux is associated with worse asthma and recurrent pneumonia.

DIAGNOSTICS

- The diagnosis may be made clinically.
- If unclear, an upper gastrointestinal series and a gastric emptying study may aid in diagnosis.
- The gold standard for diagnosis is esophageal pH monitoring, although this is often unnecessary in the setting of clinical diagnosis.

MANAGEMENT

- Nonpharmacologic interventions include raising the head of the bed, limiting exposure to acidic foods and caffeine, slowing down feeds if tube fed, or feeding postpylorically.

Medical

- H_2 antagonists and proton-pump inhibitors decrease the acidity of gastric contents but do not actually prevent reflux.
- These medications are also associated with possible increased susceptibility to infections owing to suppression of the acidity of gastric contents.
- Promotility agents such as erythromycin, metoclopramide, and bethanechol may speed up transit time in the stomach and reduce reflux; however, each medication is also associated with its own side effects, and tachyphylaxis can develop, particularly in response to erythromycin.

Surgical

- Surgical options include placement of a gastrostomy tube, a gastrostomy tube with fundoplication, or a gastrojejunostomy tube.
- The need for fundoplication versus gastrojejunostomy tube should be discussed with the family, the surgeon who may perform the procedure, and other specialty providers.

ENTERAL NUTRITION

GENERAL PRINCIPLES

- Tube feeding provides enteral nutrition when oral feeding is not adequate to meet a child's caloric demands and support appropriate growth and development.
- Enteral nutrition refers to any feeding method that can deliver nutrition via the gastrointestinal tract (orally or through a feeding tube), whereas parenteral nutrition delivers nutrients intravenously, usually via central venous access.
- The goal of tube feeding is to preserve nutritional status, support growth, and/or treat malnutrition.
- Enteral nutrition is preferable to parenteral nutrition because it is more physiologic and helps prevent mucosal atrophy and promotes motility of the GI tract.

• Absolute contraindications to enteral nutrition include total bowel obstruction, ischemic bowel, and some situations of hemodynamic instability.

CLINICAL INDICATIONS

• Inadequate oral intake due to malabsorption (e.g., cystic fibrosis, pancreatic insufficiency, short bowel syndrome, inflammatory bowel disease)
• Increased metabolic demand (e.g., congenital heart disease, hyperthyroidism, recurrent infection)
• Oral motor dysfunction (e.g., neuromuscular disease such as spinal muscular atrophy)
• Gastrointestinal tract dysfunction (e.g., intestinal pseudo-obstruction, congenital malformation)
• Acute metabolic stress (e.g., sepsis, trauma, burns)

DIAGNOSTICS

• Decision for method of enteral administration is based on several factors, including:
  ✓ Motility and function of the GI tract
  ✓ Risk of aspiration
  ✓ Projected duration

• Upper GI radiographic series can help assess for anatomic obstruction (stricture, malrotation, mass) and may show reflux with aspiration from below (though does not rule it out if not seen)
• Swallow study with fluoroscopy may also help assess aspiration risk from above.
• See **Figure 16-1**.

TYPES OF TUBES

• Several types of tubes are used to administer enteral nutrition, including nasogastric (NG), nasoduodenal (ND), nasojejunal (NJ), gastrostomy (G), and gastrojejunostomy (GJ) tubes.
• Indications for use, the patient's underlying medical conditions, and projected duration of use are important factors when determining the right method of tube feeding for the patient.

NG Tubes

• NG feeding is indicated for children in whom enteral nutrition is projected for short-term support.
• The child should have a functional GI tract and low risk of aspiration from below.
• Benefits: NG tube is easy to place and can be replaced at home by a trained caregiver if the tube becomes dislodged.
• Initial placement should be verified with an x-ray or by acidity testing to ensure that the tube is placed properly in the stomach.
• Risks: Misplacing tube into lungs resulting in feeds or medications being delivered directly to the lungs and causing respiratory compromise.

Gastrostomy Tube

• A gastrostomy tube is preferred for a child who is likely to need longer-term enteral nutrition (>3 months).
• There are three methods of placing a gastrostomy tube: surgical, endoscopic (percutaneous endoscopic gastrostomy), and radiologic (percutaneous radiologic gastrostomy [PRG]).

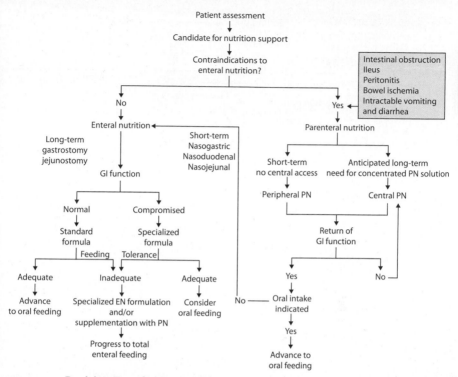

FIGURE 16-1 Decision Tree for Route of Enteral Nutrition. Reproduced with permission from Ukleja A, Freeman KL, Gilbert K, et al: Standards for nutrition support: adult hospitalized patients, *Nutr Clin Pract* 2010 Aug;25(4):403-414.

- In patients who cannot undergo general anesthesia, percutaneous endoscopic gastrostomy and PRG may be preferable.
- Surgically placed tubes can be helpful in children who need another simultaneous procedure (e.g., fundoplication).
- An attachment between the abdominal wall and stomach is created at the time of surgical placement, reducing the risk of dislodgment, whereas percutaneous endoscopic gastrostomy and PRG tube require more time for tract maturation.
- Most gastrostomy tube are secured by a pigtail (looped end), balloon, or bulb in the stomach to prevent dislodgment.
- After surgical placement, when the tract has matured, the primary gastrostomy tube can be replaced with a low-profile device (MIC-KEY, Bard button) in 6–8 weeks.
- The two main types of low-profile (skin level) tubes, fluid filled balloon and mushroom-shaped cap, both help to prevent the tube from migrating out of the stomach.
- Advantages of the balloon tube are that it can be easily replaced and comes in multiple sizes; however, balloons are easier to dislodge.
- The nonballoon type of low-profile tube is harder to dislodge and less likely to break but is more challenging to replace.
- When a gastrostomy tube is no longer needed, it can be removed, and the stoma site typically heals on its own.
- See **Figure 16-2.**

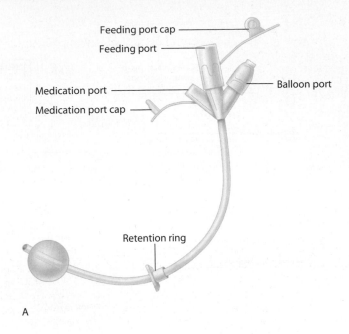

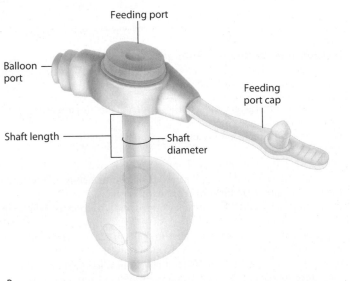

FIGURE 16-2 Typical gastrostomy tube and Low-Profile gastrostomy tube. A, Typical gastrostomy tube. Note the inflated balloon at the tip, which helps prevent the tube from being dislodged. B, Typical low-profile gastrostomy tube device. Reproduced with permission from Zaoutis LB, Chiang VW: *Comprehensive Pediatric Hospital Medicine*, 2nd ed. New York, NY: McGraw Hill; 2018.

Intestinal Tubes

- Feeding through the stomach is preferred because of its more physiologic properties and enhanced digestion.
- Postpyloric feeding (into the duodenum or jejunum) may be needed if: severe GERD, aspiration pneumonia, recurrent vomiting, or gastroparesis.
- Nasointestinal tubes (ND or NJ) are helpful for short-term enteral delivery of nutrition past the stomach.
- NJ tubes require endoscopic or radiologic placement for reliable positioning.
- ND tubes can be placed at the bedside by medical personnel, often with the aid of a dose of metoclopramide during insertion to promote movement past the stomach.
- If a child has a gastrostomy tube with persistence of reflux and aspiration, the gastrostomy tube can be converted into a GJ-tube with an extension that moves through the pylorus into the small intestine.
- Jejunostomy tubes (J-tubes) can also be placed directly into the jejunum with a surgical or endoscopic procedure, though patients must be of a certain size to have a straight J-tube placed.

ADMINISTRATION OF FEEDS

- Commercial formulas are most commonly used.
- There has recently been a resurgence in the use of blenderized tube feeds (BTF)
- Literature on the efficacy and risks of BTF as compared with formula is limited.
  - ✓ Small studies have suggested that BTF required more calories for growth than did formula.
  - ✓ Prevalence of GI upset may be lower with BTF.
  - ✓ The process can be labor-intensive and may be prohibitively expensive for many families.
- It is important that a dietitian be available to help families with meal planning to ensure adequate caloric and micronutrient intake with BTF.

Bolus versus Continuous Feed

- Enteral nutrition can be administered in bolus feeds, intermittently over a specified duration, or continuously over many hours.
- Bolus feeds can be given only to patients with intragastric feeds because only the stomach can tolerate large volumes.
- Bolus feeds are typically given over a short period (15–60 minutes) at set intervals during the day via syringe, gravity, or pump.
- Bolus feeds are preferable for ease of administration, flexibility for the patient and family, and more physiologic secretion of gut hormones.
- If a child is not tolerating bolus feeds, one option is to try continuous feeds overnight with smaller daytime boluses.
- Continuous feeds are delivered with an infusion pump at a set rate and range from 6 to 24 hours per day.
- Cycled continuous feeds refers to feeding for most of the day (e.g., 20 hours continuously with a 4-hour break), which can help with abdominal discomfort.
- Postpyloric feeds are always given over continuous or cycled continuous feeds to ensure appropriate intestinal absorption.
- See **Table 16-1**.

TABLE 16-1	Initiation and Advancement of Tube Feeds, Outlining Advancement of Feeding Schedule by Age			
	Drip Feeds		**Bolus Feeds**	
Age	**Initiation**	**Advancement**	**Initiation (mL)**	**Advancement**
Preterm	1–2 mL/kg/h	5–10 mL/kg every 8–12 hours over 5–7 days as tolerated	10–20 mL/kg	20–30 mL/kg/day as tolerated
Birth-12 mo	5–10 mL/hr	5–10 mL every 2–8 hours	10–60	20–40 mL every 3–4 hours
1–6 years	10–15 mL/hr	10–15 mL every 2–8 hours	30–90	30–60 mL per feed
6–14 years	15–20 mL/hr	10–20 mL every 2–8 hours	60–120	60–90 mL per feed
>14 years	20–30 mL/hr	20–30 mL every 2–8 hours	60–120	60–120 mL per feed

Reproduced with permission from Hay WW Jr, Levin MJ, Abzug MJ, et al: *Current Diagnosis & Treatment: Pediatrics*, 25th ed. New York, NY: McGraw Hill; 2020.

COMPLICATIONS

Infectious Complications

Cellulitis
Infection of the skin around the stoma site is often polymicrobial, including common skin bacteria such as staphylococci and streptococci, as well as enteral gram-negative bacteria and yeast.

Clinical Manifestations
• Signs of cellulitis include pain at the site, erythema, ulceration, and purulent discharge.
• If satellite lesions are visible, fungal infection should be considered.

Management
• Often requires enteral or intravenous antibiotics.
• Include methicillin-resistant *Staphylococcus aureus* (MRSA) coverage depending on the patient's medical history and frequency of hospitalization.
• Nystatin powder applied under a dressing or nystatin ointment applied under the tube can treat superficial fungal infections.

Peritonitis
• A serious complication due to leakage of gastrointestinal contents into the peritoneal cavity

Pathophysiology
• Caused by perforation of the stomach or intestines or due to extrusion of tube into false tract
• Gram-positive organisms (including coagulase-negative staphylococci and *S. aureus*) are common, as well as gram-negative bacteria, including *Pseudomonas, Enterobacter, Escherichia coli,* and *Klebsiella.*
• Fungal peritonitis is rare.

Clinical Manifestations
• Fever, vomiting, and peritoneal signs on examination (guarding, rebound tenderness)
• Fungal peritonitis may present with rapid deterioration.

Management

- Treatment requires rapid administration of broad-spectrum antibiotics and bowel rest.
- Surgical repair of perforations may be required.

Mechanical Complications

Clogging

- If a tube no longer flushes easily, it should be replaced.
- Forcing fluids through a tube is often unsuccessful and can cause perforation.
- Using liquid medications helps to avoid tube blockage from crushed pills.
- Using small-volume water flushes after all medication and feed administration limits risk of clogging.

Dislodgment

- If a tube becomes dislodged <1 month after placement, the patient should be sent back to the primary team that inserted the original tube (general surgery, gastroenterology, or radiology).
- The tube should *not* be immediately replaced by a nonmedical caregiver, given the risk of creation of a false luminal tract and insertion into the peritoneum.
- If a tube has a well established tract (>2 months after insertion), a gastrostomy tube may be replaced by the family or caregiver.
- GJ- or J-tube must always be replaced by radiology staff or another trained health care provider.

Leakage

- Leakage around the tube site can cause skin breakdown, pain, and increased risk of infection.
- If the tube is too loose, external fasteners can help decrease motion and irritation.
- If the tube is too small, it should be upsized to better fit the tract.
- If the tract continues to enlarge (often due to frequent movement of the tube by the patient), consider removing the tube from a well-healed tract for a few hours each day to help the tract shrink back to a more appropriate size.

Granulation Tissue

- Treat visible granulation tissue around the ostomy site with triamcinolone ointment applied to the site daily for 2 weeks.
- Granulation tissue that is large or bleeding can be cauterized with silver nitrate, with repeat administration if necessary.
- Occasionally, what is initially thought to be granulation tissue is actually protruding gastric or intestinal tissue; this situation may require surgical intervention.

GASTRIC-OUTLET OBSTRUCTION

Pathophysiology

- Gastric-outlet obstruction can occur if the tube or balloon migrates within the stomach toward the pylorus, blocking entrance to the duodenum.
- Children with GJ-tubes may frequently have movement of the J portion of the tube, which requires replacement.

Clinical Manifestations

- Emesis can indicate that the tube is coiled in the stomach or has migrated to block the pylorus.

Diagnostics

• An abdominal x-ray or contrast study can be obtained to confirm position.

Management

• Gastric-outlet obstruction can be alleviated by repositioning the tube or balloon and ensuring correct balloon inflation.

INTUSSUSCEPTION

Clinical manifestations

• Often present with abdominal pain and emesis
• Patients may present only with irritability.
• GJ-tubes are at increased risk of intussusception around the J portion of the tube.

DIAGNOSTICS

• An ultrasound should be obtained to rule out intussusception.

Management

• Treatment involves removal of the tube and bowel rest.
• Timing of replacement ranges from 48 hours to 1 week.
• In cases of frequent intussusception of GJ-tube, a separate gastrostomy tube and separate J-tube can be considered (though patient typically needs to weigh ≥15 kg).

FEEDING INTOLERANCE

• Some children experience abdominal pain and bloating with tube feeds, which may be alleviated by slowing the infusion rate and monitoring for constipation or, alternatively, diarrhea.
• Diarrhea can be indicative of intolerance to an ingredient in the formula or rate of infusion.
• Occasionally, the osmolality of the formula causes intolerance, and a change in formula may improve symptoms.
• Children who have undergone tube placement as well as fundoplication (surgical procedure that wraps the fundus of the stomach around the gastroesophageal junction) may experience worse retching and bloating.
• Often slowing the rate of infusion, more frequent venting of the tube, and lower osmolality of formula may improve the retching and bloating.

DUMPING SYNDROME

• Dumping syndrome can occur after fundoplication due to food moving too quickly from the stomach into the small bowel, causing fluid to move rapidly into the bowel.
• Patients may present with hyperglycemia or hypoglycemia, retching, and watery diarrhea.
• This can most often be treated with slowing of the infusion and a more gradual condensing of feeds.
• Occasionally, octreotide is also useful.

AUTONOMIC STORMING (PAROXYSMAL SYMPATHETIC HYPERACTIVITY OR CENTRAL DYSAUTONOMIA)

Autonomic storming is often seen after traumatic brain injury and in children with encephalopathy due to genetic or congenital disorders. Autonomic storming is thought to be due to dysregulation of the autonomic nervous system. However, the pathophysiology

of autonomic storming is poorly understood; thus, treatment is aimed at controlling the symptoms.

CLINICAL MANIFESTATIONS

- Symptoms include tachycardia, hyperthermia, hypertension, agitation, increased tone, dystonic posturing, tachypnea, and diaphoresis.
- Review the patient's medication list when these symptoms arise, as many medication side effects are also symptoms of autonomic storming.
- If a patient is on one of these medications and symptoms of autonomic storming develop, the medication should be discontinued and the patient observed for resolution of the symptoms.
- Common medications with side effects that mimic paroxysmal sympathetic hyperactivity include:

  ✓ Phenytoin—high fevers
  ✓ Haloperidol and chlorpromazine—neuroleptic malignant syndrome
  ✓ H_2 blockers—extrapyramidal symptoms such as dystonia, akathisia, and tremor

MANAGEMENT

- Benzodiazepines, propranolol, intrathecal baclofen, and gabapentin may be used to try to improve symptoms.
- Antihistaminergic antipsychotics such as hydroxyzine and clonazepam may also be useful in controlling symptoms; however, they may cause increased oral secretions, which can worsen agitation, and should therefore be monitored closely.

SPASTICITY

Spasticity is a condition causing certain muscle groups to become contracted. It is commonly seen in patients with neurologic devastation due to brain injury or congenital/genetic disorders. Spasticity can be a major source of pain for patients and limitation of mobility.

MANAGEMENT

Nonpharmacologic

- Physical therapy and splints may be helpful in preventing spasticity.

Pharmacologic

- Enteral medications such as diazepam, baclofen, or tizanidine are often used to decrease spasticity.
- The most common side effect is excessive drowsiness.
- Dantrolene sodium may be an alternative because it works directly in the muscle cells themselves as opposed to acting within the central nervous system (CNS), thus decreasing the sedative effect.
- Intrathecal baclofen tends to cause less sedation because of lower dose administration; however, it requires surgical implantation of a pump for continuous medication infusion.
- Botulinum toxin may be injected into specific muscles to decrease focal spasticity.
- In cases of severe contractures due to significant spasticity, surgical interventions such as tendon releases may be required.

PRESSURE INJURY

A pressure injury is a localized area of damage to the skin and underlying soft tissue. Injuries are often located over a bony prominence or in areas of high friction or tension.

EPIDEMIOLOGY

Prevalence of pressure injuries of any stage among pediatric patients in children's hospitals ranges from 4 to 35% and may be even higher among medically complex children.

PATHOPHYSIOLOGY

- The most significant risk factor is immobility.
- Other risk factors include loss of sensation, increased moisture (e.g., urinary or fecal incontinence, perspiration, drainage), malnutrition, inability to self-reposition, and cognitive impairment.
- Infants have more fat and less muscle mass and are thus more susceptible to deformation and injury.
- In infants, the occiput and ears are the most common ulceration sites.
- In adolescents and adults, the sacrum, buttocks and heels are the more common sites of injury.

CLINICAL MANIFESTATIONS

Staging

- If any pressure injury is identified, documentation should include location, size, drainage, presence of necrotic tissue, and stage of the ulcer based on National Pressure Ulcer Advisory Panel (NPAUP) guidelines.
- The NPAUP staging framework categorizes pressure ulcers in one of six stages, which are described in **Table 16-2** (also see, **Figures 16-3** and **16-4**).

MANAGEMENT

Prevention

- Neonates and children should have a documented skin exam and risk assessment for pressure injury on admission.
- The Braden Q scale incorporates measures of mobility, activity, sensory perception, moisture, friction or shear, nutrition, and tissue oxygenation and perfusion.
- Strategies for prevention include:
  ✓ Reposition at regular intervals (every 2–6 hours) to relieve frictional forces.
  ✓ Draw sheets and other devices prevent friction when skin moves against support surfaces.
  ✓ Floating heels
  ✓ Seat cushions for chair-bound patients
  ✓ Higher-density mattresses redistribute pressure more effectively than standard mattresses.
- Closely examine medical equipment devices at regular intervals, including blood pressure cuffs, nasal cannulas, masks for supplemental oxygen and noninvasive ventilation, arm boards, casts, and any other orthopedic devices.
- Devices most commonly associated with injury in the pediatric ICU are noninvasive positive-pressure face masks, casts, and tracheostomy tubes and ties.
- Proper skin care ensures good hygiene, without excessive moisture or dryness.

Treatment Options

- Local wound care, debridement if necessary, and placement of proper dressing
- Moisture retentive dressing (e.g., hydrogel) should be covered by absorptive, occlusive dressing (e.g., polyurethane foam) to help absorb any exudate and encourage "autolytic debridement" (the body's own endogenous enzymes breaking down dead tissue).

TABLE 16-2	Pressure Ulcer Staging System

- **Suspected deep-tissue injury**

  - Purple or maroon localized area of discolored intact skin or blood-filled blister due to damage of underlying soft tissue from pressure and/or shear. The area may be preceded by tissue that is painful, firm, mushy, boggy, warmer, or cooler as compared to adjacent tissue.

- **Stage I**

  - Intact skin with nonblanchable redness of a localized area usually over a bony prominence. Darkly pigmented skin may not have visible blanching; its color may differ from that of the surrounding area.

- **Stage II**

  - Partial thickness loss of dermis presenting as a shallow open ulcer with a red pink wound bed, without slough. May also present as an intact or open/ruptured serum-filled blister.

- **Stage III**

  - Full thickness tissue loss. Subcutaneous fat may be visible but bone, tendon, or muscle is not exposed. Slough may be present but does not obscure the depth of tissue loss. May include undermining and tunneling.

- **Stage IV**

  - Full thickness tissue loss with exposed bone, tendon, or muscle. Slough or eschar may be present on some parts of the wound bed. Often includes undermining and tunneling.

- **Unstageable**

  - Full thickness tissue loss in which the base of the ulcer is covered by slough (yellow, tan, gray, green, or brown) and/or eschar (tan, brown, or black) in the wound bed.

Used with permission from National Pressure Injury Advisory Panel (NPIAP). Copyright 2021 NPIAP

- See **Table 16-3.**
- Antibiotic ointment can be used sparingly every 8–12 hours (mupirocin, polymyxin B, or bacitracin zinc–polymyxin B), although there is no clear evidence to suggest that this improves outcomes.
- Systemic antibiotics should be given for clinical signs of spreading cellulitis, sepsis, or underlying osteomyelitis.

COMPLICATIONS

- The most serious complication of pressure injury is sepsis due to seeding of bacteria directly from the wound site into the bloodstream.
- Skin bacteria including staphylococci and streptococci are most common, although pressure injuries can be polymicrobial.
- Empiric antibiotics to treat these organisms should be started while awaiting culture results, with consideration for MRSA and pseudomonal coverage based on patient's prior wound cultures, immune status, and duration/frequency of hospitalization.

TRACHEOSTOMY

Many medically complex children have home tracheostomy and/or home ventilation as part of the management of their chronic illnesses or in the setting of respiratory failure.

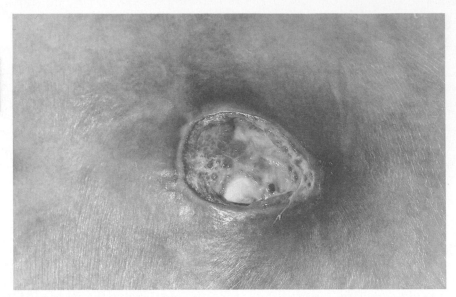

FIGURE 16-3 Stage 3 Pressure Ulcer. Well-demarcated crateriform ulcer with full-thickness skin loss extending down to fascia over greater trochanteric region. Reproduced with permission from Wolff K, Johnson RA, Saavedra AP, et al: *Fitzpatrick's Color Atlas and Synopsis of Clinical Dermatology*, 8th ed. New York, NY: McGraw Hill; 2017.

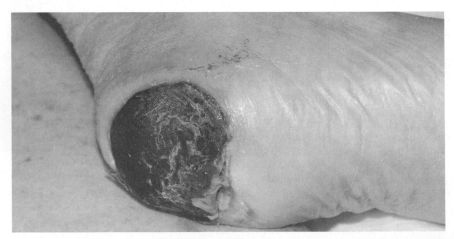

FIGURE 16-4 Stage 4 Pressure Ulcer on the Heel. Black necrosis extended in to the calcaneal bone, which also had to be debrided. Reproduced with permission from Wolff K, Johnson RA, Saavedra AP, et al: *Fitzpatrick's Color Atlas and Synopsis of Clinical Dermatology*, 8th ed. New York, NY: McGraw Hill; 2017.

TABLE 16-3	Dressing Recommendation Based on Stage of Ulceration
Injury Type	**Dressing Type and Considerations**
Stage 1 and deep tissue injury	Polyurethane film
	Hydrocolloid wafer
	Semipermeable foam dressing
Stage 2	Hydrocolloid wafers
	Semipermeable foam dressing
	Polyurethane film
Stages 3 and 4	For highly exudative wounds, use highly absorptive dressing or packing, such as calcium alginate.
	Wounds with necrotic debris must be debrided.
	Debridement can be autolytic, enzymatic, or surgical.
	Shallow, clean wounds can be dressed with hydrocolloid wafers, semipermeable foam, or polyurethane film.
	Deep wounds can be packed with gauze; if the wound is deep and highly exudative, an absorptive packing should be used.
Heel injury	Do not remove eschar on heel ulcers because it can help promote healing (eschar in other locations should be debrided).
Unstageable	Debride before deciding on further therapy.
Deep tissue injury	Avoid pressure to the area.

Reproduced with permission from Papadakis MA, McPhee SJ, Bernstein J: *Quick Medical Diagnosis & Treatment 2021*, New York, NY: McGraw Hill; 2021.

Underlying conditions prompting tracheotomy include neurodegenerative conditions, as well as congenital heart and lung diseases.

GENERAL PRINCIPLES

- A tracheotomy is a surgically created incision in the front of the neck into the trachea, below the cricoid cartilage.
- It is performed to relieve upper airway obstruction or for children requiring long-term mechanical ventilation due to underlying lung disease or neuromuscular conditions.
- The majority of children with tracheostomies have sustained reliance on the tube and its related technology for long-term survival.
- The majority of children with a tracheostomy tube had it placed at <1 year of age, decannulation among this population is extremely low.
- Tracheostomy does not prevent pulmonary infection and lung damage from aspiration; however, it does help with suctioning and clearance of secretions.
- Tracheostomy facilitates home care outside the hospital if prolonged invasive ventilation is required.
- Children generally tolerate intubation longer than adults; thus, tracheostomy is usually done later in the patient's hospital course and there is variation in timing based on hospital, provider, and joint decision making with the patient's family.

CLINICAL MANIFESTATIONS

- The three main indications are
  - ✓ bypass airway obstruction,
  - ✓ facilitating long-term mechanical ventilation, and
  - ✓ assisting in airway clearance for children with impaired clearance mechanisms.
- Airway obstruction occurs at, above, or below the level of the glottis.
- Obstruction above the glottis can be due to craniofacial abnormalities.
  - ✓ Examples include Treacher Collins syndrome, Pierre Robin sequence, Beckwith–Wiedemann syndrome, Nager syndrome, and CHARGE (coloboma, heart defects, atresia of choanae, retardation of growth and development, ear abnormalities and/or hearing loss) association.
  - ✓ It may also be related to severe laryngomalacia.
- Obstruction at the level of the glottis may be due to vocal-cord palsy that is congenital or acquired.
  - ✓ Arnold–Chiari malformation is the most common congenital CNS disease causing vocal-cord paralysis.
  - ✓ Congenital paralysis is most commonly idiopathic.
- Obstruction below the glottis:
  - ✓ Acquired subglottic stenosis in the setting of prolonged neonatal endotracheal tube intubation
  - ✓ Congenital subglottic stenosis as an isolated finding
  - ✓ Associated with other genetic conditions (including trisomy 21)

MANAGEMENT

Percutaneous versus Surgical Placement

- Most pediatric tracheotomies are performed surgically through various operative techniques.
- Percutaneous tracheostomy technique is rarely performed in children.
- The standard surgical procedure involves a vertical tracheal incision with stay sutures placed on either side to create gentle retraction around the tracheostoma.
- In the event of accidental decannulation requiring rapid tube replacement, these sutures are helpful for maintaining easy identification of the incision site.

TRACHEOSTOMY TUBES

Material

- Most pediatric tracheostomy tubes are made of polyvinyl chloride (PVC) (e.g., Shiley™) or silicone (e.g., Bivona™)
- PVC has the advantage of softening with a patient's body temperature and molding well to the anatomy of the trachea.
- Silicone may have more resistance to colonization and biofilm formation and is generally used for longer durations than PVC tubes before replacement.
- Unlike adult tubes, pediatric tubes are always single lumen.
- A neonatal tube should be used for infants under 5 kg.

Cuffed versus Uncuffed Tubes

- In children, without requirement for mechanical ventilation, an uncuffed tube is preferable for
  - ✓ prevention of mucosal injury.
  - ✓ decreased airway resistance with larger-diameter tube.
  - ✓ offers opportunity for vocalization around the tube.

- Cuffed tubes are helpful for mechanically ventilated patients to prevent air leak.
- Some cuffs are inflated with sterile water, which seals the trachea during ventilation but can be deflated and still rest tightly to the shaft of the tube to allow for periods of vocalization with a speaking valve.

Humidification

- Airway entry through the tracheostomy tube bypasses natural mechanisms of filtration and humidification that typically occurs when air moves through the nose and pharynx.
- This creates thicker and dryer secretions in children with tracheostomies and increases the risk of pulmonary infections.
- Most effective mechanisms to reduce mucus plugging and tube blockage are suctioning and humidification.
- Many home ventilators have a built-in humidification system.
- Sterile saline drops can also be placed directly in the tube if secretions are so thick that they become hard to suction.
- Similarly, saline nebulizer treatments may help loosen secretions.

Heat-and-Moisture Exchangers (HMEs)

- Devices that contain a filter to assist with warming and moisture exchange
- Upon exhalation, heat and moisture are deposited onto the filter; subsequently, during inhalation the heat and moisture are then returned to the lungs as opposed to being exhaled into the surrounding atmosphere.
- HME filters can assist with thinning secretions and preventing mucous plugging and coughing; however, they can also increase the work of breathing.
- Important to monitor for shortness of breath and desaturation when first trying the HME device.

Mist Collar

- Device that provides humidification
- It is helpful for children who cannot tolerate an HME device or who have extremely problematic thick secretions.
- The mist collar is attached to an air compressor via aerosol tubing.
- The air compressor moves air through a bottle of water to pick up moisture, which then flows through the tubing into the tracheostomy to increase humidification.

Speaking Valves

- Speaking valves are helpful in facilitating communication.
- A Passy–Muir valve is a one-way speaking valve that attaches to the outside of the tracheostomy tube.
- The valve opens as the patient inhales and closes upon exhalation so that air flows around the tube and up through the vocal cords to generate phonation.
- A speaking valve trial can be considered in a medically stable child who is alert, responsive, and can tolerate cuff deflation if he or she has a cuffed tube.
- Contraindications include severe upper airway obstruction, severe neurologic impairment, and inflated cuffed tube.

COMPLICATIONS

Complications of a tracheostomy can be divided by intraoperative, early postoperative, and late complications.

Intraoperative

- Hemorrhage
- Hypoxia
- Damage to the recurrent laryngeal nerve
- Pneumothorax
- Creation of a false track
- Infection

Early Postoperative

- Tube obstruction or displacement
- False passage formation
- Pooling of secretions leading to aspiration and lower respiratory infections
- Pneumothorax
- Bleeding from the tracheotomy site
- Stomal breakdown

Late Complications

- Stomal granuloma
- Tube occlusion
- Tracheocutaneous or tracheoesophageal fistula formation
- Subglottic stenosis
- Bacterial tracheitis

Decannulation Risk

- Caregivers must be well trained in tracheostomy care as well as tube replacement in case their child accidentally becomes decannulated.
- Proper training is important to prevent incorrect placement with formation of a false passage and subsequent airway obstruction.

Troubleshooting Complications

Discharge

- Yellow or green malodorous secretions can be indicative of infection.
- Stomal skin infection and tracheitis are often polymicrobial, including *S. aureus, Pseudomonas,* and *Candida.*
- Secretions from the lower airway can be sent for bacterial and viral studies.
- While awaiting culture results, review prior culture results for pathogens and antibiotic sensitivities to guide prophylactic treatment.
- If the patient is not systemically ill, empiric options include amoxicillin–clavulanate, quinolones (ciprofloxacin or levofloxacin) or clindamycin for MRSA coverage if there is a concern for MRSA.
- IV antibiotics such as piperacillin–tazobactam, vancomycin, and a fluoroquinolone for pseudomonal coverage should be given to unstable patients.

Stertor

- Worsening stertor and noisy breathing may suggest that the patient has an obstruction due to increased or thicker secretions.
- Try suction and sterile saline drops.

Thick Secretions
- Increase humidity from air–oxygen humidification source or increase frequency of use of a high humidity source such as an HME or a mist collar.

Blood-Tinged Secretions
- Can be due to mucosal irritation from suctioning, granulation tissue, or infection
- Try decreasing frequency of suctioning and increasing humidity.
- Evaluation by an ear, nose, and throat specialist can help if symptoms persist.

Inability to Pass a Suction Catheter
- Can be due to an oversized catheter or a buildup of mucus within the tracheostomy tube
- Try a smaller suction catheter as well as instilling 3–5 mL of normal saline into the tube prior to suctioning.
- If this doesn't work, consider tube replacement.

Increased Work of Breathing
- May be a sign of tube occlusion
- First try repositioning both the tracheostomy tube and the patient's neck, followed by suctioning.
- If this does not help, change the tracheostomy tube.

CEREBROSPINAL FLUID SHUNTS

Cerebrospinal fluid (CSF) shunts are used to treat hydrocephalus or increased intracranial pressure to prevent neurologic deterioration that will occur if the underlying condition is not treated effectively.

SHUNT STRUCTURE

- Shunts contain three segments: a proximal catheter, a valve and reservoir(s), and a distal catheter.
- Shunts are named according to their proximal and distal insertion locations.
- The proximal portion is most often placed in the lateral ventricle but may also be located in the third or fourth ventricle or a cyst within the CNS.
- The distal catheter usually ends in the peritoneal cavity but may also be located in the right atrium, pleural cavity, or even the gallbladder or ureters.
- Valve allows for one-way flow when a specific pressure differential is achieved.
- Reservoir allows for sampling of CSF.

COMPLICATIONS

SHUNT MALFUNCTION

Epidemiology
- The majority of patients with CSF shunts will have a malfunction at some point in their lifetime.

Clinical Manifestations
- Symptoms are due to increased intracranial pressure and are listed in **Table 16-4**.
- Physical exam findings may include altered mental status, bulging fontanel, increased head circumference, papilledema, increased blood pressure, and bradycardia.

TABLE 16-4	Symptoms of Shunt Malfunctions
Sleepiness or lethargy	
Hypotonia	
Macrocephaly	
Split sutures	
Bulging fontanelle	
Sunsetting	
Sixth cranial nerve palsy	
Papilledema (late finding)	
Decreased visual acuity	
Palpable kinks, fluid collections, or disconnections along the shunt	
Abdominal mass or tenderness (suggesting distal CSF fluid collection that impedes resorption)	

Reproduced with permission from Zaoutis LB, Chiang VW: *Comprehensive Pediatric Hospital Medicine*, 2nd ed. New York, NY: McGraw Hill; 2018.

SHUNT INFECTION

Epidemiology

- Infections include cellulitis, wound infections, and CNS infection.
- Infection is most likely to happen within the first few months of placement or after revision of the shunt.

Etiology

- Infections in the perioperative period are often due to coagulase-negative staphylococci, *S. epidermidis,* and *S. aureus.*
- Late shunt infections (those occurring 6–9 months after manipulation) may be associated with bacteria causing meningitis such as pneumococcus and *Haemophilus influenzae.*
- Other gram-negative bacilli are also more likely in late infections.
- Peritonitis can occur in ventriculoperitoneal shunts. These infections may be caused by enteric organisms or by *Staphylococcus* species.

Clinical Manifestations

- Symptoms of shunt infection are similar to those seen in shunt malfunctions, in addition to fever, erythema, or edema of skin overlying shunt.

Management

- Immediate Neurosurgery consult
- Tap the shunt for CSF cell count, total protein, glucose, and culture.
- Vancomycin and third-generation cephalosporin for empiric antibiotic coverage.

OVERDRAINAGE

Clinical Manifestations

- Overdrainage most commonly causes symptoms in the upright position, such as nausea, emesis, and postural headache.
- The ventricles become diminished in size.

- The shunt catheter lies against the side of the ventricle, blocking the holes within the catheter and contributing to shunt malfunction.

OTHER COMPLICATIONS

- If a ventriculoatrial shunt is present and systemic sepsis symptoms are present, consider endocarditis, hypocomplementemia, glomerulonephritis, and thromboembolic events.
- Other rare complications include inguinal hernia, perforation of intraabdominal organs, development of abdominal pseudocyst, and intussusception or volvulus around the catheter tip.

DIAGNOSTICS

- Manual assessment of the shunt and tapping of the shunt is often done by neurosurgery.
- CSF fluid can be obtained from the reservoir and analyzed for markers of infection or inflammation; however, cutoffs for white blood cells and protein levels remain controversial.
- Both elevated CSF pressure and low CSF flow can indicate malfunction.
- A shunt series is a series of x-ray exams that assess the continuity of the catheters and assess for kinks or disconnections in the catheter.
- Head CTs are often obtained to assess ventricular size and thus shunt function.
  ✓ Head CT should be compared to baseline CT, looking for signs of increased intracranial pressure.
- If abdominal pain is present with a ventriculoperitoneal shunt, a dedicated abdominal x-ray may be obtained to look for free air.
- Abdominal ultrasonography may be used to assess for pseudocyst, which can become secondarily infected.

MANAGEMENT

- If there is concern for a shunt infection, empiric therapy should be started with vancomycin and a third-generation cephalosporin.
- Often the hardware must be replaced to fully eradicate the infection.
- In some cases, the shunt is removed and an external ventricular drain is placed until treatment is completed, and then a new shunt is placed.
- The typical length of therapy is dependent on the organism but may be 2–3 weeks of IV antibiotics.
- If the shunt is malfunctioning, then at least the disturbed portion must be replaced.
- Perioperative antibiotics are used to prevent infection during manipulation and sometimes continued for 24 hours postoperatively.

PALLIATIVE CARE FOR MEDICALLY COMPLEX CHILDREN

GENERAL PRINCIPLES

- The goal of palliative care is to minimize the amount of suffering a child experiences through effective communication and aggressive symptom control.
- There is a misconception that a divide exists between palliative care and curative intention of treatment. Palliative care can simultaneously help improve quality of life even as a child is receiving treatment aimed at extending life or even providing a potential cure.
- Identifying patients who may benefit from palliative care can help maximize quality of life and provide enhanced support to patients, their families, and medical providers.

- Involving the palliative care team can also assist with decision making in alignment with the family and patient's core values to establish firm goals of care.
- Palliative care can start anytime a child is given a diagnosis of a life-limiting illness.
- Many medically complex pediatric patients may benefit from palliative care support for symptom management, quality of life discussions, and end-of life care.
- Palliative care may help the team assess the family's understanding of the diagnosis and help facilitate clearer communication between the family and other physicians and care providers when involved early.

CHAPTER 17

Metabolism

Amanda Barone Pritchard, MD
Rebecca D. Ganetzky, MD

WHEN TO SUSPECT A METABOLIC DISORDER

GENERAL PRINCIPLES

Inborn errors of metabolism (IEMs) are generally defined as disorders resulting from pathogenic genetic variants affecting the enzymes or transport proteins involved in metabolizing specific nutrient-derived substrates.

- Most frequently, these are due to pathogenic variants that decrease enzyme activity, resulting in backup of a toxic substrate or production of an abnormal toxic substrate, an inefficiency of energy production, loss of necessary intermediates, and/or abnormal storage of substrate.
- IEMs vary in their timing of onset and symptomatology.
- Newborn screening has allowed for early identification of many individuals with IEMs; however, many IEMs are not part of the newborn screen.
- Several clinical scenarios in which IEMs may be suspected are detailed in **Table 17-1.** This chapter provides a broad overview of types of IEMs and their common presentations; however, it is not an exhaustive exploration of all of these ultrarare diseases.
- IEMs should be on the differential diagnosis for patients with almost any unexplained symptoms, especially if multiple organ systems are involved. Early involvement of a biochemical geneticist is recommended for any confirmed or suspected inborn error of metabolism.

TABLE 17-1 Clinical Presentations of IEMs

Clinical Symptom or Lab Abnormality	Associated Features or Timing	Metabolic Diagnoses
Hypoglycemia	Postprandial	Glycogen storage diseases, hereditary fructose intolerance, galactosemia
	Fasting, without ketosis	FAODs
		HMG-CoA lyase deficiency
	Fasting, with significant ketosis	Ketotic hypoglycemia, ketone body utilization defects
Hyperammonemia	Metabolic acidosis (hyperammonemia is secondary in these conditions)	Organic acidemias (propionic acidemia, methylmalonic acidemia, isovaleric acidemia), severe mitochondrial defects
	Neonatal or episodic	Urea-cycle defects, severe FAODs
Metabolic acidosis	Altered mental status, maple syrup smell to urine and cerumen, ketonuria	Maple syrup urine disease (note: acidosis may not always be present)
	Hyperammonemia	Organic acidemias (propionic acidemia, methylmalonic acidemia, isovaleric acidemia)

(Continued)

TABLE 17-1 Clinical Presentations of IEMs (*Continued*)

Clinical Symptom or Lab Abnormality	Associated Features or Timing	Metabolic Diagnoses
Lactic acidosis	Other organ system pathology, childhood onset (ophthalmoplegia, neutropenia, etc.)	Electron transport chain defects (mitochondrial disease)
	Neonatal lactic acidosis, may have hypotonia, IUGR, respiratory failure	Electron transport chain defects, pyruvate dehydrogenase deficiency, pyruvate carboxylase deficiency
	Seizures, developmental delay, hypotonia	Pyruvate dehydrogenase deficiency, pyruvate carboxylase deficiency
Epileptic encephalopathy	Neonatal	Molybdenum cofactor deficiency, pyridoxine responsive seizures, glycine encephalopathy
Failure to thrive	Vomiting after high-protein meal	Urea-cycle defect, organic acidemias
	Vomiting after fructose-containing foods	Hereditary fructose intolerance
	Diarrhea, abdominal distension	Lysosomal acid lipase deficiency (Wolman disease), congenital disorders of glycosylation (MPI-CDG), Fanconi–Bickel syndrome
	History of hyperbilirubinemia, hearing loss, dysmorphic features	Peroxisomal disorders
Liver Symptoms	Neonatal onset liver failure	Galactosemia, hereditary tyrosinemia type 1, mitochondrial depletion syndromes, transaldolase deficiency, congenital disorders of glycosylation
	Neonatal cholestasis	Galactosemia, tyrosinemia type 1, Niemann–Pick disease type C, citrin deficiency, peroxisomal biogenesis defects
	Liver failure at time of introduction of fructose-containing foods	Hereditary fructose intolerance
	Late infantile or childhood onset liver failure	GSD type 4, transaldolase deficiency
	Hepatomegaly or hepatosplenomegaly with or without other organ system symptoms (skeletal abnormalities, bone pain, neurological deterioration)	Lysosomal storage diseases (Gaucher disease, Niemann–Pick disease type C, lysosomal acid lipase deficiency)

TABLE 17-1	Clinical Presentations of IEMs (*Continued*)	
Clinical Symptom or Lab Abnormality	**Associated Features or Timing**	**Metabolic Diagnoses**
Stroke-like episode	During intercurrent illness, with subsequent movement disorder symptoms (dystonia)	Glutaric aciduria type 1, more rarely other organic acidemias, mitochondrial disease (Leigh syndrome)
	Lactic acidosis	MELAS, other mitochondrial diseases
Dysmorphic features	Structural brain differences, renal cysts, cholestasis, wide anterior fontanelle, epiphyseal stippling on X-ray	Peroxisomal biogenesis disorders
	Dysostosis multiplex (skeletal abnormalities on x-ray), coarse facies, hepatosplenomegaly, and/or corneal clouding	Mucopolysaccharidoses
	Hypotonia, other congenital malformations, abnormal fat distribution	Congenital disorders of glycosylation
Cardiomyopathy	Hypoglycemia, rhabdomyolysis, elevated transaminases	FAODs
	Hypotonia, classic ECG findings (short PR interval, large QRS), large tongue	Pompe disease
	Hypotonia, dysmorphic facies and neutropenia in males	Barth syndrome (X-linked)
	Cardiac valve thickening, coarse facial features, hepatomegaly	Mucopolysaccharidoses(Hunter syndrome, Hurler syndrome), oligosaccharidoses
	Hypotonia, other structural organ differences, liver dysfunction	Congenital disorders of glycosylation (PMM2-CDG)

ECG = electrocardiographic; FOADs = fatty acid oxidation defects; GSD = MELAS = mitochondrial myopathy, encephalopathy, lactic acidosis, and stroke-like episodes glycogen storage disease HMG-CoA = 3-hydroxy-3-methylglutaryl coenzyme A; IUGR = intrauterine growth restriction; MPI-CDG = Mannosephosphate Isomerase-Congenital Disorder of Glycosylation; PMM2-CDG = Phosphomannomutase 2-Congenital Disorder of Glycosylation.

DIAGNOSTICS

IEMs can be classified in varying manners. The most common is to differentiate on the basis of the pathway affected: disorders of intermediary metabolism (e.g., organic acidurias, urea-cycle disorders), disorders resulting in inadequate energy production (e.g., mitochondrial disease), and disorders affecting macromolecules (e.g., glycogen storage disease, lysosomal storage diseases).

- Intermediary and energy metabolic disorders can cause acute decompensation.
- In acutely ill patients, initial metabolic screening and diagnostic lab tests should focus on manifestations of those disorders, including the following:
  - ✓ Glucose
  - ✓ Comprehensive metabolic panel (assess acid–base status, anion gap, transaminases, electrolytes)
  - ✓ Ammonia
  - ✓ Creatine phosphokinase (CPK)
  - ✓ Lactate (if lactate is elevated, determine lactate:pyruvate ratio)
  - ✓ Urinalysis (assess for ketonuria)
  - ✓ Plasma amino acids
  - ✓ Urine organic acids
  - ✓ Plasma acylcarnitine profile
- Although many of these tests are specific enough to be diagnostic, the sensitivity may be limited, especially if the results are not obtained until a patient is completely metabolically stabilized.
- If there is a strong clinical suspicion, genetic testing is considered the diagnostic gold standard.
- In the United States, it is generally the standard of care to confirm any IEM diagnosis genetically in addition to biochemically. This is important for counseling regarding recurrence risk and identifying other at-risk family members.

MANAGEMENT

Suspected Defects in Intermediary Metabolism or Defects in Energy Production

- Management of most IEMs, especially those of intermediary metabolism or defects in energy production, involves prevention of catabolism to divert the body from using an impaired metabolic pathway.
- In a critically ill patient in whom there is suspicion for metabolic disease without a known diagnosis, general management principles include the following:
  - ✓ Provision of large amounts of dextrose (typically, IV fluids containing D10 or higher) as a safe initial management strategy for the vast majority of these conditions
  - ✓ For acidotic patients, IV sodium bicarbonate may be needed, and can be given as a 1 mEq/kg bolus initially followed by a continuous infusion.
  - ✓ For severely acidotic patients, the bicarbonate deficit should be calculated: (circulating volume correction factor [0.5 in neonates; 0.4 in other patients]) × (weight in kg) × ([desired HCO_3^- in mmol/L] − measured HCO_3^-] = bicarbonate deficit). Half the bicarbonate deficit should be repleted within the first hour and the remaining half over 24 hours. Sodium bicarbonate should be used, as buffering agents such as acetate or citrate may not be well metabolized by patients with specific IEMs. Vital signs and lab results should be monitored closely in any critically ill patient who requires bicarbonate administration; excess administration can cause hypercapnia.
  - ✓ Lactated Ringer's should never be given to patients with elevated lactate and should be used with caution in patients with suspected organic acidopathies, as lactate competes with other organic acids for renal excretion.
  - ✓ Fasting should be avoided, especially in neonates with limited reserve. Dextrose should not be decreased in unstable patients; insulin may be needed to control hyperglycemia.
  - ✓ Specific dietary interventions are detailed throughout this chapter, but for patients with high concern for a disorder of intermediary metabolism (e.g., large anion gap metabolic acidosis, hyperammonemia, nonketotic hypoglycemia and/or rhabdomyolysis), protein

and lipids should be held for up to 24 hours pending diagnostic evaluation while providing excess dextrose.

✓ Consider echocardiography and/or electrocardiography (ECG) on the basis of clinical exam and vital signs, given that many disorders can cause cardiomyopathy or rhythm disturbances.

✓ Consider a trial of nitrogen-scavenging agents ("Urea Cycle Disorders" section) for patients with hyperammonemia; hemodialysis may be needed for medically refractory hyperammonemia or if nitrogen scavengers are not available.

Suspected Defects in Macromolecule Metabolism

• Most of the macromolecule defects (e.g., mucopolysaccharidoses [MPSs]) do not result in acute metabolic decompensation, but rather in chronic, progressive disease due to buildup of these large molecules.

• These patients may require specific enzyme-replacement therapy if available, but they do not typically require dietary interventions or measures to prevent catabolism when ill.

NEWBORN SCREENING (NBS)

• Using tandem mass spectrometry, it is feasible to quickly and easily screen dried blood spots for multiple IEMs.

• There is a Recommended Uniform Screening Panel (RUSP) with both core and secondary conditions.

• However, screening does vary from state and changes over time.

• As of 2018 the RUSP core list includes:

✓ Organic acidemias: Propionic acidemia, methylmalonic acidemia and related disorders, isovaleric acidemia, 3-methylcrotonyl carboxylase deficiency, glutaric acidemia type 1 and the rare disorders 3-hydroxy-3-methlglutaryl coenzyme A (HMG-CoA) lyase deficiency, holocarboxylase synthase deficiency, beta-ketothiolase deficiency

✓ Fatty acid oxidation disorders: Carnitine uptake defect, medium chain acyl-CoA dehydrogenase deficiency, very long chain acyl-CoA dehydrogenase deficiency, long chain hydroxy-acyl-CoA dehydrogenase deficiency and trifunctional protein deficiency

✓ Amino acid disorders: Argininosuccinic aciduria, citrullinemia type I, maple syrup urine disease, homocystinuria, phenylketonuria, tyrosinemia; the common urea-cycle disease ornithine transcarbamylase (OTC) deficiency is a notable exclusion, because of the absence of a good screening test.

✓ Biotinidase deficiency

✓ Galactosemia

✓ Lysosomal storage disorders: Pompe disease and MPS I (Hurler syndrome)

✓ X-linked adrenoleukodystrophy

✓ Nonmetabolic disorders: Hypothyroidism, congenital adrenal hyperplasia, hemoglobinopathies, critical congenital heart disease, cystic fibrosis, hearing loss, severe combined immunodeficiency and spinal muscular atrophy

DIAGNOSTICS

• The core of NBS methodology is tandem mass spectrometry analysis of acylcarnitines and amino acids; this test makes many inborn errors of intermediary metabolism significantly less likely in the setting of a normal newborn screen.

• NBS is a screening test, meaning that the cutoffs for a "positive" screen are often low to ensure that as many affected infants as possible are captured and to minimize false negative results.

- Diagnostic testing is required to follow-up all screening tests.
- Common scenarios causing false positives include transient tyrosinemia of the newborn due to immature liver function resulting in elevated tyrosine, abnormal values in prematurity causing abnormal congenital adrenal hyperplasia testing, and total parental nutrition causing elevated methionine and/or tyrosine.
- All abnormal NBS results warrant critical review.
- False negative results can also occur, albeit more rarely, especially in fatty acid oxidation defects, as abnormalities on acylcarnitine profile can normalize when an infant is well.
- When an abnormal NBS result occurs follow the instructions from the state.
- The ACT (ACTion) sheets and algorithms published by the American College of Medical Genetics and Genomics are freely available online resources; these also include important history details to ascertain regarding patient status if a NBS is positive (available at https://www.ncbi.nlm.nih.gov/books/nbk55827/).

FATTY ACID OXIDATION DISORDERS

GENERAL PRINCIPLES

Class of metabolic diseases in which enzyme deficiencies in mitochondrial fatty acid import or β-oxidation limit the ability of mitochondria to use fat as an energy source

EPIDEMIOLOGY

- Overall incidence about 1:10,000; autosomal recessive inheritance
- Medium-chain acyl-CoA dehydrogenase (MCAD) deficiency is the most common fatty acid oxidation (FAO) defect.

PATHOPHYSIOLOGY

The most significant danger is hypoketotic hypoglycemia, leading to failure of multiple organ systems.

General considerations:

- FAO provides energy for heart and liver at baseline, and for skeletal muscle during prolonged exercise.
- FAO produces ketones used by brain as energy source during prolonged fast.
- FAO supports gluconeogenesis by providing adenosine triphosphate (ATP), acetyl-CoA, and reduced electron carriers.
- The risk for hypoketotic hypoglycemia is highest when relying on FAO for energy (e.g., prolonged fast, infection).
- Buildup of long-chain fats is toxic to the liver, heart, and muscle cells and can result in acute liver injury, cardiomyopathy, or episodic rhabdomyolysis in times of catabolism or excess fat consumption.

CLINICAL MANIFESTATIONS

- Varies with syndrome
- Initial presenting symptoms include hypoketotic hypoglycemia, neonatal neurologic symptoms, coma, Reye-like syndrome, cardiac arrhythmia, cardiomyopathy, sudden death, rhabdomyolysis

DIAGNOSTICS

Decompensated Patient

- Dextrose stick, basic metabolic panel (BMP), hepatic function panel, ammonia (secondary hyperammonemia can be seen), CKP, plasma acylcarnitine profile, total and free carnitine
- Blood gas if concern for metabolic acidosis
- Urine for ketones, myoglobin (if blood is found on urinalysis), and organic acid profile
- Consider ECG, echocardiography.

Other Diagnostic Studies

- Acylcarnitine analysis as part of NBS may identify FAO disorders (FAOD) in many presymptomatic patients, but a normal NBS does not rule out FAOD.
- Molecular (DNA) diagnosis
- Enzyme assays on fibroblasts for some disorders

MANAGEMENT

Initial Acute Stabilization

Goals are to reverse hypoglycemia immediately, curtail anabolism, and treat associated morbidities:

- Place largest-gauge IV catheter possible immediately. Some patients require central access to enable sufficiently high dextrose infusion rates.
- Dextrose bolus if hypoglycemic, then start dextrose infusion with D10 plus age-appropriate electrolytes at $1.5\times$ the maintenance rate. Insulin surge after dextrose infusion inhibits further lipolysis.
- Use caution with fluid volumes if patient has a known history of cardiomyopathy or exam findings are consistent with heart failure.
- Saline boluses if dehydrated, but should not delay establishing euglycemia
- Do *not* use intralipids.

Chronic Management

- Carnitine supplementation for primary carnitine deficiency (e.g., carnitine transporter defect). Sometimes used in other FAODs, but benefit is controversial.
- For disorders affecting long-chain FAO: Low-fat, high-carbohydrate diet, limit long-chain fatty acid intake. Diet is unrestricted in medium- and short-chain disorders.
- For disorders affecting long-chain FAO: Supplement diet with medium-chain triglycerides (2–3 g/kg/day for infants; 1 g/kg/day in older children).
- Strategies to avoid hypoglycemia include frequent or continuous feeds, evening snacks with glucose polymers (e.g., corn starch), and close clinical monitoring during intercurrent illness.
- Immunizations are not contraindicated, but frequent feeds and prophylactic antipyretics are recommended to reduce catabolism associated with febrile reactions. Particularly fragile patients may need IV fluids before and after immunizations.
- Any procedure requiring sedation and a period of nothing by mouth requires admission for IV fluids before the procedure.

SPECIFIC DISORDERS

Important diagnostic laboratory studies for each entity are given in Table 17-2.

TABLE 17-2 Diagnostic Values of FAODs and Disorders of Ketone Metabolism

Disorder	Acylcarnitine Profile	Urine Organic Acids	Plasma-Free Carnitine
Short-chain acyl-CoA dehydrogenase deficiency	↑ C4	Ethylmalonate, methylsuccinate, butyrylglycine	Normal or ↓
Short-chain L-3-hydroxyacyl-CoA dehydrogenase deficiency	↑ C4-OH	Usually normal or 3-hydroxybutyric acid	Usually normal
Medium-chain acyl-CoA dehydrogenase deficiency	↑ C6:0, C8:0, C10:1	Hexanoylglycine medium-chain dicarboxylic acids and acylglycines	Normal to ↓
Carnitine/acylcarnitine translocase deficiency	↑ Esters of 16–18 carbons	Normal or ↑ dicarboxylic acids	↓
Carnitine transporter defect	↓ all species, especially C2	Normal or ↑ dicarboxylic acids	↓ (with paradoxical ↑ urine carnitine)
Carnitine palmitoyltransferase I deficiency	↓ Long-chain esters	Normal	Normal or ↑ with high free carnitine: (C16+C18) ratio
Carnitine palmitoyltransferase II deficiency	↑ Esters of 16–18 carbon length	Normal or ↑ dicarboxylic acids	↓
Mitochondrial trifunctional protein deficiency and long-chain-3-hydroxyacyl-CoA dehydrogenase deficiency	↑ C16OH, C18OH +/− C16, C18	Normal or ↑ dicarboxylic acids	Usually ↓
Very-long-chain acyl-CoA dehydrogenase deficiency	↑ C14:1	Normal or ↑ dicarboxylic acids	Normal or ↓
Multiple acyl-CoA dehydrogenase deficiency*	Multiple increased species, including a subset of C4, C6, C8, C10:1 and C14:1 in conjunction with C5DC	Subset of findings in SCAD, MCAD, VLCAD plus at least one of: glutarate, 2-hydroxyglutarate, isovalerylglycine and/or isobutyrylglycine	Normal or ↓
Beta-ketothiolase deficiency†	↑ C5:1, ↑ C5-OH or normal	Variable, but may have increased 2-methylacetoacetate, 2-butanone, 2-methyl-3-hydroxybutyrate	Usually normal
Succinyl-CoA: 3-ketoacid-CoA transferase deficiency	Normal	Normal or ↑ ketones, may have dicarboxylic acids	Normal

*Also known as glutaric aciduria type II.
†Also known as methylacetoacetyl-CoA thiolase deficiency and T2 deficiency.

MEDIUM-CHAIN ACYL-CoA DEHYDROGENASE (MCAD) DEFICIENCY

A mitochondrial FAOD affecting β-oxidation of medium-chain (e.g., 4–12 carbon length) fatty acids, causing fasting- or stress-induced episodes of hypoketotic hypoglycemia associated with emesis/lethargy.

- Patients who are diagnosed on newborn screen are typically asymptomatic between episodes of hypoglycemia.
- Exclusively breastfed neonates with MCAD have had increased rates of perinatal death; supplementing with formula or pumped breast milk to ensure adequate caloric intake is recommended.
- Unchecked catabolism may lead to severe hypoglycemia, arrhythmia and death, especially in undiagnosed patients.
- Hepatic steatosis generally improves after resolution of decompensation, but acylcarnitine profile is abnormal between episodes in some patients
- Long-term manifestations are unusual, but may include developmental disabilities and seizure disorder resulting from recurrent hypoglycemia especially in patients with delayed diagnosis.
- Newborn screen acylcarnitine analyses detect MCAD deficiency in presymptomatic individuals.

SHORT-CHAIN ACYL-CoA DEHYDROGENASE (SCAD) DEFICIENCY

A mitochondrial FAOD affecting β-oxidation of short-chain (e.g., 4–6 carbon length) fatty acids. The clinical course is incompletely defined. Patients diagnosed on newborn screen are almost exclusively asymptomatic.

- No specific dietary interventions are recommended.

SHORT-CHAIN L-3-HYDROXYACYL-CoA DEHYDROGENASE (SCAHD) DEFICIENCY

A mitochondrial FAOD affecting β-oxidation of short-chain (e.g., 4–6 carbon length) fatty acids. Although the FAOD itself is asymptomatic, hyperinsulinemic hypoglycemia results from a secondary function of the SCHAD enzyme in the insulin secretory pathway. See "Hyperinsulinism" section.

LONG-CHAIN FATTY ACID OXIDATION DISORDERS

Included in this category are disorders that affect metabolism of all chain lengths because the majority of dietary fats are long-chain.

CARNITINE/ACYLCARNITINE TRANSLOCASE DEFICIENCY

A mitochondrial FAOD affecting transport of acylcarnitines across the inner mitochondrial membrane, limiting ability to use fat as an energy source. Long-chain fatty acylcarnitine and free fatty acid accumulation may contribute to the clinical picture.

- Two clinical subtypes exist:
  - ✓ Severe: Neonatal onset hypoketotic hypoglycemia, hypertrophic cardiomyopathy, ventricular arrhythmias, hyperammonemia, myoglobinuria
  - ✓ Mild: Fasting- or stress-induced hypoketotic hypoglycemia

CARNITINE TRANSPORTER DEFECT

The transporter defect impairs transport of carnitine across cytoplasmic membranes into the cell. This results in reduced renal conservation of carnitine (leading to reduced serum carnitine levels) and decreased intracellular carnitine levels (especially muscle cells), both of which contribute to the impairment of FAO.

• Clinical manifestations include hypertrophic cardiomyopathy, progressive cardiac failure, skeletal muscle weakness, and hypoketotic hypoglycemia

CARNITINE PALMITOYLTRANSFERASE I DEFICIENCY

A mitochondrial FAOD affecting conversion of fatty acyl-CoA esters to acylcarnitine. Defective mitochondrial fatty acid import reduces or abolishes ability to use fat as an energy source. The first episode of decompensation usually occurs in infancy or early childhood.

• Manifestations include hypoketotic hypoglycemia, hepatomegaly, and hepatic encephalopathy (Reye syndrome).

CARNITINE PALMITOYLTRANSFERASE II DEFICIENCY

A mitochondrial FAOD affecting mitochondrial import of long-chain fatty acids, resulting in defective conversion of acylcarnitines to fatty acyl CoA.

• Three clinical subtypes are defined by age at onset of symptoms:
  ✓ Myopathic: Episodic muscle weakness, myalgia and rhabdomyolysis after prolonged exercise or other stressors, starting variably in the first to sixth decade; CKP may normalize between episodes.
  ✓ Lethal neonatal: Fatal multiorgan system disease, including hypoglycemia, hepatic and renal insufficiency, congenital malformations (including neuronal migration defects), and death, often in the neonatal period
  ✓ Infantile: Hypoglycemia, hypotonia, hepatic dysfunction, hepatomegaly, cardiomegaly, and seizures

MITOCHONDRIAL TRIFUNCTIONAL PROTEIN DEFICIENCY AND LONG-CHAIN-3-HYDROXYACYL CoA DEHYDROGENASE DEFICIENCY

Mitochondrial FAOD affecting β-oxidation of long-chain fatty acids. For long-chain (12–16 carbon length) fatty acids, one protein (mitochondrial trifunctional protein) carries out the hydratase, 3-hydroxyacyl-CoA dehydrogenase, and thiolase reactions. Some variants affect all three activities, while others affect only the dehydrogenase. Impaired ability to oxidize long-chain fatty acids severely compromises use of fat as an energy source.

• Isolated long-chain 3-hydroxyacyl-CoA dehydrogenase (LCHAD) deficiency is associated with hypoketotic hypoglycemia, fulminant hepatic disease, hypertrophic cardiomyopathy, episodic rhabdomyolysis, peripheral neuropathy, and pigmentary retinopathy.
• Mitochondrial trifunctional protein (TFP) deficiency manifests as hypoketotic hypoglycemia, dilated cardiomyopathy, episodic rhabdomyolysis, and hypotonia.
• Pregnant mothers carrying fetuses affected with TFP and/or LCHAD deficiencies have an increased incidence of acute fatty liver of pregnancy and HELLP (hemolysis, elevated liver enzymes, and low platelets) syndrome.

MULTIPLE ACYL CoA DEHYDROGENASE DEFICIENCY (GLUTARIC ACIDURIA TYPE II)

Multiple acyl-CoA dehydrogenase deficiency (MADD) affects transfer of electrons from fatty acyl-CoA to the electron-transport chain, resulting in FAOD. The block also affects oxidation of branched-chain amino acids (leucine, isoleucine, valine) and of glutaryl-CoA (an oxidation product of tryptophan, lysine, hydroxylysine).

• Three clinical subtypes exist:
  ✓ Neonatal onset with congenital anomalies: Prematurity, hypoglycemia, metabolic acidosis, hypotonia, hepatomegaly, cardiomegaly, polycystic kidneys, and genitourinary, skeletal, and craniofacial abnormalities

✓ Neonatal onset without congenital anomalies: Severe metabolic decompensation in first few days of life

✓ Later onset: Variable phenotype including metabolic decompensations and myopathy

VERY LONG-CHAIN ACYL-CoA DEHYDROGENASE DEFICIENCY

Pathogenic variants in *ACADVL*, the gene implicated in Very Long Chain AcylCoA Dehydrogenase (VLCAD) Deficiency, result in an impaired ability to oxidize fatty acids longer than 14 carbons in mitochondria and severely compromises use of fat as an energy source.

- Different clinical subtypes exist:
  ✓ Severe: Neonatal- or infantile-onset hypertrophic cardiomyopathy, hypoketotic hypoglycemia, and/or Reye-like syndrome
  ✓ Mild: Episodic hypoketotic hypoglycemia during stress or fasting, absent or later-onset cardiomyopathy
  ✓ Late-onset: Presentation in the second to third decade of life with muscle weakness and rhabdomyolysis after prolonged exercise or other stressors
- NBS acylcarnitine analyses have detected VLCAD in presymptomatic individuals; however, it is important to note that "late-onset" forms may be missed.

KETONE UTILIZATION DEFECTS

GENERAL PRINCIPLES

Class of disorders impairing the ability to utilize and clear ketone bodies.

EPIDEMIOLOGY

- Overall incidence about 1 in 1 million; autosomal recessive inheritance
- These conditions are likely underdiagnosed.

PATHOPHYSIOLOGY

Ketones that are synthesized are cleared inefficiently and unable to be utilized, resulting in energy failure in the fasted state and episodic ketoacidosis.

CLINICAL MANIFESTATIONS

- Stresses associated with ketosis (fasting, infection, dehydration) cause severe ketoacidosis
- Ketosis with or without hypoglycemia. Ketosis may persist in the absence of hypoglycemia and even in the face of hyperglycemia. These diseases are important to consider in the differential diagnosis for diabetic ketoacidosis as well as ketotic hypoglycemia.
- Ketoacidosis with Kussmaul respirations and anion gap metabolic acidosis
- Symptoms of ketoacidosis: Lethargy, fatigue, malaise, nausea, vomiting, anorexia
- Hypoglycemia-related complications: Seizures, mental status changes

DIAGNOSTICS

- BMP/anion gap, glucose, ketones
- Fasting is not necessary for diagnosis, but supervised safety fasts may be performed to determine the length of time patient can safely fast without developing dangerous ketoacidosis.
- Molecular (DNA) testing confirms suspicion.

MANAGEMENT

- Avoidance of fasting
- Ketogenic diet is absolutely contraindicated

- Sodium bicarbonate may be necessary for normalizing pH
- Any procedure requiring sedation and a period of nothing by mouth requires admission for IV fluids before procedure.

β-KETOTHIOLASE DEFICIENCY (METHYLACETOACETYL-CoA THIOLASE DEFICIENCY, T2 DEFICIENCY)

A rare defect affecting the interconversion of acetyl-CoA and acetoacetyl-CoA. Often there is clearing of ketones and absence of symptoms between episodes. Onset is typically in infancy or early childhood.

- Beta-ketothiolase deficiency is characterized by episodic ketoacidosis associated with headaches and malaise.
- Basal ganglia involvement including chorea and MRI abnormalities consistent with metabolic stroke have been reported in multiple patients.
- Urine organic acids may show subtle elevations in tiglylglycine and 2-methyl-3-hydroxybutyrate in some patients, but absence does not rule out disease.
- Rare cases may be identified by NBS.

SUCCINYL-CoA:3-OXOACID-CoA TRANSFERASE (SCOT) DEFICIENCY

A defect affecting the addition of a CoA body to acetoacetate to make acetoacetyl-CoA. This is the first step in ketolysis and is necessary for any ketolysis to occur. Half of patients present in the neonatal period, with the remainder presenting mostly in early childhood.

- Permanent ketosis/ketonuria is pathognomonic, but not universal
- Even patients with permanent ketosis are asymptomatic between episodes of deterioration.

UREA-CYCLE DEFECTS (UCDS)

GENERAL PRINCIPLES

Class of metabolic diseases in which an enzyme deficiency compromises activity of the urea cycle, which normally functions to remove waste nitrogen as urea. Commonly present with hyperammonemia.

ETIOLOGY

- Pathogenic variants in urea-cycle enzymes, including carbamoyl phosphate synthetase (CPS), OTC, argininosuccinic acid synthetase (ASAS), argininosuccinic acid lyase (ASAL), and arginase
- Pathogenic variants in the transporters necessary for urea cycle substrates entering and exiting the mitochondrion: hyperornithinemia-hyperammonemia-homocitrullinuria (HHH) syndrome (mitochondrial ornithine transporter deficiency); citrin deficiency (aspartate–glutamate transporter)
- OTC deficiency is an X-linked disease. Other UCDs are autosomal recessive.

EPIDEMIOLOGY

- Overall prevalence of UCDs: About 1 in 30,000
- Most common is OTC deficiency: About 1 in 40,000

PATHOPHYSIOLOGY

- The urea cycle is a major mechanism for ammonia (NH_3) clearance by converting it to water-soluble urea.

- Decompensation states occur during "nitrogen imbalance," when the nitrogen load exceeds excretion ability, resulting in hyperammonemia.
- Conditions of increased nitrogen load include high-protein diets, muscle catabolism (induced by fasting, stress, or exercise), and medicines that increase protein turnover.
- Ammonia-stimulated hyperventilation causes respiratory alkalosis.
- Hyperammonemia increases tryptophan transport across the blood–brain barrier, enhancing serotonin production. Intracerebral glutamine also accumulates, contributing to cerebral edema. The overall effect is an encephalopathy that can include somnolence and coma.

CLINICAL MANIFESTATIONS

- Great variability in clinical spectrum
- Episodic decompensations with hyperammonemia; cerebral edema, encephalopathy (lethargy, seizures, coma), respiratory alkalosis, other acid–base disturbances
- Neonatal clinical presentation may mimic sepsis.
- Older patients: Poor appetite, cyclical vomiting, psychosis
- On exam, focus on airway, breathing, circulation (ABCs), hydration status, mental status, neurologic exam, and possible sources of infection.
- Unexplained tachypnea may be due to hyperammonemia.

DIAGNOSTICS

- NBS programs detect some UCDs in presymptomatic patients; however, OTC and CPS are *not* detected by this screening. Additionally, decompensation in severe cases typically precedes the results of the newborn screen.
- Neonatal presentation is similar to that for sepsis or meningitis, so it is important to check ammonia levels in septic-appearing newborns.

Decompensated Patient (Initial Hyperammonemic Episode)

- NH_3 should be checked urgently; sample should be drawn on free-flowing blood, without a tourniquet, and placed on ice.
- The initial approach to the differential diagnosis of hyperammonemia includes ruling out sepsis, organic acidopathies, and FAO defects. Send for CBC and differential counts, blood culture, inflammatory markers, measurement of arterial blood gases (ABG); dextrose stick; BMP/anion gap; liver-function tests (LFTs); prothrombin/partial thromboplastin (PT/PTT); plasma amino acids; plasma lactate/pyruvate; plasma acylcarnitine profile, total and free carnitine. These studies help determine the cause of hyperammonemia and evaluate for comorbidities of diseases in the differential diagnosis.
- Urine for urinalysis, organic acids, and orotic acid; urine amino acid analysis
- If UCD is confirmed, brain MRI should be performed once stable to ascertain degree of neurologic damage.

Decompensated Patient (Known UCD)

- NH_3, dextrose stick, basic metabolic panel/anion gap, plasma amino acids

Definitive Diagnostics

- Amino acid profile is diagnostic in some UCDs (ASAL, ASAS deficiency), urine orotic acid, molecular (DNA) analysis, enzyme analysis

	Children (mg/kg)			Adolescents/Adults (g/m²)		
Diagnosis	**Sodium Phenylacetate**	**Sodium Benzoate**	**Arg-HCl**	**Sodium Phenylacetate**	**Sodium Benzoate**	**Arg-HCl**
Presumed UCD	250	250	600			
CPS/ OTC	250	250	200	5.5	5.5	4.0
ASAS/ ASAL	250	250	600	5.5	5.5	12

TABLE 17-3 IV Nitrogen-Scavenging Agents*

*Dose size is same for load and maintenance infusion. Deliver loading dose over 90 minutes, then start every 24-hour continuous infusion.

Arg-HCl = arginine-HCl; ASAL = argininosuccinic acid lyase deficiency; ASAS = argininosuccinic acid synthetase deficiency; CPS = carbamoyl phosphate synthetase deficiency; OTC = ornithine transcarbamylase deficiency; UCD = urea-cycle disorder.

MANAGEMENT (DECOMPENSATED PATIENT)

- ABCs/fluid management: Ventilatory and pressor support, wide-gauge IV (consider central access), start IV infusion with 12.5% dextrose in water for neonates (add half or normal saline and potassium in older patients) at 1.5× maintenance rate. Titrate dextrose concentration or rate of infusion upward as necessary until ammonia decreases to stop catabolism. As high as 15–20% dextrose at 1.5× maintenance may be necessary. Do not decrease glucose-infusion rate (GIR) in the acutely ill patient. If hyperglycemia develops (glucose persistently >150 mg/dL), begin insulin drip at 0.05–0.1 unit/kg/hr and titrate to target glucose of 100–150 mg/dL.
- Bulk NH_3 removal: Dialysis may be necessary, especially if ammonia exceeds 500 umol/L or is rising despite medical management. Consider consults with nephrology and critical care and IV nitrogen-scavenging agents (Table 17-3).
- Reversal of catabolic state: Stop protein feeds. dextrose infusion as above. consider insulin drip. consider intralipids. Amino acids must be provided within 24–48 hours or protein turnover will persist. For total parenteral nutrition, start with 1–1.5 g amino acids/kg/day; if tolerating enteral feeds, use protein-free formula with gradual reintroduction of protein (may need nasogastric tube).
- Laboratory monitoring during critical phase: ABGs every 4 hours or as indicated for intubated patients; BMP every 4 hours; NH_3 every hour until <300 umol/L; plasma amino acids may be helpful daily or every few days if rapid turnaround time is available (use to determine adequate citrulline/arginine as below, monitor protein intake status); other laboratory studies as indicated for dialysis patients
- Transition/home management: Enteral nitrogen scavengers include sodium phenylbutyrate or glycerol phenylbutyrate and sodium benzoate; some patients require citrulline (CPS, OTC deficiency) or arginine (ASAS, ASAL deficiency) therapy; routine monitoring of nutritional markers, plasma amino acids, NH_3; consider gastric tube (G-tube) placement, especially for neurologically impaired patients; normal immunization schedule with prophylactic antipyretics. For procedures requiring sedation and period of nothing by mouth, consider admission for IV fluids before procedure; liver transplantation is curative for some patients.

SPECIFIC UREA-CYCLE DEFECTS

ARGINASE DEFICIENCY (ARGININEMIA)

Arginase catalyzes the cytoplasmic production of ornithine and urea from arginine. Arginase deficiency causes arginine elevation and increases risk for hyperammonemia as well as toxic effects of arginine and its derived compounds. Unlike other UCDs, arginase deficiency presents primarily as a chronic neurologic disorder with progressive spastic diplegia/quadriplegia, ataxia, and choreoathetosis.

- Episodic hyperammonemic episodes can occur, but are less prominent than those in other UCDs.
- Diagnosis is confirmed by plasma amino acid profile, which shows elevated arginine.
- Urinary orotic acid is also increased.

ARGININOSUCCINIC ACID LYASE DEFICIENCY

ASAL catalyzes the cytoplasmic production of arginine from argininosuccinic acid. In ASAL deficiency, citrulline accumulates and arginine becomes an essential amino acid.

- Hepatomegaly and hepatic dysfunction/fibrosis may develop.
- Diagnosis is confirmed by plasma amino acid profile, which shows elevated citrulline and argininosuccinate with decreased arginine.
- Many patients have developmental delay and cognitive impairment (independent of control of hyperammonemia) as well as trichorrhexis nodosa (coarse, brittle hair that breaks easily).
- The presence of argininosuccinate esters on plasma or urine amino acids is pathognomonic.
- Urinary orotic acid is also increased.

ARGININOSUCCINIC ACID SYNTHETASE DEFICIENCY (CITRULLINEMIA TYPE I)

ASAS catalyzes the cytoplasmic production of argininosuccinic acid from citrulline and aspartic acid. In ASAS deficiency, citrulline accumulates (hence, its historic name of citrullinemia) and arginine becomes an essential amino acid.

- Plasma amino acids reveal elevated citrulline and decreased arginine.
- Urinary orotic acid is also increased.

CARBAMOYL PHOSPHATE SYNTHETASE DEFICIENCY

CPS catalyzes production of carbamoyl phosphate from NH_3, HCO_3^-, and ATP. Citrulline and arginine, downstream urea-cycle products, become essential amino acids.

- Diagnosis is confirmed by plasma amino acid profile, which shows elevated glutamine with decreased citrulline and arginine.
- Urinary orotic acid is normal; this key feature distinguishes CPS deficiency from OTC deficiency.
- Carglumic acid, a CPS activator, should be considered as a treatment option.

ORNITHINE TRANSCARBAMYLASE DEFICIENCY (ORNITHINE CARBAMOYLTRANSFERASE DEFICIENCY)

OTC is an enzyme encoded on the X chromosome, which catalyzes the entry step into the urea cycle. Citrulline and arginine, downstream urea-cycle products, become essential amino acids.

- Classic presentation is a male neonate, well at birth, with progressive emesis, feed refusal, and encephalopathy within a few days. Seizures occur in approximately 50% of patients.

Female OTC deficiency carriers have varying degrees of symptomatology depending on X-inactivation pattern in hepatocytes. Older patients may present with cyclic vomiting or behavior disturbances rather than frank metabolic decompensation
- Diagnosis is confirmed by plasma amino acid profile, which shows elevated glutamine and decreased citrulline and arginine.
- Urinary orotic acid is also increased.

DEFECTS OF AMINO ACID METABOLISM

HEREDITARY TYROSINEMIA TYPE 1

Hereditary tyrosinemia type 1 (HT1) is an inborn error of tyrosine (tyr) metabolism causing progressive liver and renal failure. It is due to mutations in the *FAH* gene, which encodes fumarylacetoacetate hydrolase, the terminal enzyme in tyr metabolism.

EPIDEMIOLOGY

- Incidence about 1 in 100,000; autosomal recessive inheritance
- Incidence much higher in the Lac-St. Jean region of Quebec

PATHOPHYSIOLOGY

- Tyr metabolism is both ketogenic (producing acetoacetate) and gluconeogenic (producing fumarate). Tyr metabolism occurs in the hepatocyte and the proximal renal tubule.
- Elevated tyr is due to inhibition of downstream biochemical steps and does not contribute to liver or renal injury.
- Blockade at the fumarylacetoacetate hydrolase (FAH) step causes an accumulation of fumarylacetoacetate (FAA), an alkylating agent that promotes apoptosis and alters gene expression, resulting in hepatocyte damage.
- Accumulation of succinylacetone, a byproduct of FAA, contributes to renal Fanconi syndrome.
- Hypoglycemia may result from hepatic dysfunction, reduced availability of gluconeogenic precursors, and decreased expression of genes required for glucose production.
- Porphyria crises may occur because succinylacetone inhibits δ-aminolevulinic acid dehydratase in the heme synthetic pathway.
- FAA's mutagenic activity may contribute to the development of hepatocellular carcinoma.

CLINICAL MANIFESTATIONS

- Hepatic failure is progressive if untreated, usually beginning in the neonatal period or early infancy. Patients may present with acute hepatic crises, with hypoalbuminemia, ascites, and jaundice.
- High risk for cirrhosis and hepatocellular carcinoma if untreated
- Coagulopathy due to compromised liver synthetic function may be the first symptom, sometimes manifested by gastrointestinal bleeding.
- Proximal renal tubular dysfunction often presents as a renal Fanconi syndrome.
- Symptoms due to attacks of porphyria include painful peripheral neuropathy, hypertonia, abdominal pain, and autonomic instability.
- Causes of death include liver failure, hemorrhage, respiratory arrest (during porphyria episodes), and hepatocellular carcinoma

DIAGNOSTICS

- Plasma amino acids may reveal elevated tyr, phenylalanine (phe), and methionine. Definitive diagnosis requires demonstration of succinylacetone on urine organic acid quantitation or on filter-paper blood specimens. FAH enzyme activity and genetic testing can be used for confirmation.
- There are multiple other conditions (e.g., transient tyrosinemia of the newborn) that can cause elevated tyr; it is important not to make a diagnosis of tyrosinemia 1 on the basis of elevated tyr on NBS alone.
- Elevation in alpha-fetoprotein may predate elevated tyr levels
- Tyr is often not severely elevated, so the sensitivity of newborn screening is poor in the several states that do not measure succinylacetone
- Check coagulation studies and other markers of liver synthetic function. Hepatic transaminases may or may not be elevated.

MANAGEMENT

- 2-(2-nitro-4-trifluoromethyl-benzoyl)-1,3-cyclohexanedione (NTBC, nitisinone) inhibits 4-HPPD, an upstream step in tyr metabolism, reducing production of FAA and succinylacetone. NTBC decreases risk of liver failure and hepatocellular carcinoma. Starting dose is 1 mg/kg/day orally divided twice daily, adjusted for biochemical control
- NTBC treatment increases blood tyr and phe levels, so treated patients require dietary restriction of these amino acids.
- NTBC can cause corneal erosions and other ocular abnormalities, especially if dietary control is poor, so baseline and routine ophthalmologic exams are indicated.
- Liver transplantation is an option for NTBC-nonresponders.

MAPLE SYRUP URINE DISEASE

Maple syrup urine disease (MSUD) is caused by autosomal recessive mutations in branched-chain ketoacid dehydrogenase, resulting in decreased ability to process branched-chain amino acids (leucine, isoleucine, and valine). Inheritance is autosomal recessive.

EPIDEMIOLOGY

- Overall incidence is 1 in 185,000; however, it is as common as 1 in 400 in certain Mennonite populations.

PATHOPHYSIOLOGY

- Three genes (*BCKDHA, BCKDHB, DBT*) are known to cause MSUD.
- Accumulation of branched-chain amino acids interferes with entry of other large neutral amino acids into the brain.
- Accumulated branched-chain ketoacids result in depletion of brain glutamate and glutamine.

CLINICAL MANIFESTATIONS

Patients may be diagnosed on NBS before symptoms develop. Even when detected on screening and infant is placed on good dietary control, episodic deterioration may occur, especially with intercurrent illness.

- Episodic encephalopathy or coma is associated with cerebral edema; it is related to elevated leucine levels.

- Characteristic "maple syrup" odor (due to branched-chain ketoacid production) is detectable in urine and cerumen when there is poor dietary control.
- Mild intellectual impairment in comparison to family, even when well-controlled.

DIAGNOSTICS

- Most patients are detected on NBS.
- Plasma amino acids show elevations of leucine, isoleucine, and valine, as well as alloisoleucine, whose presence is pathognomonic for MSUD.
- Urine organic acids show branched-chain ketoacids.

MANAGEMENT

- Dietary management with restriction of branched-chain amino acids.
- May require hospital admission for dextrose-containing IV fluids and close dietary management during intercurrent illness or with symptoms of elevated leucine levels (altered mental status, lethargy, ataxia).
- Patients experiencing leucine encephalopathy *may not* exhibit any abnormalities on routine labs (e.g., no acidosis, ketonuria, or hyperammonemia). In centers where plasma amino acids cannot be checked rapidly, treatment should be initiated on the basis of clinical symptoms.
- Urine dipsticks can be provided to families to monitor at home for ketonuria, which can indicate increased branched-chain amino acids and metabolic decompensation. Note that point-of-care blood ketone monitors typically detect only beta-hydroxybutyrate, so are not useful in this setting.
- Thiamine: 25–100 mg/day. Cofactor for branched-chain ketoacid decarboxylase. Few patients respond; trial for approximately 4 weeks
- Liver transplantation is used for severe or refractory cases.

PHENYLKETONURIA

Phenylketonuria (PKU) is an inborn error of phe metabolism associated with intellectual disability. Mutations in the gene encoding phe hydroxylase (PAH) account for most cases. Inheritance is autosomal recessive.

EPIDEMIOLOGY

- Overall incidence in American children is 1 in 15,000

PATHOPHYSIOLOGY

- Increased phe interferes with large neutral amino acid transport in both directions across the blood–brain barrier.
- Altered amino acid transport probably affects central nervous system (CNS) protein and neurotransmitter (especially dopamine, serotonin) synthesis.
- Phe is hydroxylated to form tyr, a precursor of melanin. Relative underpigmentation (lighter hair and skin than family members) of PKU patients reflects decreased tyr availability.

CLINICAL MANIFESTATIONS

Due to newborn screening, PKU patients are now diagnosed before symptoms develop. Historically, abnormalities included seizures, infantile spasms, increased tone/spasticity, and microcephaly.

- Patients detected on screening and put on lifelong good dietary control may still have subtle learning-style and behavioral differences, including increased incidence of attention-deficit/hyperactivity disorder.
- Tics, parkinsonism, and behavior abnormalities occur in poorly controlled patients.
- Light pigmentation of hair, skin, eyes
- Eczema in 20–40%
- Urinary phenylacetic acid causes the classic "mousy odor."

DIAGNOSTICS

- All U.S. neonates are now screened for elevated phe levels.
- Confirmatory testing requires plasma amino acid quantitation to verify elevated phe and to determine the phe:tyr ratio. A phe:tyr ratio greater than 3:1 reflects a state of hyperphenylalaninemia.

MANAGEMENT

- Early treatment is associated with better neurodevelopmental outcomes. Dietary therapy should begin immediately after diagnosis, by the end of the first week of life if possible. Dietary management is recommended in patients with phe levels persistently above 6 mg/dL (360 mcmol/L). Phe-reduced formulas and foods form the basis of dietary therapy. Patients also take a small amount of complete protein to provide requisite amounts of phe and tyr.
- Goal phe level is controversial, but many experts agree that 2–6 mg/dL (120–360 mcmol/L) are acceptable levels.
- Phe restriction is lifelong. Previous liberalization of diet in adults was hypothesized to result in mild cognitive changes.
- Kuvan (sapropterin) is a synthetic cofactor for the PAH enzyme, which also acts as a chaperone to stabilize the protein and increase enzyme activity. It is most effective in patients who have residual enzyme activity and may allow liberalization of diet.
- A new injectable enzyme replacement therapy (Palynziq, pegvaliase-pqpz) has been approved by the Food and Drug Administration (FDA) for adults with PKU, but requires careful initiation and monitoring because of the high risk of anaphylaxis.
- Mothers with PKU need strict dietary control before and during pregnancy. Poor first-trimester control increases fetal risk for microcephaly, mental retardation, and congenital heart disease.

DEFECTS OF CARBOHYDRATE METABOLISM

GALACTOSEMIA

Galactosemia is an inborn error of galactose metabolism resulting in toxicity after ingestion of lactose or galactose. Mutations may occur in any of three genes involved in galactose metabolism: galactokinase, galactose-1-phosphate uridyltransferase (GALT), and uridine diphosphate-galactose 4′ epimerase. GALT deficiency accounts for the majority of cases. "Classical" galactosemia is caused by severe GALT deficiency (<5% activity). Partial, or Duarte, GALT deficiency (10–25%) is more common and is benign.

EPIDEMIOLOGY

- Prevalence of classical galactosemia is 1 in 50,000.
- Inheritance is autosomal recessive.

PATHOPHYSIOLOGY

- Symptoms appear in neonates fed breast milk or cow's-milk formulas, both of which contain lactose, a disaccharide of glucose and galactose.
- In patients with GALT deficiency, galactose-1-phosphate (gal-1-P) accumulates. Hypoglycemia occurs because galactose cannot be converted to glucose and gal-1-P inhibits phosphoglucomutase, an enzyme required for glycogenolysis.

CLINICAL MANIFESTATIONS

- NBS has allowed for detection of presymptomatic individuals.
- Affected children are well at birth, with symptoms appearing in a few days.
- In a U.S. series following galactosemic neonates: 89% had symptoms from hepatocellular damage (jaundice, hepatomegaly, ascites, transaminitis, hyperammonemia, and coagulopathy), 76% had food intolerance (poor feeding, emesis), 29% had failure to thrive, 16% had lethargy, 10% had sepsis (usually *Escherichia coli*), and 1% had seizures.
- Other neonatal manifestations include hypoglycemia, renal Fanconi syndrome, and cataracts. Early death by sepsis, hepatic failure, or renal failure may occur unless patient is diagnosed and treated.
- Long-term sequelae include developmental delay, speech dyspraxia, cataracts, and premature ovarian insufficiency even in children with disorder well-controlled on diet.

DIAGNOSTICS

- While NBS may be highly sensitive for galactosemia, in some states, the methodology precludes diagnosis in children on lactose-free formulas. Additionally, many newborns become symptomatic before the diagnosis is reported by the laboratory, underscoring the need to recognize the clinical picture.
- Evaluation of a sick neonate in whom galactosemia is suspected: Dextrose stick, BMP, blood culture, LFTs, PT/PTT, ammonia, urine for reducing substances, urine galactitol, erythrocyte gal-1-P, GALT activity (whole blood or dried sample on filter paper)
- Evaluation of an asymptomatic neonate referred because of a presumptive positive NBS result: Urine galactitol, erythrocyte gal-1-P, GALT activity
- Interpretation of GALT activity: <5% = classical galactosemia; 10–25% = Duarte/galactosemia (D/G); 50% = galactosemia carrier (benign); 75–90% = Duarte carrier (benign)

MANAGEMENT

- In sick neonates, discontinue feeds, reverse hypoglycemia if present, and begin dextrose infusion. Fresh-frozen plasma may be needed to correct coagulopathy.
- In asymptomatic neonates with a NBS positive for galactosemia (decreased GALT *and* increased galactose level), consider stopping galactose-containing feeds pending confirmation and start non–galactose-containing formula (e.g., soy-based). If the screen is equivocal (e.g., in states that test both GALT activity and galactose, a finding of elevated galactose with normal GALT activity), it may be permissible to continue breastfeeding while awaiting confirmation. Feeding decisions are best made in consultation with a geneticist.
- Long-term management of classical galactosemia includes avoidance of dietary galactose (dairy products and some other foods). Calcium supplementation is important. International guidelines for management of classical galactosemia have been published (*J Inherit Metab Dis* 2017;40:171–176). Consultation with a clinical nutritionist is helpful.

- In galactokinase deficiency, which causes isolated cataracts, elimination of dairy products alone is sufficient treatment.
- Severe epimerase-deficiency galactosemia is difficult to treat because deficiency impairs not only production of glucose from galactose, but also galactose biosynthesis, which is necessary for processing of some proteins and lipids.
- The Duarte allele (specific known sequence changes within the *GALT* gene) reduces the enzyme activity of the GALT enzyme, but not as severely as classic disease. Many centers do not modify diet for children with a Duarte allele with or without a classic allele (D/D or D/G galactosemia).

HEREDITARY FRUCTOSE INTOLERANCE

Hereditary fructose intolerance is an inborn error in metabolism resulting in toxicity after fructose ingestion. It is due to a pathogenic variant in the gene encoding aldolase B, an enzyme required for conversion of fructose to glucose. Exposure to fructose, sucrose (a glucose–fructose disaccharide), or sorbitol causes symptoms to occur.

EPIDEMIOLOGY

- In the United Kingdom, about 1% carry a common disease-causing allele and 1 in 20,000 are homozygous.
- Inheritance is autosomal recessive.

CLINICAL MANIFESTATIONS

- Most affected infants are asymptomatic until solid foods are initiated, when they are exposed to sucrose or fructose, usually around 6 months of age. However, some formula contains fructose, so symptoms may present earlier.
- Symptoms include abdominal pain, vomiting, severe hypoglycemia (diaphoresis, lethargy, seizures, coma), hepatotoxicity (jaundice, coagulopathy, ascites), elevated uric acid, and renal Fanconi syndrome.
- Untreated disease progresses to chronic hepatic and renal failure.

PATHOPHYSIOLOGY

- Aldolase B deficiency primarily affects hepatocytes, mucosa of the small intestine, and the proximal renal tubules, major sites of aldolase B expression. Aldolase B cleaves fructose-1-phosphate (F-1-P) into 3-carbon products that can be used for glycolysis, glycogen synthesis, or gluconeogenesis.
- Aldolase B deficiency leads to accumulation of F-1-P and depletion of phosphate sources, especially inorganic phosphate (P_i) and ATP P_i depletion activates purine degradation, resulting in hyperuricemia. F-1-P accumulation prevents glycogen breakdown and gluconeogenesis, contributing to hypoglycemia. Inhibition of gluconeogenesis causes precursors (e.g., lactate, pyruvate) to accumulate, resulting in metabolic acidosis, which is compounded by proximal renal tubular dysfunction.

DIAGNOSTICS

- Blood glucose; comprehensive metabolic panel (assess K, HCO_3, BUN, Cr), phosphate, liver-function tests; PT/PTT; uric acid
- Urine for reducing substances (sugars) and amino acids
- Definitive diagnosis is based on DNA analysis. The IV fructose challenge test is dangerous and therefore no longer recommended.

MANAGEMENT

- Sick patient after fructose exposure: ABCs; establish IV access; treat hypoglycemia, metabolic acidosis, and electrolyte abnormalities (especially hypophosphatemia)
- Long-term management: Avoid fructose and fructose-containing sugars, including sucrose and sorbitol. Consultation with a clinical nutritionist is helpful.
- Sources of sucrose (table sugar) include candies/desserts, canned foods, and soft drinks,
- Sources of fructose include fresh fruits, raw vegetables, new potatoes, whole flour, brown rice, and some infant formulas.
- Sources of sorbitol include some medications and diabetes products.

ORGANIC ACIDEMIAS

Organic acidemias (also known as organic acidurias) are a group of metabolic disorders due to inborn enzyme deficiencies in metabolism of amino acids to allow entrance to the tricarboxylic acid (TCA) cycle, leading to accumulation of non-amino organic acids. Mutations in the genes encoding a variety of enzymes cause these disorders.

- Propionyl-CoA carboxylase (propionic acidemia [PA])
- Methylmalonyl-CoA mutase (methylmalonic acidemia [MMA])
- Isovaleryl-CoA dehydrogenase (isovaleric acidemia [IVA])
- 3-methylcrotonyl-CoA carboxylase (3-methylcrotonyl-CoA carboxylase deficiency [3-MCCD])
- Glutaryl-CoA dehydrogenase (glutaric acidemia type 1 [GA1])

EPIDEMIOLOGY

- Prevalence: PA, 1 in 100,000; MMA, 1 in 80,000; IVA, 1 in 100,000; 3-MCCD, 1 in 40,000; GA1, 1 in 100,000
- Autosomal recessive inheritance

DIFFERENTIAL DIAGNOSIS

In patients with acidosis and neurologic dysfunction, consider:

- Nonmetabolic causes: Sepsis, renal tubular acidosis, congenital cardiovascular or pulmonary malformation, hypocalcemia, other electrolyte abnormalities, toxins, intracranial bleed
- Metabolic causes: Biotinidase deficiency and holocarboxylase synthetase deficiency (which have secondary effects on the carboxylases above), cobalamin metabolism disorders (intersects with MMA pathway), primary lactic acidosis syndromes

PATHOPHYSIOLOGY

- Enzyme deficiency causes organic acid accumulation and, consequently, a variety of toxic effects on cellular function.
- Organic acid accumulation inhibits metabolic pathways, including ketogenesis, gluconeogenesis, and ureagenesis.
- Some organic acids also interfere with hematopoiesis.
- Decompensation occurs during states of catabolism (infection, fasting, exercise, other stress) or increased protein turnover (excess dietary protein, general anesthetics, steroids).

CLINICAL MANIFESTATIONS

Perform a comprehensive history and physical exam focusing on ABCs; hydration status; tachypnea (may be due to acidosis or hyperammonemia); complete neurologic exam, including

mental status; cardiac exam; epigastric tenderness (vomiting may be due to pancreatitis); superficial skin desquamation; source of infection (if febrile); and unusual odor in urine or breath.

Neonatal Presentation

Similar to sepsis; typically a full-term baby, well for the first few days, then with dramatic decompensation:

- Lethargy and progressive neurologic dysfunction (seizures, abnormal tone, unusual movements, coma)
- Poor feeding, hypoglycemia, metabolic acidosis, ketonuria (which is never a normal finding in a neonate), hyperammonemia
- Stroke-like episodes, typically of the bilateral basal ganglia, presenting as choreoathetoid or dystonic movements (especially GA1)
- Bone marrow suppression, pancreatitis
- Unusual odor of body fluids (such as "sweaty feet" odor in IVA)

Later Presentation

- Poor appetite, failure to thrive, preference for nonprotein foods
- Episodic vomiting, hypotonia, seizures
- Cardiomyopathy (especially PA)
- Chronic renal failure (especially MMA)
- Macrocephaly is seen in GA1 at birth or shortly thereafter; these patients can also present with spontaneous subdural hemorrhage (widening of Sylvian fissures and cerebral volume loss increases risk for tearing bridging veins).
- Global developmental delay, especially with regression

Episodic Decompensation

- Catabolic states can cause appearance, recurrence, or exacerbation of any of the previous signs or symptoms.

DIAGNOSTICS

- Newborn screening programs include an acylcarnitine profile.

Decompensated Patient (Initial Presentation)

- General sepsis workup: CBC with differential, blood culture, inflammatory markers
- NH_3, ABG with lactate, dextrose stick, basic metabolic panel/anion gap, LFTs, amylase/lipase in vomiting patient, plasma lactate/pyruvate
- Metabolic tests: Plasma amino acids; plasma acylcarnitine profile and total/free carnitine; urine for urinalysis, organic acids, and methylmalonic acid level
- Consider head CT if cerebral edema is suspected.
- Perform ECG and echocardiography for signs of cardiac failure.

Decompensated Patient (Known Organic Acidemia)

- Dextrose stick; BMP/anion gap; NH_3; CBC with differential; LFTs and lipase/amylase for vomiting/abdominal pain; plasma amino acids; urine for urinalysis, ABGs if unstable vital signs or clinical concern

Definitive Diagnostics

- Genetic testing

MANAGEMENT

- ABCs/fluid management: Ventilatory and pressor support as needed. Place widest-gauge IV. Most patients will need multiple access sites and some will require central venous access; start infusion with D10-based solution at 1.5× maintenance rate; monitor urine output.
- Reverse acidosis: Maintain HCO_3 at 22–25. If severely acidotic (pH <7.22 or HCO_3^- <14 mEq/L), give $NaHCO_3$ based on bicarbonate deficit. The bicarbonate deficit can be calculated as follows: (circulating volume correction factor [0.5 in neonates; 0.4 in other patients]) × (weight in kg) × ([desired HCO_3^- in mmol/L] – measured HCO_3^-] = bicarbonate deficit). Half of the bicarbonate deficit should be repleted within the first hour (typically as 1–2 mEq/kg boluses) and the remaining half over 24 hours. Minimize other sodium sources to prevent hypernatremia. Hemodialysis may be necessary for refractory acidosis or hyperammonemia. Tris(hydroxymethyl)aminomethane is contraindicated.
- Reverse catabolic state: Stop protein feeds; in patients unable to tolerate enteral feeds, start total parenteral nutrition *without amino acids,* with goal intake 20% above maintenance nutrition. Use 10% dextrose (1.5× maintenance rate) and intralipids (1–3 g/kg/day). Avoid decreasing GIR; dextrose concentration may be increased if volume needs to be decreased. Alternatively, should hyperglycemia develop (glucose persistently >150 mg/dL), begin insulin drip at 0.05–0.1 unit/kg/hr and titrate to a target glucose of 100–150 mg/dL. Hold amino acids for 24 hours, and then start gradual reintroduction; if tolerating enteral feeds, use protein-free formula with gradual reintroduction of protein using medical foods to supplement.
- Reverse hyperammonemia: Carglumic acid (Carbaglu), if available, is the preferred ammonia-targeting agent; otherwise, nitrogen-scavenging agents (as in UCDs) may be used. In severely ill patients, immediate consultations with nephrology to arrange dialysis and critical care are warranted.
- Laboratory monitoring during critical phase: ABGs at least every 4 hours; BMP every 4 hours; NH_3 every 2–4 hours until less than 300 mcmmol/L; daily plasma amino acids (if turnaround time is rapid, can use to adjust protein intake); daily CBC count with differential; other laboratory studies as indicated for dialysis patients
- Medication therapy:
  - ✓ Carnitine: 50–200 mg/kg/day if carnitine deficient (MMA, PA, GA1)
  - ✓ Glycine: 10%: 250–600 mg/kg/day. Favors formation of rapidly excreted isovalerylglycine (IVA)
  - ✓ Hydroxycobalamin: 1 mg intramuscular injection daily. Cofactor for methylmalonyl-CoA mutase (MMA)
- Transition/chronic care: Choose appropriate home formula and daily protein allowance with metabolic dietitian; routine monitoring of nutritional markers, plasma and urine organic acids, acylcarnitine profile/carnitine levels, electrolytes, LFTs, CBC with differential; may require long-term medication and alkalinization therapy; consider gastrostomy-tube placement, especially for patients with failure to thrive or feeding aversion; early intervention services; yearly developmental assessment; yearly bone density scans after age 4; normal immunization schedule with immunization followed by 24 hours of prophylactic antipyretics and protein-free diet; for procedures requiring a period of nothing by mouth, consider admission for IV fluids before procedure.

PRIMARY LACTIC ACIDOSIS

MITOCHONDRIAL RESPIRATORY CHAIN DEFECTS

Inborn errors in assembly, structure, or function of the protein complexes necessary for oxidative phosphorylation. Respiratory-chain defects (RCDs) are a large family of rare

and typically incurable mitochondrial disorders. **Within the family are recurrent named clinical syndromes such as mitochondrial encephalomyelopathy with lactic acidosis and stroke (MELAS); myoclonic epilepsy with ragged red fibers (MERRF); neuropathy, ataxia, and retinitis pigmentosa (NARP); chronic progressive external ophthalmoplegia (CPEO); myoneurogastrointestinal disorder and encephalomyopathy (MNGIE); Barth syndrome; Pearson syndrome; Kearns–Sayre syndrome; Leigh syndrome. However, the majority of pediatric RCD patients have a rare/private disease that is not easily categorized, but has multisystem manifestations that may overlap the named syndromes.**

ETIOLOGY

- The respiratory chain of the inner mitochondrial membrane contains five multisubunit protein complexes.
- Complete assembly and maintenance of the respiratory chain requires proteins from the mitochondrial genome and hundreds of nuclear genes.
- Mutations in nuclear or mitochondrially encoded genes can lead to RCD.
- Mutations in mitochondrial DNA are maternally inherited.
- RCD resulting from mutations in nuclear genes is inherited in an autosomal recessive, autosomal dominant, or X-linked fashion—mostly autosomal recessive.

EPIDEMIOLOGY

- Estimated prevalence of childhood RCD is 1 in 10,000.

PATHOPHYSIOLOGY

- RCD leads to inability to produce ATP from reduced electron carriers. This affects the efficiency of energy production from essentially all fuel sources.
- Decreased ATP production is associated with damage in tissues with high metabolic demand. Failure to reoxidize electron carriers decreases TCA efficiency and leads to lactic acidosis.
- Increased generation of toxic reactive oxygen species occurs.
- Note that lactic acidemia indicates an elevation in blood lactate without causing concomitant acidosis; lactic acidosis indicates a metabolic acidosis caused by an elevated lactate (typically requiring a lactate >5 mmol/L).

CLINICAL MANIFESTATIONS

Phenotypes in RCD are variable, even within the same family. The presence of progressive dysfunction in seemingly unrelated organ systems should raise suspicion for an RCD. Tissues with high requirements for oxidative phosphorylation tend to be the most severely affected. These include:

- Skeletal muscle: Weakness, myopathy, rhabdomyolysis, ophthalmoplegia
- Central nervous system: Seizure, hearing loss, basal ganglia dysfunction, developmental delay, abnormal tone, retinopathy, stroke-like events
- Liver: Steatosis, transaminitis, fulminant or neonatal hepatic failure
- Bone marrow: Neutropenia, sideroblastic anemia
- Pancreas: Diabetes mellitus, exocrine insufficiency
- Heart: Arrhythmias (Wolff–Parkinson–White syndrome or heart block), cardiomyopathy
- Proximal renal tubule: Renal tubular acidosis

A wide range of findings is possible on physical exam:

- Eyes: Evaluate for ophthalmoplegia and retinal abnormalities.
- Respiratory: Kussmaul respirations suggest metabolic acidosis, which can be due to lactic acidemia or ketonemia

- Cardiac: Irregular rhythms, new murmurs/gallops, signs of congestive heart failure
- Gastrointestinal: Hepatomegaly
- Neurologic: Evaluate tone, mental status, and focal deficits

DIAGNOSTICS

In patients in whom a respiratory-chain defect is suspected:

- BMP, LFTs, CBC, and CKP
- Elevated lactate and lactate:pyruvate ratio may be present at baseline or may be uncovered after glucose loading. The most sensitive and specific time to test is ~2 hours postprandially.
- Plasma beta-hydroxybutyrate: Beta-hydroxybutyrate may be disproprotionately higher than acetoacetate, therefore urinalysis may underestimate or fail to detect ketosis.
- Plasma amino acids: May have elevations in alanine if lactic acidemia has been longstanding
- Urine organic acids: May reveal elevated lactate, ketones, and TCA cycle intermediates (e.g., α-ketoglutarate)
- Urine amino acids: A generalized aminoaciduria reflecting proximal renal tubular dysfunction occurs in some patients. (Generalized aminoaciduria is typical in healthy neonates, limiting the diagnostic utility of urine amino acids in this age group.)
- In patients with CNS disease, cerebrospinal fluid (CSF) lactate and pyruvate; typically best interpreted if plasma lactate and pyruvate are obtained at the same time.
- MRI of brain for structural or degenerative abnormalities
- MR spectroscopy to detect lactate, especially in basal ganglia
- ECG if rhythm abnormalities are suspected; consider echocardiography

For definitive diagnosis:

- DNA analysis via whole-exome sequencing plus mitochondrial genome sequencing is the preferred first line of testing.
- For patients in whom suspicion is high and molecular testing is unrevealing, functional assays of electron transport chain activity in liver or muscle can be used.

MANAGEMENT

- There is no definitive management for RCDs. Supportive therapies vary according to organ system involved.
- A variety of cofactors, antioxidants, and other agents have been attempted. These include coenzyme Q10, vitamin C, vitamin E, thiamine, carnitine, creatine, alpha lipoic acid, riboflavin, and others. No therapy has been conclusively shown to be effective in improving outcome with exception of arginine in cases of metabolic stroke (MELAS and others). Most patients opt to take a mitochondrial "cocktail" of a combination of the above vitamins/supplements, given their minimal risk, in attempt to maximize mitochondrial function.

MITOCHONDRIAL DEPLETION SYNDROMES

Inborn errors in mitochondrial DNA replication, or maintenance of mitochondrial nucleotide pools, resulting in inability to replicate mitochondrial DNA. There are 15 described genes, each with a slightly different presentation.

ETIOLOGY

- Mitochondria maintain an independent genome, with their own polymerase, helicase, and nucleotide pools.
- Each of these genes for maintenance of the mitochondrial genome is nuclear-encoded.

EPIDEMIOLOGY

• Incidence of at least 1 in 50,000; varies by ethnic group

PATHOPHYSIOLOGY

• Decreased efficiency of mitochondrial DNA replication results in decreasing numbers of mitochondria and rapid accumulation of mitochondrial mutations over time.
• There is secondary loss of ATP production resulting from depletion of mitochondria and accumulation of errors affecting the respiratory chain

CLINICAL MANIFESTATIONS

Phenotypes in mitochondrial depletion vary by gene involvement, but typical symptoms include:

• Rapid developmental regression in a previously typical patient.
• Seizure, especially epilepsia partialis continua (EPC) (persistent, focal motor seizure)
• Rapidly progressive cerebral volume loss
• Steatosis, transaminitis, decreased synthetic function, hepatic failure, especially in response to valproic acid
• Hypoglycemia may occur.

DIAGNOSTICS

• BMP, LFTs, and CKP
• Elevated lactate and lactate:pyruvate ratio in blood or CSF or evidence seen on MR spectroscopy.
• Electroencephalography will differentiate EPC from other movement abnormalities.
• Urine organic acids may reveal elevated lactate, ketones, and TCA cycle intermediates (e.g., fumarate)
• Quantitation of mitochondrial DNA in muscle and liver is diagnostic.
• Molecular DNA testing targeted to the depletion syndromes provides a definitive diagnosis.

MANAGEMENT

• Disease is almost always inevitably progressive; treatment symptoms.
• As in RCDs, a mitochondrial cocktail may be tried and continued if it provides symptomatic relief, but there is no evidence as to its efficacy.
• Valproic acid is strictly contraindicated; its use in these cases may result in fatal hepatic failure.

PYRUVATE DEHYDROGENASE DEFICIENCY

Pyruvate dehydrogenase (PDH) deficiency is an inborn error resulting in decreased activity of PDH, a mitochondrial enzyme complex that converts pyruvate to acetyl-CoA. Inefficient oxidation of carbohydrates and a propensity for lactic acidosis occurs. Assembly and activity of PDH require products of at least nine genes, but the vast majority of patients have mutations affecting the E1β subunit.

EPIDEMIOLOGY

• Several hundred cases have been described; incidence is unknown.
• Despite its X-linked inheritance, PDH E1α deficiency has a similar incidence in males and females. The random nature of X-inactivation may lead to a different phenotype in females.

PATHOPHYSIOLOGY

- PDH, the biochemical step between glycolysis and the TCA cycle, is exclusively involved in carbohydrate metabolism.
- Inability to generate acetyl-CoA from glucose severely limits the amount of energy (ATP) produced per mole of glucose.
- Involvement of the CNS reflects the exquisite dependence of the brain on aerobic glucose oxidation for cellular functions.
- Lactic acidosis results from the conversion of excess pyruvate to lactate by lactate dehydrogenase.

CLINICAL MANIFESTATIONS

- Severity is variable and is determined both by residual enzyme activity and, for females, the pattern of X-inactivation.
- Involvement of the CNS is universal and can cause poor feeding, hypotonia, lethargy, and coma in neonates.
- Two general phenotypes exist: A "metabolic" presentation of overwhelming, refractory neonatal lactic acidosis (especially in boys with profound E1α deficiency), and a chronic "neurologic" presentation causing developmental delay, seizures, and ataxia (typical in affected girls).
- Severely affected patients may have prenatal symptoms or abnormalities at birth including low birth weight, decreased fetal movements, facial dysmorphism (resembling fetal alcohol syndrome), and dysgenesis of the corpus callosum.
- Degenerative changes in the CNS, including subacute neurodegeneration of the brainstem and basal ganglia (Leigh disease), occur in some patients. Apnea and sudden death may occur as a result of brainstem dysfunction.
- Hepatomegaly is uncommon and suggests alternative diagnoses.

DIAGNOSTICS

- Plasma lactate and pyruvate: Elevations of both with a normal or near-normal ratio are strongly suggestive; however, these elevations may be intermittent.
- Plasma amino acids often reveal an elevated alanine in PDH deficiency and other inborn forms of lactic acidosis.
- Lactate may also be elevated in other body fluids, including urine and CSF. Lactate and pyruvate in the CSF are helpful diagnostic aids in children with neurologic symptoms in whom a metabolic disease is suspected (though CSF lactate elevations can be seen in patients with seizures regardless of etiology).
- Brain MRI to evaluate structural or degenerative CNS abnormalities. Concurrent MR spectroscopy to measure lactate peaks is very helpful.
- Genetic testing may confirm the diagnosis, but mutations can be mosaic and not always detectable in blood. PDH enzymology is complementary to genetic testing and provides residual enzyme activity, which can be predictive of prognosis. Virtually any tissue can be used for PDH enzymology, including skin fibroblasts, lymphocytes, and muscle. Various PDH components are examined separately in the assays, often allowing for precise biochemical diagnosis.

MANAGEMENT

- Bicarbonate therapy to treat chronic acid load
- Use caution with dextrose-containing fluids, because glucose loads exacerbate lactic acidosis. Generally safe to start with D5-based solutions if necessary, unless patient is stabilized on a ketogenic diet. Dextrose should be used only very conservatively to treat hypoglycemia once the ketogenic diet has been initiated.

- Medications: Alpha-lipoic acid can be used. A minority of patients respond to thiamine (0.5–2 g/day). The PDH activator dichloroacetate is being studied.
- Ketogenic (low-carbohydrate) diets have been associated with improved development and improved seizure management; these bypass the lack of PDH complex activity to generate acetyl-CoA. Involvement of a biochemical geneticist is recommended prior to initiation of the ketogenic diet, as this is contraindicated in related disorders (e.g., pyruvate carboxylase deficiency).

PYRUVATE CARBOXYLASE DEFICIENCY

Pyruvate carboxylase (PC) deficiency is an inborn error resulting in decreased activity of PC, an enzyme that converts pyruvate to oxaloacetate, an important TCA cycle intermediate.

EPIDEMIOLOGY

- Estimated prevalence of 1 in 250,000; however, increased rates have been noted in certain Native American and European groups.
- Inheritance is autosomal recessive, though at times, due to the size of the gene and intronic mutations, clinical sequencing may not identify mutations.

PATHOPHYSIOLOGY

- PC deficiency impairs carboxylation of pyruvate to oxaloacetate, resulting in accumulation of pyruvate that is then converted to lactate and alanine.
- Acetyl-CoA cannot enter the TCA cycle, so excess ketone bodies are produced.
- Inadequate oxaloacetate results in impaired gluconeogenesis and fasting hypoglycemia.
- Secondary urea-cycle dysfunction occurs because of inadequate production of aspartic acid, which can result in elevated plasma citrulline and hyperammonemia.

CLINICAL MANIFESTATIONS

- Three phenotypes have been recognized; common features include metabolic acidosis, failure to thrive, developmental delay, and seizures:
  ✓ Type A (infantile): Mild metabolic acidosis with developmental delays, hypotonia, seizures, failure to thrive with episodes of metabolic decompensation during intercurrent illness. More common in Native American populations.
  ✓ Type B (neonatal lethal): Hypoglycemia, hyperammonemia, ketosis, citrullinemia, tremor, abnormal eye movements, seizures, developmental delay, and at times early death. Described as more common in French population.
  ✓ Type C ("benign"/intermittent): episodic metabolic acidosis, variable developmental delay
- Brain MRI may show abnormalities in types A and B, including hypomyelination, ventricular dilation, cystic lesions or gliosis (in brain stem, cerebellum, basal ganglia)
- Hepatomegaly is sometimes seen.

DIAGNOSTICS

- Plasma lactate and pyruvate. Elevations of both with an elevated (especially in type B) or normal lactate:pyruvate ratio may be seen.
- Check glucose and ammonia levels.
- Plasma amino acids may reveal elevated alanine, citrulline, and lysine; aspartic acid and glutamine may be low.
- Blood ketones may be elevated; paradoxical ketosis (increased ketones following dextrose administration) is nearly pathognomonic.

- CSF lactate and pyruvate may be elevated; also check CSF amino acids for elevated glutamic acid and proline; decreased glutamine. CSF studies should be obtained at the same time as plasma lactate:pyruvate ratio and amino acids when possible. CSF studies are not mandatory for diagnosis.
- Brain MRI and MR spectroscopy may be helpful.
- Genetic testing of the *PC* gene can be sent; deep intronic mutations and mosaic mutations frustrate a molecular diagnosis in ~1% of alleles. PC enzyme activity (fibroblasts or lymphoblasts) is a complementary diagnostic technique and also provides residual enzyme activity (which does not correspond to prognosis).

MANAGEMENT

- During acute decompensation: place large-gauge IV; check comprehensive metabolic panel, ammonia, glucose, IV dextrose-containing fluids (D5–10%) for hypoglycemia or if not tolerating feeds, IV sodium bicarbonate for acidosis (1 mEq/kg; may be repeated if needed) followed by continuous infusion (2–4 mEq/kg/day), may need ammonia scavengers for hyperammonemia similar to dosing in UCDs (see **Table 17-3**), consider citrate supplementation of IV sodium or potassium citrate (1000 to 1500 mg/kg/day).
- Anticipate that dextrose will raise lactate and ketones in the short term, worsening acidosis.
- Fasting should be avoided, patients should have a high-carbohydrate, high-protein diet and frequent feedings to avoid utilizing gluconeogenesis.
- Medications: Bicarbonate therapy to treat chronic acid load, citrate supplementation may help provide a substrate for the TCA cycle, and aspartic acid may aid urea-cycle function; biotin is often given to maximize PC activity but its efficacy is not proven.
- Ketogenic diet is absolutely contraindicated.

PEROXISOMAL DISORDERS

PEROXISOMAL BIOGENESIS DISORDERS (PBDs)

Peroxisomes are an essential organelle, which have the key function of controlling metabolism of very-long-chain fatty acids and the synthesis of complex lipids, such as plasmalogens from dietary fats.

EPIDEMIOLOGY

- Overall incidence is 1 in 50,000.
- The previously recognized entities Zellweger syndrome, infantile Refsum disease, and neonatal adrenoleukodystrophy are now more properly understood to be points along a spectrum.

PATHOPHYSIOLOGY

- Complex lipid metabolism is important for generating myelin and bile acids.
- Peroxisomes are also important in detoxification of reactive-oxygen species.
- All peroxisomal proteins must be targeted into the peroxisome using a very complex process. Targeting errors result in disease.

CLINICAL MANIFESTATIONS

- Disease represents a spectrum from mild to severe.
- Dramatic hypotonia may be noted in infancy.
- Dysmorphic facies include large fontanelle, broad forehead, hypertelorism, and epicanthal folds.

- Brain anomalies include cerebellar abnormalities (most common), heterotopias, and cerebral dysplasia.
- Seizures
- Retinal degeneration or cataracts
- Sensorineural hearing loss
- Renal cysts
- Transaminitis, jaundice, and hepatic synthetic failures
- Patients with severe disease usually have developmental regression and death within the first few years of life. Patients with more mild disease may escape clinical attention for a few years.

DIAGNOSTICS

- DNA testing (peroxisomal gene panel of the *PEX* genes) is diagnostic.
- Very-long-chain (branched) fatty acid (VLCFA) profile is a good initial diagnostic/screening test for PBD.
- Some cases may be incidentally identified by NBS programs performing VLCFA as a screen for X-linked adrenoleukodystrophy.
- In a patient with abnormal VLCFA: Plasmalogens, pipecolic acid, phytanic acid, pristanic acid, and bile acids may help differentiate the location of the pathogenic variant.
- Epiphyseal stippling on x-rays is highly suggestive.
- Brain MRI to look for structural defects

MANAGEMENT

- Management is largely supportive; multiple specialists are typically involved in care.
- Gastrostomy tube may be needed for nutritional support.

X-LINKED ADRENOLEUKODYSTROPHY

The exact etiology of X-linked adrenoleukodystrophy is unknown. It is thought to be involved with the importation of fats into peroxisomes for further processing.

EPIDEMIOLOGY

- Overall incidence is 1 in 21,000 (males); 1 in 17,000 (males and females)
- X-linked adrenoleukodystrophy is the most common peroxisomal disease.

PATHOPHYSIOLOGY

- Not fully understood
- Very-long-chain fatty acids accumulate, likely because they cannot be imported into the peroxisome
- Very-long-chain fatty acids are directly adrenotoxic.
- Errors in complex fat metabolism likely are partially responsible for leukodystrophy.
- Inflammatory component to leukodystrophy with lymphocyte infiltration in the CNS

CLINICAL MANIFESTATIONS

- Phenotypes of patients affected with X-linked adrenoleukodystrophy vary among adrenoleukodystrophy, with onset either in childhood, adolescence, or adulthood; adrenomyeloneuropathy; and isolated adrenal insufficiency.
- Female carriers can be symptomatic with either adrenomyeloneuropathy or isolated Addison disease but do not have leukodystrophy.
- Deterioration of handwriting is the classic harbinger of disease progression.

DIAGNOSTICS

- VLCFA profile
- Cases can be identified presymptomatically by NBS analysis of VLCFA.
- *ABCD1* gene sequencing confirms disease.
- Brain MRI with gadolinium to assess degree of leukodystrophy.

MANAGEMENT

- Bone marrow transplantation ideally before the onset of neurologic symptoms; usually considered at the earliest sign of radiographic changes.
- Physiologic adrenal replacement and periodic monitoring of adrenal function.
- For those identified presymptomatically, close follow-up with a neurologist and serial MRIs are also indicated to allow prompt bone marrow transplantation.
- The "Lorenzo's Oil" diet, replacing normal dietary fats with a mix of oleic acid and erucic acid has been studied but not found to be effective.

CONGENITAL DISORDERS OF GLYCOSYLATION (CDG)

GENERAL PRINCIPLES

Glycosylation is the addition of sugars to proteins and lipids. This step is important for trafficking of proteins to the right organelles, protein folding, and therefore, ultimately correct enzyme functioning.

EPIDEMIOLOGY

- Overall incidence—at least 1 in 10,000; the most common form PMM2-CDG is 1 in 20,000; likely underdiagnosed; true prevalence may be higher.
- PMM2-CDG is especially high in the Dutch population, with a carrier frequency of 1 in 70.
- The number of recognized disorders of glycosylation is increasing exponentially.

PATHOPHYSIOLOGY

- Abnormalities in adding sugars to proteins and lipids cause abnormal molecular targeting.
- Disease results from the loss of function of the abnormally glycosylated enzymes.

CLINICAL MANIFESTATIONS

Each disease has unique features, related to the particular defect in glycosylation. The full phenotypic spectrum is not well known and a high index of suspicion is required. Testing should be considered in any patient with neurologic or multisystemic disease without other etiology. Common symptoms include:

- Hypotonia
- Structural brain anomalies, especially cerebellar hypoplasia
- Abnormal fat-pad distribution
- Inverted nipples
- Hyperinsulinemic hypoglycemia
- Protein-losing enteropathy
- Coagulopathy
- Liver dysfunction
- Eye malformations
- Congenital myasthenia

DIAGNOSTICS

- Transferrin isoelectric-focusing (carbohydrate-deficient transferrin) is a good initial screen.
- N-linked glycan and O-glycan analysis is complementary and should be used in cases in which the index of suspicion is high; can be used to differentiate among CDGs.
- DNA testing (panel or whole exome sequencing) may be most definitive.

MANAGEMENT

- Management is largely supportive.
- Supplemental sugar therapy may be beneficial in specific conditions: common treatments include mannose for Mannosephosphate isomerase (MPI)-CDG and galactose for Phosphoglucomutase 1(PGM1)-CDG; similar rational therapies may be applicable to other rare CDGs.

GLYCOGEN STORAGE DISEASES (GSDs)

GENERAL PRINCIPLES

A family of inherited disorders affecting glycogen metabolism. Glycogen is a highly branched polymer of glucose and is stored in liver and muscle. The glycogen found in these disorders is abnormal in quantity, quality, or both.

- Conversion of glycogen into pyruvate to enter the TCA cycle occurs in two parts: Glycogenolysis from glycogen to glucose-6-phosphate and glycolysis from glucose-6-phosphate to pyruvate.
- Some enzyme defects are localized in liver, others in muscles; a few are generalized.

EPIDEMIOLOGY

- Frequency (all forms): About 1 in 20,000 live births
- Autosomal recessive inheritance (except the X-linked *PHKA2* gene encoding a subunit of phosphorylase kinase causing type IX GSD)
- Types I, II, III, and IX most commonly present in early childhood; type V (McArdle disease) most common in adults.
- Common mutations in GSD Ia have been reported in Ashkenazi Jewish, Chinese, Japanese, and Mexican populations.

ETIOLOGY

- More than 12 types; can be classified by organ involvement and clinical manifestations into liver and muscle glycogenoses (Table 17-4).
- Hepatic glycogen storage disease: Type 0, type I (von Gierke disease), type III, type IV, type VI, and type IX;
  ✓ Typically cause hepatomegaly (except type 0) and fasting hypoglycemia
  ✓ Types III and IV are also associated with hepatic cirrhosis.
- Muscle glycogen storage disease: Types II, V, VII, and IX
  ✓ Progressive skeletal muscle weakness, cardiomyopathy, or both (type II)
  ✓ Muscle pain, exercise intolerance, myoglobinuria, and fatigue (types V, VII, and IX)

DIAGNOSTICS

- Initial workup for GSDs should include glucose, lactate, uric acid, plasma ketones, triglycerides, CKP, LFTs

TABLE 17-4	Classification of Glycogen Storage Diseases		
Type	**Deficient Enzyme**	**Tissue**	**Main Clinical Features**
0	Glycogen synthase	Liver	Postprandial hyperglycemia with elevated lactate, fasting ketosis, hypoglycemia
Ia	Glucose-6-phosphatase (von Gierke disease)	Liver, kidney	Hypoglycemia with inappropriate hypoketonemia, hepatomegaly, lactic acidosis, hypertriglyceridemia, hyperuricemia, round "doll" face
Ib-d	Glucose-6-phosphatase-related transport	Liver	Above + neutropenia, infections, inflammatory bowel disease (Ib/c)
II	Acid α-glucosidase (Pompe disease)	Muscle	Infant form: cardiomyopathy and hypotonia Later form: myopathy
III	Debranching enzyme (Cori disease)	Liver, muscle	Ketotic hypoglycemia, hepatomegaly, proximal myopathy (normal lactate and uric acid), cardiomyopathy
IV	Branching enzyme (Andersen disease)	Liver	Perinatal form with fetal akinesia deformation sequence, arthrogryposis, hydrops, and neonatal death
			Congenital neuromuscular type with hypotonia, respiratory distress, cardiomyopathy
			Later onset types with hepatosplenomegaly, cirrhosis, myopathy
V	Phosphorylase (McArdle disease)	Muscle	Exercise intolerance, elevated CKP, myalgia, rhabdomyolysis, "second wind" phenomenon after brief cessation of exercise
VI	Phosphorylase	Liver	Hepatomegaly; mild fasting ketotic hypoglycemia
VII	Phosphofructokinase, phosphoglycerate kinase, phosphoglycerate mutase (Tauri disease)	Muscle	Exercise intolerance without "second wind", hemolysis causing jaundice with sustained exercise, elevated CKP, rhabdomyolysis
IX	Phosphorylase b kinase	Liver, muscle, blood	Hepatomegaly; mild fasting ketotic hypoglycemia, hemolysis, myalgia, progressive weakness

- Genetic diagnosis is now the gold standard and should be performed in all patients in whom GSD is suspected.
- Hepatic glycogen storage disease: Enzyme defects can be detected only in tissue acquired by liver biopsy.
- Muscle glycogen storage disease: Exercise test can be used to demonstrate the failure of venous lactate and pyruvate to rise and the production of uric acid, inosine, hypoxanthine, and ammonia to increase excessively; myopathy should be verified by enzyme assay from muscle biopsy.

MANAGEMENT

- Prevention of hypoglycemia while avoiding storage of even more glycogen in the liver and muscle
- Hepatic glycogen storage disease:
  - ✓ Nasogastric tube feedings at night; frequent feedings every 2–3 hours during the day using a lactose-free and sucrose-free formula
  - ✓ Uncooked cornstarch (1.75–2.5 g/kg) mixed in water, soy formula, or soymilk is given every 4 hours in infants and every 6 hours in older children (GSD I) or at bedtime (GSD 0, VI, IX)
  - ✓ Restrict intake of fructose and galactose (GSD I)
  - ✓ Supplementation with calcium and multivitamins
  - ✓ Allopurinol may be used to lower the concentration of uric acid (GSD I).
  - ✓ Liver transplantation has been successful.
  - ✓ May require admission for dextrose-containing IV fluids when ill (for those with hypoglycemia)
  - ✓ GSD IV treatment is symptomatic; liver transplantation may be used in those with limited other comorbidities
- Muscle glycogen storage disease: Avoidance of strenuous exercise to prevent rhabdomyolysis

LYSOSOMAL STORAGE DISEASES (LSDs)

GENERAL PRINCIPLES

A group of over 50 disorders related to abnormal lysosomal function, characterized by abnormal accumulation of undegraded substrates within the lysosome. These diseases typically have multiorgan system involvement, which can include the skeleton, liver, spleen, eyes, heart, connective tissue, and brain. Mucopolysaccharidoses (MPSs) are a subset of LSD.

EPIDEMIOLOGY

- In total, estimated prevalence of 1 in 8000 births
- Majority autosomal recessive inheritance, some X-linked (Hunter syndrome/MPS II, Fabry disease)
- Ashkenazi Jewish population has increased carrier frequency of Gaucher disease (1 in 13) and Tay–Sachs disease (1 in 30), and others.

PATHOPHYSIOLOGY

- Many LSDs are caused by mutations in genes that encode acid hydrolases, membrane proteins, transporter proteins, and activator proteins involved in lysosomal function
- Results in buildup of abnormal or undegraded substrates in multiple organs and tissues

- LSDs include the MPSs, oligosaccharidoses, mucolipidoses, sphingolipidoses, and lipofuscinoses.
- Pompe disease is both an LSD and a GSD (abnormal lysosomal accumulation of glycogen).

CLINICAL MANIFESTATIONS

- Timing of onset of symptoms can vary from neonatal presentations to adult onset.
- Symptoms can occur in multiple organ systems, including visceral (e.g., hepatosplenomegaly), ocular (e.g., cherry red spot, retinal dystrophy), skeletal (e.g., dysostosis multiplex), neurologic (e.g., seizures, cognitive impairment, behavioral differences), and hematologic (e.g., thrombocytopenia, substrate-filled vacuoles in lymphocytes)
- LSDs typically are not at risk of acute metabolic decompensation requiring specific IV fluid or dietary management.

DIAGNOSTICS

- Diagnostic testing typically depends on which category of LSDs is being considered.
- General testing strategies include enzyme assay or enzyme panels, biomarker testing (e.g., urine glycosaminoglycans for MPS, plasma oxysterols for Niemann–Pick type C), and confirmatory genetic testing.
- Many individuals may be identified presymptomatically or early in disease course with expansion of NBS. Some states have begun screening for MPS I, Pompe and/or Krabbe disease. Further LSDs may likely be added to NBS in the future.

MANAGEMENT

- Management is disease-specific; however, many LSDs (including MPS I, MPS II, MPS IVA, MPS VII, Pompe disease, Gaucher disease, Fabry disease, and lysosomal acid lipase deficiency) have FDA-approved enzyme-replacement therapies available; these are best initiated early in the course of symptoms.
- Some disorders are amenable to substrate reduction therapy (e.g., oral eliglustat in Gaucher disease).
- Gene therapies are in development

MUCOPOLYSACCHARIDOSES (MPSs)

A group of 7 disorders (MPS I, II, III, IV, VI, VII, and IX) caused by defects in the lysosomal degradation of mucopolysaccharides. They share progressive multiorgan involvement due to abnormal accumulation of glycosaminoglycans.

EPIDEMIOLOGY

- In total, estimated prevalence of 1 in 20,000 births
- All are autosomal recessive, with the exception of MPS II (Hunter syndrome), which is X-linked.

PATHOPHYSIOLOGY

- MPSs are caused by mutations in genes that encode enzymes involved in the degradation of mucopolysaccharides.
- Lack of enzyme activity results in abnormal accumulation of glycosaminoglycans (GAGs), which deposit in multiple tissues, including brain and connective tissue.

CLINICAL MANIFESTATIONS

- Coarsening of facial features over time is common in many patients, as classically described in MPS I (Hurler syndrome) patients.
- "Red flags" for MPS patients include coarse facial features, skeletal dysplasia (dysostosis multiplex), recurrent upper respiratory infections and/or recurrent episodes of otitis media, hearing loss, hepatomegaly, valvular heart disease, umbilical or inguinal hernia, joint stiffness (especially "trigger finger"), median neuropathy (due to GAG storage around the carpal tunnel), corneal clouding and developmental delay and/or aggressive behavior.
- Given the rarity of these diseases, many patients face a delay of a year or more for diagnosis; it is crucial to consider MPS in patients with a combination of the above symptoms without a clear explanation.
- Variable spectrum of severity and age of onset

DIAGNOSTICS

- Enzyme assay or enzyme panels can be performed.
- Urine GAGs (e.g., heparan sulfate, dermatan sulfate, keratan sulfate) can also be a good screen and may narrow the differential diagnosis.
- Confirmatory genetic testing

MANAGEMENT

- MPS I, MPS II, MPS IVA, and MPS VII have FDA-approved enzyme-replacement therapies available.
- Hematopoietic stem-cell transplantation has been effective in Hurler syndrome (MPS I) if performed within the first 12 months of life.
- MPS patients are at high risk for complications during anesthesia because of upper airway obstruction, odontoid hypoplasia, cardiac disease, and skeletal abnormalities. Interventions requiring anesthesia should be performed at centers with experience caring for patients with MPS.

Neonatology 18 CHAPTER

Kelley Kovatis, MD
Nicole Pouppirt, MD
Jennifer M. Brady, MD

BIRTH AND NEONATAL RESUSCITATION

NEONATAL RESUSCITATION

EPIDEMIOLOGY

- Each year in the United States, approximately 4 million infants are born.
- Approximately 10% of infants will require some form of resuscitation at birth.
- Less than 1% of infants require advanced resuscitation at birth (intubation, chest compressions, cardiac medications).

PATHOPHYSIOLOGY

- In newborns, the need for resuscitation is most commonly caused by inadequate ventilation.
- Failure to breathe at birth is most commonly caused by a period of hypoxia related to birth asphyxia, maternal drug use, or maternal anesthesia.
- Primary apnea is the absence of respiratory effort in the perinatal period that responds to stimulation. This is often the result of a short period of mild hypoxia immediately prior to birth.
- Secondary apnea is the absence of respiratory effort in the perinatal period that does not respond to stimulation and requires positive pressure ventilation to resolve. This is more indicative of a longer period of in utero hypoxia.
- Newborns with primary and secondary apnea will present similarly at birth with apnea. Assessing response to stimulation is the only way to distinguish between the two.

MANAGEMENT

The Neonatal Resuscitation Program (NRP) periodically updates the algorithm used for clinical decision-making at deliveries, the most recent recommendations are explained below.

- **Preparation for Birth**
  - ✓ Personnel: Every delivery should have at least one person trained in neonatal resuscitation present. Additional personnel should be available if the need for advanced resuscitation is expected. Team roles should be assigned prior to birth.
  - ✓ Equipment: Necessary equipment should be present and checked to be sure that it is functioning. Equipment available should include a warmer bed, blankets, hat, stethoscope, bulb and wall suction, bag and mask device, oxygen with blender, pulse oximeter, laryngoscope with blade, and endotracheal tubes.
- **Initial Routine Evaluation and Care**
  - ✓ Following delivery, the term infant should be warmed, dried, and stimulated.
  - ✓ If secretions are blocking the airway, they should be suctioned.
  - ✓ Simultaneously one should assess the infant's muscle tone and respiratory effort.
  - ✓ In a term infant who does not appear to need resuscitation, the above steps can occur while the neonate is lying on the mother's abdomen.

TABLE 18-1	Goal Preductal Oxygen Saturations Based on Infant's Minute of Life
Age	Targeted Preductal Oxygen Saturation
1 minute	60–65%
2 minutes	65–70%
3 minutes	70–75%
4 minutes	75–80%
5 minutes	80–85%
10 minutes	85–95%

Need for Resuscitation

- For infants who are still apneic or gasping despite above steps, or in whom the heart rate is <100 beats/minute, positive pressure ventilation should be given by 1 minute of life with an appropriately sized mask covering both the infant's nose and mouth, ensuring an adequate seal.
- Positive pressure ventilation should be initiated at peak inspiratory pressures of 20 cm H_2O, at a rate of 40–60 breaths per minute, and at 21% FiO_2 for term infants.
- Concurrently, a pulse oximeter should be placed on the infant's right hand (preductal saturation) and application of cardiac leads should be considered for accurate heart rate assessment.
- FiO_2 should be titrated as needed to meet goal target oxygen saturations based on minute of life, as described in Table 18-1.
- Signs of achieving effective ventilation include effective chest rise, adequate breath sounds, improving pink color, improving tone, improving oxygen saturations, heart rate >100 beats/minute, and spontaneous respirations.
- If effective ventilation is not achieved after 30 seconds of positive pressure ventilation, steps to correct inadequate assisted ventilation should be taken.
- The mnemonic MR. SOPA can be used to proceed through corrective measures: M = mask adjustment, R = reposition airway, S = suction nose and mouth, O = open mouth, P = pressure increase, and A = airway alternative
- If effective ventilation is unable to be achieved with corrective steps, an alternative airway should be placed.

Need for Advanced Resuscitation

- The most common alternative airway is endotracheal intubation. However, in certain circumstances a laryngeal mask airway (LMA) may also be considered.
- Because ineffective ventilation is a more common cause of depressed heart rate in an infant than a primary cardiac cause, an infant with a heart rate <60 beats/minute despite positive pressure ventilation should be intubated to attempt to achieve adequate ventilation prior to initiating chest compressions.
- If after intubation the infant's heart rate remains <60 beats/minute, chest compressions should be initiated. FiO_2 should be increased to 100% if it hasn't been already.
- Chest compressions can be given by the thumb technique (thumbs depressing sternum with hands encircling chest) or the two-finger technique (depressing sternum with index and middle finger). The 7th edition of NRP defines the thumb technique as the preferred method of providing chest compressions to a neonate. Chest compressions should depress the lower third of the sternum, depressing one-third of chest circumference.

- Chest compressions should be coordinated with breaths, three chest compressions to one breath, with a goal of 90 chest compressions and 30 breaths every minute.
- If heart rate remains <60 beats/minute, IV access should be obtained, most commonly through emergent placement of an umbilical venous catheter (UVC). Epinephrine should be given if asystole is present or heart rate remains <60 beats/minute after 60 seconds of coordinated chest compressions and ventilation.
- IV epinephrine is preferred to endotracheal epinephrine if IV access is available. Epinephrine dosage (1:10,000 solution, 0.1 mg/mL) is 0.1–0.3 mL/kg given IV or 0.5–1mL/kg given via endotracheal tube. Dosage can be repeated every 3–5 minutes if heart rate remains <60 beats/minute.
- Stopping resuscitative efforts can be considered if after 10 minutes of adequate resuscitation there is still no detectable heart rate.

Special Resuscitation Considerations

- Preterm infants:
  - ✓ Special consideration should be given to temperature regulation in preterm infants. This includes increasing the ambient temperature in the delivery room, placing the infant in a plastic bag or under plastic wrap after delivery, rather than drying the infant immediately at birth.
  - ✓ Initial resuscitative efforts for preterm infants should start with an FiO_2 of 21–30%. Titrate FiO_2 as per infant saturation goal guidelines based on minute of life (similar to term infant) (see **Table 18-1**).
- Meconium-stained fluid:
  - ✓ In the past, infants who were born through meconium-stained fluid and not vigorous at birth were immediately intubated, with suctioning of their airway. This is no longer recommended.
  - ✓ Resuscitation of an infant born through meconium-stained fluid should take the same approach as for any other infant, following the initial steps of warming, drying, and stimulating at birth while assessing respiratory effort.

APGAR SCORES

The Apgar score was designed to provide a quick, reproducible way to evaluate a newborn's condition following delivery at 1 and 5 minutes of life (Table 18-2). If the 5-minute score is less than 7, additional scores are assigned every 5 minutes until the newborn has a score of 7 or more, up to 20 minutes of age.

- The Apgar score itself does not determine the need for resuscitation.
- The 1-minute score has not been shown to have predictive value, but a 5-minute score of 0–3 is associated with increased mortality in both preterm and full-term infants.
- Change in scores at 1 and 5 minutes may reflect effectiveness of resuscitation efforts.

ROUTINE NEWBORN CARE

NEWBORN ASSESSMENT

DEFINITIONS

- Gestational age (completed weeks): time elapsed between the first day of the last menstrual period and the day of delivery
- Chronologic age (days, weeks, months, or years): time elapsed since birth

TABLE 18-2	Apgar Score		
	0	**1**	**2**
Appearance (color)	Blue or pale	Pink body, blue extremities	Completely pink
Pulse (heart rate)	Absent	<100 bpm	>100 bpm
Grimace (reflex irritability)	No response	Grimace	Sneeze, cough
Activity (muscle tone)	Limp, flaccid	Some flexion	Active movements
Respiratory effort	Absent	Gasping; slow, irregular	Regular; good, lusty cry

bpm = beats per minute.

- Postmenstrual age (weeks): gestational age plus chronologic age
- Corrected age (weeks or months): chronologic age reduced by the number of weeks born before 40 weeks of gestation

CLINICAL MANIFESTATIONS

History

- Medical history of the newborn should include mother's past medical and pregnancy history, the current pregnancy, and the family history.
- Information about the delivery and the delivery room stabilization should be documented.
- Psychosocial risk factors should be determined.
- Presence or absence of risk factors for sepsis should be assessed.

Physical Examination

- The Ballard score was designed to assess a newborn's gestational age through a scoring system that combines physical characteristics with neuromuscular development. (See "Prematurity" section for defining degree of prematurity by gestational age and birth weight.)
- Weight, length, and head circumference should be plotted on a nomogram to determine percentiles.
  ✓ Intrauterine growth restriction: deviation and reduction in expected fetal growth pattern
  ✓ Small for gestational age: birth weight <10th percentile for gestational age or more than 2 standard deviations from the mean
  ✓ Average for gestational age: birth weight is between 10th and 90th percentile for infant's gestational age
  ✓ Large for gestational age: birth weight >90th percentile for gestational age
  ✓ Measurements that are symmetrically small suggest chronic exposure, congenital infection, or genetic abnormality.
  ✓ Measurements that spare the head circumference relative to the other measurements suggest placental insufficiency.

DIAGNOSTICS

- Glucose: See "Hypoglycemia" section.
- Newborn metabolic screening:
  ✓ Each year, 4.1 million newborns are screened for congenital disorders in the United States. Of these, 4000 are diagnosed with a condition tested for on the screening test.
  ✓ Newborn metabolic screening tests screen for disorders that are detectable before the onset of significant symptoms and have a treatment to prevent adverse clinical consequences of the disease. These conditions include inborn errors of metabolism, endocrine disorders, hemoglobinopathies, immunodeficiencies, and cystic fibrosis.

✓ The American Academy of Pediatrics (AAP) and the American College of Obstetricians and Gynecologists recommend that all states screen newborn infants for a core panel of 29 treatable congenital conditions and an additional 25 conditions that may be detected by screening. However, newborn screening varies from state to state.

✓ Newborn screening should be performed 24–48 hours after birth.

✓ The most commonly diagnosed conditions are hearing loss, primary congenital hypothyroidism, cystic fibrosis, sickle cell disease, and medium-chain acyl–coenzyme A dehydrogenase deficiency.

✓ For more detailed information refer to Chapter 17 on Metabolism.

- Hearing screen
  ✓ Hearing loss is a common condition, affecting 6 in 1000 live births.
  ✓ There is a two-step screen for hearing loss:
    ▪ Automated otoacoustic emissions (OAE): Sound is presented to the cochlea through a speaker inserted into the ear canal; it stimulates the cochlea to making a specific response, which is picked up and recorded by a microphone and recorder within the ear canal insert. OAE testing is inexpensive, does not require sedation, and can be performed quickly. It can be affected by external and middle ear conditions.
    ▪ Auditory brain-stem response (ABR): Electrodes placed on the scalp record the resulting electrographic activity of sound impulses as it propagates along the auditory nerve and brain stem. Outer ear and middle ear disease affect ABR to a lesser extent than OAE, but the testing requires a calm, resting infant.

- Car-seat trials: The AAP recommends that babies born at less than 37 weeks' gestation and more mature babies with respiratory or neurologic abnormalities have a period of observation in a car seat before discharge to monitor for apnea, bradycardia, or oxygen desaturation.

- Congenital heart disease (CHD)screen:
  ✓ Critical congenital heart disease is a group of congenital heart defects (hypoplastic left heart syndrome, pulmonary atresia, tetralogy of Fallot, total anomalous pulmonary venous return, tricuspid atresia, truncus arteriosus communis, coarctation of aorta, double-outlet right ventricle, Ebstein's anomaly, interrupted aortic arch, and single ventricle) that affect newborns and is one of the leading causes of infant deaths in the United States. Approximately 18 in 10,000 babies are born with a critical congenital heart defect that requires intervention during infancy.
  ✓ Universal newborn screening is endorsed by the AAP, the American Heart Association (AHA), and the American College of Cardiology.
  ✓ Screening should occur on the right hand (preductal) and either foot (postductal).
  ✓ The baby passes screening if the oxygen saturation is 95% or greater in the right hand and the foot and the difference is <3% between the right hand and the foot.
  ✓ Screen is failed if the oxygen saturation is <90% in the right hand and the foot.
  ✓ A repeat screen should be performed in 1 hour if the oxygen saturation is 90–95% in the right hand and the foot or there is ≥3% difference between the right hand and the foot.
  ✓ If an infant fails the CHD screen, he or she should be examined to rule out noncardiac causes of hypoxemia. If an alternative cause is not identified, a cardiologist or neonatologist should be consulted, and echocardiography should be performed.

MANAGEMENT

Preventive treatment

- Prevention of ophthalmia neonatorum and conjunctivitis:
  ✓ Neonatal conjunctivitis is an acute mucopurulent infection occurring in the first 4 weeks of life and affects 1.6–12% of all newborns.

✓ Neonatal conjunctivitis may be caused by chemical irritation, non–sexually transmitted bacteria, sexually transmitted bacteria, and viruses.

✓ *Neisseria gonorrhoeae* is the most concerning cause of conjunctivitis and can cause blindness. Infection causes purulent conjunctivitis with profuse exudate and swelling of the eyelids. Treatment consists of single dose of cefotaxime or ceftriaxone for symptomatic infants or for asymptomatic infants of untreated mothers.

✓ Administration of topical antibiotic ointment (erythromycin or tetracycline) within a few hours after birth has been effective in reducing the incidence of blindness secondary to gonococcal conjunctivitis.

✓ Neonates presenting with signs of conjunctivitis should have a conjunctival swab sent for Gram stain and culture.

- Prevention of vitamin K–deficiency bleeding
  ✓ Vitamin K is required for biologic activation of coagulation factors II, VII, IX, and X.
  ✓ Placental transfer and neonatal synthesis of vitamin K is limited. Therefore, newborn infants are deficient in vitamin K and are at increased risk of bleeding.
  ✓ There are three presentations of vitamin K-deficiency bleeding:
  ✓ Early vitamin K-deficiency bleeding: Manifests in the first 24 hours and usually occurs in infants born to mothers who are taking medications that inhibit vitamin K (e.g., anticonvulsants). Frequently associated with intracranial and intraabdominal hemorrhage.
  ✓ Classic vitamin K-deficiency bleeding: Manifests in the first week of life. The clinical presentation is often mild, but significant blood loss and intracranial hemorrhage have been reported.
  ✓ Late vitamin K-deficiency bleeding: Manifests in infants 2–12 weeks of age, and symptoms are usually severe. The mortality rate is approximately 20%, and 50% of children have intracranial hemorrhages. Late vitamin K-deficiency bleeding is associated with exclusive breastfeeding.
  ✓ The AAP recommends that all newborns receive vitamin K 0.5–1 mg IM at birth.
  ✓ There is no approved oral preparation of vitamin K in the United States.
- Circumcision
  ✓ The surgical removal of the prepuce (foreskin) of the penis
  ✓ Neonatal circumcision is controversial among professional societies, health care professionals, and parents.
  ✓ Benefits: Lower rates of urinary tract infection, penile cancer, penile inflammation, penile dermatoses, and sexually transmitted infections; easier hygiene
  ✓ Disadvantages: Procedure-related complications (inadequate skin removal, bleeding, infection, urethral complications, glans injury, excessive removal of skin, adhesions, anesthetic complications), sexual dissatisfaction, pain
- Hepatitis B virus (HBV): see "Hepatitis B" in "Congenital and Perinatal Infections" section.

Common Problems in the Nursery

- Hypothermia and hyperthermia: See "Temperature Regulation" section.
- Voiding
  ✓ 95% of newborns void by 24 hours of age.
  ✓ Delayed voiding may be secondary to neonatal stress during delivery.
  ✓ No output by 48–72 hours may be due to renal (renal agenesis, renal vascular thrombosis, cystic kidney disease) or postrenal (neuropathic bladder dysfunction, obstruction of urinary flow) causes.
  ✓ Ultrasound of bladder, kidneys, and posterior urethra should be performed.

✓ Fewer than four wet diapers on day 4 of life is concerning for inadequate milk intake in breastfed infants.
- Stooling
  ✓ 99.7% of newborns pass meconium by 24 hours of life.

COMMON NEWBORN PROBLEMS

HYPERBILIRUBINEMIA

Defined as an elevation of total serum bilirubin

EPIDEMIOLOGY

- Neonatal jaundice affects up to 84% of term newborns.
- Severe hyperbilirubinemia (total serum bilirubin of >20 mg/dL occurs is less than 2% of term infants.
- Hyperbilirubinemia is more common and more severe in preterm infants.

PATHOPHYSIOLOGY

- Hemoglobin is released during red blood cell (RBC) hemolysis.
- Unconjugated bilirubin binds to albumin and is transported to the liver.
- Unbound, unconjugated bilirubin can cross the blood–brain barrier and is toxic to the central nervous system.
- Uridine diphosphate glucuronosyltransferase conjugates the unconjugated bilirubin in the liver.
- Conjugated bilirubin collects in the gallbladder and bile duct and is excreted in the stool.
  ✓ Unconjugated (indirect) hyperbilirubinemia:
  - Increased production:
    ▷ Hemolytic anemia: ABO or Rh incompatibility, minor blood-group incompatibility
    ▷ ABO incompatibility: Most common cause of neonatal hyperbilirubinemia.
      - Hemolysis caused by maternal–fetal ABO blood-group incompatibility and transplacental passage of maternal immunoglobulin (Ig) G to the fetus.
      - Usually, the mother is group O and the newborn group A or B. Mothers with type O blood do not have A or B antigens and produce anti-A and anti-B antibodies throughout life.
      - Maternal anti-antibodies cross the placenta and attach to fetal RBCs, resulting in hemolysis and release of unconjugated bilirubin.
      - Hyperbilirubinemia is often mild because A and B antigens are expressed on many tissues in addition to RBCs, allowing other sites for maternal antibodies to attach to.
    ▷ Rh incompatibility: Hemolysis caused by maternal–fetal blood-group incompatibility of the rhesus D antigen (Rh) and resultant transplacental passage of IgG antibodies from a previously sensitized mother to her fetus.
      - Occurs in mothers who are RhD-negative who carry fetuses with paternally derived Rh antigens.
      - Rh D-positive fetal RBCs cross into maternal circulation during pregnancy or delivery.
      - Maternal antibodies are produced against foreign Rh antigen and, during subsequent pregnancies, maternal IgG anti-Rh antibodies cross the placenta and attach to fetal RBCs. This results in fetal hemolysis and release of unconjugated bilirubin. Rh disease is usually more severe than ABO incompatibility because Rh antigens are expressed only on RBCs.

- Mothers should be screened, and anti-D immunoglobulin should be given to RhD-negative mothers at 28–36 gestational weeks and at delivery to try to prevent maternal sensitization. An additional dose of anti-D should be given to mothers when transplacental hemorrhage is suspected.
  - ▷ Enzyme deficiency: Glucose-6-phosphate dehydrogenase (G6PD) deficiency, pyruvate kinase deficiency
  - ▷ Membrane defects: Hereditary spherocytosis, elliptocytosis
  - ▷ Other: Cephalohematoma, significant bruising, polycythemia
  - ▪ Decreased clearance: Crigler–Najjar syndrome, Gilbert syndrome
  - ▪ Increased enterohepatic circulation: Gastrointestinal obstruction, breastfeeding/breast milk jaundice
  - ▪ Multifactorial: Physiologic jaundice, congenital hypothyroidism, hypopituitarism, metabolic disorders, sepsis
- ✓ Conjugated (direct) hyperbilirubinemia (conjugated bilirubin concentration >1 mg/dL when the total serum bilirubin (TSB) concentration is ≤5 mg/dL, or ≥20% of the TSB concentration)
  - ▪ Anatomic: Biliary atresia, Alagille syndrome, tumors of the liver and biliary tract, intrahepatic and periductal lymphadenopathy
  - ▪ Infectious: Urinary-tract infection, hepatitis, TORCH (toxoplasma, rubella, cytomegalovirus, and herpes simplex) infections
  - ▪ Genetic/inborn errors of metabolism: α_1-antitrypsin deficiency, galactosemia, tyrosinemia, fructosemia, glycogen storage disease, lipid storage disease, idiopathic hypopituitarism
  - ▪ Miscellaneous: Total parenteral nutrition–induced cholestasis, medications, hypothyroidism, hemochromatosis

CLINICAL MANIFESTATIONS

- Jaundice: Clinically visible at bilirubin levels of 5–7 mg/dL; first apparent in the face and descends as level increases (visual inspection has limited reliability)
- Early neurologic findings in context of extremely high bilirubin levels (bilirubin encephalopathy): hypertonia, arching, retrocollis, opisthotonos, fever, and high-pitched cry.
- Later neurologic findings/kernicterus: athetoid cerebral palsy, auditory dysfunction, dental dysplasia, paralysis of upward gaze, and variable intellectual disability

DIAGNOSTICS

- If hemolytic anemia is suspected in utero, Doppler blood flow in the middle cerebral artery should be assessed (increased velocity is associated with anemia). There is an increased risk of fetal hydrops.
- Transcutaneous bilirubin or TSB should be obtained in any infant who develops jaundice in the first 24 hours after birth.
- The result should be interpreted on the basis of the bilirubin nomogram. Reassessment should be based on the zone in which the bilirubin falls on the nomogram (this is for infants born at >35 weeks without risk factors)
- If the cause of hyperbilirubinemia is not evident, a complete blood count (CBC) with smear, reticulocyte count, G6PD level, thyroid function, liver function, prothrombin/partial thromboplastin time, urine culture, serum amino acids, urine organic acids, urine-reducing substances may be considered.
- A liver ultrasound, hepatobiliary imaging (e.g., diisopropyl iminodiacetic acid scan), or percutaneous liver biopsy may also be considered.

MANAGEMENT

Unconjugated hyperbilirubinemia

- Ensure adequate hydration
- Phototherapy: Light energy converts unconjugated bilirubin to a structural isomer, which can be excreted without conjugation. Blue lamps (460–490 nm) are most effective. Infant should be placed as close as possible to the light.
  - ✓ The AAP recommends initiating phototherapy in healthy, term, or near-term infants based on day of life and risk factors (**Figure 18-1**). Note that nomogram values are based on total serum bilirubin levels.
  - ✓ Phototherapy should be initiated at lower levels for premature infants.
  - ✓ Discontinuation of phototherapy is not standardized.
- Intravenous gamma globulin is recommended for infants who have isoimmune hemolytic disease if the TSB is rising despite phototherapy or the TSB is within 2–3 mg/dL of the level for an exchange transfusion. A second dose can be administered in 12 hours, if needed.
- Exchange transfusion: Double-volume exchange transfusions are reserved for infants at high risk of kernicterus and should be performed only in a neonatal intensive care unit (NICU) by a trained physician. The procedure rapidly removes the circulating bilirubin and any antibodies that may be contributing to ongoing hemolysis.
  - ✓ Consider exchange transfusion in healthy, term infants with total bilirubin levels of 25–30 mg/dL.

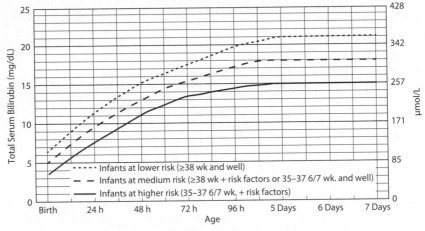

- Use total bilirubin. Do not subtract direct reacting or conjugated bilirubin.
- Risk factors = isoimmune hemolytic disease, G6PD deficiency, asphyxia, significant lethargy, temperature instability, sepsis, acidosis, or albumin <3.0g/dL (if measured)
- For well infants 35–37 6/7 wk can adjust TSB levels for intervention around the medium risk line. It is an option to intervene at lower TSB levels for infants closer to 35 wks and at higher TSB levels for those closer to 37 6/7 wk.
- It is an option to provide conventional phototherapy in hospital or at home at TSB levels 2–3 mg/dL (35–50mmol/L) below those shown but home phototherapy should not be used in any infant with risk factors.

FIGURE 18-1 Bilirubin nomogram. In infants born at ≥35 weeks' gestation age, this nomogram designates the total serum bilirubin level at which to initiate phototherapy (based on risk factors and hours of life). Reproduced with permission from American Academy of Pediatrics Subcommittee on Hyperbilirubinemia: Management of hyperbilirubinemia in the newborn infant 35 or more weeks of gestation, *Pediatrics* 2004 Jul;114(1):297-316.

✓ In infants with specific risk factors, consider exchange transfusion at lower bilirubin levels.

✓ Complications of exchange transfusions include infection, portal venous thrombosis, thrombocytopenia, necrotizing enterocolitis, electrolyte imbalance, graft-versus-host disease, and death.

Conjugated Hyperbilirubinemia

• Management is aimed at treating the underlying cause.

• Phenobarbital, cholestyramine, and ursodiol may promote bile flow and decrease serum bilirubin levels.

• Dietary management: Formulas containing medium-chain triglycerides are better absorbed, supplement with fat-soluble vitamins (A, D, E, and K)

• Kasai procedure (hepatoportoenterostomy) is used to bridge to transplantation in infants with biliary atresia.

HYPOGLYCEMIA

There is much debate on the definition of neonatal hypoglycemia. Per the AAP, hypoglycemia is defined as a glucose level of <45 mg/dL in the first 24 hours.

EPIDEMIOLOGY

• Hypoglycemia may occur in up to 10% of healthy term newborns in the first 24–48 hours.

• Hypoglycemia is more common in premature infants.

PATHOPHYSIOLOGY

The fetus receives a steady supply of glucose via facilitated diffusion across the placenta. The fetus produces its own insulin to permit euglycemia. Postnatally, the constant transplacental supply of glucose ceases, and the glucose concentrations in the healthy term newborn fall during the first 2 hours after delivery and stabilizes by 4–6 hours of life.

• Inadequate glucose supply

✓ Inadequate glycogen stores: Prematurity, fetal growth restriction

✓ Impaired glucose production: Inborn errors of metabolism, endocrine disorders (e.g., cortisol and growth hormone), other (maternal treatment with beta-sympathomimetic agents, hypothermia, severe hepatic dysfunction)

• Increased glucose utilization

✓ Excessive insulin secretion: Infant of a diabetic mother (see "Infant of a Diabetic Mother" section), congenital hyperinsulinism, fetal growth restriction, Beckwith–Wiedemann syndrome, perinatal asphyxia or stress, maternal intrapartum treatment with glucose, abrupt interruption of an infusion of a solution with high glucose concentration, meconium aspiration syndrome, hypothermia, polycythemia

✓ Other causes: Poor perfusion/oxygenation, perinatal asphyxia, sepsis

CLINICAL MANIFESTATIONS

• Often asymptomatic

• Jitteriness/tremors, sweating, irritability, tachypnea, pallor, poor feeding, weak or high pitched cry, change in level of consciousness, seizures, hypotonia, apnea, bradycardia, cyanosis, and hypothermia

DIAGNOSTICS

• The AAP recommends that the initial feed occur within 1 hour after birth and a glucose level obtained 30 minutes after the first feed for infants with risk factors. Symptomatic infants with a glucose of <40 mg/dL should be given IV glucose. Asymptomatic infants

<4 hours of age with a screening glucose of <25 mg/dL should be refed. After 1 hour, if rechecked glucose is <25 mg/dL, infant should receive IV glucose, or if rechecked glucose concentration is 25–40 mg/dL, infant may be fed again. Infants should be fed every 2–3 hours. Asymptomatic infants 4–24 hours of age with a screening glucose of <35 mg/dL should be fed. After 1 hour, if rechecked glucose is <35 mg/dL, infant should receive IV glucose, or if rechecked glucose concentration is 35–45 mg/dL, infant may be fed again. The target glucose is >45 mg/dL prior to routine feeds
- The Pediatric Endocrine Society recommends a blood glucose of >50 mg/dL in the first 48 hours and then a blood glucose of >60 mg/dL beyond the first 48 hours of life.

MANAGEMENT

- Enteral feedings, IV glucose bolus (D10 at 2 mL/kg), IV glucose infusion (D10 at 3 mL/kg/hr)
- The use of buccal dextrose gel in term infants may be effective (40% dextrose gel 200 mg/kg).
- Glucagon and diazoxide/octreotide may be considered for persistent hypoglycemia.
- Alternative causes of hypoglycemia should be considered if hypoglycemia persists. A "critical sample" is collected during a period of hypoglycemia and includes plasma glucose, insulin, C-reactive peptide, beta-hydroxybutyrate, free fatty acids, acylcarnitine profile, lactate, ammonia, and urine organic acids. A basic metabolic panel and hepatic panel should be obtained.

INFANT OF A DIABETIC MOTHER

An infant born to a mother with diabetes

EPIDEMIOLOGY

- Infants born to diabetic mothers (IDMs) are at increased risk of morbidity and mortality. IDMs have a 2–3× higher risk of congenital malformations than infants of nondiabetic mothers. Perinatal mortality is 3–10× higher than in the general population.
- Gestational diabetes occurs in 2–10% of pregnancies in the United States.

PATHOPHYSIOLOGY

- Maternal hyperglycemia results in fetal hyperglycemia and subsequently increased fetal insulin production during the second half of pregnancy.
- Elevated insulin levels result in fat production (leads to macrosomia) and increased glycogen content in the liver, kidney, skeletal muscle, and heart (contributes to ventriculomegaly).
- Elevated insulin levels also delay fetal lung maturation.
- Chronic fetal hyperinsulinism increases fetal metabolic rates and subsequent oxygen consumption, leading to fetal hypoxia.
- Hypoxia stimulates erythropoietin production, which may result in polycythemia. These changes result in an increased risk of fetal asphyxia and intrauterine demise in IDMs.

CLINICAL MANIFESTATIONS

- Hypoglycemia (see "Hypoglycemia" section): IDMs may have earlier, more profound and persistent hypoglycemia than non-IDMs.
- Macrosomia/large for gestational age: Macrosomia results from increased adiposity and increased liver and skeletal mass due to insulin stimulated fetal growth. Macrosomia and maternal diabetes are independent risk factors for shoulder dystocia and brachial plexus injury. Clavicle and humerus fractures are also associated complications.
- Congenital malformations: The most common malformations involve the heart, central nervous system, kidneys and urinary tract, skeletal system, and gastrointestinal system. Presenting signs and symptoms vary depending on the anomaly/anomalies present.

Clinicians should maintain a high index of suspicion for underlying anomalies, particularly in infants of mothers with known poor glycemic control.

- Respiratory distress syndrome (RDS): IDMs born at <38 weeks' gestation have $6\times$ higher risk of RDS than gestational age–matched non-IDMs owing to decreased surfactant. RDS typically presents as increased work of breathing and/or hypoxia.
- Perinatal asphyxia: The increased risk of perinatal asphyxia is greatest in offspring of mothers with preexisting diabetes, most notably those with renal and atherosclerotic disease and/or a long history of unstable glucose control. Clinical findings of asphyxia include hypotonia and poor respiratory effort at birth and seizures in the neonatal period.
- Hypocalcemia: Hypocalcemia is a consequence of transient hypoparathyroidism that results from fetal and maternal hypomagnesemia. Hypocalcemia may result in irritability and decreased myocardial function.
- Hematologic manifestations: IDMs are at increased risk of polycythemia, hyperbilirubinemia, and venous thrombosis.
- Hypertrophic cardiomyopathy: The cardiomyopathy typically seen in IDMs is characterized by septal hypertrophy. In severe cases, there may be marked hypertrophy of the myocardium. Hypertrophy typically resolves over first few months of life, some infants may be critically ill in the newborn period because of outflow-tract obstruction and cardiac dysfunction.
- Gastrointestinal issues: Small left colon and intestinal hypomotility are the most commonly encountered gastrointestinal issues.
- Long-term outcomes: There is a possible delay in intelligence and psychomotor development independent of perinatal complications in IDMs. There is also an increased risk of obesity, impaired glucose tolerance, blunted insulin secretion, and hypertension in IDMs.

DIAGNOSTICS

- See "Hypoglycemia" section.
- Consider hematocrit and bilirubin monitoring if there is concern for polycythemia and jaundice.

MANAGEMENT

- See "Hypoglycemia" section.
- Symptomatic or severe hypocalcemia should be treated with calcium gluconate. Coexisting hypomagnesemia should be treated with magnesium to allow for effective correction of hypocalcemia.
- A cardiology consult may be beneficial for patients with cyanotic heart disease.
- Hyperbilirubinemia and polycythemia should be managed (see "Polycythemia" section).
- IDMs should be monitored for symptoms of birth injury and congenital malformations.

NEONATAL ABSTINENCE SYNDROME (NAS)

Constellation of symptoms that occurs when an infant is exposed to opioids in utero.

EPIDEMIOLOGY

- The incidence of NAS has been increasing in the United States and varies by region from a low of 1 per 1000 (District of Columbia) to a high of 56 per 1000 (West Virginia) in 2017 (https://www.hcup-us.ahrq.gov/faststats/NASMap)
- Of infants with prenatal exposure to opioids, reported rates of NAS requiring pharmacotherapy ranges from 42% to 94%.

PATHOPHYSIOLOGY

- NAS is a consequence of the abrupt discontinuation of chronic fetal exposure to substances that were used or abused by the mother during pregnancy.
- Several factors can affect the accumulation of opioids in the fetus. Opiate drugs have low molecular weights, are water-soluble, and are lipophilic. Therefore, they are easily transferable across the placenta to the fetus.
- The pathophysiologic mechanism of opioid withdrawal in neonates is not known.
- Opioids mostly act through opioid receptors (μ, κ, and δ), which are extensively distributed across the nervous system. A lack of opioids in a chronically stimulated state increases activity in opioid receptors and results in increased production of various neurotransmitters. These neurotransmitters result in the symptoms associated with NAS.

CLINICAL MANIFESTATIONS

- Presentation is highly variable in timing of onset and severity of symptoms.
- Preterm infants <35 weeks' gestation have a less extensive expression and incidence of NAS than term infants.
- Tremors, irritability, excessive crying, sleep and wake disturbances, alterations in tone or movement, feeding difficulties, gastrointestinal disturbances (vomiting, loose stools, gassiness), autonomic dysfunction (sweating, sneezing, mottling, fever, yawning, nasal congestion), seizures

DIAGNOSTICS

- NAS is a clinical diagnosis based on maternal history and infant's symptoms.
- Toxicologic confirmation is necessary to identify the type of substance used during the pregnancy. Analysis of the urine or meconium is recommended. Meconium testing is more sensitive and has a longer window of detection (from 20 weeks of gestational age until delivery).

MANAGEMENT

Several abstinence scoring methods (Lipsitz tool, Finnegan Neonatal Abstinence Scoring System, Neonatal Withdrawal Inventory) have been developed and validated for clinical use. These tools measure the severity of neonatal withdrawal symptoms and are used to initiate, adjust, and wean pharmacologic therapy.

- The eat, sleep, console approach recommends no pharmacologic interventions if the infant can eat ≥1 ounces per feed, sleep >1 hour, and be consoled within 10 minutes
- The length of hospitalization should be sufficient to detect signs of withdrawal and should be a minimum of 4–5 days for infants exposed to any opioid.
- The initial treatment of all infants exposed to substances in utero is nonpharmacologic and includes small frequent feeds of high-calorie milk, minimal stimulation practices and swaddling. Kangaroo care and pacifiers are also included. Music therapy and massage therapy may be considered.
- There are currently no uniformly accepted standard pharmacologic regimens for management of NAS. Morphine is the most commonly preferred medication. Methadone and buprenorphine are alternatives to morphine.
- Phenobarbital is the drug of choice for nonopiate NAS and is often used as an adjunctive agent for opioid NAS.
- Clonidine has been studied, but no large-scale studies have proven its efficacy for NAS.
- Breastfeeding should be encouraged in mothers who are not taking illicit drugs, have no polydrug abuse, or are not infected with human immunodeficiency virus.

NEWBORN SEPSIS AND SCREENING

A clinical syndrome characterized by systemic signs of infection frequently accompanied by bacteremia

EPIDEMIOLOGY

- The overall incidence of neonatal sepsis ranges from 1 in 1000 to 5 in 1000 live births.
- Sepsis accounts for approximately 15% of all neonatal deaths.
- Rates of neonatal sepsis increase with decreasing gestational age. The estimated incidence of sepsis in term neonates is 1 in 1000 to 2 in 1000 live births. The estimated incidence of early-onset sepsis in preterm infants (<37 weeks) is 3.71 in 1000 live births and 10.96 in 1000 live births in very-low-birth-weight (VLBW) infants.

PATHOPHYSIOLOGY

- Early-onset sepsis (EOS): blood and/or cerebrospinal fluid (CSF) culture-proven infection occurring in a newborn <7 days of age. For continuously hospitalized VLBW infants, EOS is defined as culture-proven infection occurring at <72 hours of life.
  - ✓ EOS is usually due to vertical transmission by ascending contaminated amniotic fluid or during vaginal delivery from bacteria in the mother's lower genital tract. *Listeria monocytogenes* is the exception; it occurs via hematogenous spread.
  - ✓ Group B *Streptococcus* (GBS) is the leading cause of EOS in term infants. However, the incidence of GBS has decreased by 87% due to the implementation of intrapartum antibiotic prophylaxis. *Escherichia coli* is the second leading cause of EOS in all infants, but it is the leading cause of EOS in preterm infants.
  - ✓ Other organisms that cause EOS are *Enterococcus; Staphylococcus aureus*, coagulase-negative *Staphylococcus, Listeria, Bacteroides* spp., *Klebsiella*, Non-typeable Haemophilus Influenzae.
- Late-onset sepsis (LOS): Definition is variable. Some clinicians define LOS as a positive blood culture occurring 72 hours after birth, any time from 4 to 7 days after birth, or up to 30 days of life with or without clinical symptoms.
  - ✓ LOS is usually secondary to vertical transmission in which an initial neonatal colonization evolves into a later infection, or horizontal transmission in which transmission occurs from an infected care provider or environmental source.
  - ✓ Gram-positive organisms are primarily responsible for LOS. The most common isolated organism is coagulase-negative staphylococci (CoNS). Because of its low virulence, the diagnosis of true CoNS bacteremia relies on two cultures obtained from different sites within 24 hours growing the same organisms with the same sensitivities. Methicillin-resistant *Staphylococcus aureus* (MRSA) is becoming an increasingly prevalent cause of LOS.
  - ✓ LOS due to gram-negative organisms is associated with higher mortality. *E. coli* is the most common gram-negative rod causing LOS. Other gram-negative organisms commonly reported include *Klebsiella, Enterobacter*, and *Serratia. Pseudomonas aeruginosa* is less common but carries the highest mortality risk among premature infants.
  - ✓ Yeast bloodstream infections are less common but carry significant mortality.
- Culture-negative sepsis: Occurs when infants have signs and symptoms of physiologic dysregulation ascribed to a bacterial etiology but in whom an organism has not been isolated in properly collected cultures of blood, cerebral fluid, or urine.

CLINICAL MANIFESTATIONS

- Signs and symptoms of sepsis are often subtle. Symptoms include temperature instability (usually hyperthermia in term infants and hypothermia in preterm infants), irritability,

lethargy, respiratory distress, cyanosis, poor feeding, tachycardia, apnea, bradycardia, poor perfusion, and hypotension. Other findings include jaundice, hepatomegaly, vomiting, abdominal distention, and diarrhea. Fetal and delivery room signs and symptoms include intrapartum tachycardia, meconium-stained amniotic fluid, and Apgar score ≤6.
- VLBW infants who develop sepsis are significantly more likely to die and to have impaired neurodevelopmental outcomes than those who are not infected

DIAGNOSTICS

- A positive blood culture is the gold standard to confirm the diagnosis of neonatal sepsis.
- The Centers for Disease Control and Prevention and the AAP advocate evaluation of infants who are born with signs of illness, well-appearing infants born in the setting of maternal chorioamnionitis, and infants born to women who do not receive adequate GBS intrapartum antibiotic prophylaxis when indicated, with consideration given to gestational age at birth and duration of rupture of membranes. EOS calculators are tools that can be used to estimate the risk of early-onset sepsis in individual patients based on risk factors
- EOS:
  ✓ Review of pregnancy, labor, and delivery risk factors: GBS infection, chorioamnionitis, membrane rupture ≥18 hours
  ✓ Blood culture
  ✓ Lumbar puncture: Blood cultures may be negative in as many as 38% of infants with meningitis. Therefore, lumbar puncture is indicated if there is a positive blood culture, laboratory data suggestive of sepsis, and/ or worsening clinical status while taking antibiotics.
  ✓ CBC with differential
  ✓ CBCs obtained at 6–12 hours of life are more predictive of sepsis.
  ✓ Immature:total neutrophil (I:T) ratio: an elevated I:T ratio (≥0.2) has the best sensitivity for predicting neonatal sepsis.
  ✓ Consider chest radiography, tracheal aspiration, and measurement of C-reactive protein and/or procalcitonin levels
- LOS:
  ✓ Workup similar to that for EOS, with the exception that blood cultures should be obtained from central catheter if present.

MANAGEMENT

- EOS:
  ✓ Ampicillin and gentamicin are widely used empirical antibiotics.
  ✓ Ampicillin and a third-generation cephalosporin
  ✓ Ceftriaxone is not recommended for use in the first week after birth because it can displace bilirubin from albumin and can precipitate when used with calcium-containing products
- LOS:
  ✓ Controversial and dependent on hospital-specific resistance patterns.
  ✓ Oxacillin(or nafcillin) and gentamicin may be reasonable for empirical antibiotic therapy. The use of vancomycin should be initiated if the infant is critically ill and the postulated infecting organism is MRSA. Third-generation cephalosporins should be discouraged outside of suspected meningitis.
  ✓ Consider amphotericin B if there is concern for *Candida* infection
  ✓ Choice of antibiotic should be narrowed as much as possible once an organism has been identified.

POLYCYTHEMIA

A hematocrit that exceeds expected value for gestational and postnatal age

EPIDEMIOLOGY

- Polycythemia occurs in 1–2% of healthy newborns born at sea level and up to 5% of infants born at high altitude.
- More common in small for gestational age neonates (10–15% affected)

PATHOPHYSIOLOGY

- Polycythemia results from an increase in RBC mass.
- An increased RBC mass may be observed in chronic intrauterine hypoxia (IUGR, maternal diabetes, maternal smoking) and increased fetal blood volume (delayed cord clamping, maternal–fetal transfusion, twin-to-twin transfusion).
- Other causes of polycythemia include large for gestational age, congenital hypothyroidism, neonatal thyrotoxicosis, congenital adrenal hyperplasia, Beckwith–Wiedemann syndrome, and trisomies 13, 18, and 21.
- Viscosity is directly proportional to hematocrit (HCT) but rises logarithmically above an HCT of 60%. When viscosity increases, blood flow is impaired and tissue perfusion is decreased.

CLINICAL MANIFESTATIONS

- Most neonates with polycythemia are asymptomatic.
- Plethora, delayed capillary refill, lethargy, apnea, tremors/jitteriness, poor feeding, hypotonia, exaggerated startle reflex, tachypnea, cyanosis, tachycardia, respiratory distress, cardiomegaly, prominent vascular markings on chest radiograph, elevated pulmonary vascular resistance, renal dysfunction (oliguria, proteinuria, or hematuria), hypoglycemia, hypocalcemia, and hyperbilirubinemia
- Seizures, congestive heart failure, thrombosis, thrombocytopenia, disseminated intravascular coagulation, and necrotizing enterocolitis are possible but rare.

DIAGNOSTICS

- Characterized by an HCT or hemoglobin concentration >2 SD above the normal value for gestational and postnatal age. For a term infant, polycythemia is defined as an HCT $>65\%$ on a peripheral venous sample.
- Capillary hematocrits are significantly higher than venous values and should be used as a screening test. If the capillary value is $>65\%$, repeat with a venous stick (HCT level varies by sample site: arterial HCT$<$venous HCT$<$capillary HCT).

MANAGEMENT

- Asymptomatic neonates with HCT 60–70% can be treated by liberalizing fluid intake and serial monitoring of HCT.
- Partial-exchange transfusion (PET) should be considered for symptomatic neonates with an HCT $>65\%$ or any neonate with a venous HCT $>70\%$ (although this is controversial). There is no evidence that PET improves long-term outcomes in neonates.
  - ✓ The goal for PET is to decrease HCT to 50–55%.
  - ✓ The volume to exchange is calculated as (estimated blood volume = 100 mL/kg):

$$\frac{\text{Blood volume} \times (\text{Observed HCT} - \text{Desired HCT})}{\text{Observed HCT}}$$

✓ Normal saline is the replacement fluid of choice.
✓ Repeat the HCT at the end of the exchange and 4–6 hours later.

TEMPERATURE REGULATION

Maintenance of body temperatures within a desired range

EPIDEMIOLOGY

- Both hypothermia and hyperthermia are associated with increased mortality and morbidity.
- The World Health Organization and other scientific organizations recommend that axillary temperature be maintained between 97.7 and 99.5°F (36.5 and 37.5°C).
- As many as 40% of extremely preterm infants have temperatures <95°F (35°C) at the time of NICU admission.

PATHOPHYSIOLOGY

- Hypothermia:
  ✓ Thermoreceptors on the newborn's skin are stimulated by cool external temperatures. After birth, there is a rapid fall in surrounding temperatures, and a newborn must rely primarily on nonshivering mechanisms to maintain body temperature. Nonshivering mechanisms involve chemical thermogenesis, which depends on brown fat. When brown fat is metabolized, the heat that is produced warms the organ and blood directly, leading to an elevation in body temperature.
  ✓ Preterm infants are at high risk for hypothermia. Preterm infants have less brown fat and a larger skin-surface area, resulting in more radiant heat loss and insensible losses. Once brown fat is depleted, it cannot be replaced.
  ✓ Infant can lose heat by four routes:
    - Evaporation: Heat loss due to evaporation of water (most common)
    - Radiant: Heat loss due to being near but not in direct contact with cold surfaces (prominent route of heat loss in infants >28 weeks)
    - Conduction: Heat loss due to direct contact with cold surfaces
    - Convection: Heat loss due to cold air
- Hyperthermia
  ✓ Most often occurs because of environmental factors leading to overheating
  ✓ May also be caused by sepsis, dehydration, medications or abnormal nervous system response

CLINICAL MANIFESTATIONS

- Lethargy, irritability, abnormal respirations, abnormal tone, abnormal heart rate, apnea, dehydration, poor feeding, blood pressure instability

DIAGNOSTICS

- Hypothermia
  ✓ Cold stress (96.8–97.5°F [36–36.4°C])
  ✓ Moderate hypothermia (89.6–96.6°F [32–35.9°C])
  ✓ Severe hypothermia (<89.6°F [<32°C])
- Hyperthermia (>99.5°F [>37.5°C])

MANAGEMENT

- Hospitals should optimize the ambient temperature of the delivery room. The NRP recommends that delivery room temperatures should be 73.4–77°F.

- The use of warm weighing scales, warm blankets, and hats reduce heat loss. Drying infants in the delivery room also reduces heat loss.
- Skin servo control, where the incubator temperature is controlled by the infant's skin temperature, is preferable to air-temperature control for infants who require incubators.
- Humidity has become an essential component of care in extremely preterm infants, but there is no standard for percentage of humidity or length of exposure.
- Plastic wraps and plastic bags should be used for infants born at <28 weeks' gestation and/or <1500 grams. The use of thermostable gel mattresses may be considered in this patient population.

CONGENITAL AND PERINATAL INFECTIONS

Congenital and perinatal infections, historically referred to as TORCH infections, comprise a group of diseases that affect the fetus and newborn. Classically, the term TORCH represented toxoplasmosis, Other (traditionally syphilis), Rubella, Cytomegalovirus (CMV), and Herpes simplex virus (HSV). The "other" category has expanded to include human immunodeficiency virus (HIV), enterovirus, parvovirus, varicella, and most recently, Zika virus. These infections share many clinical manifestations and can be difficult to differentiate. Insufficient information exists about the management and outcomes of severe acute respiratory syndrome coronavirus-2 (SARS-CoV-2), the cause of coronavirus disease 2019 (COVID-19) in congenital or perinatal infections.

CONGENITAL INFECTIONS

- See Table 18-3 for further details.

CYTOMEGALOVIRUS (CMV)

Epidemiology
- The most common human intrauterine infection
- 1% of all liveborn infants in the United States have congenital CMV; however, only 5–10% of infected infants are symptomatic at birth.

Etiology
- Double-stranded DNA virus

Pathophysiology
- Can be transmitted to fetus after maternal primary infection or recurrent infection
- Sequelae are more common in infants after maternal primary infection (25%) than after reactivation of maternal infection (8%)
- Infant is more likely to be symptomatic or to have sequelae if maternal infection occurs during the first half of pregnancy.
- Can also be acquired postpartum from infected breast milk or blood products.

Clinical Manifestations
- The most common clinical finding is hepatomegaly.
- Other findings include microcephaly with periventricular calcifications, chorioretinitis, sensorineural hearing loss, thrombocytopenia, hepatosplenomegaly, hyperbilirubinemia, intrauterine growth retardation, pneumonitis, mental impairment (IQ ≤70)

TABLE 18-3 Congenital Infections

Infection	Epidemiology/ Transmission	Clinical Characteristics	Diagnosis	Treatment	Outcome
CMV	Most common intrauterine infection Sequelae more common if infected during first half of pregnancy, though transmission more likely in third trimester	Leading cause of deafness (moderate to profound sensorineural hearing loss) and learning disability Hepatomegaly (most common), splenomegaly, jaundice, IUGR Microcephaly with periventricular calcifications	Positive viral culture or PCR (urine, saliva, blood, CSF, or respiratory secretions) within 3 weeks after birth	Ganciclovir or valganciclovir in symptomatic congenital infection with moderate to severe disease Significant toxicities include neutropenia and thrombocytopenia Treatment not recommended in asymptomatic infants	Symptomatic infants at birth: 20–30% mortality, 66% of survivors have sequelae. Asymptomatic infants at birth: 5–15% risk of later sequelae
Rubella	Transmission is most likely in the first or third trimester of pregnancy Sequelae more common if infected before 20 weeks' gestation	Most common defects: Sensorineural deafness, eye (cataracts); CNS (microcephaly); cardiac (PDA, pulmonary artery or valvular stenosis)	Viral culture from nasopharynx, urine, blood, or CSF Serial IgG levels or rubella-specific IgM	Supportive Infants with congenitally acquired rubella considered contagious for 1 year	75% of infected infants who are asymptomatic at birth develop sequelae years later.

Syphilis	Highest risk of transmission in primary and secondary disease. Transmission can occur at any point in pregnancy	Fetal or perinatal death in 40–50%. Early: Hydrops, IUGR, hepatosplenomegaly, mucocutaneous lesions, snuffles, leptomeningitis. Late (>2 years old): Hutchinson teeth, saddle nose, mental impairment, seizure disorder	Nontreponemal (VDRL or RPR) and treponemal (FTA-ABS or MHA-TP) tests on infant serum. Identify spirochetes by dark-field microscopy or direct fluorescent antibody tests of lesions, exudate, or tissue	Treatment options depend on how likely congenital syphilis infection is. Penicillin G is the drug of choice.	Treatment of early-stage infection can prevent late manifestations.
Toxoplasmosis	More severe disease if acquired earlier in pregnancy. Increasing risk of transmission with increasing gestational age	Approximately 75% are asymptomatic. Classic triad: hydrocephalus, chorioretinitis (most common), intracranial calcifications	Positive infant IgM or IgA. Positive infant IgG after 12 months of age. *Toxoplasma* serum, urine, and CSF PCR	Pyrimethamine and sulfadiazine with folinic acid supplementation	Good prognosis with treatment
Zika	Transmitted to mother via *Aedes* spp. mosquito or sexual intercourse. Transmitted to fetus during maternal infection	Severe microcephaly. Eye anomalies, contractures, neurologic dysfunction, hearing loss	Zika virus RNA nucleic acid testing in serum and urine, IgM antibody. Plaque reduction neutralization test	No treatment exists. Obtain head ultrasound, ABR testing and refer to early intervention services	Can result in motor impairment, vision abnormalities and hearing loss

ABR = auditory brainstem response; CNS = central nervous system; CSF = cerebrospinal fluid; FTA-ABS = fluorescent treponemal antibody absorption; IUGR = intrauterine growth restriction; MHA-TP = microhemagglutination assay–*Treponema pallidum*; PCR = polymerase chain reaction; PDA = patent ductus arteriosus; RPR = rapid plasma reagin; VDRL = Venereal Disease Research Laboratory.

Diagnostics

- Proof of congenital infection requires positive viral culture or polymerase chain reaction (PCR) from specimen (urine, saliva, blood, CSF, or respiratory secretions) within 3 weeks after birth.
  - ✓ For positive results after 4 weeks of life, neonate must also have intracranial calcifications, chorioretinitis, or other signs of intrauterine disease.
- Presumptive diagnosis can be made by fourfold rise in IgG titer in paired serum samples or a positive IgM (infrequently used method).

Management

- Ganciclovir (and oral valganciclovir) is the treatment of choice for symptomatic infants with moderate to severe congenital disease.
- Neonates with congenital CMV disease (with or without CNS involvement) have improved hearing and neurodevelopmental outcomes at 2 years of age when treated with oral valganciclovir.
- Ganciclovir has significant toxicity (neutropenia and thrombocytopenia).
- Consult a pediatric infectious disease specialist to aid in treatment and management.

RUBELLA

Epidemiology

- Rubella is no longer endemic in the United States.

Etiology

- RNA virus causing a very mild, but extremely contagious disease; referred to as "German measles"

Pathophysiology

- Transmission to the fetus can occur at any point in pregnancy, but is more likely in the first and third trimesters (particularly in the last month of pregnancy).
- Congenital defects are more likely if infection occurs prior to 20 weeks of gestation.

Clinical Manifestations

- Can result in spontaneous abortion, fetal death, or congenital rubella syndrome.
- Most common manifestation is sensorineural deafness, followed by neurologic impairment.
- Cardiac malformations (patent ductus arteriosus[PDA] most common; also, pulmonary artery stenosis, pulmonary valvar stenosis, aortic valve stenosis, tetralogy of Fallot)
- Ocular abnormalities (cataracts, glaucoma, pigmented retinopathy, microphthalmia)
- Microcephaly, meningoencephalitis
- Blueberry muffin lesions (extramedullary dermal hematopoiesis), thrombocytopenia, and hemolytic anemia can also occur.
- Delayed manifestations occur in >20% of individuals with congenital rubella infection. These include insulin-dependent diabetes and thyroid disease.

Diagnostics

- Viral culture of specimens from blood, CSF, urine, and nasopharynx
- RNA PCR from nasopharynx or urine
- Detection of rubella-specific IgM in first 6 months of life
- Serial serum rubella IgG levels demonstrate an increase over several months

Congenital Infections

Management

- Treatment is solely supportive. Isolate neonate from other newborns, as infant may be contagious.

SYPHILIS

Epidemiology

- Rates of syphilis infection and, thus, congenital infection, have been increasing since the early 2000s.

Etiology

- Syphilis is caused by a mobile spirochete, *Treponema pallidum.*

Pathophysiology

- *Treponema pallidum* can cross the placenta at any point during pregnancy.
- Infection of the fetus can also occur if there is contact with active genital lesions during delivery.
- Infection can be transmitted to the fetus at any stage of maternal disease; rate of transmission is highest (60–90%) with primary and secondary syphilis.

Clinical Manifestations

- Preterm delivery, nonimmune hydrops, congenital infection, fetal or perinatal death (occurs in 40–50% of cases).
- Two-thirds of infected liveborn neonates are asymptomatic.
- Overt infection can manifest in the fetus, newborn, or later in childhood.
- Early congenital manifestations (detected before 2 years of age, typically before age 3 months): Nonimmune hydrops, IUGR, failure to thrive, hemolytic anemia, jaundice, hepatomegaly, bullous lesions and desquamation on palm and soles, copper-colored maculopapular rash, condyloma lata, chorioretinitis, uveitis, snuffles (copious nasal secretions), osteochondritis, periostitis, meningitis, parrot pseudoparalysis (decreased movement of one or both upper extremities due to painful periostitis)
- Late congenital manifestations: typically detected after 2 years of age

Diagnostics

- Presumptive diagnosis: Nontreponemal (Venereal Disease Research Laboratory [VDRL] or rapid plasma reagin [RPR]) and treponemal (fluorescent treponemal antibody absorption [FTA-ABS] or microhemagglutination assay–*T. pallidum* [MHA-TP]) tests on infant serum
- Definitive diagnosis: Identify spirochetes by dark-field microscopy or direct fluorescent antibody tests of lesions, exudate, or tissue
- CSF evaluation for leptomeningitis (VDRL, cell count, and protein)
- CBC with differential and platelet count
- Chest x-ray, long-bone radiographs, liver function tests, ophthalmologic examination, auditory brain stem response, and neuroimaging as clinically indicated

Management

- Penicillin G remains the drug of choice for any stage of syphilis.
- Treatment recommendations depend on whether it is confirmed, possible, or probable that the neonate has congenital syphilis.

435

TOXOPLASMOSIS

Epidemiology

- An estimated 1.1 in 1000 women experience acute infection during pregnancy.

Etiology

- Toxoplasmosis is caused by an intracellular parasite, *Toxoplasma gondii.*

Pathophysiology

- Maternal infection with *Toxoplasma gondii* occurs via ingestion of cysts from infected meat or from contact with cat excrement. Transmission ensues if primary infection occurs during pregnancy.
- The risk of transmission to the fetus increases with advancing gestational age at time of maternal infection, with an overall risk of 20–50%.
- The severity of disease in the infant is inversely proportional to the gestational age at the time of infection; therefore, the disease is most severe if infection occurs in the first trimester.

Clinical Manifestations

- 70–90% are asymptomatic at birth.
- Visual impairment, learning disabilities, or intellectual disability become apparent several months to years later. The most common clinical finding is chorioretinitis.
- Other findings include hydrocephalus with generalized calcifications, microcephaly, seizures, opisthotonos, microphthalmia, deafness, lymphadenopathy, hepatosplenomegaly, jaundice

Diagnostics

- Serologic diagnosis is based on positive IgM or IgA assay within first 6 months of life or persistently positive IgG titers beyond 12 months.
- *Toxoplasma* PCR should be performed on serum, urine, and CSF as soon as possible if suspicion is high.
- May detect intracranial calcifications or ventriculomegaly on head ultrasound

Management

- Pyrimethamine combined with sulfadiazine for a prolonged (>1 year) course decreases disease severity. Must supplement with folinic acid.
- Shorter treatment duration for asymptomatic infants

ZIKA VIRUS

Epidemiology

- Geographical areas with Zika virus include Africa, Asia, the Caribbean, Central America, North America, the Pacific Islands and South America.
- Outbreak in the Americas began in 2014; decreasing prevalence since 2017

Etiology

- Single-stranded RNA virus

Pathophysiology

- Transmitted via the bite of an infected *Aedes* species mosquito or via sexual intercourse with an infected person
- Can also be transmitted from a pregnant woman to her fetus

Clinical Manifestations

- Can be asymptomatic. Symptoms outside of congenital infection include fever, rash, arthralgia, conjunctivitis, myalgia, and headache.
- Congenital Zika syndrome is a pattern of birth defects in infants born to mothers infected with the virus.
  - ✓ Clinical findings include severe microcephaly and other brain anomalies (calcifications, ventriculomegaly), eye anomalies (cataracts, microphthalmia, optic nerve atrophy), congenital contractures and neurologic abnormalities (alterations in tone, swallowing dysfunction, hearing loss, and visual impairment).

Diagnostics

- The following infants should be tested for congenital Zika virus infection:
  - ✓ Infants with birth defects consistent with congenital infection born to mothers with possible exposure, regardless of maternal testing results
  - ✓ Infants without birth defects born to mothers with laboratory evidence of possible Zika infection during pregnancy
- Testing is not recommended in infants without defects born to mothers without laboratory evidence of possible Zika infection during pregnancy.
- Zika virus RNA nucleic acid testing of serum and urine, Zika virus IgM antibody
- Plaque reduction neutralization test can be used to determine false positive results.
- CSF testing for IgM and RNA, if available
- Testing within the first few days after birth is recommended.

Management

- No antiviral treatment exists.
- Infants with defects consistent with congenital Zika syndrome and infants born to mothers with laboratory evidence of infection (regardless of birth defects) should undergo head ultrasonography, comprehensive ophthalmologic exam, and automated ABR by 1 month of age (also needs to pass OAE test) and should be referred to early intervention services.
- Consultation with infectious disease, genetic, and neurologic specialists should be considered.

PERINATAL INFECTIONS

HEPATITIS B

Epidemiology

- Every year in the United States, approximately 25,000 infants are born to maternal HBV carriers. Without prophylaxis, 90% of these infants will acquire HBV infection.
- Up to 90% of infected patients under 1 year of age will develop chronic HBV infection, 25% of these patients will experience early death due to cirrhosis and liver cancer.

Etiology

- Hepatitis B virus (HBV) is a partially double-stranded DNA virus.

Pathophysiology

- Perinatal transmission usually occurs as the result of blood exposure during delivery. In utero transmission is rare, occurring less than 2% of the time.
- Risk of perinatal infection is 70–90% for infants born to hepatitis B surface antigen (HBsAg)–and hepatitis B e antigen (HBeAg)–positive mothers; 5–20% if the mother is HBsAg-positive and HBeAg-negative.
- Transmission risk factors: High viral load, HBeAg-positive

Clinical Manifestations

- Usually asymptomatic in infants <1 year of age
- Symptoms can be nonspecific or can present with hepatitis and jaundice.

Diagnostics

- Infants born to HBsAg-positive mothers should be tested for anti-HBs and HBsAg at 9–12 months of age.

Management

- Hepatitis B immunization (HepB) prevents hepatitis B infection with 90% efficacy.
- Hepatitis B immunoglobulin (HBIG) consists of donor plasma with a high concentration of anti-HBs, used for postexposure prophylaxis. Postexposure prophylaxis with HBIG in addition to HepB vaccine affords greater protection than HepB vaccine alone; transmission can be prevented in 95% of infants born to hepatitis B–positive mothers.
- It is recommended that all infants, regardless of maternal hepatitis B status, receive the HepB vaccine series.
- For infants born to hepatitis B–positive mothers, administer the initial dose of HepB vaccine within 12 hours of birth and HBIG concurrently at a different site (HBIG efficacy decreases with increasing time from exposure; unlikely to be effective after 7 days).
  - ✓ If the infant is <2 kg, the HepB vaccine and HBIG should be administered within 12 hours after birth.
- For infants born to mothers with unknown hepatitis B status, administer HepB vaccine within 12 hours after birth, and the mother should be tested as soon as possible.
  - ✓ For infants ≥2 kg: If the mother is found to be HBsAg-positive, the infant should receive HBIG as soon as possible, within 7 days after birth.
  - ✓ For infants <2 kg: HBIG should be administered within 12 hours of life if maternal status cannot be determined.
- If a birth dose of HepB vaccine is administered in infants <2 kg, it is not counted toward the vaccine series. These infants require three additional doses of the vaccine.
- HBV infection is not a contraindication to breastfeeding.

HEPATITIS C

Epidemiology

- An estimated 1.3% of the U.S. population has chronic hepatitis C virus (HCV) infection.

Etiology

- HCV is a small single-stranded RNA virus.

Pathophysiology

- Transmission primarily through parenteral exposure to infected blood (i.e., IV drug use, needlestick injuries). Transmission via blood transfusion and sexual intercourse is rare.
- Risk of perinatal transmission from an HCV RNA–positive mother to her infant ranges from 4 to 7% per pregnancy.
- Transmission risk factors: Vaginal lacerations, internal fetal monitoring, maternal coinfection with HIV, and prolonged rupture of membranes

Clinical Manifestations

- Can be asymptomatic or have nonspecific signs of illness
- Chronic infection can cause severe hepatitis, cirrhosis, and hepatocellular carcinoma.

Diagnosis

- Perform anti-HCV IgG testing in perinatally exposed infants at 18 months of age, after mother's passive antibodies have disappeared.
- Nucleic acid amplification test for HCV RNA may be performed at 1–2 months of age if desired, but should be repeated regardless of result.

Management

- No available antiviral therapies for individuals under 2 years old
- Antiviral therapies, as well as interferon- and ribavirin-based therapies, are available for older children.
- Not a contraindication to breastfeeding, unless the mother's nipples are cracked or bleeding

HERPES SIMPLEX VIRUS (HSV)

Epidemiology

- U.S. incidence of neonatal HSV infection: 1 in 2000 to 1 in 30000 live births

Etiology

- HSV is a double-stranded DNA virus.

Pathophysiology

- Transmission via exposure to infected maternal genital tract or ascending infection
- Less common forms of transmission include congenital and postnatal infection.
- Can be transmitted from mother to neonate during primary or recurrent infections; much higher rate of transmission in maternal primary infection (25–60%) than in recurrent maternal infection (2%)
- Majority of infected neonates born to women without history of HSV or clinical findings

Clinical Manifestations

- Neonatal forms of HSV disease:
  - ✓ Skin, eye, and mouth disease: 45%, involves skin, eye, and/or mouth; usually presents at 1–2 weeks of life
  - ✓ Localized CNS disease: 30%,;usually presents at 2–3 weeks of life
  - ✓ Disseminated disease: 25%, involves multiple organs (i.e., liver dysfunction, coagulopathy) and can involve CNS; usually presents at 1–2 weeks of life
- High morbidity and mortality
- Consider in differential diagnosis for neonate with fever in first 3 weeks of life.
- The majority of infected neonates demonstrate disease within first month of life, asymptomatic disease in neonates is very rare.
- Vesicular rash is present in 80% of neonates with skin, eye, and mouth disease and approximately 60% of neonates with other forms of disease. Recurrent skin lesions are also common.

Diagnostics

- HSV culture or PCR assay of swabs from mouth, nasopharynx, conjunctivae, anus and vesicular rash, if present
- CSF and serum HSV DNA PCR assay
- Serum alanine transaminase

Management

- Consider consultation with a pediatric infectious disease specialist

- Parental acyclovir is the treatment of choice for neonatal HSV disease
- Oral acyclovir suppression therapy after parenteral treatment is recommended for all forms of disease.
- Neonates with ocular involvement should receive topical ophthalmic treatment.
- Brain imaging and ophthalmologic evaluation recommended for all forms of disease.
- Repeat lumbar puncture for CSF HSV DNA PCR is recommended at treatment completion in patients with CNS disease to confirm negativity; if positive, further treatment is required.
- For evaluation and management of asymptomatic neonates born to mothers with active genital lesions, refer to the AAP Statement "Guidance on Management of Asymptomatic Neonates Born to Women with Active Genital Herpes Lesions."
- Contact precautions should be used for women with active HSV lesions before, during, and after delivery and for neonates born to mothers with active genital lesions.
- Breastfeeding is allowed if no breast lesions are present.
- Neonates born to mothers with a history of recurrent HSV infection but without genital lesions should be observed for signs of illness.

HUMAN IMMUNODEFICIENCY VIRUS (HIV)

Epidemiology

- The risk of HIV infection in an infant born to an untreated HIV-positive mother, without breastfeeding, is 25%.

Etiology

- HIV types 1 and 2 are retroviruses. Low HIV2 prevalence in the United States; predominantly present in West Africa.
- Contain reverse transcriptase enzyme that transforms single-stranded viral RNA into double-stranded DNA

Pathophysiology

- Present in blood, semen, vaginal secretions, and breast milk
- Transmission from mother to infant can occur in utero, perinatally, or via breastfeeding.
- Maternal viral load is an important factor in mother-to-baby transmission.

Clinical Manifestations

- Untreated children who acquire HIV from their mother can be symptomatic in the first months of life but usually are asymptomatic until after 12–18 months of age.
- Clinical manifestations are rare since the advent of testing and aggressive treatment, but they can include fever, lymphadenopathy, failure to thrive, hepatosplenomegaly, oral and diaper dermatitis, recurrent invasive bacterial infections, and CNS disease.

Diagnostics

- Routine HIV testing for every pregnant woman is the standard of care in the United States.
- Infants born to HIV-infected mothers acquire passive antibodies; thus, antibody testing is not useful in the first 2 years of life..
- Preferred test for infants born to HIV-infected mothers is HIV DNA PCR assay.
  ✓ HIV quantitative RNA PCR assays can also be used, but low viral loads may result in false negative results. Used as a complementary test to determine the initial viral load.
- For HIV-exposed infants, DNA or RNA PCR testing is recommended at 14–21 days and again at 1–2 months and 4–6 months of age if negative.
  ✓ An infant is considered infected if two different samples from two different time points are positive.

Management

- Consultation with an HIV infection specialist is recommended; recommendations may vary over time.
- Pregnant women should receive antiretroviral therapy with a goal of achieving viral suppression during pregnancy, as well as postpartum.
- Interventions to avoid mother-to-baby transmission: Antiretroviral prophylaxis and cesarean section (in women with viral load >1000 copies/mL prior to 38 weeks' gestation); avoidance of breastfeeding, procedures which compromise the fetus' skin (i.e., fetal scalp electrodes) and procedures that increase maternal bleeding (instrumented vaginal delivery)
- An exposed infant should be bathed soon after birth and started on antiretroviral prophylaxis as soon as possible after birth (ideally within 6–12 hours).
  - ✓ Usual recommended regimen is zidovudine for 6 weeks.
  - ✓ A two- or three-drug regimen should be used when there is a higher risk of transmission, such as a high maternal viral load at time of delivery.
- If a mother's HIV status is unknown at birth, the mother or infant should undergo rapid antibody HIV testing.

PREMATURITY

Premature birth, defined as delivery prior to 37 weeks of gestation, is a common occurrence, with approximately 15 million infants born preterm worldwide each year. Prematurity increases an infant's risk of morbidity and mortality, with increasing risk associated with decreasing gestational age at birth.

- The World Health Organization further categorizes the degree of prematurity based on gestational age at birth:
  - ✓ Extremely preterm (<28 weeks of gestation)
  - ✓ Very preterm (28 weeks to 31 weeks 6 days of gestation)
  - ✓ Moderate to late preterm (32 weeks to 36 weeks 6 days' gestation)
- Preterm infants are also commonly categorized by their birth weight, with lower weight associated with increased risk of morbidity and mortality:
  - ✓ Extremely low birth weight: <1 kg
  - ✓ Very low birth weight (VLBW): 1–1.5 kg
  - ✓ Low birth weight: 1.5–2.5 kg

APNEA OF PREMATURITY

A prolonged pause in breathing in a preterm infant

EPIDEMIOLOGY

- Incidence of apnea of prematurity is inversely related to gestational age, with approximately 100% of infants born at <28 weeks and 20% of those born at 34 weeks affected.
- Apnea caused by mechanisms related to prematurity are uncommon in infants born at term, and other etiologies should be explored.
- Time to resolution of apnea is inversely related to gestational age. For infants born at <28 weeks' gestation; symptoms can persist until approximately 43 weeks postmenstrual age.

PATHOPHYSIOLOGY

- Apnea can be caused by central, obstructive, or mixed causes
  - ✓ Central: Immaturity of the central respiratory drive with decreased responsiveness to hypoxia and hypercapnia
  - ✓ Obstructive: Upper airway obstruction caused by nasal obstruction or upper airway collapse related to low pharyngeal muscle tone
  - ✓ Mixed: A combination of central and obstructive causes (apnea of prematurity is most commonly mixed)

CLINICAL MANIFESTATIONS

- Prolonged cessation of breathing >20 seconds or shorter pause associated with desaturations and/or bradycardia
- Apnea of prematurity is a diagnosis of exclusion.

DIAGNOSTICS

- Consider testing to rule out other cases of apnea: infections (CBC, blood culture; consider urine, CSF, respiratory culture), anemia (CBC), respiratory insufficiency (blood gas), and airway anomaly (airway evaluation)

MANAGEMENT

- Methylxanthine therapy: Treatment for central component of apnea
  - ✓ Caffeine is the most widely accepted methylxanthine treatment due to long half-life and low risk of adverse effects.
  - ✓ Caffeine inhibits adenosine receptors, which results in stimulation of the central respiratory drive.
- Continuous positive airway pressure (CPAP): Treatment for obstructive component of apnea
  - ✓ CPAP helps distend the upper airway in premature infants, decreasing the effect of the hypotonic pharynx contributing to obstruction.
  - ✓ In severe/recurrent apnea, intubation and mechanical ventilation may be necessary.

BRONCHOPULMONARY DYSPLASIA (BPD)

Also known as chronic lung disease, BPD is a form of lung disease seen in preterm infants. Definitions of the severity of BPD continue to evolve over time. Timing of evaluation for diagnostic categorization depends on gestational age. For infants born at <32 weeks' gestation, need for respiratory support is evaluated at 36 weeks' postmenstrual age, whereas for infants born at >32 weeks, evaluation occurs at <56 days postnatal age or time of discharge, whichever is sooner.

- Mild BPD: Oxygen requirement >21% for at least 28 days of life
- Moderate BPD: Need for oxygen at time of evaluation, but <30% FiO_2
- Severe BPD: Need for >30% FiO_2 and/or positive-pressure ventilation at time of evaluation

EPIDEMIOLOGY

- Most common respiratory morbidity of prematurity. Associated with significant morbidity and mortality
- Incidence is inversely related to gestational age. In infants born <1500 g, the incidence of BPD is approximately 25%.
- Additional risk factors include low birth weight, need for mechanical ventilation at a week of life, patent ductus arteriosus, and sepsis.

PATHOPHYSIOLOGY

- The pathophysiology of BPD has changed since the invention of exogenous surfactant. Descriptions are listed below, but in clinical practice, BPD is a continuum between these descriptions
  - ✓ Old BPD (seen prior to surfactant era): Inflammation, fibrosis, airway injury; lung injury caused by mechanical ventilation and oxygen toxicity
  - ✓ New BPD: Decreased septation and alveolar hypoplasia causing a reduction in surface area for gas exchange; caused by a disruption of lung development

CLINICAL MANIFESTATIONS

- Physical exam: Variable, but infant is often tachypneic with accessory muscle use. Expiratory wheeze can be present.
- Prolonged need for respiratory support

DIAGNOSTICS

- Chest x-ray: In mild to moderate BPD, often coarse interstitial pattern, pulmonary edema, and low to normal lung volumes; in severe BPD, heterogeneous lung fields with both cystic areas and streaky densities and hyperinflation
- Blood gas: Hypercarbia, often chronic

MANAGEMENT

Prevention

- Antenatal corticosteroids have not been shown to decrease the incidence of BPD. However, results may be skewed by antenatal corticosteroids, decreasing mortality of the most extremely preterm infants at highest risk for developing BPD.
- After birth, avoid of mechanical ventilation when possible. Utilize noninvasive CPAP immediately after birth when possible.
- Caffeine reduces the incidence of BPD (Caffeine for Apnea of Prematurity Trial)
- Postnatal systemic corticosteroids have been shown to reduce the incidence of BPD. Concerns exist with increased risk of gastrointestinal perforation, cerebral palsy, and neurodevelopmental impairment. In general, steroids are not recommended in the first 1–2 weeks of life. Reasonable to consider low-dose steroids in infants still on mechanical ventilation at a few weeks of life who are at significantly higher risk for developing BPD.
- Vitamin A has been shown to decrease the incidence of BPD in VLBW infants. However, drug shortages have limited clinical use.

Management

- Optimize nutrition, consider mild fluid restriction if thought to be a contributing component of pulmonary edema.
- Supportive care. If noninvasive support is not adequate, mechanical ventilation is needed to provide sufficient support. Infants often require higher tidal volumes with longer inspiratory times and lower rates. Airway evaluation and tracheostomy may be needed.
- Diuretics, inhaled bronchodilators, and inhaled and systemic steroids are often used in treatment of BPD; however, little evidence exists supporting long-term benefit, data on safety are limited. Caution should be used when using these treatments.

INTRAVENTRICULAR HEMORRHAGE (IVH)

IVH is intracranial hemorrhage associated with prematurity in which bleeding into the ventricular system of the brain originates from the germinal matrix. Bleeding can occur unilaterally or bilaterally. Severity of IVH ranges from grade I to grade IV, as defined below.

- Grade I: Bleeding confined to the germinal matrix
- Grade II: Bleeding in the germinal matrix that extends into the lateral ventricle without dilation
- Grade III: Bleeding in the germinal matrix and lateral ventricle with associated ventricular dilation
- Grade IV: Hemorrhagic infarction of the periventricular white matter associated with coexisting IVH

EPIDEMIOLOGY

- Most common type of intracranial hemorrhage in preterm infants; associated with significant morbidity and mortality
- Inversely related to gestational age. 25% of VLBW infants experience IVH.
- 90% of intraventricular hemorrhages occur within the first 3 days after birth.

PATHOPHYSIOLOGY

- Preterm infants are born with a complex collection of highly vascularized cells, called the germinal matrix, located in the periventricular area bilaterally. The germinal matrix involutes prior to term and is not routinely present in term infants.
- The germinal matrix is highly susceptible to impaired cerebral autoregulation, which can result in capillary rupture and bleeding.
- Grade I–III IVH represent progressive severity of bleeding from the germinal matrix.
- Grade IV IVH is thought to result from impaired venous drainage of the medullary veins, resulting in associated hemorrhagic infarction in the periventricular white matter.
- Periventricular leukomalacia (PVL) is another form of periventricular white matter injury that can occur in preterm infants. The exact mechanism is unknown, but it is thought to be associated with ischemia and inflammation. PVL is associated with IVH, but can also occur in the absence of IVH.

CLINICAL MANIFESTATIONS

- IVH can have varying presentations in preterm infants.
  - ✓ 25–50% of infants are asymptomatic; discovered on screening head ultrasonography
  - ✓ Some infants present with nonspecific findings of decreased activity and hypotonia.
  - ✓ A subset of infants will present with an acute clinical decompensation that can include hypotension, bradycardia, acidosis, acute severe drop in hematocrit, and bulging fontanelle.

DIAGNOSTICS

- Head ultrasonography is sufficient for diagnosis of IVH. Further head imaging is usually not needed.
- Routine head ultrasonography should be performed in infants born at <32 weeks' gestation at 7–14 days of life to screen for IVH.
- In symptomatic infants, consider hematocrit to assess for anemia and blood gas to assess for metabolic acidosis.

- In infants with known IVH who have rapidly increasing head circumference, repeat head ultrasonography should be obtained to assess for ventricular dilation and posthemorrhagic hydrocephalus.
- All infants born at <30–32 weeks' gestation, regardless of presence of IVH, should undergo repeat head ultrasonography close to term and/or at >4 weeks of age to assess for the presence of PVL). PVL changes take approximately 4 weeks from the time of insult to be visualized on head ultrasonography.

MANAGEMENT

Prevention

- Maternal antenatal corticosteroids prior to preterm birth, transport of pregnant mother to higher-level NICU to avoid transport of preterm infant, delayed cord clamping in vigorous infants, and avoidance of acute changes in blood pressure

Management

- Largely supportive care of associated symptoms. Correction of metabolic acidosis, management of blood pressure, transfusions as needed. No immediate surgical therapy is available.
- Posthemorrhagic hydrocephalus: If this occurs, it requires consultation with pediatric neurosurgery and assessment for possible need for surgical intervention, most commonly a ventriculoperitoneal shunt.

NECROTIZING ENTEROCOLITIS (NEC)

NEC is a gastrointestinal disease mainly of prematurity associated with inflammation and necrosis of the bowel wall.

EPIDEMIOLOGY

- Most common gastrointestinal complication of prematurity; associated with significant morbidity and mortality
- Incidence inversely proportional to gestational age, with >90% of cases occurring in infants born <1500 grams.
- Postnatal age at presentation varies based on gestational age. Infants born closer to term present sooner.
  ✓ For infants born at >31 weeks' gestation, mean age at presentation is 11 days of life.
  ✓ For infants born at <26 weeks' gestation, mean age at presentation is 23 days of life.

PATHOPHYSIOLOGY

- Exact mechanism of NEC unknown. Mechanism thought to involve inflammation of the gut wall, often leading to necrosis, and in severe cases perforation of the bowel wall.
- Thought to be multifactorial, with risk factors including immunologic immaturity in preterm infants and disruption of the normal gut microbiome, possibly predisposing the infant gut to pathologic bacteria.
- Approximately 20–30% of cases of NEC associated with a positive blood culture, suggesting some association with infection

CLINICAL MANIFESTATIONS

- The Bell Criteria described in **Table 18-4** defines severity of NEC based on clinical presentation and radiographic findings.
- Staging consists of stage I (suspected NEC), stage II (proven NEC), and stage III (advanced NEC). See Table 18-4 for further details.

TABLE 18-4	Staging of Necrotizing Enterocolitis		
Stage	**Clinical Symptoms**	**Radiographic Findings**	**Management**
I (suspected)	Nonspecific findings of feeding intolerance, abdominal distention Can present with bloody stools, emesis, apnea/bradycardia, lethargy	Abdominal distention No radiographic pathology	Brief period of discontinuation of enteral feeds with close monitoring of abdominal exam and x-ray To consider bowel decompression and infectious workup
II (proven)	Feeding intolerance, abdominal tenderness and distention, absent bowel sounds Can present with metabolic acidosis, thrombocytopenia, bloody stools, lethargy	Dilated bowel loops with pneumatosis intestinalis and/or portal venous gas	Serial abdominal exams and x-rays Bowel rest, nothing by mouth for 10–14 days, and bowel decompression Blood culture, broad-spectrum antibiotics (based on local antibiogram) for 7–14 days
III (advanced)	In addition to symptoms in stages I and II, presents with symptoms of shock. Can present with leukopenia, thrombocytopenia, coagulopathy, hyponatremia, and hyperkalemia	Evidence of free intraperitoneal air (pneumoperitoneum)	Similar management of stage II with following additions: Transfer to facility where pediatric surgical intervention is available. Two possible surgical interventions: exploratory laparotomy with bowel resection or placement of a peritoneal drain Length of antibiotic and NPO course of nothing by mouth dictated by surgical course

DIAGNOSTICS

- Abdominal x-ray to assess for radiographic findings discussed in Table 18-4 (dilated bowel loops, pneumatosis intestinalis (air tracking within the bowel wall), portal venous gas, pneumoperitoneum)
- Often follow serial abdominal x-rays to assess progression of disease
- Evaluate for infection (blood and urine culture), cytopenias (CBC with differential), electrolyte anomalies (basic metabolic panel), and acidosis (blood gas).
- Depending on severity of symptoms, consider coagulation studies to screen for coagulopathy.

MANAGEMENT

Prevention

- Factors shown to decrease incidence of NEC: Maternal antenatal corticosteroids, feeding with human milk, a defined NICU feeding protocol (No one specific protocol has shown benefit over others.), and avoidance of prolonged antibiotics courses when possible
- Although some studies have shown that probiotics have been associated with a decreased incidence of NEC, further evidence of safety is needed prior to recommending clinical use.

Management

- Bell Criteria discussed in "Clinical Manifestation": section can help tailor management. See Table 18-4.

RETINOPATHY OF PREMATURITY (ROP)

Abnormal retinal vascular growth occurring after preterm birth

EPIDEMIOLOGY

- Incidence inversely related to gestational age at birth.
- Greater than half of infants born <28 weeks' gestation have some degree of ROP, with 15% having severe disease.

PATHOPHYSIOLOGY

- Retinal vascularization begins at 15–18 weeks gestation and is complete by 40 weeks.
- In preterm birth, changes in blood pressure and oxygenation at birth contribute to a disruption of normal angiogenesis.
- When angiogenesis resumes, abnormal vascular growth can occur.
- Abnormal vascular growth can cause traction on the retina, and in severe cases it can lead to retinal detachment and blindness.
- Vascularization starts in the central portions of the eye at the optic disk and near the macula.
- As vascularization progresses, it proceeds towards the periphery of the eye.

CLINICAL MANIFESTATIONS

- Although severe ROP results in blindness, no signs of ROP can be detected without specialized screening eye exams conducted by ophthalmologists.

DIAGNOSTICS

- Screening eye exam by an ophthalmologist in all infants born <1500 grams or <30 weeks' gestation. Timing of first exam to occur is determined on the basis of gestational age.
  - ✓ For infants born at <27 weeks' gestation, the first exam occurs at 30 weeks postmenstrual age.
  - ✓ For infants born at >27 weeks' gestation, the first exam occurs at 4 weeks of life
- Classification of ROP is based on zone, stage, and presence or absence of plus disease.
  - ✓ Zone: Three zones. Zone 1 is central, where vascularization begins, and 3 is the peripheral eye, where vascularization is completed. ROP in zone 1 has a lower threshold for intervention because of its proximity to the macula.
  - ✓ Stage: Five stages proceeding from least severe to most severe. Stage 4 and 5 define partial and complete retinal detachment.
  - ✓ Plus disease: Dilated tortuosity of the retinal arterioles and venules

MANAGEMENT

Prevention

- No known prevention outside of preventing preterm birth
- Higher targeted oxygen limits have been associated with an increased incidence of ROP, but lower target oxygen saturation limits have been associated with increased incidence of mortality.

Management

- Ophthalmologic screening (see "Diagnostics" section)
- If infants is at high risk for progression to retinal detachment, intervention is recommended.
  - ✓ Laser photocoagulation
  - ✓ Intraventricular injection of anti–vascular endothelial growth factor
- Close ophthalmologic follow-up with reassessment of need for repeat intervention

RESPIRATORY DISTRESS

MECONIUM ASPIRATION SYNDROME/ PERSISTENT PULMONARY HYPERTENSION

A common cause of neonatal respiratory pathology characterized by in utero or perinatal aspiration of meconium-stained amniotic fluid (MSAF) that causes respiratory distress.

EPIDEMIOLOGY

- Approximately 13% of all deliveries are associated with MSAF and 5–12% of neonates who are delivered through MSAF develop meconium aspiration syndrome
- Risk factors: Post term (born after 42 weeks gestation), small for gestational age, placental insufficiency, cord compression, fetal distress

PATHOPHYSIOLOGY

- Passage of meconium seldom occurs before 34 weeks' gestation. It occurs most commonly in full-term and post term infants.
- It is related to fetal distress, which leads to a hypoxia-induced vagal response, causing passage of meconium.
- Meconium is aspirated during gasping in utero and/or perinatally, causing airway obstruction by the ball-valve mechanism.
- This results in simultaneous atelectasis and overexpansion, potentially leading to air leaks.
- Chemical inflammation (pneumonitis) causes alveolar collapse and parenchymal damage.
- Inhibition of surfactant causes alveolar collapse and decreased lung compliance.
- Persistent pulmonary hypertension of the newborn (PPHN) can occur as a result of hypoxia-induced pulmonary artery vasoconstriction and failure to transition to postnatal circulation.

CLINICAL MANIFESTATIONS

- Meconium staining of nails, skin, umbilical cord, placenta
- Often presents with initial respiratory depression followed by tachypnea, retractions, grunting, flaring, prolonged expiratory phase, rales, rhonchi, barrel chest with increased anteroposterior diameter, and cyanosis.

DIAGNOSTICS

- Chest x-ray: Classic appearance is coarse, streaky, nodular pulmonary densities, often distributed asymmetrically. May see hyperinflation with flattening of the diaphragms. Other

possible findings include pneumothorax, pneumomediastinum, pleural effusion, and cardiomegaly secondary to hypoxia.

- Arterial blood gas: Hypoxemia, respiratory and/or metabolic acidosis from hypoxia. Can also show respiratory alkalosis from hyperventilation.
- Preductal and postductal pulse oximetry: Used to evaluate right to left shunting through a PDA. A difference in saturations of >5% suggests the presence of PPHN; however, if it is absent, it does not exclude PPHN. An echocardiogram is needed in those situations.

MANAGEMENT

Prevention

- In 2015, the AHA, AAP, and International Liaison Committee on Resuscitation released guidelines that no longer recommend routine endotracheal suctioning in nonvigorous neonates born through MSAF, as the literature does not demonstrate a clear benefit to this practice. (see "Birth and Neonatal Resuscitation" section).

Management

- Monitoring in the NICU, as patients can rapidly decompensate
- Noninvasive supplemental oxygen or mechanical ventilation with chest physiotherapy and suctioning
- Minimal stimulation to prevent hypoxia
- Correction of acidosis.
- Antibiotic therapy for possible pneumonia
- Maintenance of normal body temperature (unless asphyxia and encephalopathy that meets criteria for therapeutic hypothermia is present)
- Treatment: Oxygen supplementation (risks of hyperoxia should be considered), adequate lung recruitment, acidosis avoidance, nitric oxide, vasopressors, fluid resuscitation, maintain adequate blood pressure for age
- Additional therapies: Surfactant, high-frequency mechanical ventilation, sedation, paralysis, and in severe cases, extracorporeal membrane oxygenation

NEONATAL PNEUMONIA

Neonates can become infected in utero, during delivery, or postnatally. Definitions are based on timing of symptom onset.

- Early-onset pneumonia: presents within 3 days after birth.
  - ✓ Congenital pneumonia is a subtype, acquired from the mother, and presents at birth.
  - ✓ Routes of transmission: Transplacental hematogenous spread; ascending infection through ruptured membranes; aspiration of infected amniotic fluid, meconium, or vaginal organisms
- Late-onset pneumonia: Occurring during hospitalization or after discharge, arises due to prior microbe colonization or nosocomial infection
  - ✓ Routes of transmission: Hematogenous spread, inhalation, invasion of injured tracheal or bronchial mucosa

EPIDEMIOLOGY

- Pneumonia occurs in <1% of full-term infants and approximately 10% of preterm infants
- Diagnosed in 20–60% of stillbirths and liveborn neonatal deaths upon autopsy
- Early-onset pneumonia is a major cause of mortality in extremely-low-birth-weight infants

- Risk factors for early-onset pneumonia: Prolonged rupture of membranes (>18 hours), maternal chorioamnionitis, preterm delivery, maternal GBS colonization, and maternal intrapartum fever
- Risk factors for late-onset pneumonia: Mechanical ventilation, airway anomalies, neurologic impairment resulting in aspiration, prolonged hospitalization, and presence of a central venous line, severe underlying disease

PATHOPHYSIOLOGY

- Bacterial infections:
  - ✓ GBS: Most common cause of early pneumonia, although decreased incidence since the introduction of intrapartum prophylaxis, produces ground glass appearance similar to RDS on chest x-ray
  - ✓ E. coli: Most significant pathogen in preterm infants following decline of GBS sepsis, may cause pneumatoceles
  - ✓ Streptococcus pyogenes, Streptococcus pneumoniae: Common causes of late-onset pneumonia, S. pneumoniae may cause pneumatoceles.
- Viral infections:
  - ✓ HSV: Most common cause of viral early-onset pneumonia, high mortality
  - ✓ Respiratory syncytial virus: Most common cause of late-onset pneumonia, declining incidence with introduction of immunoprophylaxis for high-risk infants

CLINICAL MANIFESTATIONS

- Symptoms can be nonspecific: Tachypnea, retractions, temperature instability, lethargy, apnea, poor feeding, poor perfusion, abdominal distension, tachycardia, metabolic acidosis, hyperglycemia, neurologic depression
- Increased oxygen requirement or respiratory support

DIAGNOSTICS

- Chest x-ray: Nonspecific findings, unilateral or bilateral, irregular patchy infiltrates, streaky densities, diffuse "ground glass" appearance with air bronchograms, pleural effusions
- CBC with differential
- Consider tracheal Gram stain and culture in mechanically ventilated patients. Typically, infants' tracheas are colonized, so may not be reliable for diagnosis.
- Pleural fluid analysis, if adequate amount
- Viral studies or specific bacterial studies, if high suspicion

MANAGEMENT

- Ampicillin and gentamicin may be adequate for early-onset pneumonia, but local antibiograms should be consulted because of the increasing incidence of gram-negative organisms
- Broad-spectrum empiric therapy for late-onset pneumonia
- 10–14 days treatment usually adequate

RESPIRATORY DISTRESS SYNDROME (RDS)

Caused by surfactant deficiency in immature lungs. Formerly known as "hyaline membrane disease."

EPIDEMIOLOGY

- Incidence is inversely proportional to gestational age; affecting 95–98% of neonates born at 22–24 weeks 'gestation

- Risk factors: Extreme prematurity, late preterm delivery, low birth weight, male sex (slight predominance), White race, elective delivery without labor, maternal diabetes, perinatal hypoxia–ischemia
- Rare genetic causes of RDS: Mutations in genes for surfactant protein (SP-B, SP-C, ABCA3, NKX2-1)

PATHOPHYSIOLOGY

- Surfactant decreases alveolar surface tension, aiding in alveolar expansion and preventing collapse. Composed of phospholipids and proteins. Produced by alveolar type II cells beginning at approximately the 20th week of gestation. Quantity and function decreases with decreasing gestational age.
- Surfactant deficiency results in decreased lung compliance, atelectasis, and ventilation/perfusion mismatch, which leads to impaired gas exchange.
- Lung inflammation and injury results. Proteinaceous membrane composed of cellular debris, "hyaline membrane," forms and lines air spaces

CLINICAL MANIFESTATIONS

- Symptoms can present minutes to hours after birth; often progressive respiratory failure in following 48–72 hours, if untreated
- Respiratory exam: Tachypnea, grunting, nasal flaring, costal retractions, cyanosis, increased oxygen requirement, decreased and/or coarse breath sounds

DIAGNOSTICS

- Chest x-ray: Diffuse "ground glass" appearance, air bronchograms (aerated airways adjacent to collapsed alveoli), low lung volumes
- Arterial blood gas: Hypoxemia, hypercapnia, respiratory acidosis

MANAGEMENT

Prevention

- Antenatal corticosteroids increase synthesis of surfactant and augment maturation of lung architecture, thus improving lung function and decreasing the severity of RDS.
  - ✓ Recommended in mothers 23 weeks to 33 weeks 6 days' gestation, with a single course recommended in mothers 34 weeks to 36 weeks 6 days' gestation, suspected to be in preterm labor
  - ✓ Most effective when administered at least 24 hours and no longer than 7 days before delivery

Postnatal Management

- Treatment of RDS: Noninvasive respiratory support, administration of surfactant therapy, intubation and mechanical ventilation. For infants with RDS not experiencing respiratory failure, nasal CPAP is the preferred first treatment.
- Additional therapies: consider antibiotics (RDS can be indistinguishable from pneumonia); supportive care including cardiovascular support, blood transfusion for anemia, and acid–base management

TRANSIENT TACHYPNEA OF THE NEWBORN (TTN)

Delayed clearance of fetal lung fluid after birth

EPIDEMIOLOGY

- Occurs in 1% of all term infants, 5–10% of preterm infants
- Risk factors: Prematurity or early term, cesarean section without labor, precipitous delivery, maternal diabetes, maternal sedation, fetal distress

PATHOPHYSIOLOGY

- Fetal lungs secrete alveolar fluid during gestation, allowing for normal lung growth.
- Alveolar fluid production decreases and clearance begins prior to delivery.
  - ✓ Fluid is resorbed via amiloride-sensitive epithelial sodium channels (ENaC), present in alveolar type II pneumocytes. Channels are activated by maternal hormones (epinephrine and glucocorticoids), which are released at the onset of labor.
  - ✓ Sodium is passively transported through ENaC and actively transported into the pulmonary interstitium; chloride and water follow via osmotic gradient, fluid is then reabsorbed via pulmonary circulation and lymphatics.
- In transient tachypnea of the newborn (TTN), delayed fluid clearance results in pulmonary edema, causing reduced pulmonary compliance, air trapping, and impaired ventilation and/or oxygenation.

CLINICAL MANIFESTATIONS

- Benign, self-limited condition
- Onset of symptoms at birth, generally persists for less than 72 hours.
- Respiratory exam: Typically, clear breath sounds, tachypnea, increased work of breathing, less commonly cyanosis

DIAGNOSTICS

- Usually a diagnosis of exclusion
- Chest x-ray findings: Increased lung volumes with flat diaphragms, prominent vascular markings, fluid in interlobar fissures
- Arterial blood gas: Mild respiratory acidosis and hypoxemia

MANAGEMENT

Supplemental oxygen or CPAP may be required; intubation and mechanical ventilation are rarely needed.

19 Nephrology

Joann Spinale Carlson, MD
Rebecca L. Ruebner, MD, MSCE

HEMATURIA

Microscopic hematuria: >5 RBCs per high-power field in a urine sample

EPIDEMIOLOGY

• Microscopic hematuria: 3–4% incidence on single urine sample; falls to 1% or less for two or more positive samples

DIFFERENTIAL DIAGNOSIS

Red Urine with a Negative Dipstick for Blood

• Medications: Chloroquine, deferoxamine, metronidazole, nitrofurantoin, pyridium, rifampin, salicylates, doxorubicin
• Dyes: Fruits/vegetables (beets, blackberries, food coloring)
• Metabolites: Melanin, methemoglobin, porphyrin, urates, tyrosinosis
• Bacteria: *Serratia* urinary-tract infection (UTI) (some strains produce a red/burgundy pigment)

Positive Urine Dipstick for Blood, but Absence of Red Blood Cells (RBCs)

• Hemoglobin: Suggests a hemolytic process
• Myoglobin: Associated with rhabdomyolysis from trauma, infection, prolonged seizures, or severe electrolyte abnormalities

Repeatedly Positive Urine Dipstick for Blood and Presence of RBCs (Hematuria)

• Urinary tract: Cystitis/urethritis, hypercalciuria, urolithiasis, trauma, coagulopathy, sports hematuria (may be traumatic or nontraumatic, the latter due either to increased filtration pressure or to increased glomerular permeability as a result of hypoxic damage to the nephron as blood is redistributed to contracting skeletal muscles)
• Kidney, nonglomerular: Acute tubular necrosis (ATN), interstitial nephritis, pyelonephritis, sickle cell disease or trait, cysts, tumors (e.g., Wilms), trauma, vascular anomalies (e.g., renal vein thrombosis)
• Kidney, glomerular: Glomerulonephritis (GN) (see "Glomerulonephritis" section)

PATHOPHYSIOLOGY

• Lesions in the glomerulus, renal interstitium, vasculature, or urinary tract result in bleeding or leakage of RBCs into the urinary tract.

CLINICAL MANIFESTATIONS

• Glomerular hematuria typically presents with brown or cola-colored urine with RBC casts, dysmorphic RBCs, and proteinuria.
• Urinary tract or vascular causes present with gross hematuria, occasionally with blood clots, eumorphic RBCs (normal appearing), and absent or minimal proteinuria.

- Hypertension, edema, and/or acute kidney injury (AKI) suggest acute GN.
- Abdominal mass suggests tumor, hydronephrosis, polycystic kidney disease, or obstruction.
- Certain rashes are associated with Henoch–Schönlein purpura (HSP) or systemic lupus erythematosus (SLE).
- Fever and dysuria suggest a UTI.

DIAGNOSTICS

The diagnostic pathway depends on whether there is gross or microscopic hematuria as well as other abnormal findings. Begin with a urinalysis with microscopy as well as a thorough history and physical exam.

- Microscopic hematuria: In the absence of RBC casts, proteinuria, hypertension, AKI, or other concerning clinical signs, repeat urinalysis weekly for 2 weeks (without exercise)
- Gross hematuria with proteinuria, dysmorphic RBCs, RBC casts, hypertension, or AKI indicates glomerular origin: Send serum electrolytes, blood urea nitrogen (BUN), creatinine, CBC with differential, and serum complement (C3, C4) (see **Table 19-1**). If postinfectious GN is suspected, send anti–streptolysin O (ASO) and/or anti-DNase B titers. Consider further evaluation such as antineutrophil antibody and antineutrophil cytoplasmic antibody based on clinical presentation
- Gross hematuria without proteinuria or RBC casts: Suggests an extraglomerular origin. Send for urine culture if symptoms of infection; renal/bladder ultrasound always indicated to evaluate for stones, tumors, and other structural lesions; consider abdominal CT without contrast if strong suspicion for urolithiasis not detected on ultrasound; consider spot urine calcium:creatinine ratio (values >0.2 raise suspicion for stones or hypercalciuria).

MANAGEMENT

- Patients with gross hematuria or persistent microscopic hematuria should be referred to a pediatric nephrologist.
- Further management depends on etiology. If no cause is found for hematuria, patients should still be monitored for the development of proteinuria and hypertension as long as hematuria is present. If hematuria completely resolves, follow-up depends on the extent of hematuria and clinical suspicion of underlying renal disease.
- Patients with acute onset of GN often need hospitalization to manage hypertension and AKI.

TABLE 19-1	Typical Complement Patterns in GN	
	C3	**C4**
Postinfectious GN	Low	Normal
SLE	Low	Low
Membranoproliferative glomerulonephritis*	Low	Low
Alport syndrome	Normal	Normal
IgA/HSP	Normal	Normal
Anti-neutrophil cytoplasmic antibody–associated vasculitis	Normal	Normal

*Complement levels can be variable.
GN, Glomerulonephritis; SLE, Systemic lupus erythematosus; HSP, Henoch-Schonlein purpura

PROTEINURIA

- Normal excretion <100 mg/m²/day or <100 mg/m²/day or 150 mg/day.
- Proteinuria defined by urine protein:creatinine ratio >0.2 on first morning urine sample in children ≥2 years of age and >0.5 in children <2 years old
- Urine protein: creatinine >2 consistent with nephrotic range proteinuria

EPIDEMIOLOGY

- Proteinuria is present in up to 10% of school-age children with routine urine screening.
- Persistent or pathologic proteinuria ranges from 0.1 to 2%.

TYPES

- Glomerular (most common, usually albumin)
- Tubular
- Overflow

ETIOLOGY

- Transient proteinuria: Most common cause. Can be due to fever, stress, exercise, etc. Often improves on repeat testing.
- Orthostatic proteinuria: Common in adolescents. Increased protein in the upright position. Evaluate with first morning urine. Overall, the prognosis is benign.
- Persistent proteinuria: Can be glomerular or tubular. Needs additional workup.
- Nephrotic syndrome: See "Nephrotic Syndrome" section.

DIAGNOSIS

- Check first morning urine when well, 1 week after menses, if applicable.
- Consider 24-hour urine output if first morning samples are variable.
- If proteinuria is fixed or persistent, further evaluation is required.
  - ✓ Renal ultrasound with history of UTI, congenital abnormality, concern for parenchymal damage or scarring
  - ✓ Labs (based on clinical scenario): Comprehensive metabolic panel (CMP), lipid panel, C3, C4, antinuclear antibody (ANA), double-stranded DNA (dsDNA). Consider antineutrophil cytoplasmic antibody (ANCA), hepatitis panel, other infectious workup such as human immunodeficiency virus (HIV)
  - ✓ Kidney biopsy if proteinuria persists or with other concerning clinical findings such as active urinary sediment, hematuria, hypocomplementemia, or elevated creatinine

TREATMENT

Depends on etiology of proteinuria. No treatment for transient or orthostatic proteinuria. If glomerular disease is present, treat the underlying disease. If the proteinuria is related to chronic kidney disease (CKD), consider angiotensin-converting enzyme (ACE) inhibitor.

HYPERTENSION

Systolic blood pressure (SBP) or diastolic blood pressure (DBP) at 95th percentile or greater for height, age, and sex or ≥130/80 mmHg (for children >13 years of age) measured on at least three separate occasions. For children <1 year, high systolic BP defines hypertension.

- Normotensive: SBP and DBP less than 90th percentile for age, height, and sex or <120/80 mmHg
- Elevated blood pressure (formerly called prehypertension): SBP and DBP between 90th and 95th percentiles or 120/80 mmHg to <95th percentile (see **Table A-1c** in Appendix A)
- Stage 1 hypertension: ≥95th percentile to <95th percentile + 12 mmHg or >130/80 mmHg to 139/89 mmHg (for children >13 years of age)
- Stage 2 hypertension: ≥95th percentile + 12 mmHg or ≥140/90 mmHg (for children >13 years of age)

EPIDEMIOLOGY

- Primary (essential) hypertension is more common in adolescents and adults.
- Secondary hypertension (caused by underlying disease process) is more common in younger children.
- Overall prevalence: ~3.5%, but as high as 11% with body mass index >95th percentile

DIFFERENTIAL DIAGNOSIS

- Inaccurate measurement due to improper technique or cuff size:
  ✓ Ideal cuff size: Bladder covers 80% of the upper arm circumference (goal, >50%). Width of cuff spans at least 40% of the distance between the olecranon and acromion. (Overestimation of BP may occur when cuff is too small.)
- Anxiety, white coat hypertension, pain
- Primary (essential) hypertension: Genetics, obesity, and diet contribute to risk
- Secondary hypertension:
  ✓ Renal: Acute GN, AKI, CKD, renal scarring
  ✓ Renovascular: Renal artery thrombosis or stenosis (ask about history of umbilical lines as a neonate), vasculitis, renal artery stenosis (fibromuscular dysplasia)
  ✓ Cardiac: Coarctation of the aorta
  ✓ Endocrine: Pheochromocytoma, Cushing disease, neuroblastoma, hypothyroidism or hyperthyroidism
  ✓ Drugs/medications: Cocaine, oral contraceptives, corticosteroids, amphetamines, sympathomimetics, cyclosporine, tacrolimus, heavy metals
  ✓ Central/autonomic nervous system: Increased intracranial pressure, dysautonomia

PATHOPHYSIOLOGY

- Hypertension is caused by dysregulation of one or more of the following mechanisms of blood pressure regulation: Sodium and water balance, renin–angiotensin–aldosterone system (RAAS), sympathetic nervous system, vascular tone

CLINICAL MANIFESTATIONS

- In children, hypertension is often asymptomatic.
- If there is a prolonged and persistent increase in blood pressure or an acute onset of severe hypertension, patients may develop headache, vision changes, nausea, epistaxis, or seizures.
- Hypertensive emergency: Severe hypertension (BP >99th percentile for age + 5 mmHg) associated with a life-threatening complication or end-organ damage; may present with encephalopathy (stroke, focal deficits), acute heart failure or myocardial infarction, pulmonary edema, aortic aneurysm, or AKI.
- Hypertensive urgency: Severe hypertension without end-organ damage. May progress to hypertensive emergency.

- Important physical exam findings when evaluating patients with hypertension:
  - ✓ Four-extremity blood pressures: BP lower in legs than arms is suggestive of coarctation (along with diminished femoral pulses).
  - ✓ General: Growth failure, obesity
  - ✓ Skin: Café-au-lait spots or neurofibromas (suggestive of neurofibromatosis), rashes or flushing (suggestive of endocrine etiologies)
  - ✓ HEENT: Moon facies (Cushingoid), blurred disk margins on fundoscopic exam, proptosis (hyperthyroidism)
  - ✓ Chest/CV: Rales; hyperdynamic chest; rub, gallop, or murmur; decreased lower-extremity pulses
  - ✓ Abdomen: Hepatosplenomegaly, renal bruit, abdominal mass
  - ✓ Neurologic: Focal deficits such as Bell's palsy

DIAGNOSTICS

Because hypertension is often asymptomatic, BP screening is an important part of the well visit. If it is >90th percentile, follow with two to three readings over at least 6 weeks to document a sustained elevation and to rule out anxiety or issues with technique. If persistently above the 95th percentile:

- Basic metabolic panel with BUN and creatinine, urinalysis to screen for proteinuria or hematuria, which would be concerning for glomerular disease, lipid profile, renal ultrasound with Doppler (recommended in children <6 years old or those with abnormal urinalysis or renal function). In obese patients, add hemoglobin A_{1c} (HBA$_{1c}$), aspartate aminotransferase (AST) and alanine aminotransferase (ALT). Consider echocardiography to look for left ventricular hypertrophy (LVH).
- 24-hour ambulatory blood pressure may be helpful to differentiate white coat hypertension from sustained hypertension.

  If indicated by initial studies or concern for specific etiology, consider:

- Imaging: CT or magnetic resonance (MR) angiography for renal artery stenosis, dimercaptosuccinic acid (DMSA) scan to evaluate for renal scarring
- Labs: CBC (in patients with growth delay or abnormal renal function), plasma renin activity and aldosterone levels, thyroid function, serum metanephrines (if concern for pheochromocytoma), drug screen
- Other studies: Sleep study (with history of snoring, daytime sleepiness, or apnea)

  If the blood pressure remains between the 90th and 95th percentiles:

- Monitor every 6 months before initiating an extensive evaluation.
- If the child is obese, institute lifestyle intervention with a weight control plan. Consider Dietary Approaches to Stop Hypertension (DASH) diet. For more information, see the 2017 AAP guidelines on hypertension.
- If no improvement, additional evaluation may be warranted, with referral to nephrology

MANAGEMENT

General Management Issues

Management depends on the severity of the blood pressure, presence of end-organ damage, and the underlying etiology. The overall goal is to prevent long-term sequelae of hypertension, including cardiac disease, retinal damage, and CKD.

- Nonpharmacologic: For management of mild essential hypertension and for prevention, encourage weight reduction, sodium restriction in diet, minimize caffeine, exercise, and smoking cessation.

- Pharmacologic: Initiate when nonpharmacologic efforts fail or if severe elevation of blood pressure or signs of end-organ damage. Type of medication (**Table 19-2**) depends on age, comorbid conditions, mechanism of hypertension (e.g., ACE inhibitor for renin-mediated hypertension), and tolerability of side effects

Hypertensive Emergency

- Obtain IV access and admit to intensive care unit.
- Goal is to lower BP promptly (within 1 hour) to prevent a life- or organ-threatening injury, but then gradually to preserve cerebral perfusion
- Reduce mean arterial pressure by one-third of planned reduction over 6 hours, additional third over next 24–36 hours, and final third over next 48 hours

TABLE 19-2 Medications to Treat Hypertension			
Antihypertensive Class	**Examples of Medications**	**Mechanism of Action**	**Side Effects**
ACE inhibitors	Captopril, enalapril, lisinopril	RAAS blockade, also have renoprotective and antiproteinuric effects (beneficial in CKD)	AKI, hyperkalemia, cough, angioedema, birth defects
ARBs	Losartan, valsartan	RAAS blockade, also have renoprotective and antiproteinuric effects (beneficial in CKD)	AKI, hyperkalemia, birth defects
Calcium-channel blockers	Amlodipine, nifedipine	Peripheral vasodilation	Flushing, peripheral edema, gingival hyperplasia
Diuretics	Loop diuretics (furosemide, bumetanide), thiazide diuretics (chlorothiazide, hydrochlorothiazide), potassium-sparing diuretics (spironolactone)	Promote salt and water excretion	Dizziness, dehydration, muscle cramps, cardiac dysrhythmias
Beta-blockers	Atenolol, propranolol, labetalol (combined alpha-beta blocker)	Decreased cardiac output, decreased systemic vascular resistance	Bradycardia, bronchoconstriction, insulin resistance, alteration in lipid profiles, contraindicated in asthma
Central alpha-2 agonists	Clonidine, guanfacine	Centrally acting alpha-2 agonists that result in peripheral vasodilation	Fatigue, rebound hypertension if withdrawn quickly

- IV medications: Labetalol and esmolol (avoid with asthma, bronchopulmonary dysplasia, and heart failure), hydralazine (avoid with increased intracranial pressure), nitroprusside (monitor cyanide levels with prolonged use), nicardipine (may cause reflex tachycardia)

Hypertensive Urgency

- Requires prompt but gradual and controlled reduction in blood pressure over 24 hours
- Medications: Hydralazine orally/IV/IM, nifedipine orally, labetalol IV, clonidine orally, enalapril IV

ACUTE KIDNEY INJURY

Decrease in renal function over hours to days that results in failure to excrete nitrogenous wastes and regulate electrolyte and water homeostasis
- Anuria: Complete cessation of urine output
- Oliguria: Excretion of <1 mL/kg/hr in infants, less than 0.5 mL/kg/hr in children, and less than 500 mL/day in adults

ETIOLOGY

- Prerenal: Dehydration most common; bleeding; decrease in effective circulating blood volume (shock, hypoalbuminemia, burns, heart failure, liver failure); renal artery or venous occlusion
- Intrarenal:
  ✓ Glomerular: Acute GN (see "Glomerulonephritis" section), hemolytic–uremic syndrome (HUS)
  ✓ Tubular: ATN—dehydration, medications (aminoglycosides), toxins (myoglobin in setting of rhabdomyolysis, uric acid in setting of tumor lysis syndrome, IV contrast)
  ✓ Interstitial: Acute interstitial nephritis—medications (Nonsteroidal anti-inflammatory drugs, antibiotics including penicillins, cephalosporins, Bactrim, ciprofloxacin, and proton pump inhibitors), infections
- Postrenal: Bladder-outlet obstruction (posterior urethral valves, occluded catheter); bilateral ureteral obstruction; intraabdominal tumor obstructing urinary flow

CLINICAL MANIFESTATIONS

- Depends on etiology of AKI
- Prerenal: May have signs/symptoms of dehydration, hypotension; typically oliguric
- Renal: May have hypertension; can be oliguric (e.g., GN) or nonoliguric (e.g., ATN, acute interstitial nephritis)
- Postrenal: May have intrabdominal mass (bladder obstruction); will be oliguric/anuric if there is a complete obstruction

DIAGNOSTICS

Urinary Sediment and Indexes

- Obtain urine before fluid resuscitation or diuretic administration
- Calculate the fractional excretion of sodium (FENa):

$$\text{FENa} = ([\text{Na}_{urine}] / [\text{Na}_{plasma}]) \times 100 / ([\text{Creatinine}_{urine}] / [\text{Creatinine}_{plasma}])$$

  ✓ Can only be interpreted in the presence of oliguria

- Prerenal etiologies: High specific gravity; hyaline and fine granular casts; cellular casts unusual; urine Na less than 20 mmol/L; FENa less than 1%
- Renal etiologies: May see brown granular casts in ATN; RBC casts in GN; FENa >1%

Laboratory Studies

- Elevated BUN and creatinine, decreased glomerular filtration rate (GFR)
- Bedside The Chronic Kidney Disease in Children Study equation for estimation of GFR:

$$GFR(mL/min/1.73\,m^2) = 0.413 \times (Height/Serum\,Creatinine)$$

(Note: Height measured in cm; serum creatinine measured in mg/dL)

This formula was developed in a cohort of children with CKD, and it likely underestimates GFR in children with normal kidney function.

- Hyponatremia or hypernatremia, hyperkalemia, hyperphosphatemia, hypocalcemia, acidosis

Imaging/Other Studies

- Ultrasonography for intrinsic and postrenal causes; additional imaging as indicated
- ECG: If electrolyte abnormalities

MANAGEMENT

Fluid Management

- Daily weights, strict input and output
- If volume depleted/prerenal: Fluid replacement with isotonic fluid (normal saline 10–20 mL/kg IV, may repeat if clinically warranted)
- If oliguric and not responding to fluid resuscitation and/or fluid overloaded: Restrict fluids to insensible losses (300 ml/m²/day) + replacement of urinary and gastrointestinal (GI) losses
- Bladder catheterization may be indicated if there is outlet obstruction or for better quantification of urine output.

Electrolyte Management

- Metabolic acidosis should be treated with sodium bicarbonate; correction of acidosis with bicarbonate can further lower the ionized calcium and precipitate tetany. If hypocalcemic, give calcium before correcting acidosis.
- Hyperkalemia: No potassium in fluids; (see "Management" in "Hyperkalemia" section in Chapter 9). Treatment should include calcium gluconate for cardiac protection.

Other Management Issues

- Cardiovascular: Antihypertensive medications may be indicated.
- Renal: Avoid nephrotoxic medications including but not limited to NSAIDs, ACE inhibitors, immunosuppressants (e.g., cyclosporine and tacrolimus), chemotherapeutic agents (e.g., cisplatin), antivirals (i.e., acyclovir), antibiotics (e.g., aminoglycosides, vancomycin, and gentamicin). Avoid IV contrast. Adjust dosing/schedule of medications for GFR.
- Indications for dialysis (failure of conservative management of fluid and electrolyte imbalance or cardiopulmonary compromise): Hyperkalemia and/or acidosis unresponsive to medications (HCO_3^- <10 mmol/L); symptomatic uremia (symptoms such as seizure, altered mental status, pericarditis); volume overload (congestive heart failure [CHF], pulmonary edema); dialyzable toxins (isopropyl alcohol, methanol, ethylene glycol, salicylates, lithium)

- Postrenal failure secondary to obstruction: Place bladder catheter, may require surgical intervention and urology consultation

CHRONIC KIDNEY DISEASE

- Pediatric CKD:
  ✓ GFR <60 ml/min/1.73 m² for >3 months with implications for patient health
  ✓ GFR>60 ml/min/1.73 m² accompanied by structural kidney abnormalities, proteinuria, tubular dysfunction, or pathologic abnormalities on histology
- GFR calculated using the bedside The Chronic Kidney Disease in Children Study equation: 0.413 × height (in cm) / serum creatinine
- Stages of CKD:
  ✓ Stage 1: GFR ≥90 ml/min/1.73 m²
  ✓ Stage 2: GFR 60–89 ml/min/1.73 m²
  ✓ Stage 3: GFR 30–59 ml/min/1.73 m²
  ✓ Stage 4: GFR 15–29 ml/min/1.73 m²
  ✓ Stage 5: GFR <15 ml/min/1.73 m²
- Staging for CKD is not applicable to children under 2 years of age.

ETIOLOGY

- Congenital anomalies of the kidney and urinary tract (CAKUT): Accounts for approximately 60% of cases of CKD in children; includes renal dysplasia/hypoplasia, obstructive uropathy
- Glomerular disorders: Focal segmental glomerulosclerosis, systemic lupus erythematosus, IgA nephropathy, Alport syndrome, etc.
- Cystic/tubular disorders: Autosomal dominant and autosomal recessive polycystic kidney disease, nephronophthisis, cystinosis, oxalosis, etc.

CLINICAL MANIFESTATIONS

- Nonglomerular disorders:
  ✓ Poor growth, failure to thrive
  ✓ Polyuria, polydipsia
  ✓ Urinary tract infections in patients with urologic abnormalities
- Glomerular disorders:
  ✓ Gross hematuria
  ✓ Proteinuria
  ✓ Edema
  ✓ Hypertension

DIAGNOSTICS

- Urinalysis: Dilute urine can be seen in CAKUT and tubular disorders; gross hematuria and/or fixed proteinuria is suggestive of glomerular disease.
- Electrolytes: tubular wasting of electrolytes can occur in patients with CAKUT or tubular disorders, so hyponatremia, hypokalemia, and acidosis may be present. Hyperkalemia may be present with glomerular diseases or progressive CKD. Hyperphosphatemia occurs with progressive CKD due to ineffective renal excretion of phosphate.
- CBC and iron studies: Anemia is common in CKD due to inadequate erythropoietin production, iron deficiency, and anemia of chronic disease.
- Parathyroid hormone and 25-hydroxyvitamin D level: Vitamin D deficiency is common, and secondary hyperparathyroidism develops as a result of hyperphosphatemia and impaired conversion of 25-hydroxyvitamin D to 1,25-dihydroxyvitamin D (1α-hydroxylation occurs in the kidney).

- Renal ultrasound: Helpful to identify etiology and chronicity of kidney disease; may show small, echogenic kidneys in renal dysplasia/hypoplasia or hydronephrosis in obstructive uropathy
- Voiding cystourethrogram: To evaluate for obstructive uropathy or in patients with recurrent UTIs
- Renal biopsy: May be indicated in certain glomerular disorders, if creatinine is rapidly increasing, or if diagnosis is unknown
- Genetic testing: May be indicated to evaluate for inherited forms of CKD (GeneReviews* is a good reference for genetic diseases.)

MANAGEMENT

- Congenital abnormalities, tubular disorders, and hereditary kidney diseases usually have no specific treatment, and management is targeted at treating CKD complications and preventing additional kidney injury. Glomerular diseases may be treated with immunosuppressive medications depending on the specific diagnosis.
- Preventing additional kidney injury: Avoid dehydration, avoid nephrotoxins, including NSAIDs, prevent UTIs
- Managing CKD complications:
  ✓ Hypertension: Strict BP control may slow CKD progression.
  ✓ Anemia: Treat with iron supplementation and erythropoiesis-stimulating agents
  ✓ Hyperlipidemia: Dietary modifications; consider statins in older children (Good resources include the American Heart Association and American Academy of Family Physician websites.)
  ✓ Metabolic bone disease: Dietary phosphate restriction, phosphate binders, vitamin D supplementation (cholecalciferol, ergocalciferol), and activated vitamin D supplementation (calcitriol)
  ✓ Growth failure: (defined as height less than 3rd percentile or failure to reach adequate height after 3–6 months of optimal medical care and supplemental nutrition) may require recombinant growth hormone
- Renal replacement therapy (dialysis or kidney transplantation) may be required with refractory fluid overload, hyperkalemia, acidosis, and poor growth/nutrition.

GLOMERULAR DISEASES

GLOMERULONEPHRITIS

Nephritic syndrome: Hematuria with RBC casts, proteinuria, hypertension, and AKI; due to glomerular injury with glomerular inflammation
- Classification according to complement (see Table 19-1)
- Perform thorough history of any recent precedent infections.
- If you suspect glomerulonephritis, consider sending CMP, CBC with differential, first morning urinalysis with protein:creatinine, C3, C4. Based on clinical suspicion, send ANA, dsDNA if concerned for lupus and ANCA panel if concerned for vasculitis.

POSTINFECTIOUS GLOMERULONEPHRITIS

EPIDEMIOLOGY

- Most common cause of GN in children. Peak age, 2–12 years; males:females = 2:1
- May occur sporadically or as part of an epidemic

ETIOLOGY

- Most common after group A streptococcal pharyngitis or skin infection. Also staphylococci; gram-negative bacteria; viruses such as coxsackievirus, hepatitis, cytomegalovirus (CMV), Epstein–Barr virus (EBV), HIV, and varicella (these viruses can also be associated with other GN types). Parasitic and fungal infections have also been reported.

PATHOPHYSIOLOGY

- Deposition of circulating immune complexes
- Autoimmune response to a self-antigen with molecular mimicry
- Pathology characterized by an acute diffuse proliferative GN with neutrophilic infiltrate in the glomeruli with immune complex deposition in the glomeruli

CLINICAL MANIFESTATIONS

- Typically presents 7–21 days after streptococcal pharyngitis and 14–21 days after skin infection
- Hematuria (microscopic or gross) with RBC casts, dysmorphic RBCs, proteinuria, hypertension, and AKI
- Hypertension: Commonly occurs secondary to salt and fluid overload
- Edema: Typically in face and upper extremities; related to urinary sodium and fluid retention
- Encephalopathy (headache, mental status change, seizure): May be related to a concomitant central nervous system (CNS) vasculitis or severe acute hypertension
- Orthopnea, dyspnea, rales, and gallops may be associated with CHF
- Pharyngeal erythema or impetigo has usually resolved.
- Resolution of disease: Hypertension and edema typically resolve in 1–2 weeks. Microscopic hematuria may persist for up to a year. Persistence of proteinuria longer than 1 year may indicate more severe disease or an alternative diagnosis.

DIAGNOSTICS

- Urinalysis: Urine may have rusty or tea color; presence of heme and protein. Microscopic evaluation reveals RBC casts or dysmorphic RBCs, occasional hyaline or granular casts
- Electrolytes, BUN, creatinine: Patients may have elevated creatinine and hyperkalemia.
- ASO titer, anti-DNase B titer: Doubling of ASO titer is highly indicative of recent streptococcal infection (70% sensitive). The peak value is found at 3–5 weeks. Anti-DNase B titer increases earlier than ASO; therefore, sending cultures for both increases sensitivity of detecting streptococcal infections.
- Streptozyme: 95% sensitive; no correlation with disease severity; positive in skin infection
- Complement levels (specifically C3): Reduced in the early acute phase and usually return to normal in 6–8 weeks
- Renal biopsy: If unclear diagnosis, rapidly progressive renal failure, or if complement levels fail to normalize
- Renal ultrasound: If gross hematuria or AKI
- Chest x-ray: To evaluate for pulmonary edema if severe fluid overload or CHF

MANAGEMENT

- Fluids: Restrict fluids if patient has edema or hypertension; consider diuretics (Loop diuretics are commonly used in the setting of edema and/or hypertension.)
- Electrolytes: Salt restriction if edema or hypertension; avoid potassium if AKI present

- Treat hypertension due to fluid overload with loop diuretics. Calcium-channel blockers can also be used. Avoid ACE inhibitors and angiotensin-receptor blockers (ARBs) in the setting of AKI and hyperkalemia
- The presence of AKI is not associated with worse prognosis. Children rarely require dialysis for AKI associated with postinfectious GN.
- Infectious diseases: If pharyngitis or skin infection persists, treat with a penicillin antibiotic or clindamycin or azithromycin if allergic to penicillin
- Long-term prognosis is generally good, with full renal recovery. A small proportion of patients will have persistent proteinuria, hypertension, and/or CKD.

IgA NEPRHOPATHY

EPIDEMIOLOGY

- Most common cause of primary GN worldwide. 10–20% of cases of primary GN in the United States
- Prevalence: 25 in 100,000 to 50 in 100,000 individuals; male:female = 2–6:1
- Onset: Usually 15–35 years of age; uncommon before 10 years of age

ETIOLOGY

- Etiology unknown. Genetic factors may lead to an increased susceptibility.
- Upper respiratory infection (URI) or mucosal infections often precedes onset by a few days.

PATHOPHYSIOLOGY

- Circulating IgA immune complexes and, to a lesser extent, other immune complexes are deposited in the glomerular mesangium.

CLINICAL MANIFESTATIONS

- Most children present with gross hematuria or with asymptomatic microscopic hematuria on screening urinalysis. Children with macroscopic hematuria often have a history of a URI or gastroenteritis 1–2 days before onset. Gross hematuria is typically recurrent. Proteinuria, hypertension, and elevated creatinine may be present.
- Generally has a benign course in children; however, up to 30% of patients may develop progressive CKD.
- Indicators of poor prognosis: Hypertension and elevated creatinine at time of presentation; persistent proteinuria >1 g/day; biopsy with crescents or tubulointerstitial fibrosis

DIAGNOSTICS

- Urinalysis: RBCs, proteinuria, RBC casts. Consider 24-hour urine protein collection.
- Renal biopsy is diagnostic. Consider for patients with persistent proteinuria, elevated creatinine, or in patients with recurrent gross hematuria without clear etiology.

NEPHROTIC SYNDROME

Composite of clinical findings: Proteinuria, hypoalbuminemia, edema, hypercholesterolemia

EPIDEMIOLOGY

- 2 in 100,000 to 7 in 100,000 in children; 70–80% younger than 6 years old

- About 80% of children with nephrotic syndrome (NS) have minimal change disease, 8% membranoproliferative glomerulonephritis (MPGN), 7% focal segmental glomerulosclerosis

DIFFERENTIAL DIAGNOSIS

- Minimal change disease: Most common cause of nephrotic syndrome in children. Characterized by normal glomerulus on light microscopy, loss of epithelial foot processes on electron microscopy; possibly related to allergic triggers, atopy; often triggered by URI, allergies, or immunizations
- Focal segmental glomerulosclerosis: More common in adolescents, Black race; may be primary (idiopathic), genetic, or secondary (infections, medications); more likely to be unresponsive to steroids and progress to end-stage kidney disease
- Membranous glomerulopathy: Primary (idiopathic) or secondary (SLE, infections)
- MPGN: May be immune-complex–mediated or complement-mediated (C3 glomerulopathy). Most commonly idiopathic in children; can also be secondary to infections (e.g., hepatitis), malignancy, and autoimmune disorders. C3 glomerulopathy typically caused by dysregulation of the alternative complement cascade.

PATHOPHYSIOLOGY

- Nephrotic syndrome arises from a permeability defect in the glomerular capillaries that allows protein to be lost from the plasma into the urine.

CLINICAL MANIFESTATIONS

- Facial, periorbital, and pretibial edema; anasarca or ascites
- Vomiting or diarrhea secondary to bowel wall edema; abdominal pain due to reduced blood flow to the splanchnic bed
- Tachycardia if intravascular volume depleted
- Foamy, frothy urine
- Rales, dyspnea, and orthopnea in severe cases of fluid extravasation and pulmonary edema
- Urinary loss of antithrombin III, increased fibrinogen, and hemoconcentration predispose to hypercoagulability. Lower leg pain or swelling may signify a deep venous thrombosis. Homan sign (calf pain when ankle is forcibly dorsiflexed while knee is flexed) has poor sensitivity (<50%) and specificity (<50%).
- Urinary loss of IgG may predispose to infection. If abdominal pain present, consider spontaneous bacterial peritonitis.

DIAGNOSTICS

- Initial studies: Urinalysis, serum chemistries, lipids, albumin, CBC; consider C3 and C4
- Urinalysis: Large protein, possible microscopic hematuria (about 25%)
- 24-hour urine collection: >40 mg/m^2/hr or >1000 mg/m^2/day of protein
- Urine protein:creatinine ratio >2 mg protein/mg creatinine in first morning void
- Hypoalbuminemia (usually <2 g/dL)
- Serum cholesterol >200 mg/dL: Related to increased liver production of cholesterol and urinary losses of lipoprotein lipase
- Hyponatremia, hypocalcemia (related to hypoalbuminemia)
- Hemoconcentration causes elevated hemoglobin, platelets
- Consider renal biopsy if: Older age at presentation, <1 year of age at diagnosis, disease has not responded to 4–6 weeks of steroid treatment (steroid-resistant), progressive renal failure, clinical suspicion for diagnosis other than minimal change disease

MANAGEMENT

- Fluids: Because of low oncotic pressure, patients may appear to be fluid-overloaded while they are actually intravascularly depleted. If vomiting, diarrhea, hypotension, or tachycardia present, give normal saline bolus IV and maintain on IV fluids to replace losses (monitor strict inputs/outputs)
- Albumin: May be used to increase oncotic pressure in severe cases of edema; use with extreme caution if patient has respiratory compromise or elevated creatinine; follow infusion with diuretics
- Prednisone: 60 mg/m^2 or 2 mg/kg daily for 4–6 weeks followed by taper over 2–3 months. If condition is steroid-resistant or there are frequent relapses, consider alternative immunosuppressive therapy.
- Loop diuretics: Consider loop diuretics to increase urine output if patient is severely edematous.
- Nutrition: Low-sodium diet to reduce fluid retention
- Infectious considerations: Blood culture and empiric antibiotic coverage for fever and/or severe abdominal pain

OTHER COMMON CONDITIONS

DIARRHEA-ASSOCIATED HEMOLYTIC–UREMIC SYNDROME

Microangiopathic hemolytic anemia, thrombocytopenia, and AKI following a prodromal illness of acute gastroenteritis, typically with Shiga toxin–producing *Escherichia coli*

EPIDEMIOLOGY

- Incidence in the United States: 1 in 100,000 to 3 in 100,000 population/year
- Peak age: 6 months–4 years; seasonal peak during summer months

ETIOLOGY

- Diarrheal HUS caused by infection with Shiga toxin–producing *E. coli* (STEC), especially O157:H7 (90% of cases), which can be found in undercooked hamburger meat, farm animals, alfalfa sprouts; may occur in outbreaks
- Other Shiga toxin-producing etiologies: Non-O157 strains of *E. coli*, *Salmonella dysenteriae*
- Differential diagnosis includes *Streptococcus pneumoniae* HUS (which accounts for 5% of all cases); classically associated with complicated pneumonia; atypical HUS (associated with genetic mutations; consider with atypical presentations without diarrhea or with recurrent episodes of HUS); secondary HUS (bone marrow transplantation, SLE, malignancy, posttransplantation); thrombotic thrombocytopenic purpura (TTP)

PATHOPHYSIOLOGY

- Shiga toxin crosses gastrointestinal epithelium, enters bloodstream, and binds neutrophils, which carry the toxin to endothelial cells in other organs.
- Shiga toxin preferentially binds to endothelial cell receptors, causing a cascade of intracellular events leading to cell death, tissue ischemia, local activation of coagulation and fibrinolytic reactions and release of inflammatory cytokines, and resulting in multiorgan injury.

CLINICAL MANIFESTATIONS

- Typical course: Fever, diarrhea (90% with bloody stools), abdominal pain, vomiting 24–72 hours after exposure to *E. coli*

- ~15% of children with enterohemorrhagic *E. coli* gastrointestinal infection will develop HUS about 5–10 days after infection
- Present with pallor, petechiae, jaundice, oliguric AKI; can have volume overload, hypertension
- Gastrointestinal manifestations: Severe colitis; risk for bowel ischemia; pancreatitis
- Neurologic symptoms: Irritability, lethargy, restlessness, seizures, ataxia, tremors
- Cardiac failure from myocarditis; cardiomyopathy in rare cases

DIAGNOSTICS

- Stool testing: Stool culture for *E. coli* O157:H7 or direct assay for Shiga toxin
- CBC: Thrombocytopenia often first manifestation of HUS; hemolytic anemia with schistocytes on peripheral-blood smear; leukocytosis
- Serum chemistries and electrolyte panel
- Elevated amylase/lipase and glucose insensitivity if pancreas involved
- Hypoalbuminemia secondary to enteropathy

MANAGEMENT

- Early consultation with nephrology and possible admission to intensive care unit
- Once HUS is diagnosed, fluids should be restricted to insensible losses + urine output + stool output
- Meticulous management of electrolytes
- Provide sufficient calories with parenteral nutrition if needed
- Transfuse packed RBCs only if hemoglobin <6–7 g/dL or cardiovascular compromise
- Transfuse platelets only if active bleeding or before surgery
- Avoid antimotility medications and, if possible, antibiotics (i.e., when no coexisting bacterial infection)
- May require dialysis

RENAL TUBULAR ACIDOSIS (RTA)

Failure of the kidneys to maintain normal plasma concentration of bicarbonate due to impaired bicarbonate reabsorption or hydrogen ion (urinary acid) excretion, which results in a nonanion gap hyperchloremic metabolic acidosis

An overview of RTA is found in **Table 19-3**.

TABLE 19-3	Overview of RTA			
Type of RTA	**Primary Defect**	**Urine Studies**	**Serum K**	**Characteristics**
Type 1	Distal tubule; impaired distal acidification	pH >5.5; urine anion gap (UAG) is positive	Low to normal	Acidosis can be severe, associated with nephrocalcinosis
Type 2	Proximal tubule; reduced bicarbonate reabsorption	Distal acidification of urine is intact. UAG is negative	Low to normal	Can be associated with Fanconi syndrome; may require larger doses of bicarbonate to treat
Type 4	Distal tubule; decreased aldosterone secretion or resistance	Urine pH can be variable; UAG is positive	High	Can be associated with UTIs or obstructive uropathy

RTA = Renal tubular acidosis; UAG = Urine anion gap; UTI = Urinary tract infection
We can then just use UAG for type 1 if we define it in legend.

467

ETIOLOGY

All forms may be either primary (sporadic or hereditary) or secondary to other conditions:

- Type I: Distal RTA
  - ✓ Primary: Inherited autosomal dominant or sporadic
  - ✓ Secondary: Obstructive uropathy, sickle cell nephropathy, autoimmune disorders (Sjögren syndrome, SLE, thyroiditis, chronic hepatitis), toxins/medications
- Type II: Proximal RTA
  - ✓ May be an isolated defect in bicarbonate reabsorption or global proximal tubular dysfunction (Fanconi syndrome)
  - ✓ Isolated: Sporadic, hereditary (autosomal recessive), carbonic anhydrase deficiency
  - ✓ Fanconi syndrome: Proximal tubular dysfunction with proteinuria, glycosuria, phosphaturia, and aminoaciduria; in children, most commonly inherited (e.g., cystinosis, Lowe syndrome, Wilson disease, galactosemia, tyrosinemia) or secondary to toxins (heavy metals, medications)
- Type IV: Hyperkalemic RTA
  - ✓ Hypoaldosteronism due to adrenal insufficiency, congenital adrenal hyperplasia
  - ✓ Pseudohypoaldosteronism (aldosterone resistance) due to obstructive uropathy; pyelonephritis, interstitial nephritis, hereditary disorders

CLINICAL MANIFESTATIONS

All forms present with nonanion gap acidosis, may present with growth failure within first few years of life.

DIAGNOSTICS

- Basic metabolic panel; blood gas/pH via venipuncture
- Confirm type of metabolic acidosis (anion gap versus non-anion gap):

$$\text{Anion gap} = [Na^+] - [Cl^- + HCO_3^-]$$

  - ✓ If anion gap greater than 20, acidosis is most likely NOT due to RTA
- Urinalysis: In distal RTA, unable to acidify urine in setting of acidosis, so urine pH will be >.5. In proximal RTA, urine pH may be appropriately <5.5 in setting of acidosis as distal acidification is still intact.
- Urine anion gap (UAG):

$$UAG = [Urine\,Na^+] + [Urine\,K^+] - [Urine\,Cl^-]$$

  - ✓ Negative UAG: Normal, GI bicarbonate losses, possible proximal RTA
  - ✓ Positive UAG: Suggests type I; falsely positive UAG if there is low urine volume and/or low urine Na in the setting of dehydration

MANAGEMENT

- Bicarbonate replacement is the most important therapeutic step:
  - ✓ Usually as sodium bicarbonate, sodium citrate (Bicitra), or sodium–potassium citrate (Polycitra). Divide replacement into 3–4 doses per day. Titrate dose to maintain normal bicarbonate levels. Proximal RTA usually requires higher daily doses of alkali. Consider phosphate replacement for Fanconi syndrome. Give mineralocorticoids for hypoaldosteronism.

UROLITHIASIS

Stones can be found in the lower (bladder, urethra) or upper (kidney, ureter) urinary tract.

EPIDEMIOLOGY

- Incidence has been increasing in the United States over the past 25 years.
- In children, most due to metabolic and genitourinary abnormalities or infection

ETIOLOGY

- Calcium stones (calcium oxalate and calcium phosphate): Most common stones in children
  - ✓ Normocalcemic hypercalciuria: Distal RTA, loop diuretics, formulas high in calcium or parenteral calcium
  - ✓ Hypercalcemic hypercalciuria: Increased absorption from bone (hyperparathyroidism, immobilization) or increased absorption of calcium from the gut
  - ✓ Promoters of calcium stone formation: Hypocitraturia, hyperuricosuria, hyperoxaluria, hyperphosphaturia
- Uric acid stones:
  - ✓ Urinary pH <5.8 promotes uric acid crystal precipitation
  - ✓ Idiopathic: Normal serum uric acid concentration
  - ✓ Inborn errors of metabolism that cause hyperuricemia (i.e., Lesch–Nyhan syndrome)
  - ✓ High cell turnover from myeloproliferative, lymphoproliferative, or chronic hemolytic disorders can cause hyperuricemia.
  - ✓ Ketogenic diet, inflammatory bowel disease, chronic diarrheal conditions
- Cystinuria:
  - ✓ Autosomal recessive disorder characterized by the failure of the renal tubules to reabsorb cystine, ornithine, lysine, and arginine
  - ✓ pH <7 precipitates cystine
- Struvite stones:
  - ✓ Related to UTI with organisms that can split urea and increase NH_4, resulting in increased urinary pH
  - ✓ *Proteus* (70%), *Pseudomonas, Klebsiella, Streptococcus, Serratia* spp.
  - ✓ Tend to grow rapidly and form staghorn calculi
  - ✓ More common in children with anatomic abnormalities of the urinary tract

CLINICAL MANIFESTATIONS

- Sudden onset of severe, crampy abdominal or flank pain that radiates to scrotum or labia
- May have nausea, vomiting, dysuria, frequency, urinary retention
- Hematuria (microscopic or gross) in 90%
- May have fever if associated with UTI

DIAGNOSTICS

- Urinalysis: Hematuria, signs of concomitant UTI
- Urine microscopy: May reveal crystals; normal RBC morphology
- If febrile, send blood and urine cultures
- Urine calcium: urine creatinine ratio
- Serum electrolytes and creatinine
- Abdominal film may pick up radio-opaque stones
- Renal/bladder ultrasound can reveal shadowing of stones, nephrocalcinosis, and obstruction

- Gold standard for diagnosis is CT without IV contrast
- Attempt to obtain stone by straining urine stream
- If first episode, every child should undergo renal and bladder ultrasonography and CMP. Children <3 years old should have spot urine for calcium, oxalate, uric acid, citrate, and creatinine. Once potty trained, children should have 24-hour urine collection. Further testing and follow-up based on initial evaluation.

MANAGEMENT

- If unable to drink or vomiting, institute nothing-by-mouth regimen. Use IV fluids at 1.5–2× maintenance dose in the absence of renal failure and/or obstruction.
- Pain relief with anti-inflammatory drugs like ketorolac or narcotics if needed.
- Uric acid stones: Increase fluid intake, alkalinization (pH >6.5), allopurinol (consider with confirmed hyperuricemia and hyperuricosuria)
- Hypercalciuria: Increase fluid intake, dietary sodium restriction. Dietary calcium restriction is NOT recommended. Thiazide diuretics will decrease urinary calcium excretion. Consider citrate. Consider dietary oxalate restriction if calcium oxalate stones are found
- Cystinuria: Urinary alkalinization (pH >7) with potassium citrate; low methionine and sodium diet. If this fails, consider penicillamine and Thiola
- Stone removal by urology department may be needed if stone is obstructing the urethra and causing hydronephrosis, is causing a chronic UTI, or is a struvite stone.
  ✓ Stones below the pelvic brim: Ureteroscopy with direct stone removal or lithotripsy
  ✓ Upper tract stones: Extracorporeal shock-wave lithotripsy

RHABDOMYOLYSIS

DEFINITION

- Syndrome associated with muscle breakdown, release of intracellular components into the circulation and elevated creatine phosphokinase (CKP) levels. Can cause renal injury.

ETIOLOGY

- Includes physical and nonphysical causes. See **Table 19-4**.

PATHOPHYSIOLOGY

- Regardless of etiology, muscle-cell membrane integrity is compromised. There is a decrease in available intracellular adenosine triphosphate necessary for Na–K exchanger and calcium-exchanger, and calcium moves from the extracellular to intracellular space. This results in sustained contraction, energy depletion, and cell death as well as the release of enzymes and oxygen-free radicals.

TABLE 19-4	Possible Causes of Rhabdomyolysis
Physical	**Nonphysical**
Compression and trauma	Infection (e.g., influenza, coxsackievirus)
Occlusion or hypoperfusion of vasculature	Drug induced (e.g., antipsychotics, statins)
Muscle overuse	Electrolyte abnormalities
Electric current	Metabolic myopathies
Hyperthermia	Endocrinopathies
	Inflammatory myopathy (rarely)

- Myoglobin, released in large amounts, is unbound in serum and is filtered by the kidney. When urine flow is decreased (hypotension) myoglobin can precipitate, leading to ATN, tubular obstruction, and AKI.
- Release of intracellular potassium and phosphorus
- Damage and cell death of muscle also results in large fluid shifts into the affected areas with ensuing shock and AKI

CLINICAL MANIFESTATIONS

- Myalgias, weakness, pain, muscle tenderness. Urine can be dark/brown/red.
- Fluid shifts may result in hypotension, shock, tachycardia, or hypernatremia.
- Oliguric or nonoliguric AKI
- May progress to compartment syndrome
- Electrolyte abnormalities: Hypocalcemia initially; hypercalcemia during recovery phase; hyperkalemia; hyperphosphatemia
- Seizure, cardiac arrhythmia from electrolyte abnormalities

Chronic Rhabdomyolysis

- In metabolic myopathies: Low-grade chronic muscle pain, episodic dark urine with exercise
- Muscle cramps precipitated by exercise, followed by weakness

DIAGNOSTICS

- Lab results show elevated CKP (MM fraction): From striated muscle breakdown; peak concentrations >50,000–100,000 U/L; elevated lactate dehydrogenase; elevated uric acid; basic metabolic panel can have multiple electrolyte abnormalities; anion gap acidosis; hematologic parameters may reflect disseminated intravascular coagulation
- Urine shows myoglobinuria. Urinalysis, positive dipstick for blood, no or few RBCs, reddish-golden pigmented granular casts
- ECG: Changes consistent with electrolyte abnormalities

MANAGEMENT

- Strict monitoring of intake and output, daily weights, chemistries, urine pH with each void
- Mainstay of therapy is aggressive fluid resuscitation with isotonic fluid. Use of bicarbonate-based fluid to alkalinize the urine is controversial, but may be indicated in patients with low urine pH (<6.5) and/or severe rhabdomyolysis.
- Frequent neurovascular exams of affected muscle groups to detect compartment syndrome
- Consider dialysis if severe renal failure or refractory electrolyte abnormalities

Jennifer McGuire, MD, MSCE
Marissa Di Giovine, MD

ACUTE WEAKNESS

Acute loss of strength, measured by the force of maximal contraction. Acute weakness can further be characterized by time course (fixed, fluctuating, or fatigable), pattern of muscle involvement, muscle bulk and tone, deep tendon reflexes (DTRs), sensory symptoms, muscle fasciculations, and bowel and bladder symptoms. Be sure to assess for common mimics, such as joint or bone pain causing refusal to walk or move, fatigue, and ataxia.

- Muscle bulk: Assess symmetry of muscle bulk
- Muscle tone: Assess by passive movement of limbs with patient relaxed; may be normal, increased (hypertonic: spastic or rigid), or decreased (hypotonic)
- Strength and deep tendon reflexes: See Table 20-1.

ETIOLOGY (BY LOCALIZATION)

- Central nervous system (CNS), brain: Acute arterial ischemic stroke or transient ischemic attack, sinus venous thrombosis, inflammatory/demyelinating lesion (such as acute disseminated encephalomyelitis (ADEM) or multiple sclerosis), encephalitis, metabolic stroke, unilateral or bilateral
- CNS, spinal cord (anterior horn-cell body): Cord infarction, cord compression (abscess, mass, venous malformation), trauma, contusion, infection (e.g., enterovirus), inflammatory/demyelinating lesions (transverse myelitis, ADEM, acute flaccid myelitis), spinal epidural abscess, syringomyelia
- Spinal root of peripheral nerve: Acute inflammatory demyelinating polyneuropathy (Guillain–Barré syndrome [GBS])
- Peripheral nerve (axon): Intensive care unit (ICU) neuropathy, human immunodeficiency virus (HIV) or zidovudine and certain antiretroviral therapies (zalcitabine, didanosine, lamivudine, stavudine), hereditary tyrosinemia, acute intermittent porphyria, medication-related (e.g., phenytoin, vincristine, nitrofurantoin, isoniazid), toxins (heavy metals, glue), metabolic (uremia-mixed sensory and motor, or pure motor after dialysis), autoimmune (lupus), other vasculitis, chronic juvenile rheumatoid arthritis

TABLE 20-1	Scales for Strength and DTRs		
Scale	Strength	Scale	Deep Tendon Reflexes
5	Full, normal strength	5+	Increased with sustained clonus
4	Meets some resistance	4+	Increased with non-sustained clonus
3	Overcomes gravity, but not resistance	3+	Increased with spread across one joint
2	Moves in a plane, but does not overcome gravity	2+	Normal
1	Flicker of movement only	1+	Diminished
0	No movement	0	Absent

TABLE 20-2	Summary of Examination for Weakness by Localization				
Examination Summary	**Strength**	**Tone**	**DTRs**	**Sensory Loss**	**Fasciculations**
Spinal cord	↓	↓ then ↑	↓ then ↑	+	+/−
Anterior horn cell	↓	↓	—	—	+
Spinal root	↓	↓	—	—	—
Peripheral nerve	↓	↓	↓/−	+	—
Neuromuscular junction	↓	↓	+ (nl)	—	—
Muscle	↓	↓	+ (nl)	—	—

+ (nl) indicates that the finding is present and its presence is what is normally expected in healthy children.
DTRs = deep tendon reflexes

- Neuromuscular junction: Myasthenia gravis, botulism, tic paralysis, pharmacologic block-ade, aminoglycoside toxicity
- Muscle: Myositis (infectious, dermatomyositis, polymyositis), metabolic (hypocalcemia, hypokalemia, hypothyroid state), medication-related (especially steroids), ICU myopathy, familial periodic paralysis (primary or secondary hypo/hyperkalemic)

CLINICAL MANIFESTATIONS

- See **Table 20-2** for expected examination findings by location.
- CNS, brain: Unilateral or bilateral (depending on etiology and distribution) weakness, some-times in a cerebrovascular distribution (e.g., arterial ischemic stroke), but not always. May have concomitant encephalopathy, language, cranial nerve, or sensory changes; initial low tone then spastic; extensor plantar response ("upgoing toe") on affected side (**Table 20-2**).
- CNS, spinal cord: Acute flaccid paralysis ("spinal shock"; spasticity develops over time), bowel or bladder symptoms, incontinence, evolving spasticity, sensory level, back pain or trauma, with or without fasciculations, fever (epidural abscess), hypotension (infarction), decreased rectal tone, extensor plantar response ("upgoing toe")
- Spinal root of peripheral nerve: Symmetric length-dependent weakness, often concomitant sensory disturbance, distal more than proximal weakness, areflexia, with or without back pain, normal to decreased tone
- Peripheral nerve: Weakness and sensory loss in distribution of specific nerve, in several discrete nerve distributions (mononeuritis multiplex), or diffusely in polyneuropathy (may be painful); may have decreased DTRs
- Neuromuscular junction: Hypotonia, normal to decreased DTRs, no sensory loss (see "Myasthenia Gravis" and "Botulism" sections)
- Muscle: Proximal more than distal weakness, normal tone, myalgias, normal to decreased DTRs, no sensory loss.

ETIOLOGY (BY LOCALIZATION)

- CNS, brain: Arterial ischemic stroke or transient ischemic attack, sinus venous thrombosis, inflammatory/demyelinating lesion (such as ADEM or multiple sclerosis), encephalitis, metabolic stroke.
- CNS, spinal cord (anterior horn-cell body): Cord infarction, cord compression (abscess, mass, venous malformation), trauma, contusion, infection (e.g., enterovirus), inflammatory/demyelinating lesions (transverse myelitis, ADEM, acute flaccid myelitis), syringomyelia
- Spinal root of peripheral nerve: Acute inflammatory demyelinating polyneuropathy (Guillain–Barré syndrome)

- Peripheral nerve (axon): ICU neuropathy, HIV or certain antiretroviral therapies (zalcitabine, didanosine, lamivudine, stavudine), hereditary tyrosinemia, acute intermittent porphyria, medication-related (e.g., phenytoin, vincristine, nitrofurantoin, isoniazid), toxins (heavy metals, glue), metabolic (uremia-mixed sensory and motor, or pure motor after dialysis), autoimmune (lupus), other vasculitis, chronic juvenile rheumatoid arthritis
- Neuromuscular junction: Myasthenia gravis, botulism, tic paralysis, pharmacologic blockade, aminoglycoside toxicity
- Muscle: Myositis (infectious, dermatomyositis, polymyositis), metabolic (hypocalcemia, hypokalemia, hypothyroid state), medication-related (especially steroids), ICU myopathy, familial periodic paralysis (primary or secondary hypokalemia or hyperkalemia)

DIAGNOSTICS

Imaging

- Immediate brain imaging if stroke or hemorrhage is suspected
  - ✓ Noncontrast head computed tomography (CT) or magnetic resonance imaging (MRI), depending on availability for emergency imaging. CT is typically more readily available and is good for ruling out hemorrhage, but it can miss early ischemia or other subtle structural changes. MRI provides better structural resolution but may not be available for emergency use. If CT is performed and gives reassuring results but clinical suspicion for a brain lesion persists, follow-up MRI should be obtained.
- MRI of spine if concern for spine pathology; may be able to support a diagnosis of Guillain–Barré syndrome by demonstration of enhancement of nerve roots after administration of gadolinium (but this is neither sensitive nor specific to Guillain–Barré syndrome).

Electrophysiology (Electromyography and Nerve Conduction Velocities)

- Distinguishes anterior horn, peripheral-nerve axon, neuromuscular junction, or muscle process; may show evidence of demyelination. Repetitive stimulation for suspected myasthenia gravis.
- Abnormalities frequently appear >1 week after symptom onset, so this is rarely used for short-term diagnosis.

Laboratory Studies

- Creatine phosphokinase (CKP), electrolytes, thyroid function if myopathy is suspected
- Lumbar puncture (LP) to look for cytoalbuminemic dissociation (high protein, low cerebrospinal fluid [CSF] white blood cell [WBC] count) if Guillain–Barré syndrome is suspected or to look for evidence of inflammation.
- Lyme titers for mononeuritis multiplex, a painful, asymmetrical, and asynchronous sensory and motor peripheral neuropathy that involves at least two separate nerves
- Aminolevulinic acid for porphyria
- Consider screening metabolic evaluation (serum amino acids, urine organic acids, lactate, pyruvate, acylcarnitine profile, ammonia) if clinically indicated
- Muscle biopsy: Performed as needed to evaluate for evidence of myopathy

MANAGEMENT

Management depends on clinical setting and diagnosis.

- Stroke: Prompt recognition and management are important.
- Spinal-cord emergencies: Early steroids may stem evolution to compression; neurosurgical intervention may be needed; antibiotics if abscess is suspected
- Uremic neuropathy: May respond to dialysis early in course

- Neuromuscular weakness: Close monitoring of respiratory status with frequent vital capacity and negative inspiratory force measurements. Consider intubation if vital capacity is <15 mL/kg or for rapid deterioration. Specific treatments for Guillain–Barré syndrome, botulism, myasthenia (see the sections for these disorders).
- Elevated CKP: Monitor for rhabdomyolysis, monitor renal function, and maintain hydration.

ALTERED MENTAL STATUS

Decreased alertness or consciousness, acute behavioral changes (agitation, confusion, delusions, hallucinations), or altered cognition resulting from a pathologic process affecting the brain, whether an intrinsic central nervous process or diffuse metabolic derangement

- Altered mental status results when there is dysfunction in both cerebral hemispheres, both thalami, and/or the ascending reticular activating system.

Definitions:

- Normal: Awake, easy to arouse, and maintain alertness
- Lethargic: Difficult to maintain alertness
- Obtunded: Decreased alertness, responsive to pain, or other specific stimuli
- Stuporous: Decreased alertness, responsive only to pain
- Comatose: Unresponsive to voice, pain, or any other stimuli, Glasgow Coma Scale score <8 (**Table 20-3**).

TABLE 20-3	The Glasgow Coma Scale		
Response	**Score**	**Infants**	**Children**
Ocular	4	Open spontaneously	Open spontaneously
	3	To sound	To sound
	2	To pain	To pain
	1	Not at all	Not at all
Verbal	5	Coos, babbles	Oriented
	4	Cries but consolable	Confused
	3	Cries to pain, irritable	Inappropriate words
	2	Moans to pain, inconsolable	Nonspecific sounds
	1	None	None
Motor	6	Normal spontaneous movement	Follows commands
	5	Withdraws from touch	Localizes pain
	4	Withdraws from pain	Withdraws from pain
	3	Decorticates (abnormal flexion) to pain	Decorticates (abnormal flexion) with pain
	2	Decerebrates (abnormal extension) to pain	Decerebrates (abnormal extension) with pain
	1	Flaccid	Flaccid

ETIOLOGY

- Metabolic derangement: Low or high glucose, Na^+ or Ca^{2+}, low Mg^{2+}, thyroid dysfunction, hypoparathyroidism, hepatic or renal encephalopathy, hypotension, hypertensive encephalopathy, hyperammonemia, sepsis, hypoxemia, hypercarbia, adrenal insufficiency, inborn error of metabolism
- Drugs or toxins: Alcohol, common drugs of abuse, narcotics, benzodiazepines, barbiturates, glues, solvents, antihistamines, anticholinergics, neuroleptics, supratherapeutic anticonvulsants, steroids, CO, cyanide, acetaminophen, others
- Seizure: Nonconvulsive seizures or postictal state
- Infection: Meningitis, encephalitis, CNS abscess, or sepsis; may also see altered mental status with common infections like urinary tract infection, pneumonia, or others in a child with underlying neurodevelopmental disability
- Structural: Space-occupying lesion, obstructed ventriculoperitoneal (VP) shunt, cerebral edema and increased intracranial pressure, large demyelinating lesions, posterior reversible encephalopathy syndrome, autoimmune encephalitis
- Vascular: Subarachnoid hemorrhage subdural hemorrhage, intracerebral hemorrhage, large territory arterial ischemic stroke, migraine, anoxic encephalopathy, cerebral sinus venous thrombosis
- Trauma: Concussion, contusion, hemorrhage, abusive head trauma
- Psychiatric: Delirium, catatonia, akinetic mutism, conversion
- Other: Intussusception

CLINICAL MANIFESTATIONS

Physical exam Findings

- Evaluate using the Glasgow Coma Scale (see **Table 20-3**).
  - ✓ Normal aggregate Glasgow Coma Scale score, based on age: Birth–6 months: 9; older than 6–12 months: 11; older than 1–2 years: 12; older than 2–5 years: 13; and older than 5 years: 14
- Vital signs and breathing pattern (Cushing's triad: bradycardia, hypertension, and abnormal breathing pattern—suggests elevated intracranial pressure).
- Possible loss of brain-stem reflexes, including pupillary, corneal, vestibulo-ocular, others
- Fundoscopic exam
- Full neurologic exam
- The presence of vesicular dermatologic lesions suggest herpes simplex virus.

DIAGNOSTICS

- Glucose, electrolytes, liver function tests, ammonia, arterial blood gas, complete blood count, thyroid function tests, toxicology screen, blood culture, urinalysis and urine culture, erythrocyte sedimentation rate, C-reactive protein
- Electrocardiogram (ECG) to evaluate for arrhythmia
- Head CT to evaluate for mass lesions if focal neurologic deficits or clinical concern for increased intracranial pressure (ICP)
- LP unless obvious cause identified and if no clinical or radiographic concern for increased intracranial pressure and impending herniation
  - ✓ Opening pressure, routine studies with cell counts, protein, glucose, gram stain, bacterial culture, CSF herpes simplex virus (HSV) polymerase chain reaction (PCR)
  - ✓ consider other infectious and autoimmune studies as indicated by history
- Electroencephalography (EEG) to evaluate for subclinical seizures, postictal state (or if normal, to suggest brain-stem pathology—e.g., a "locked-in" state that may be present with a pontine lesion and create the appearance of altered mental status)

MANAGEMENT

- Treat reversible causes:
  - ✓ Correct electrolyte; acid–base; airway, breathing, and circulation (ABCs); glucose disturbances
  - ✓ Antibiotics (see "Meningitis: section in Chapter 15); consider empiric acyclovir for HSV meningoencephalitis
  - ✓ Anticonvulsants when seizures are ongoing clinically or subclinically
  - ✓ Maintain normal body temperature
  - ✓ Consider naloxone and other specific antidotes as clinically indicated.
- Neurosurgical consultation for decompression of space-occupying lesion, acute hydrocephalus, or to monitor intracranial pressure

ATAXIA

Impaired control of coordination, movement, and balance

- Cerebellar ataxia: Intrinsic cerebellar disturbance; cause of most pediatric cases of ataxia
- Sensory ataxia: Disturbance of input to cerebellum (from frontal lobes, posterior columns, and/or spinocerebellar tracts)
- Vestibular ataxia: vestibular system dysfunction

ETIOLOGY

- Acute ataxia
  - ✓ Postinfectious or immune-mediated: Acute cerebellar ataxia, acute disseminated encephalomyelitis, Miller Fisher variant of Guillain–Barre syndrome
  - ✓ Infectious: viral cerebellitis, meningitis, labyrinthitis
  - ✓ Drug ingestion: Alcohol, phenytoin, carbamazepine, phencyclidine, thallium, antihistamines, benzodiazepines, barbiturates, antihistamines, lithium, chemotherapeutic agents, heavy metal poisoning, bromide intoxication
  - ✓ Other: Head trauma, cerebellar hemorrhage, neuroblastoma (opsoclonus-myoclonus-ataxia), hydrocephalus, seizure or post-ictal state, basilar migraine, posterior circulation stroke, conversion
- Intermittent ataxia: Metabolic disorder (e.g., pyruvate dehydrogenase deficiency, mitochondrial disorders), seizure or post-ictal state, recurrent genetic ataxias, migraine syndromes (like acute paroxysmal vertigo)
- Subacute, chronic, or progressive ataxia: Structural brain injury or congenital anomaly, brain tumor, metabolic disorders, genetic ataxias, degenerative spinocerebellar diseases (e.g., Friedreich ataxia, ataxia–telangiectasia)

CLINICAL MANIFESTATIONS

- Manifestations depend on location of the lesion:
  - ✓ Cerebellar vermis: Truncal ataxia
  - ✓ Cerebellar hemispheres: Gait veers toward involved side, dysmetria with or without tremor of ipsilateral extremity
  - ✓ Sensory ataxia (peripheral nerve or posterior columns): Symptoms worse when eyes closed with a positive Romberg test); may have abnormal sensation of light touch, proprioception, vibration, difficulties with fine motor movements

PHYSICAL EXAM FINDINGS

- Cerebellar exam: Coordination, truncal ataxia, limb ataxia

- Cranial nerves: Lower brain-stem abnormalities raise concern for tumor or vascular insufficiency; vermis lesions cause direction-changing nystagmus; opsoclonus (concern for neuroblastoma)
- Motor: Unilateral weakness is concerning for posterior-fossa lesions; loss of DTRs suggests sensory ataxia
- Sensory: Afferent sensory input abnormalities are exacerbated by eye closure (not true of cerebellar ataxia)
- Mental status: Consider encephalitis if abnormal

DIAGNOSTICS

Radiology

- Brain imaging: CT in the short term to rule out acute hemorrhage or space-occupying lesion; MRI best for evaluation of posterior fossa, including brain stem and cerebellum.
- Body CT if concern for neuroblastoma

Laboratory Studies

- Toxicology screen
- Complete blood count (CBC), electrolytes, thyroid function (hypothyroidism can mimic ataxia)
- LP for routine cell counts and chemistries, oligoclonal bands (for inflammatory suspicion), anti-GQ1B (if concern for Miller Fisher syndrome).
- Urine vanillylmandelic acid and homovanillic acid tests (if opsoclonus–myoclonus present and there is a concern for neuroblastoma)
- Consider metabolic/genetic evaluation (especially if intermittent or progressive ataxia)

MANAGEMENT

- Treat underlying etiology
- Postinfectious cerebellitis is self-limited (begins to resolve in 1–4 weeks). Steroids are not routinely indicated, but if clinical presentation is fulminant or very aggressive, may be considered.
- Physical and occupational therapy

BRAIN DEATH

Irreversible loss of all functions of the entire brain, including the brain stem

- Protocols for brain death, or death by neurological criteria differ by institution; physicians must act in accordance with their own institution's policies.
- The American Academy of Pediatrics has an online tool kit that summarizes guidelines and provides teaching materials and a checklist, available at https://www.aap.org/en-us/Documents/socc_pediatric_bd_guideline_tool.pdf
  ✓ Protocols vary for infants ≤30 days of age, and for children >30 days of age. Neonates with an estimated gestational age of <37 weeks *cannot* be adequately assessed on physical examination, so assessment of brain death may occur in infants only if the estimated gestational age and postnatal life span in total exceeds 37 weeks.
- A comatose patient with intact circulatory function must be declared dead by neurologic criteria before organ donation can be pursued.

REQUIRED COMPONENTS OF ASSESSMENT

- Identify a cause of irreversible cessation of all brain function (e.g., hypoxic–ischemic brain injury, traumatic brain injury, intracranial tumors, herniation syndrome, others)

- Assess potentially confounding factors that would compromise the quality of the physical examination or ancillary tests, and ensure that none are present.
  - ✓ Core body temperature should be ≥35°C.
  - ✓ Sedative and anticonvulsant medication levels should not be higher than usual therapeutic range.
  - ✓ Neuromuscular blockade may not be present (test train-of-four if needed).
  - ✓ Assess injuries to the face, neck, or eyes that may preclude portions of the exam.
  - ✓ Assess for significant electrolyte, acid–base, or endocrine disturbances that could confound exam.
- Perform a physical examination at the beginning and end of the time period required by age to confirm complete loss of consciousness, vocalization, and volitional activity. The two examinations should be performed by different physicians.
  - ✓ Look for spontaneous eye opening, response to verbal stimuli, and response to painful/noxious physical stimuli to all four extremities and the head.
  - ✓ Assess cranial nerves, including pupillary response, oculocephalic testing, oculovestibular testing, facial and oropharyngeal muscle movement to stimulation, gag and cough reflexes
  - ✓ Assess absence of spontaneous or induced movements during the examination. There should be no movement except standard spinal reflexes.
  - ✓ Apnea test
  - ✓ Perform ancillary testing for all patients ≤30 days of age and for older patients with the presence of confounding factors; options include nuclear medicine cerebral blood flow study, brain death protocol EEG, cerebral angiography
- Age-specific requirements:
  - ✓ ≤30 days old: Must support for a minimum of 48 hours from the time of injury prior to the initiation of formal evaluation for brain death. Two exams and brain death protocol EEG should be performed at least 48 hours apart. This observation period may be shortened if an ancillary test (typically, a cerebral blood flow study) is performed and also consistent with brain death. In that case, a second exam is still required, but it may be performed earlier than 48 hours after the first, after the ancillary test is performed.
  - ✓ >30 days old: Consider waiting at least 24 hours between the time of brain injury and the initiation of formal evaluation for brain death, as the acute event may lead to difficulty in interpreting the exam. The two exams should be performed at least 12 hours apart. This observation period may be shorted as above if an ancillary test is also consistent with brain death. In that case, a second exam is still required, but it may be performed earlier than 12 hours after the first, after the ancillary test is performed.

MANAGEMENT

- If patient satisfies definition for death by neurologic causes, physician should explain to family that patient is dead.
- Consider organ donation, depending on the wishes of the family.

BASICS OF NEUROLOGIC ASSESSMENT

CRANIAL NERVES

Problems with cranial nerve (CN) function suggest brain-stem abnormalities. For localization, consider the Rule of Fours: CN I–IV arise at midbrain level; CN V–VIII arise at pons level; CN IX–XII arise at medulla level.

- CN I: Olfactory—Smell of nonnoxious scents (e.g., coffee)

- CN II: Optic—Pupillary response, visual acuity, visual fields, fundus exam
- CN III: Oculomotor—Eye movements: vertical and medial gaze, eyelid elevation. Palsy gives you a "down and out" eye with ptosis. A CN III nerve palsy with pupil dilation requires emergency neuroimaging, given concern for aneurysm or herniation.
- CN IV: Trochlear—Eye movements: intorsion with adduction (down and in)
- CN V: Trigeminal—Facial sensation (three distributions)
- CN VI: Abducens—Eye movements: lateral gaze
- CN VII: Facial—Muscles of facial expression
- CN VIII: Vestibulocochlear—Hearing, balance, coordination of eye movements
- CN IX: Glossopharyngeal—Palate elevation, phonation
- CN X: Vagus—Palate elevation, phonation
- CN XI: Spinal accessory—Trapezius and sternocleidomastoid strength
- CN XII: Hypoglossal—Tongue symmetry, strength

DERMATOMES

The surface of the skin is divided into dermatomes, areas of skin innervated by sensory fibers derived from a single spinal nerve root (Figure 20-1)

ACQUIRED NEUROLOGIC DISEASE

ACUTE DISSEMINATED ENCEPHALOMYELITIS (ADEM)

An acute inflammatory demyelinating condition of the CNS characterized by the acute onset of encephalopathy not explained by fever/illness, multifocal neurologic symptoms, or characteristic MRI findings. ADEM is typically monophasic, though it can have fluctuations of symptoms for up to 3 months. Rarely, a child may have a second episode (multiphasic ADEM).

EPIDEMIOLOGY

- 50–75% have prodromal illness: Usually upper respiratory infection or nonspecific febrile illness
- About 90% of children recover completely over 1 week to 6 months.
- Mortality is rare (<5%), but occurs with hemorrhagic forms or with fulminant disease causing elevated intracranial pressure.

PATHOPHYSIOLOGY

- Autoimmune disorder triggered by an environmental stimulus in a genetically susceptible individual

DIFFERENTIAL DIAGNOSIS

- Bacterial or viral meningitis or encephalitis, other inflammatory demyelinating disorders (clinically isolated syndrome, multiple sclerosis (Table 20-4), neuromyelitis optica spectrum disorder, sarcoidosis), CNS vasculitis, embolic events
- A child that has three or more episodes of acute inflammatory demyelination no longer meets diagnostic criteria for ADEM; chronic relapsing/remitting demyelinating disorders should be considered.

CLINICAL MANIFESTATIONS

- Encephalopathy

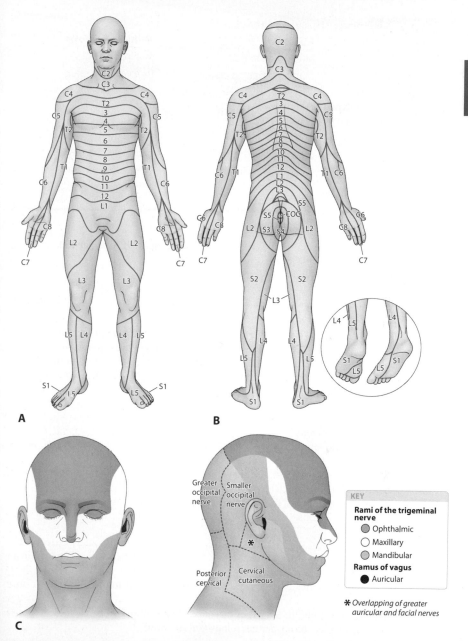

FIGURE 20-1 Dermatomes. The cutaneous fields of peripheral sensory nerves. Reproduced with permission from Wolff K, Johnson RA, Saavedra AP, et al: *Fitzpatrick's Color Atlas and Synopsis of Clinical Dermatology*, 8th ed. New York, NY: McGraw Hill; 2017.

TABLE 20-4	Distinguishing ADEM from Multiple Sclerosis	
Feature	**ADEM**	**Multiple Sclerosis**
Time course	Mostly monophasic	Multiple episodes
Encephalopathy	Must be present as part of diagnostic criteria	Rare early in disease
MRI lesion distribution	Diffuse, bilateral, white and grey matter	Periventricular white matter
Ataxia	Common	Uncommon
Longitudinal MRI	Lesions may resolve	Expect new lesions over time
Demographics	More common in younger ages (<10 years old), no sex difference	More common in adolescents and adults, girls more than boys

ADEM = acute disseminated encephalomyelitis

- Multifocal neurologic deficits (ataxia, hemiparesis, optic neuritis, CN palsies), seizures, headache, fever, nausea/emesis, meningismus
- Perform general exam to evaluate for infection.

DIAGNOSTICS

Laboratory Studies

- CSF: 50–80% have abnormal CSF profiles, including slightly increased protein and/or mild to moderately increased WBCs (usually $<50/mm^3$, lymphocyte predominance). CSF glucose is normal. Myelin basic protein is elevated. Oligoclonal bands are present in <30%.
- Serum: Consider anti-aquaporin-4 IgG antibody (to rule out neuromyelitis optica)
- Other laboratory studies as indicated by clinical situation

Radiology

- Early imaging may be normal.
- MRI brain should be done in the acute setting if available. If MRI is not available, CT may be helpful to rule out other pathological processes
  - ✓ T2-weighted MRI: Scattered increase signal in the white more than gray matter. Lesions are typically bilateral, asymmetric, patchy, and variable in size.
- Consider MRI of the spinal cord to help in differential diagnosis from other acute inflammatory demyelinating lesions.

MANAGEMENT

- May resolve over 2–4 weeks without treatment, but most neurologists will opt to treat in an acute presentation to hasten recovery.
  - ✓ Pulse methylprednisolone: Dose varies, but many use 15–30 mg/kg/dose given once daily for 3–5 days
  - ✓ Intravenous immunoglobulin (IVIG) or plasma exchange may also be useful if response to steroids is incomplete (consider neurology consultation).
- Physical and occupational therapy

ACUTE MYOPATHY

Motor dysfunction at the level of muscle that causes acute weakness; may be painful or painless

ETIOLOGY

- Inflammatory/infectious: Infectious (e.g., influenza, others), benign acute childhood myositis, idiopathic inflammatory progressive myopathies (dermatomyositis, polymyositis), vasculitis, other rheumatologic disorders. Inflammatory myopathies typically have a symmetric proximal muscle distribution.
- Electrolyte and endocrinologic: Hypocalcemia, hypokalemia, hypophosphatemia, hypothyroidism
- Genetic and metabolic: Inherited disorders of carbohydrate, lipid, or purine metabolism, critical-illness myopathy
- Drugs and toxins: illicit drugs (cocaine, heroin), alcohol, corticosteroids, others
- Rhabdomyolysis

DIFFERENTIAL DIAGNOSIS

- Joint disease, peripheral neuropathy (Guillain–Barré syndrome, axonal neuropathy), neuromuscular junction disorder (neuromuscular blockade, botulism, myasthenia gravis)

DIAGNOSTICS

- Laboratory studies: Plasma muscle enzymes (CKP, aldolase, lactate dehydrogenase, aminotransferases), blood urea nitrogen (BUN), and creatinine (if CKP is elevated). Inflammatory markers such as erythrocyte sedimentation rate (ESR) and serologic tests may be elevated/abnormal in inflammatory myopathies,(e.g. Mi-2 antibodies, which is positive in 25% of dermatomyositis patients).
- Nerve-conduction studies and electromyography (EMG): Normal conduction velocities. Myopathic features can be seen from 1 week after onset. EMG reveals small and polyphasic motor unit potentials.
- Muscle biopsy: Inflammatory changes, fiber necrosis replaces muscle by fat, dermatomyositis leads to perifascicular atrophy, polymyositis leads to endomysial inflammation, lipid myopathy
- Muscle MRI: Can help define extent of edema or fatty infiltration

MANAGEMENT

- Management is variable; consider neurology consultation.
- Generally, analgesia and systemic corticosteroids are used.
- Immunosuppression: Methotrexate, azathioprine, or cyclophosphamide (consider neurology consultation for indications and dosing)
- IVIG for refractory inflammatory myopathies (2 g/kg divided over 5 days in the short term, then monthly)
- Monitor for rhabdomyolysis and hydrate if CKP is elevated (see "Rhabdomyolysis" section in Chapter 19)
- Physical therapy to avoid contractures from inactivity
- Dermatomyositis: Consider evaluation for malignancy, especially testicular cancer in males.

BOTULISM

Neuroparalytic illness caused by neurotoxin produced by *Clostridium botulinum* (anaerobic, spore-forming bacillus)

EPIDEMIOLOGY

- *C. botulinum* is found in soil, honey, and home-canned foods.
- Four types: Infantile, foodborne, wound, and adult. Infantile is most common.

✓ Annually, 70 to 110 cases of infantile botulism are reported in the United States to the Centers for Disease Control and Prevention.
  ■ 70–90% of cases occur in breast-fed infants.
    ■ Typical age: 2 weeks–12 months, but median age at diagnosis is 10–14 weeks, and 95% of cases occur in infants younger than 6 months.
• Neurologic sequelae are rare with proper supportive care.

PATHOPHYSIOLOGY

• Infant botulism: Ingested spores germinate and colonize the gastrointestinal (GI) tract (infection) then release toxin.
• Foodborne botulism: Ingested toxin from contaminated food
• Neurotoxin binds irreversibly to presynaptic nerve endings, inhibiting acetylcholine release. Toxin does not cross the blood–brain barrier.

DIFFERENTIAL DIAGNOSIS

• Sepsis, toxin ingestion (e.g., organophosphates), Guillain–Barré syndrome, myasthenia gravis, stroke, metabolic disorders, tick paralysis

CLINICAL MANIFESTATIONS

• Symmetric, descending flaccid paralysis
• Infants classically present with constipation; they may also present with poor feeding and weak cry, followed by respiratory compromise.
• Children and adults with foodborne botulism classically present with nausea, emesis, abdominal pain, and diarrhea.
• Cranial nerves (ophthalmoparesis, ptosis, disconjugate gaze, diminished gag, difficulty swallowing, weak suck) involved initially and then descends to upper extremities and respiratory muscles
  ✓ Normal pupillary light reflex fatigues with repeated stimulation over 1–2 minutes.
• Progressive weakness and hypotonia (typically, over 1–2 weeks) with bulbar and spinal-nerve abnormalities.
• DTRs are initially normal despite profound hypotonia; hyporeflexia develops later in the course.
• Autonomic dysfunction is common, including decreased tearing and salivation.

DIAGNOSTICS

Botulism is largely a clinical diagnosis after ruling out other common disorders on the differential diagnosis.

• Consider evaluation for sepsis in infants.
• Serum toxicology screen
• EMG: Changes may lag behind clinical symptoms, so not typically used for acute diagnosis. Classic findings include an incremental response in muscle action potential with high-frequency stimulation; normal nerve-conduction velocity.
  ✓ No response to injection of edrophonium chloride or neostigmine, which distinguishes it from myasthenia gravis.
• Brain and/or spine imaging if diagnosis unclear

Confirmatory laboratory studies

• *C. botulinum* toxin identification in stool; may use water enema to facilitate sample collection if constipated. However, results take several days, so treatment should not be delayed pending results.

MANAGEMENT

- Human-derived botulinum immune globulin ("baby BIg") for infants
- Trivalent equine antitoxin for adults (risk of anaphylaxis)
- To obtain antitoxin or immune globulin (in any state), call California Department of Health Services: 510-540-2646 (www.infantbotulism.org)
  - ✓ Administration within 3 days of hospitalization is ideal, though administration within 4–7 days yields better outcomes than no treatment.
- Avoid aminoglycosides because they can potentiate neuromuscular blockade, precipitating rapid clinical deterioration.
- Contact state/local public health authorities for suspected or documented cases of botulism (except infant botulism).
- Supportive care:
  - ✓ Up to 70% may require mechanical ventilation and or nasogastric feeds.
  - ✓ Nasogastric tube feedings are usually required during course of illness to prevent aspiration of formula.
    - ▪ Small volumes of continuous enteral feeding stimulates gut motility and may obviate the need for central venous catheterization.
    - ▪ Resume oral feedings when gag, swallow, and suck reflexes return.
    - ▪ Strict monitoring of intake/output and weight given risk of syndrome of inappropriate hormone (SIADH), which complicates up to 15% of cases
- Typical hospitalization is 2–3 weeks, though full recovery may take up to 2 months.
- Case fatality rates are less than 1% with proper supportive management.

GUILLAIN–BARRÉ SYNDROME (GBS)

A spectrum of acute inflammatory polyradiculoneuropathies, that cause demyelination or axonal injury to the peripheral nerves and spinal nerve roots. GBS is the most common cause of acute flaccid paralysis in infants and children in developed countries in the post-polio period. Common subtypes include the following.

- Acute inflammatory demyelinating polyradiculoneuropathy: Rapidly progressive often ascending weakness in more than one limb, areflexia. This is the most common form of GBS in the United States.
- Miller Fisher syndrome: Cranial nerve predominant form of GBS with descending weakness, ataxia, ophthalmoparesis, and areflexia

EPIDEMIOLOGY

- Incidence: 0.34 in 100,000 to 1.34 in 100,000 children/year
- Slight male predominance; any race/ethnicity; any age, though less common under 2 years old
- 50–82% of children have an antecedent respiratory or gastrointestinal infection within 6 weeks prior to GBS presentation (common: *Campylobacter jejuni*).
- Other risk factors: surgery, parturition, hematologic malignancies, human immunodeficiency virus (HIV) seroconversion
- Seen in a higher-than-expected rate in patients with sarcoidosis, systemic lupus erythematosus (SLE), lymphoma, and solid tumors.

PATHOPHYSIOLOGY

- Immune-mediated inflammation and demyelination of spinal-nerve roots and peripheral nerves, likely instigated by molecular mimicry (anti-GM1 Ab with *C. jejuni*, anti-GQ1B antibody with Miller Fisher syndrome)

485

DIFFERENTIAL DIAGNOSIS

- Infections: Poliomyelitis and other enteroviral infections (LP with elevated WBCs), acute flaccid myelitis, diphtheria, myositis
- Inflammatory: transverse myelitis, acute cerebellar ataxia
- Drugs: Isoniazid, vincristine, amitriptyline, hydralazine, nitric oxide
- Toxins: Lead, mercury, arsenic, thallium, organophosphates, glue, acrylamide, tick paralysis
- Neuromuscular blockade: Botulism, myasthenia gravis
- Structural: Spinal cord compression, posterior fossa lesion, bilateral strokes
- Other: Porphyria, myopathy

CLINICAL MANIFESTATIONS

- Rapidly progressive, bilateral, symmetric, often ascending limb weakness and sensory changes: 50% plateau by 2 weeks, 80% by 3 weeks
  ✓ Young children often complain of pain, older children and adults of numbness, tingling, and/or pain. Pain can present as a refusal to walk and can make children appear irritable.
  ✓ Respiratory muscle weakness may lead to respiratory insufficiency and need for mechanical ventilation.
- Depressed DTRs
- CN abnormalities in up to 50%, including facial weakness (most common), ophthalmoparesis.
- Autonomic nerve dysfunction may lead to vital sign instability
- Back pain from spinal nerve root inflammation
- Preserved mental status
- Ataxia

DIAGNOSTICS

- CSF: Cytoalbuminemic dissociation (elevated CSF protein [typically 80–200 mg/dL]) in the context of a normal or mildly elevated CSF WBC (<10 mononuclear cells/mm³) is the classic finding, but this may be absent in first week of disease
- EMG: Abnormal in 50% of patients in the first 2 weeks and in 85% of patients afterward; demonstrates evidence of segmental demyelination.
- MRI: to rule out spinal-cord compression. While MRI spine may demonstrate enhancing nerve roots, this is neither sensitive nor specific to make diagnosis.

MANAGEMENT

- Admit patient for observation.
- Supportive therapy: Monitor respiratory status with serial negative inspiratory force (NIF); intubation if necessary (consider if vital capacity <15 mL/kg). Avoid aminoglycoside antibiotics (which may cause presynaptic neuromuscular blockade).
- Immune modulatory therapy: May hasten recovery. Choose either:
  ✓ IVIG 2 g/kg divided into five daily doses
  ✓ Plasmapheresis: Plasma exchange volume 200–250 mL/kg divided in three to five treatments over 7–14 days
- Other: Pain control (mostly back, limb) with gabapentin nonsteroidal anti-inflammatory drugs (NSAIDs). Bowel regimen, Foley catheter if voiding limited. Deep venous thrombosis prophylaxis if immobile.
- With good care, 90% of children will have a full recovery. Relapses may suggest the onset of a chronic inflammatory demyelinating polyneuropathy.

INCREASED INTRACRANIAL PRESSURE (OR INTRACRANIAL HYPERTENSION)

Abnormal elevation of pressure inside the skull, caused by:

- Too much spinal fluid around the brain due to a mechanical obstruction (obstructive hydrocephalus) or cerebrospinal fluid under-reabsorption (communicating hydrocephalus)
- Bleeding or swelling in the brain due to an arterial ischemic stroke, intracranial hemorrhage, cerebral sinus venous thrombosis, traumatic injury, infection, tumors, others
- Space-occupying lesions, such as tumor, abscess, hemorrhage, others
- Normal ICP varies with age
  - ✓ Neonate: <12 cmH$_2$O
  - ✓ Child <12 months: 1.5–6 cmH$_2$O
  - ✓ Child: 3–7 cmH$_2$O
  - ✓ Adolescent: <15 cmH$_2$O
  - ✓ Adult: <20 cmH$_2$O

ETIOLOGY

- Hydrocephalus (obstructive or communicating), VP shunt malfunction, arterial ischemic stroke, intracranial hemorrhage, cerebral sinus venous thrombosis, traumatic brain injury, infection, tumor, abscess, pseudotumor cerebri, intracranial hemorrhage, cerebral edema, others

PATHOPHYSIOLOGY (OF EDEMA)

- Vasogenic: Impaired blood–brain barrier; increased capillary permeability; increased capillary transmural pressure; retention of extravasated fluid in interstitial space; occurs near tumors, hemorrhages, inflammatory foci
- Cytotoxic: Impaired Na$^+$–K$^+$–ATPase pump due to decreased cerebral blood flow; causes increased extracellular K$^+$ and increased intracellular Ca^{2+}, leading to cell death secondary to membrane dysfunction; occurs near areas of ischemia and hypoxemia.
- Interstitial: High pressure obstructive hydrocephalus leading to ischemia
- Hydrostatic: Increased transmural vascular pressure resulting in increased extracellular fluid; may result from abrupt loss of cerebral autoregulation.
- Osmotic: Decreased serum osmolality and hyponatremia (Na$^+$ <125 mEq/L)

CLINICAL MANIFESTATIONS

- Mental status changes: May range from mild irritability to coma. Assess Glasgow Coma Scale score (see **Table 20-3**).
- Headache: Especially early morning and worse when supine
- Nausea, vomiting
- Acutely increasing head circumference (look for a relative increase in percentile compared to prior measurements); full or bulging fontanel or increased separation of sutures in infants
- Papilledema, though absence does not rule out elevated ICP; this is uncommon in infants.
- Visual-field loss, unilateral or bilateral abducens nerve palsies (with diplopia), other eye-movement abnormalities, including "sunsetting" (downward eye deviation with impaired upward gaze).
- Focal neurologic deficits
- Cushing's triad: Bradycardia, hypertension, irregular respirations

DIAGNOSTICS

- Clinical guideline for evaluation of suspected nontraumatic intracranial hypertension can be found at https://www.chop.edu/clinical-pathway/intracranial-hypertension-non-traumatic-clinical-pathway

- Clinical guidelines for evaluation of severe traumatic brain injury can be found at https://www.chop.edu/clinical-pathway/brain-injury-severe-traumatic-picu-clinical-pathway

Radiology

- Emergency head CT or brain MRI with and without contrast: Can have normal head CT with increased ICP, so normal head CT should be followed with MRI if clinical suspicion remains.
- Head ultrasonography usually sufficient for diagnosis in infants with open fontanel, but normal ultrasound should also be followed with MRI if clinical suspicion remains.
- If ventriculoperitoneal shunt is present:
  - ✓ The Children's Hospital of Philadelphia pathway for evaluation/treatment of suspected ventricular shunt obstruction or infection can be found at https://www.chop.edu/clinical-pathway/ventricular-shunt-obstruction-infection-clinical-pathway
  - ✓ Obtain head CT with low-dose radiation protocol. Scout lateral radiograph to include entire neck to clavicles. To evaluate shunt tubing, obtain a single anteroposterior or posteroanterior x-ray of chest and abdomen.

Laboratory Studies

- If clinically indicated, consider LP *only after* neuroimaging excludes mass lesion or effaced ventricles.
- Serum electrolytes and osmolarity
- Ammonia level if diffuse cerebral edema

ICP Monitoring (Intensive Care Unit Setting)

- Indicated if Glasgow Coma Scale score <8, rapidly deteriorating neurologic status, pharmacologic paralysis, mechanical ventilation with increased mean airway pressures or increased pulmonary end-expiratory pressure

MANAGEMENT

Resuscitation

- ABCs, control seizures
- Maintain adequate mean arterial pressure (MAP) because:
  - ✓ Cerebral perfusion pressure: $CPP = MAP - ICP$
- Low CPP results in ischemia. Goal CPP is >60 mmHg in adolescents and >50 mm Hg in infants and children.

Reduce Cerebral Blood Volume

- Elevate head of bed to 30 degrees.
- Hyperventilation to goal partial pressure of carbon dioxide ($PaCO_2$) 30–34 mm Hg, only recommended in acute setting, long-term hyperventilation is not recommended.
- Cerebral vasoconstricting sedation (thiopental, pentobarbital)
- Avoid hyperthermia, hypoglycemia.

Reduce Brain and Cerebrospinal Fluid Volume

- Osmotic agents: Must monitor blood pressures, electrolytes, serum osmolarity. Options include:
  - ✓ 3% hypertonic saline bolus 5–10 mL/kg (maximum, 500 mL/dose)
  - ✓ Mannitol 0.25 mg/kg IV every 10 minutes, up to three doses (effect seen in 10–15 minutes and lasts up to 8 hours)
- Furosemide 0.5–1.0 mg/kg IV (or 0.15–0.3 mg/kg IV when used along with mannitol)

- Acetazolamide 30 mg/kg/day IV or orally in four to six divided doses (maximum, 1 g/day) (may cause transient increased ICP due to CO_2 release, but then decreases CSF production significantly)
- Dexamethasone 1–2 mg/kg IV or orally loading dose (maximum, 10 mg) followed by 1 mg/kg/day in four divided doses (maximum, 16 mg/day) to decrease vasogenic edema
- Ventriculostomy drain or VP shunt (neurosurgery consultation)
- Consider decreasing fluid infusion to two-thirds of maintenance requirements using 0.9% normal saline rather than 0.45% normal saline

Reduce Intracranial Volume

- Surgical decompression, VP shunt for acute hydrocephalus

For Suspected Shunt Malfunction

- Emergency shunt revision (neurosurgery consultation)

IDIOPATHIC INTRACRANIAL HYPERTENSION

Clinical syndrome characterized by increased ICP with normal CSF composition and no other cause of intracranial hypertension found on neuroimaging or other evaluation. Commonly referred to as pseudotumor cerebri

EPIDEMIOLOGY

- Classically affects obese women of child-bearing age
  ✓ Before puberty: No sex difference, less commonly associated with obesity
- Associated conditions and possible risk factors include:
  ✓ Neurologic: Venous sinus thrombosis, meningitis (including Lyme disease)
  ✓ Systemic: Malnutrition, refeeding, hypertension, anemia, renal failure, significant weight gain, sleep apnea, uremia
  ✓ Rheumatologic: SLE, Behçet's disease
  ✓ Medications: Growth hormone, tetracyclines (including doxycycline, minocycline) hypervitaminosis A, retinoids (including isotretinoin), corticosteroid withdrawal, lithium, thyroxine, nalidixic acid, oral contraceptive pills
  ✓ Endocrine: Obesity, hyper/hypothyroid, hypoparathyroidism, Addison disease, pregnancy, polycystic ovarian syndrome

PATHOPHYSIOLOGY

- Etiology unknown.
- Theories include increased CSF outflow resistance at either the arachnoid granulation tissue or the CSF lymphatic drainage sites, cerebral venous outflow abnormalities, obesity-related increased abdominal and intracranial venous pressure, altered sodium and water retention, abnormalities in vitamin A metabolism.

CLINICAL MANIFESTATIONS

- Headache worse in morning or while lying flat, with or without nausea, vomiting, and photophobia
  ✓ Most common presenting symptoms in adults, but younger children may not have headache.
- Visual symptoms
  ✓ Diplopia (CN VI palsy or divergence insufficiency from increased ICP), blurry vision (common in children), loss of central vision (central scotoma), visual-field loss, may progress to blindness if untreated.

✓ Transient visual obscurations, photopsias (brief sparkles or flashes of light) likely due to optic nerve ischemia, both provoked by Valsalva maneuver or positional changes.
✓ Papilledema
• Pulsatile tinnitus
• Symptoms may improve immediately after a lumbar puncture.

DIAGNOSTICS

Idiopathic intracranial hypertension should be suspected in a patient with headaches and papilledema, but it is a diagnosis of exclusion. Secondary causes of intracranial hypertension must always be ruled out.

Radiology

• Emergency imaging with head CT or MRI brain to evaluate for mass or hydrocephalus; MRI or magnetic resonance venography (MRV) is best for venous sinus thrombosis

Laboratory

• Lumbar puncture with opening pressure, cell count, glucose, protein, cultures (should be normal except pressure; protein can be low)
   ✓ Opening pressure should be measured in the lateral recumbent position, not sitting up.
   ✓ Elevated opening pressure is >25 cmH$_2$O in adults, likely >28 cmH$_2$O in children 1–18 years old,
   ✓ Specific laboratory tests to evaluate for specific etiologies (e.g., vitamin A, serology for Lyme disease)
   ✓ Consider CBC, electrolytes, BUN, creatinine, antinuclear antibody (ANA) testing, urinalysis, hypercoagulability tests
• Vision testing: Optic disc assessment, visual acuity, and quantitative perimetry testing at diagnosis and at regular intervals thereafter

MANAGEMENT

Goals of treatment are to alleviate symptoms and preserve vision.

Medical

• Weight loss if obese
• Carbonic anhydrase inhibitors (acetazolamide, topiramate: see "Increased Intracranial Pressure" section for dosing guidelines). Watch for dose-dependent paresthesias.
• If substantial visual-field loss: admit, administer steroids such as dexamethasone (see "Increased Intracranial Pressure" section) or prednisone (1–2 mg/kg/day up to 60–100 mg/day with a gradual taper over 2 weeks), follow serial visual field exams.
• Stop any precipitating agents.
• No specific treatment if headache resolves in 24–48 hours

Surgical

• In asymptomatic patients for whom medications fail:
   ✓ Optic-nerve sheath fenestration
   ✓ Lumbar peritoneal shunt

Other

• Serial LPs to remove CSF are *not* effective long term.

MIGRAINE

The most common disabling primary headache disorder in children and adolescents. Classically characterized by a recurrent, throbbing, moderate-to-severe headache associated with photophobia, phonophobia, nausea, and/or emesis, lasting between 1 and 72 hours.

- Status migrainosus is a typical migraine attack in a person with an episodic migraine history that is debilitating and lasts for more than 72 hours.
- Chronic migraine is headache occurring at least 15 days per month for at least 3 months, at least 8 days per month meeting criteria for migraine.
  - ✓ Auras are sometimes associated with migraine. By definition, they develop gradually, last no more than 1 hour, and are completely reversible. Types of auras include visual symptoms (e.g., flickering lights, spots, lines, or loss of vision), paresthesias, numbness, or speech disturbance.
  - ✓ Motor weakness is not an aura and requires further emergency evaluation by a neurologist.

EPIDEMIOLOGY

- Migraines occur in all ages, though prevalence increases in adolescence. By age 10, approximately 5% of children have had migraine.
- Before puberty, boys and girls are equally affected. After puberty, girls are affected more often than boys.
- Most children have a family history.

DIFFERENTIAL DIAGNOSIS

- Other primary headache disorders, including tension-type headaches and trigeminal autonomic cephalalgias (cluster headache).
- A headache caused by another disorder ("secondary headache"), such as head or neck trauma, arterial ischemic stroke or venous sinus thrombosis, intracranial lesions or hemorrhage, meningitis or other systemic infection, elevated ICP, others. Consider secondary causes of headache when:
  - ✓ Systemic signs or symptoms of serious infection or rheumatologic disease, including fever, weight loss, rash, arthritis, or other chronic medical condition.
  - ✓ New neurologic signs or symptoms, particularly altered mental status, papilledema, a focal deficit on exam, or new seizure. It may be difficult to distinguish some auras from more worrisome neurologic signs or symptoms; when in doubt, rule out a secondary cause of headache.
  - ✓ Sudden onset: "Thunderclap" or "worst headache of life" suggests bleeding, vascular causes, or intermittent obstruction.
  - ✓ Occipital location is unusual in primary headache.
  - ✓ Progressive or brand new headache in the absence of family history
  - ✓ Pain worsened by Valsalva maneuver, when supine, or first thing in the morning.
  - ✓ Pain causes waking from sleep or is associated with a new neurologic deficit or seizure.
  - ✓ Child <6 years of age
- Medication overuse headache may occur with daily use of analgesics over several weeks.

PATHOPHYSIOLOGY

- Poorly understood, but likely multifactorial and polygenic.
- Cortical spreading depression (a self-propagating wave of neuronal and glial depolarization that spreads across the cerebral cortex) is likely the cause of aura and may activate head pain.

CLINICAL MANIFESTATIONS

- Premonitory phase: Affective, vegetative, and sensitivity symptoms that appear hours to a day before head pain
- Headache phase: Head pain is typically throbbing or pulsatile, though this may vary. In children, it may be bifrontal, bitemporal, or generalized, whereas unilateral pain is more common in adults. May include light/sound sensitivity (young children may not be able to verbalize this, but may seek quiet, dark rooms) and nausea and/or emesis. Most children obtain relief with sleep. Aura may occur before or during headache.
- Postdromal phase: Exhaustion, feeling drained, sometimes cognitive difficulties

DIAGNOSTICS

- Migraine diagnosis is based on clinical criteria in the context of a normal general and neurologic history and examination.
- Vital signs with orthostatics
- Consider neurology consultation if concern for secondary headache or for difficult-to-manage headaches
- Consider ophthalmology consultation if concern for papilledema

Laboratory Assessment

- Blood work is not necessary for diagnosis of migraine, but may be considered based on differential diagnosis.
- Lumbar puncture: Consider after neuroimaging if suspicion for meningitis, intracranial hemorrhage, pseudotumor cerebri (idiopathic intracranial hypertension). Check opening pressure, cell counts, protein, glucose, Gram stain, and bacterial culture, and save a sample for future testing.

Radiology

- Not always warranted if history is consistent with migraine and neurologic exam is normal.
- Consider neuroimaging if rapidly increasing headache frequency, lack of coordination, localized neurologic signs or symptoms, headache causing awakening from sleep, or with other suspicion of a secondary headache.
  - ✓ Head CT if emergent concerns for an acute intracranial process such as hemorrhage, elevated intracranial pressure, mass, stroke
  - ✓ MRI brain if nonemergent concerns or if head CT is normal but clinical suspicion remains for a secondary cause of headache.

MANAGEMENT

Acute

- Supportive measures, including hydration (oral or intravenous), lay in a darkened room with the door closed to minimize noise and allow rest, distraction and relaxation techniques
- Medication should be taken as soon as possible after symptom onset to maximize efficacy.
  - ✓ A clinical guideline for emergency department evaluation/treatment of a child with headache can be found at https://www.chop.edu/clinical-pathway/migraine-headache-emergent-care-clinical-pathway
  - ✓ A clinical guideline for inpatient management of a child with headache can be found at https://www.chop.edu/clinical-pathway/migraine-headache-inpatient-treatment-clinical-pathway

✓ Mainstays of therapy include fluids, NSAIDs (ibuprofen 10 mg/kg [maximum, 800 mg] or ketorolac 0.5 mg/kg [maximum, 30 mg]), and metoclopramide (0.2 mg/kg [maximum, 10 mg). Pain should be reassessed within 30–60 minutes after medications.

  ■ Valproic acid (15 mg/kg [maximum, 1000 mg]) and/or methylprednisolone (2 mg/kg [maximum, 200 mg) may be considered in the emergency department in conjunction with neurology consultation in specific populations if above are ineffective.

  ■ Dihydroergotamine (dosing protocols vary by institution), magnesium (50 mg/kg, [maximum, 1000 mg]), and/or levetiracetam (20 mg/kg [maximum, 1000 mg]) may be considered in conjunction with neurology consultation in specific inpatient populations.

  ■ Do *not* use opioids or nalbuphine, which are ineffective for migraine.

Chronic

• Ask the child/family to keep a calendar to track possible triggers (stress, poor sleep, dehydration, irregular meals, odors, weather changes, specific food, menstrual cycles), to clarify features of attacks and to help assess the effectiveness of treatment.

• A daily preventive medication may be considered in children who have more than three headaches monthly or who have significant time lost from school or very debilitating migraines. Effects of any prophylactic medication may take 1–2 months to be seen. Options include:

  ✓ Dietary supplements: riboflavin 5 mg/kg/day (maximum, 400 mg daily); magnesium oxide 200–400 mg daily (maximum, 1500 mg/day) divided three times daily; CoQ10 1–3 mg/kg/day (maximum, 100 mg/day); vitamin D supplementation only if deficient.

  ✓ Before puberty:

    ■ Cyproheptadine starting at 0.25 mg/kg/day (maximum, 2–12 mg/day) given at bedtime

  ✓ After puberty:

    ■ Amitriptyline starting at 0.1 mg/kg/day (up to 10 mg/day) given at bedtime (following a normal screening ECG). Dose may be slowly titrated up to 2 mg/kg/day as tolerated.

    ■ Topiramate starting at 0.2 mg/kg/day (up to 25 mg) given at bedtime. Dose may be slowly titrated to 2–3 mg/kg/day (maximum, 200 mg/day) as tolerated.

  ✓ Additional medication options should be discussed during a neurology consultation.

MULTIPLE SCLEROSIS

Multiple central nervous system demyelinating episodes separated in time and space. Multiple sclerosis (MS) is a lifelong disease with a variable course.

EPIDEMIOLOGY

• Geographic variation in prevalence: Northern United States, >30 in 100,000; Southern United States, 5–30 in 100,000; children who move before age 15 acquire risk of new environment.

• About 5% of MS presents before the age of 18; <1% of patients have onset prior to the age of 10.

• Male:female = 1:1 before puberty; 1:2.2 to 1:3 after puberty

• 25% risk of developing MS if monozygotic twin has MS

• In patients with MS, family history is positive in 10–26%.

PATHOPHYSIOLOGY

• Immune-mediated inflammation and demyelination of central white matter, possible molecular mimicry and attack of myelin basic protein

- Etiology is likely multifactorial, with a particular environmental trigger (Epstein–Barr virus, low vitamin D, others) occurring in a genetically susceptible individual (certain human leukocyte antigen haplotypes)
- Neuropathologic lesions are plaques: 1 mm–4 cm in diameter; loss of myelin, sparing of axons; T cells, macrophages; evolution to gliosis

DIFFERENTIAL DIAGNOSIS

- MS is a diagnosis of exclusion and must be distinguished from other inflammatory and demyelinating diseases of childhood, infections, metabolic disorders, and rheumatologic disorders.
  ✓ ADEM, optic neuritis, transverse myelitis, neuromyelitis optica, sarcoidosis, leukodystrophies
  ✓ CNS infections, CNS vasculitis, Lyme encephalitis, HIV encephalitis, syphilis
  ✓ Mitochondrial disorders, vitamin B_{12} deficiency, CNS malignancies
  ✓ Systemic lupus erythematosus, Sjögren syndrome, Behçet disease, antiphospholipid antibody syndrome, other collagen vascular or autoimmune disease

CLINICAL MANIFESTATIONS

Relapsing–Remitting Course

- 97–99% of children with multiple sclerosis will have a relapsing–remitting course.
- Characterized by intermittent attacks of increased disability following by either partial or complete recovery to baseline. These attacks may last days to weeks and may be precipitated by an acute infection or metabolic derangement.
- Common symptoms in relapsing–remitting disease include:
  ✓ Optic neuritis: Painful; usually unilateral loss of vision; on exam may see swollen disc, decreased color saturation, and decreased acuity with acute optic neuritis; a pale disc is seen with previous optic neuritis.
  ✓ Transverse myelitis or spinal-cord syndrome
  ✓ Ataxia, loss of coordination, nystagmus, other cerebellar dysfunction
  ✓ Bladder dysfunction
  ✓ Loss of sensation
  ✓ Weakness (acute or chronic), spasticity
  ✓ Seizures: 10–22% of children with MS, more with younger age at onset
  ✓ Mental status, energy, and mood: Usually normal at disease onset, possible cognitive difficulties, fatigue, depression over time
  ✓ L'Hermitte's phenomenon: Neck flexion causes electrical sensation down arms.
  ✓ Uhthoff's phenomenon: Symptoms worsen or brought on by heat.

Primary Progressive Multiple Sclerosis

- Characterized by a continuously worsening disability over time in the absence of discrete attacks; unusual in children.

DIAGNOSTICS

Clinical Diagnostic Criteria (May Meet Any One of the Following)

- ≥2 nonencephalopathic (i.e., unlike ADEM) clinical CNS events with presumed inflammatory cause, separated by >30 days and involving more than one area of the CNS
- One nonencephalopathic episode of typical MS associated with MRI findings that are disseminated in space, and in which a follow-up MRI shows ≥1 new enhancing or nonenhancing lesions consistent with dissemination in time

- One ADEM attack followed by a nonencephalopathic clinical event, ≥ 3 months after symptom onset, that is associated with new MRI lesions that are disseminated in space
- A first, single, acute event that does not meet ADEM criteria and whose MRI findings are disseminated in both time and space (only for children ≥ 12 years old)

Radiology

- MRI of brain and spinal cord with and without gadolinium: Callosal and periventricular white matter lesions are common and seen best on T2-weighted and fluid-attenuated inversion recovery images. Active/new lesions enhance, old lesions do not. Old lesions may look like a "black hole" on T1-weighted imaging

Laboratory

- Lumbar puncture: Oligoclonal bands, elevated IgG index
- Bloodwork to rule out other processes.
  - ✓ Antibodies: ANA, antineutrophil cytoplasmic antibodies, anti-ssA, anti-ssB, ACE, anti-scl70, anticardiolipin antibody
  - ✓ Inflammatory markers: ESR, C-reactive protein (CRP)
  - ✓ Infectious: rapid plasma reagin (RPR), HIV, Lyme disease; vitamin B_{12} level

Ancillary Testing

- Visual and somatosensory evoked potentials may support a diagnosis of demyelination, but are neither necessary nor sufficient for diagnosis.
- If history of oral and genital ulcers: Skin pathergy test for Behçet's disease

MANAGEMENT

Short-Term Management of an Attack

- Evaluate and treat any precipitating infection (temperature check, urinalysis, chest x-ray, etc.)
- If symptoms are severe and progressive (e.g., nonambulatory), consider pulse steroids (methylprednisolone 20–30 mg/kg/dose given once daily for 3–5 days [maximum, 1 g/day]) and taper to hasten recovery from attack.
  - ✓ Optic neuritis: IV steroids hasten recovery (no effect on final vision) and may slow progression of MS (IV only).
  - ✓ If symptoms do not improve with steroids, may consider IVIG 2 g/kg divided over 2–5 days.
  - ✓ If demyelination is severe and life-threatening, or a child is not responding to above therapy, may consider plasmapheresis (5–7 exchanges every other day).
- Physical and occupational therapy during admission

Prevention of Disease Progression

- Disease-modifying therapies may be considered after acute hospitalization in the outpatient setting. Commonly used therapies in pediatric multiple sclerosis include: interferon (IFN)-1α, IFN-1 β, glatiramer acetate, and less commonly fingolimod, natalizumab, and rituximab.

MYASTHENIA GRAVIS

An antibody-mediated autoimmune disease resulting in depletion of nicotinic acetylcholine (ACh) receptors at the neuromuscular junction and subsequent fatigable weakness

- Myasthenic crisis: Life-threatening respiratory weakness

EPIDEMIOLOGY

- 50–125 cases per million population (approximately 10% are children)

- Develops at any age
- After puberty, girls are affected more often than boys.
- 15% of adults with myasthenia gravis will have thymomas but rare in children; 85% of adults have thymic lymphofollicular hyperplasia.
- 10% of children will have associated autoimmune disease.

PATHOPHYSIOLOGY

- Autoantibodies cause deficit of ACh receptors at neuromuscular junctions, leading to accelerated degradation, functional blockade of the binding sites, and complement-mediated damage to the receptors.
- Abnormal ACh receptors (simplified membrane folds) and wide synaptic space also contribute
- Resulting decreased amplitude of end-plate potentials causes failure to trigger action potentials, reducing muscle power.

DIFFERENTIAL DIAGNOSIS

- Congenital myasthenic syndrome, transient neonatal myasthenia, drug-induced myasthenia, hyperthyroidism, Lambert–Eaton syndrome, botulism

CLINICAL MANIFESTATIONS

- Weakness and fatigability of skeletal muscles, ptosis, dysphagia, shortness of breath, blurred vision
- Muscles usually strongest early in the morning. Symptoms improve with rest.
- Diplopia, ptosis most often: 50% at presentation, 80–90% later. Ask the child to sustain upward gaze to bring out symptoms of ptosis.
- Generalized weakness in two-thirds of children: Bulbar, truncal, limb
- Intact DTRs, sensation, and coordination
- Closed eye rest test: Rest with eyes closed for 15 minutes. Observe degree of ptosis before and after test.

DIAGNOSTICS

Anticholinesterase Test (Edrophonium [Tensilon])

- Tensilon 0.1–0.2 mg/kg (maximum, 10 mg) IV: Start with 20% as test dose and wait 2 minutes; if no improvement, try 30% and wait 2 minutes; if still no improvement, try 50% and reassess.
- Positive if unequivocal improvement in objectively weak muscle
- Monitor for bradycardia, hypotension, respiratory compromise
- Have atropine ready immediately if patient becomes bradycardic.

Radioimmunoassay for ACh-Receptor Antibodies

- Anti–ACh-receptor antibodies positive in 50–90% of pediatric patients.
- Anti–muscle specific kinase antibodies positive in another 15%

Other

- Thyroid function studies: 3–8% will have hyperthyroidism.
- Consider screening for other autoimmune disorders, especially diabetes mellitus.
- Purified protein derivative test before immune therapy
- Serum vitamin B_{12} level
- EMG: Repetitive nerve stimulation, single fiber EMG if unclear
- Consider chest CT to evaluate thymus
- If isolated CN weakness, consider brain imaging to rule out intracranial abnormality.

MANAGEMENT

Chronic Medical Management

- Anticholinesterase agents: Pyridostigmine (Mestinon) is first-line therapy, though may be less helpful in anti–muscle specific kinase antibody–positive children:
  - ✓ Initial dosing in children is every 4–6 hours. In adults, usually given three times a day but sustained release formulations permit every day to twice-daily dosing.
  - ✓ Titrate dose to effect.
- Immunosuppression: Prednisone, azathioprine, others
- Other immunotherapy: Plasmapheresis, IVIG; used for myasthenic crisis, preparation for thymectomy, or failure to respond to medications.

Crisis

- Criteria to consider mechanical ventilation include forced vital capacity <15 mL/kg, <30% predicted for age, severe aspiration, or labored breathing; consider plasmapheresis or IVIG.

Surgical Management

- Thymectomy may accelerate time to remission in childhood generalized myasthenia gravis

SPINAL-CORD EMERGENCY

Suspected in nonencephalopathic children with progressive weakness and sensory symptoms (not involving the face), bowel/bladder dysfunction, and/or autonomic dysfunction

ETIOLOGY

- Mechanical (trauma, contusion)
  - ✓ Breech or traumatic delivery in infants
  - ✓ Motor vehicle accidents, diving, falls in older children.
    - Cervical spine injury is most common. May occur in setting of head injury or other trauma.
  - ✓ Compression from disc or fracture, hematoma, abscess, laceration, tumor, or syringomyelia.
- Infarction: Hypotension (e.g., after arrest), aortic dissection, anterior spinal artery occlusion
- Inflammation/demyelination: transverse myelitis, neuromyelitis optica, acute flaccid myelitis, MS, vasculitis

CLINICAL MANIFESTATIONS

- Motor: Sudden flaccid paralysis with areflexia (spinal shock) that later evolves over weeks to a spastic paresis or plegia
- Sensory: Level detected by pin, vibration, temperature
- Neck or back pain, fever if abscess
- Bowel and bladder compromise
- May have diaphragm paralysis if C3–C5 are involved; follow respiratory function.
- Preserved mental status and CN function unless there is concurrent head injury

DIAGNOSTICS

- Must first rule out compressive or vascular etiology that requires neurosurgical intervention
  - ✓ STAT MRI of the spine with and without contrast if available, CT spine with and without contrast if MRI not available
- Depending on clinical suspicion: Electrolytes, CBC, ESR, CRP, ANA, bone radiographs, LP

MANAGEMENT

- Emergency neurosurgical consultation if trauma or concern for cord compression. Better outcomes function is regained within 24 hours.
  - ✓ Consider immobilization of the spine, including a cervical collar if trauma
  - ✓ ABCs
- Emergency oncology consultation if neuroimaging is concerning for tumor
- Emergency stroke neurology consultation if neuroimaging is concerning for infarction
- Consider prompt glucocorticoids for trauma, tumor, or inflammatory lesion. Glucocorticoid of choice and dosing dependent on indication; discuss with consulting services.
- If cervical or progressive lesion: Monitor respiratory status with serial forced vital capacity and NIF measurements.
- Other: Supportive therapy, pain control, bowel regimen, Foley catheter, deep-vein thrombosis prophylaxis, intubation if necessary

STROKE

- Arterial ischemic stroke: Focal neurologic deficit in an arterial territory distribution with corresponding infarction on neuroimaging
- Transient ischemic attack (TIA): Brief (<24 hours) focal neurologic deficit in an arterial territory distribution, but *without* corresponding infarction on MRI of brain
- Primary intracranial hemorrhage: Includes parenchymal, intraventricular, and subarachnoid hemorrhage due to cerebrovascular disease
- Cerebral venous thrombosis: Thrombotic occlusion of cerebral venous system with or without corresponding venous infarction.

EPIDEMIOLOGY

- Arterial ischemic stroke
  - ✓ 3 in 100,000 to 13 in 100,000 children/year
    - In infants <30 days old: 1 in 4000 live births
  - ✓ 55% of childhood strokes are ischemic.
  - ✓ Mean interval to diagnosis in children is 24 hours after symptom onset. Though parents frequently do seek medical attention sooner, ischemic strokes are frequently initially mis-diagnosed.
  - ✓ 5% mortality; recurrence risk 5–15% at 2 years
- Primary intracranial hemorrhage
  - ✓ Intracranial hemorrhage: 1 in 100,000 to 3 in 100,000 children/year
  - ✓ 5–25% mortality
  - ✓ Recurrent risk from arteriovenous malformation or aneurysm 1–2% per year
- Cerebral venous thrombosis
  - ✓ 0.7 in 100,000 children/year
  - ✓ 5–10% mortality
- Long-term disability in 60% of survivors

ETIOLOGY

- Thrombosis, embolism, hemorrhage, hypoperfusion
- No cause detected in 20%.
- Risk factors for arterial ischemic stroke: Congenital heart disease, sickle cell disease, coagulation disorders, infection (e.g., endocarditis, varicella), moyamoya, arterial dissection
- Risk factors for hemorrhagic stroke: Arteriovenous malformation, cerebral aneurysm, cavernous malformations, head trauma, bleeding diathesis

- Risk factors for cerebral venous thrombosis: Severe dehydration, sepsis, hypercoagulability, intracranial infections

PATHOPHYSIOLOGY

- Arterial ischemic stroke: Decreased cerebral blood flow (due to vessel occlusion, hypoperfusion) causes ischemia. Cell death causes edema and surrounding damage. Children may have secondary hemorrhage into ischemic stroke territory,
- Primary intracranial hemorrhage: Mass effect causes local damage and may result in midline shift or herniation,
- Cerebral venous thrombosis: Venous hypertension, venous infarction with hemorrhages
- Maximal edema occurs 2–3 days after ischemic stroke supratentorially, 3–5 days after ischemic stroke infratentorially (e.g. cerebellum, brain stem). May have secondary ischemic events if another major vessel is occluded owing to surrounding edema.

CLINICAL MANIFESTATIONS

- Ischemic stroke: Focal neurologic deficit in a vascular distribution
- Primary intracranial hemorrhage: Severe acute headache ("worst headache of life"), altered mental status, focal neurologic deficit, seizure
- Cerebral venous thrombosis: headache, emesis, altered mental status (particularly lethargy).
- For all strokes, watch closely for signs and symptoms of elevated ICP, including possible impending herniation syndromes:
  ✓ Serial exams are critical
  ✓ Vital signs: Cushing's triad of hypertension, bradycardia, and abnormal respirations
  ✓ May have papilledema, double vision (VIth nerve palsies)
  ✓ Seizures
- Look for evidence of trauma or predisposing disease

DIAGNOSTICS

Radiology

- Noncontrast head CT to look for hemorrhage, edema; may see signs of early infarction (though this can be missed on CT)
- MRI brain best for early infarcts (diffusion-weighted MRI)
- MR angiography/venography (MRA/MRV) to evaluate vascular abnormalities: Include MRA of neck if suspect arterial dissection and MRV if suspect cerebral venous thrombosis
- Cerebral angiography if further information required after MRA
- Transcranial Doppler ultrasound can predict increased risk in patients with sickle cell disease.

Cardiac Evaluation

- ECG, transthoracic echocardiogram (for arterial ischemic stroke)

Laboratory Studies

- CBC, prothrombin time/partial thromboplastin time/international normalized ratio, lipid profile, HIV, RPR
- Hypercoagulability workup (see **Box 12-1**): Protein C and protein S levels, antithrombin III, factor V Leiden, homocysteine level and *MTHFR* gene, antiphospholipid, prothrombin 20210 gene mutation, lipoprotein a, β_2-glycoprotein 1
- Screen for vasculitis: ESR, C3, C4, ANA
- Toxicology screen, especially for cocaine

- Hemoglobin electrophoresis for patients with sickle cell disease
- Blood culture if suspect endocarditis
- If infarct not in typical vascular distribution, consider metabolic cause: Plasma ammonia, lactate, pyruvate, amino acids, urine organic acids, CSF lactate

MANAGEMENT

- For initial resuscitation: ABCs, treat hypoglycemia, treat seizures, maintain temperature at 36.5–37°C, institute nothing by mouth regimen.

Acute Medical Management

- Arterial ischemic stroke: Lay flat (maximize cerebral perfusion); liberal IV normal saline (avoid dextrose to minimize edema); correct electrolyte abnormalities (avoid hyperosmolality); maintain normotension (goal is upper limit of normal; do not overtreat hypertension); monitor ICP; if arterial dissection or cardiac clot, consider heparin in consultation with hematology.
- Hemorrhagic stroke: Monitor vital signs, ICP; elevate head 30 degrees; maintain normotension; correct electrolyte imbalances; correct anemia; *avoid* anticoagulation. Consider neurosurgical consultation for possible evacuation.
- Cerebral venous sinus thrombosis: Monitor vital signs, ICP; elevate head 30 degrees; liberal IV normal saline; if not contraindicated, start heparin (no bolus)

Anticoagulation

- Discuss any anticoagulation plans with neurology and hematology consultations. Potential medications and indications are:
  - ✓ Antiplatelet therapy: Consider use in cryptogenic arterial ischemic stroke, mild prothrombotic states, cerebral arteriopathy
    - Aspirin (acute and chronic therapy): Typical dose is 2–3 mg/kg/day; causes antiplatelet effect (low-dose = 1 mg/kg/day).
  - ✓ Systemic anticoagulation: consider in consultation with hematology for major prothrombotic states, intracardiac thrombus, valve disease, extracranial cerebral artery dissection, cerebral venous sinus thrombosis. Must weigh risks of bleeding with risk of recurrence or extension of ischemia and/or thrombus. Contraindications include thrombocytopenia, recent intracranial hemorrhage, active systemic hemorrhage, major surgery within previous 24 hours, uncontrolled severe hypertension. While on any of these therapies, avoid contact sports.
    - Heparin: Do *not* administer bolus. For children <12 months, start with 28 U/kg/hr; 1–11 years, 20 U/kg/hr; >12 years, 17 U/kg/hr. Rate should not exceed 1000 units/hr in any age group. Target activated partial thromboplastin time: 60–85 seconds
    - Low-molecular-weight heparin (enoxaparin): Children ≥2 months of age, start with 1 mg/kg/dose every 12 hours; <2 months use 1.5 mg/kg/dose every 12 hours. Target anti-Xa level: 0.5–1 unit/mL
    - Warfarin (Coumadin): Oral option, but harder to manage levels than with options above. Start with 0.1 mg/kg/day. Target international normalized ratio is 2.0–3.0.
- Thrombolytics have not been well studied in children with stroke and are not routinely recommended at this time.

Surgical

- Endovascular therapy may be considered for select cases of arterial ischemic stroke depending on age, clinical deficit, time from last known normal/at neurologic baseline, medical stability, and location of thrombus.
- Emergency evacuation of large hemorrhage and/or increased ICP

- May require ventriculostomy to monitor ICP.
- Consider surgery for vascular malformations, large middle cerebral artery infarcts, and hydrocephalus

TRANSVERSE MYELITIS

Acute or subacute inflammatory process involving both gray and white matter of the spinal cord, resulting in bilateral motor, sensory, and autonomic dysfunction. May be idiopathic or secondary to other broader disorders (e.g., MS, acute disseminated encephalomyelitis, others). The following discussion is directed toward idiopathic cases.

EPIDEMIOLOGY

- At least one to eight new cases per million per year; seasonal clustering (winter)
- Peak incidence at ages 10–19 and 30–39 years
- No sex or familial predisposition
- One-third recover completely, one-third have moderate permanent disability, one-third have severe persistent disability.
- Idiopathic cases are thought to largely be postinfectious.
- Recovery begins within 1–3 months, and can proceed over years. Persistent disability in ~40%.
- Disorders that cause secondary transverse myelitis
  ✓ Infections: enteroviruses, West Nile virus, others
  ✓ Rheumatologic disorders: SLE, Sjögren syndrome
  ✓ Paraneoplastic syndrome
  ✓ Multifocal inflammatory neurologic disease: MS, neuromyelitis optica, acute disseminated encephalomyelitis, sarcoidosis

DIFFERENTIAL DIAGNOSIS

- Other causes of myelopathy
  ✓ Compressive: Trauma, epidural masses or blood, vertebral body fractures, spondylosis, tuberculosis
  ✓ Vascular myelopathies
  ✓ Metabolic and nutritional myelopathies
  ✓ Neoplasm
  ✓ Radiation myelitis
- Nonmyelopathic disorders that mimic transverse myelitis
  ✓ Guillain–Barré syndrome

CLINICAL MANIFESTATIONS

- Back pain may precede neurologic symptoms
- Weakness: Flaccid initially, spastic later
- Sensory changes (numbness, pain), commonly with a sensory level (the lowest spinal cord level that still has intact sensation)
- Autonomic symptoms (bowel, bladder, sexual dysfunction) develop acutely/subacutely; typical nadir in function by 2 days
- Often fever, nuchal rigidity

DIAGNOSTICS

- MRI brain and spine with and without gadolinium

Laboratory Studies

- Lumbar puncture: Increased WBC (lymphocytic predominance), normal or increased protein, normal glucose. Send bacterial and viral cultures, oligoclonal bands, IgG index,

501

aquaporin 4 IgG. Consider cytology, specific viral studies (e.g., enterovirus, varicella–zoster virus, Epstein–Barr virus, cytomegalovirus)
- Serum: Aquaporin 4 IgG, ANA profile, vitamin B_{12}, copper, vitamin D, vitamin E, HIV, human T-cell lymphotropic virus type 1, RPR, Lyme testing, mycoplasma serology
- Urinalysis and culture if urinary retention

MANAGEMENT

- High-dose IV methylprednisolone (15–30 mg/kg/dose, maximum 1 g/day) for 5 days is standard of care
- Sphincter dysfunction: Intermittent catheterization; treat constipation
- Supportive: Physical and occupational therapy

SEIZURES AND EPILEPSY

GENERAL PRINCIPLES

A *seizure* is a paroxysmal event caused by abnormal electrical discharges in the brain.

- Focal seizures: Affect/originate in one part of the brain. Any focal motor sign, sensory, or psychic experience with or without preserved awareness. May evolve into a generalized seizure. Previously classified as either "simple" (preserved consciousness) or "complex" (impairment of awareness).
- Generalized seizures: Affect whole brain. Includes tonic–clonic, tonic, clonic, atonic, myoclonic, absence, epileptic spasms, myoclonic, myoclonic-atonic, and myoclonic–tonic–clonic

Epilepsy is recurrent unprovoked seizures or a single unprovoked seizure in the context of an epileptiform EEG or other propensity for seizure.

EPIDEMIOLOGY

- 1% of children will have an unprovoked seizure by age 14 years
- 0.4–0.9% of children, and 1.2% overall population has epilepsy

ETIOLOGY

- Fever (see "Febrile Seizures" section)
- Structural: Tumor, CNS malformation, hypoxic–ischemic injury, head trauma (accidental or nonaccidental), CNS hemorrhage, arterial ischemic stroke
- Infectious: CNS infection, sepsis
- Metabolic: Hyperammonemia, inborn error of metabolism, genetic (e.g., channelopathy), low or high glucose, Na, or Ca, low Mg
- Genetic (previously termed "idiopathic"): Includes channelopathies
- Immune: Autoimmune encephalitis
- Other: Toxin, medication, medication withdrawal, unknown

DIFFERENTIAL DIAGNOSIS

- Syncope: Brief anoxia may precipitate a provoked seizure in an otherwise healthy child ("convulsive syncope")
- Breath-holding spell, tic, cardiac dysrhythmia with collapse, myoclonus, behavioral event (e.g., staring), parasomnia, conversion disorder (non-epileptic), gastroesophageal reflux (Sandifer syndrome)

PHYSICAL EXAM

- During a seizure, the following are possible: Impaired awareness, change in vital signs, focal seizure activity. Seizure is an abnormal activation, so eyes are usually open.
- After a seizure, the following are possible: Decreased awareness and responsiveness, Todd's paresis (transient postictal paresis that resolves within 24–48 hours), eye deviation toward the side of seizure focus, eyes may be closed

MANAGEMENT

- Acute management focuses on maintaining control of ABCs and, when appropriate, cessation of seizures with benzodiazepines, for example, lorazepam (0.05–0.1 mg/kg IV); maximum dose is 4 mg for children and 8 mg for adults (see "Status Epilepticus" section)
- Chronic management consists of raising the seizure threshold and should be initiated after a second unprovoked seizure or after a first unprovoked seizure with an epileptiform EEG.
  - ✓ Outpatient anticonvulsant can be chosen based on seizure type, EEG, and side effect profile. See **Table 20-5** for a summary of commonly prescribed anticonvulsants.

FEBRILE SEIZURES

- Simple febrile seizure: A brief (<15 minute), generalized seizure in a developmentally normal 6-month to 5-year-old with fever (>38°C). No more than one seizure in 24 hours
- Complex febrile seizure: A seizure that is prolonged (>15 minutes), has focal features, or is recurrent (more than one in 24 hours) in a developmentally normal 6-month to 5-year-old child with fever

EPIDEMIOLOGY

- 2–5% of all children have had a febrile seizure.
- Peak incidence: 12–18 months
- Recurrence risk:
  - ✓ Age <12 months: 50%
  - ✓ Age ≥12 months: 30%
  - ✓ Second febrile seizure: 50% have at least one additional recurrence.
- Overall risk of epilepsy in children with simple febrile seizures is similar to 1% risk in general population. Children with multiple febrile seizures, complex febrile seizure, and the first seizure at <12 months of age have about a 2% risk.

DIAGNOSTICS

- American Academy of Pediatrics practice guidelines for the evaluation of a child with simple febrile seizures can be found at: http://pediatrics.aappublications.org/content/127/2/389
- Lumbar puncture: Should be performed:
  - ✓ Age <6 months: Always
  - ✓ Age 6–12 months: Strongly consider, particularly if *Haemophilus influenzae* type B and *Streptococcus pneumonia* immunizations are deficient (or unknown), if clinical suspicion of intracranial infection, if complex febrile seizure, if focal neurologic findings on exam, or if concurrent/previous antibiotic treatment (may mask clinical signs or symptoms of intracranial infection).
  - ✓ Age >12 months: Consider if clinical suspicion of intracranial infection, complex febrile seizure, focal neurologic findings on exam, concurrent/previous antibiotic treatment

TABLE 20-5 Common Anticonvulsants

	Contraindications	Adverse reactions	Advantages/Special considerations
Any type of epilepsy (generalized, focal, mixed)			
Levetiracetam (Keppra) • Start 10–20 mg/kg/day, divided BID		Moodiness/aggression in 10%	• Can load IV • Rapid titration • Few drug-drug interactions
Brivaracetam (Briviact) • Start (all divided BID) ✓ 4–16 years old: ✓ 11–50 kg: 1–2 mg/kg/day ✓ ≥50 kg: 50–100 mg/day ✓ ≥16 years old: 100 mg/day		Mood changes	• 2nd generation of levetiracetam; thought to have improved side effect profile as compared with levetiracetam
Phenobarbital (Luminal) • Start (all QD or divided BID): ✓ Neonates: 3–4 mg/kg/day ✓ Infants: 4–5 mg/kg/day ✓ 1–5 years old: 6–8 mg/kg/day ✓ 5–12 years old: 4–6 mg/kg/day		Sedation/respiratory depression, younger children can have paradoxical reaction (hyperactivity), cognitive concerns	• Can load IV • Levels well defined and able to be obtained quickly
Valproic acid (Depakote, Depakene, Depacon) • Start 10 mg/kg/day divided BID–TID (depends on formulation)	• Metabolic/mitochondrial disease (risk of fulminant hepatotoxicity) • Pregnancy (risk of teratogenicity) • Pancreatitis (can trigger)	Fulminant hepatotoxicity if underlying metabolic/mitochondrial disorder, thrombocytopenia, idiosyncratic pancreatitis, weight gain, tremor, teratogenicity, hair loss	• Can load IV • Rapid titration • Levels well defined and able to be obtained quickly • May stabilize mood • May also treat headaches

Lamotrigine (Lamictal)
• Start:
  ✓ Already on valproic acid:
    ✓ 2–12 years old: 0.15 mg/kg/day divided QD–BID
    ✓ >12 years old: 25 mg every other day
  NOT on valproic acid or other enzyme-inducing medications:
  • 2–12 years old: 0.3 mg/kg/day
  • >12 years old: 25 mg QD
	• History of lamotrigine-associated rash
	• Use with caution in hepatic dysfunction, renal failure, with concurrent estrogen-containing OCPs, and with concurrent valproic acid (all of which may cause changes in lamctrigine serum concentrations requiring dose adjustment).
		Serious skin rashes such as SJS if titrated up too quickly (most life-threatening rashes occur in the first 2–8 weeks of treatment, can also have TEN, benign rashes may also occur)
		
		Other: HA, insomnia, tremor, ataxia, mood changes
			• May exacerbate myoclonic epilepsy
			• May stabilize mood
			• May have to give higher end of dosing to patients <6 years old
			• Interacts with valproic acid (valproic acid increases lamotrigine levels) and carbamazepine (increases carbamazepine toxicity)
			• Interacts with estrogen-containing OCPs (decreases lamotrigine levels)

Topiramate (Topamax) • Start 1–3 mg/kg/day divided BID	Use with caution if family history of kidney stones	Cognitive slowing, weight loss, metabolic acidosis, kidney stone, anhidrosis, paresthesia, anemia	• May also treat headaches • Interacts with OCPs

Zonisamide (Zonegran)
• Start
  ✓ <16 years old: 1–2 mg/kg/day divided QD–BID
  ✓ >16 years old: 100 mg QD
	Use with caution if family history of kidney stones	Serious rashes, mood changes, bone marrow suppression, rhabdomyolysis, pancreatitis, oligiohdrosis/hyperthermia in pediatric patients, specifically, cognitive slowing/impaired memory, paresthesia	• Caution if hypersensitive to sulfonamides

Clobazam (Onfi)
• Start (divided BID–TID)
  ✓ <12.5 kg or <2 years old: 0.25 mg/kg/day
  ✓ 12.5–30 kg: 5 mg/day
  ✓ >30 kg 10 mg/day
	Avoid if concomitant opioid use: combination may result in profound sedation/respiratory depression, coma, and death	Sedation, ataxia, muscle weakness, irritability, hyperactivity, psychosis, increased salivation/secretions, weight gain, thrombocytopenia	• Long half-life
			• Watch out for paradoxical reactions to benzos, especially in younger children

(Continued)

TABLE 20-5 Common Anticonvulsants (*Continued*)

	Contraindications	Adverse reactions	Advantages/Special considerations
Focal epilepsy (these medications may worsen generalized epilepsy)			

Carbamazepine (Tegretol)
• Start (divided BID–QID)
  ✓ <12 years old: 5–10 mg/kg/day
  ✓ ≥12 years old: 400 mg/day
		Serious dermatologic reactions (SJS, TEN), especially with HLA-B*1502 allele.
		
		Risk of aplastic anemia (overall low risk, but 5–8× greater than that of general public)
		
		Other: drug interactions, idiosyncratic leukopenia and aplastic anemia, arrhythmias, dizziness, ataxia, blurry vision, teratogenicity, hyponatremia
			• Many drug interactions related to hepatic enzyme inducer (induces thus decreases levels of benzodiazepines, erythromycin increases carbamazepine levels)
			• May have some mood-stabilizing qualities

Oxcarbazepine (Trileptal)
• Start (divided BID)
  ✓ 4–16 years old: 8–10 mg/kg/day (max, 600 mg/day)
  ✓ ≥16 years old: 300–600 mg/day
		Rashes (including SJS), SIADH, ataxia, hyponatremia, agranulocytosis, aplastic anemia (less likely than carbamazepine), diplopia	• 2nd generation of carbamazepine; thought to have improved side effect profile and less drug interactions
			• May have some mood-stabilizing qualities

Eslicarbazepine (Aptiom)
• Start (all QD):
  ✓ 11–21 kg: 200 mg
  ✓ 22–38 kg: 300 mg
  ✓ >38 kg: 400 mg
		Rashes (including SJS), mood changes, dizziness/ataxia, blurred vision, hyponatremia, LFTs elevated, T_3/T_4 decreased	• 3rd generation of carbamazepine; thought to have improved side-effect profile with less risk of hyponatremia than carbamazepine/oxcarbazepine

Gabapentin (Neurontin)
• Start (divided TID)
  ✓ 3–12 years old: 10–15 mg/kg/day
  ✓ ≥12 years old: 300 mg/day
		Weight gain, sedation, mood changes, rashes, rhabdomyolysis, withdrawal if discontinued abruptly, GI upset, impotence, hostility (especially in children), hyperkinesia (especially in children)	• DEA/FDA classification varies by state
			• Also effective for neuropathic pain, postherpetic neuralgia
			• Can rapidly titrate

Pregabalin (Lyrica)
• Start (divided BID–TID)
  ✓ Children: 2.5 mg/kg/day (max, 150 mg)
  ✓ Adults: 150 mg/day
	• Use caution in patients with heart failure due to risk of increased peripheral edema.
	• Use with caution if history of angioedema
		May cause euphoric/addictive behavior, mood changes, angioedema, weight gain, thrombocytopenia, rhabdomyolysis	• 2nd generation of gabapentin
			• Not FDA-approved for children (consent required <18); may not be as benign as initially thought
			• Schedule V substance
			• Renally excreted, so good for liver failure
			• Can start immediately at full dose, but should not discontinue abruptly

Phenytoin (Dilantin)
• Start (oral or IV):
  ✓ Children: 4-5 mg/kg/day divided BID–TID
  ✓ Adults: 200–300 mg/day divided QD–BID
• IV loading: 15–20 mg/kg at specific rate (check with pharmacy); fosphenytoin is same IV load dosing
	• Heart block,
	• Sinus bradycardia
	• Use with caution if low albumin (will increase free phenytoin and effective dose)
		Cardiovascular risk with rapid infusions (severe hypotension and cardiac arrhythmias).
		
		Can cause tissue/vascular injury IV/IM, rashes/hypersensitivity reactions, hepatic enzyme inducer (so other drug interactions), gingival hyperplasia, arrhythmias/conduction disturbance, affects blood lines, toxic delirium, GI upset
			• Can load IV, though if doing so, consider fosphenytoin instead (less cardiac risk, but still a black box warning)
			• Rapid titration
			• Levels well-defined and able to be obtained quickly, but hard to maintain levels with oral dosing in infants, and unpredictable pharmacokinetics at higher doses

(Continued)

TABLE 20-5 Common Anticonvulsants (*Continued*)

	Contraindications	Adverse reactions	Advantages/Special considerations

Lacosamide (Vimpat)
• Start (divided BID)
  ✓ ≤17 years old: 2 mg/kg/day
  ✓ >17 years old: 100 mg/day
		Prolonged PR interval and other arrhythmias, dizziness/HA, diplopia, psychiatric, nystagmus, DRESS, pruritus, GI upset	• Dosing, including loading doses based on limited data in children (not approved for children)
			• Can load IV with caution
			• Consider screening ECG prior to start and after dose escalation
			• Schedule V substance

Infantile Spasms			
ACTH (Acthar) • Start 75 U/m² BID		Cushingoid appearance, weight gain, emotional lability/mood changes, insomnia, psychosis, adrenal insufficiency, immunosuppression, myopathy, DM, increased ICP/pseudotumor cerebri, pancreatitis, GI upset to GI perforation, headache	• *Very expensive* in the United States • Monitoring: Weekly BP, daily stools, daily urine dips for glucose, consider PPD placement, Bactrim prophylaxis, weekly BMPs (for K⁺) • Causes immunosuppression: hold vaccinations during and immediately after treatment, especially live vaccines
Prednisolone (Orapred) • Protocols vary. One starting point is 10 mg QID; discuss with neurology.		Similar to ACTH	• Can consider same monitoring as ACTH, but need for this not as well defined

Vigabatrin (Sabril) • Start 50 mg/kg/day divided BID	Permanent vision loss (peripheral vision), reversible MRI changes (of unknown significance), weight gain, irritability, paresthesia, peripheral neuropathy	• Prescribers much be enrolled to prescribe this; website: www.vigabatrinREMS.com • Formal serial eye exams, including visual fields, are recommended.

Other

Ethosuximide (Zarontin) • Start (divided BID) ✓ <6 years old: 10–15 mg/kg/day ✓ ≥6 years old: 500 mg/day	Decreased appetite/weight loss, bone marrow depression, mood changes, GI symptoms, irritability, sleep disturbance	• Used mainly for absence seizures, but abrupt withdrawal can cause absence status. • Not usually used for GTC or focal seizures, as may worsen convulsive seizures in mixed epilepsy
Cannabidiol (Epidiolex) • Start ✓ ≥2 years old: 5 mg/kg divided BID	Mood changes, Liver injury	No contraindications at time of publication, but only very recently FDA-approved, so this may change • Epidiolex (FDA-approved cannabidiol product) is Schedule V, but marijuana and other cannabidiol products remains schedule I substances • Interacts with other medications

ACTH = adrenocorticotropic hormone; BID = twice a day; BMP = basic metabolic panel; BP = blood pressure; DM = diabetes mellitus; DRESS = drug rash with eosinophilia and systemic symptoms; FDA = Food and Drug Administration; GTC = generalized tonic–clonic; HA = hemagglutination; HLA = human leukocyte antigen; LFT = liver function test; max = maximum; OCP = oral contraceptive pill; PPD = purified protein derivative; D = once a day; SJS = Stevens–Johnson syndrome; T_3 = triiodothyronine; T_4 = thyroxine; TEN = toxic epidermal necrolysis; TID = three times a day.

- CT/MRI:
  - ✓ Infectious Disease Society of America guidelines for when to obtain neuroimaging prior to LP can be found at https://academic.oup.com/cid/article/39/9/1267/402080
    - Head CT should be considered before LP if a child is immunocompromised, if there is clinical concern for elevated ICP, if there are focal findings on neurologic exam, or if there is congenital heart disease with right-to-left shunt.
  - ✓ Not otherwise routinely indicated for simple febrile seizure if recovery is complete and exam is normal.
  - ✓ Should be obtained for complex febrile seizures
- Laboratory studies: Electrolytes, Mg^{2+}, Ca^{2+}, CBC, glucose
- EEG: Not indicated for simple febrile seizure. Consider for complex febrile seizures as outpatient procedure with neurology.

MANAGEMENT

AAP Practice Guidelines for the long-term management of a child with simple febrile seizures can be found at: http://pediatrics.aappublications.org/content/121/6/1281

- Antipyretic medications do *not* prevent recurrent febrile seizures.
- Continuous or intermittent anticonvulsant medications are not recommended for prevention of simple febrile seizures.
- In cases of prolonged febrile seizures, it may be appropriate to prescribe rectal diazepam for use as abortive therapy. Dosing: for age less than 5 years, 0.5 mg/kg; for 5 years or older, 0.25 mg/kg, maximum 10 mg/dose in children, 20 mg/dose in adults.

INFANTILE SPASMS

Generalized epilepsy characterized by seizures with brief bilateral contractions of neck, trunk, and extremities, often occurring in clusters (flexor, extensor, or mixed). Seizures often occur upon awakening or upon falling asleep.

- Cryptogenic (10–45%): No underlying cause identified. Normal development prior to onset of spasms.
- Symptomatic (50–90%): Clearly defined underlying cause and/or significant developmental delay prior to onset of spasms. Common causes include CNS malformations (e.g., tuberous sclerosis), genetic syndromes (e.g., Down syndrome), metabolic disorders, intrauterine insults, and others.
- West syndrome: Triad of infantile spasms, developmental plateau/regression, and hypsarrhythmia on EEG

EPIDEMIOLOGY

- 1 in 4000 to 1 in 6000 live births
- 85% begin before age 1 year (peak age at onset, 3–6 months)
- Normal development following resolution of spasms occurs in about 25% of patients with cryptogenic infantile spasms (in symptomatic infantile spasms fewer patients have normal development)
- Spasms typically end by 3–5 years, but other types of seizures persist in 60%.
- Prognosis is better with early and aggressive therapy.

CLINICAL MANIFESTATIONS

- Brief symmetric contractions of head, neck, and extremities
- Often occur in clusters on falling asleep or awakening
- Often associated with loss of developmental milestones

DIAGNOSTICS

- EEG: Hypsarrhythmia (disorganized, high-amplitude multifocal epileptiform pattern); electrodecremental seizures
- Brain MRI: Evaluates for malformations, bleeds, etc.
- Laboratory studies: genetic and metabolic screening evaluations

MANAGEMENT

- Goals include disappearance of hypsarrhythmia, reduction in seizures, and stabilization of development. Initiate treatment in conjunction with neurology consultation. Options include:
  ✓ Consider pyridoxine trial (see "Neonatal Seizures" section)
  ✓ Adrenocorticotropic hormone: Unclear mechanism of action on epileptogenesis. Must be given IM; 70–80% will respond; adverse effects include hypertension, irritability, weight gain, hyperkalemia, hyperglycemia, risk of sepsis, risk of infection at injection sites
    ▪ Can consider high dose oral steroids instead with input of neurology consultant.
  ✓ Vigabatrin: First line for patients with tuberous sclerosis. Dosing per **Table 20-5**.
  ✓ Other medications: Topiramate, valproate, and benzodiazepines may be considered. Dosing per **Table 20-5**.
  ✓ Ketogenic diet
  ✓ Excision of a symptomatic focal lesion can occasionally be curative

NEONATAL SEIZURES

Seizure that occurs in the first month of life

EPIDEMIOLOGY

- 4.4 in 1000 live births; incidence increases with earlier gestational age
- Approximately 50% of infants with seizures due to hypoxic–ischemic encephalopathy have moderate to severe neurologic abnormalities at follow-up.

ETIOLOGY

- By age at presentation:
  ✓ <24 hours of life: hypoxic–ischemic encephalopathy, stroke, hemorrhage, infection (TORCH, meningitis)
  ✓ 24–72 hours of life: problems above, plus structural abnormalities
  ✓ >72 hours: problems above, plus metabolic abnormalities
- Other causes at any age: trauma, pyridoxine dependency, familial neonatal convulsions ("5th day fits"), other genetic epilepsy syndromes

PATHOPHYSIOLOGY

- Electric discharges in the neonatal brain are regional and rarely spread to contralateral hemisphere; therefore, generalized tonic–clonic seizures are rare in neonates

DIAGNOSIS

History

- Family history of neonatal seizures, metabolic disorders
- Maternal drug use, pregnancy history
- Apgar less than 5 at 5 minutes, base deficit greater than 10 at birth concerning for hypoxic-ischemic injury

EEG

- Normal EEG in term infant or mildly abnormal EEG = good prognosis
- Flat or burst-suppression pattern on EEG = poor prognosis
- EEG abnormal for >2 weeks in newborn with asphyxia = always poor prognosis
- If EEG positive for subclinical seizures, consider continuous EEG during medication loading until subclinical seizures cease

Laboratory Studies

- Glucose, electrolytes, BUN, creatinine, Ca^{2+}, Mg^{2+}, PO_4, bilirubin, ammonia
- Blood gas (rule out acidosis)
- If metabolic acidosis and increased ammonia, send urine organic acids
- Check state newborn metabolic screening results
- Consider serum amino acids, lactate, pyruvate, long-chain fatty acids
- Consider karyotype
- Consider TORCH titers
- Lumbar puncture: Cell counts in tubes 1 and 4, protein, glucose, gram stain and culture, CSF HSV PCR, metabolic laboratory studies (CSF lactate/pyruvate, amino acids)
- Serum/urine toxicology screen from mother and/or neonate

Radiology

- Head ultrasound to evaluate for intraventricular hemorrhage; brain MRI with and without contrast to evaluate for other structural lesions

Evaluate for Pyridoxine Dependency with Empiric Treatment

- Give 100 mg IV pyridoxine during EEG monitoring, then continue 100 mg orally every day for 1 week. Positive if all clinical seizures stop (minutes) and EEG normalizes (hours).

MANAGEMENT

- If identifiable, treat underlying disorder.
- Seizures due to hypoxic–ischemic encephalopathy typically improve or subside after 72 hours, regardless of therapy
- Antiepileptic drugs:
  - ✓ Phenobarbital is first-line therapy in neonates. Load 15–20 mg/kg IV, then maintenance 5–8 mg/kg/day.
  - ✓ Phenytoin is second-line therapy. Load 20 mg/kg IV to achieve level 15–20 μg/mL, then maintenance 4–6 mg/kg/day. Fosphenytoin: same dose given as phenytoin equivalents, but can be administered either IM or as a faster IV infusion than phenytoin
  - ✓ Levetiracetam and topiramate are other options for second-line therapy.
  - ✓ Benzodiazepines are useful to stop seizures in the short term while loading other medications and for breakthrough seizures.
  - ✓ Check levels after loading and check levels regularly if seizures continue or if subclinical seizures are noted on EEG.
- Review with neurology consultant if seizures do not easily respond to first-line phenobarbital.

STATUS EPILEPTICUS

A convulsive seizure lasting more than 5 minutes, a nonconvulsive seizure lasting more than 10 minutes, or multiple seizures without return to baseline in between

- A clinical guideline for the evaluation and management of status epilepticus can be found at: https://www.chop.edu/clinical-pathway/status-epilepticus-clinical-pathway

EPIDEMIOLOGY

- >50% of children presenting in status epilepticus were not previously known to have seizures.
- 10% of children with epilepsy present with status epilepticus.
- 25% of children with epilepsy will have at least one episode of status epilepticus, most within the first 5 years after diagnosis.
- Most common pediatric neurology emergency

DIAGNOSTICS

- After stabilization (ABCs), check glucose immediately.
- Electrolytes, BUN, creatinine, LFTs, ABG, anticonvulsant levels, urine toxin screen
- In a patient without known epilepsy: NH_3, metabolic screens
- Consider CT head or MRI brain once patient is hemodynamically stable if seizure did not self-resolve, if there is new focality, or if the child is not waking up as expected to look for possible structural causes.
- Consider LP if/when patient is stable; blood and urine cultures (especially if fever); also consider CSF cell counts for HSV and enterovirus, or other infectious testing, pending CSF cell count results.

MANAGEMENT

Acute management focuses on maintaining control of ABCs and cessation of seizures. It is probably most important to give medications quickly, rather than to give any specific medication. Successive doses of any anticonvulsant, particularly benzodiazepines or barbiturates, may suppress respiration and necessitate intubation

Convulsive Status Epilepticus

- ABCs
- Check glucose and give 50% glucose solution 1 mg/kg (unless on ketogenic diet)
- Anticonvulsants that may be loaded parenterally:
  1. Benzodiazepines (choose one):
     a. Ativan (lorazepam) 0.05–0.1 mg/kg IV or IM (maximum, 8 mg)
     b. Versed (midazolam) 0.2 mg/kg IV or 0.2–0.5 mg/kg per rectum
     c. Doses may be repeated every 5–10 minutes, but if seizures persist after approximately three doses, proceed to one of the following:
  2. Phenytoin 25 mg/kg IV *slowly* (no faster than 1 mg/kg/min, usually over 1 hour) in non–dextrose-containing solution; monitor for cardiac arrhythmia
     a. Alternative: Fosphenytoin (same dose, but can be given either IM or as a faster IV infusion than phenytoin with less risk of cardiac arrhythmia)
  3. Phenobarbital 20 mg/kg IV; monitor for hypotension and respiratory suppression
  4. Valproic acid 40 mg/kg IV if patient is >2 years old and there is no suspicion for metabolic disease
  5. Levetiracetam 50 mg/kg IV (maximum, 2500 mg/dose; good for patients on chemotherapy as there are fewer interactions.
- If these are ineffective, coma agents should be considered with concurrent EEG monitoring and neurology consultation.
  ✓ Pentobarbital loading dose of 5–10 mg/kg once over 1–2 hours, then infusion starting at 1 mg/kg/hr; bump and bolus to titrate to EEG burst suppression.

✓ Midazolam bolus of 0.1 mg/kg once, then infusion starting at 0.1 mg/kg/hr; bump and bolus to titrate to EEG burst-suppression.
- If there is concern for ongoing subclinical seizures after convulsive seizures have stopped, an EEG should be obtained.
- Consider empiric antibiotics and acyclovir if concern for CNS infection.

Nonconvulsive Status Epilepticus

- ABCs
- Check glucose and give 50% glucose solution 1 mg/kg (unless on ketogenic diet).
- Similar medications may be used as for convulsive status. The longer these seizures continue, the harder it may be to stop them, but these seizures do not pose the same immediate danger as convulsive status epilepticus. Therefore, anticonvulsants should be given judiciously.

UNPROVOKED SEIZURE, FIRST

A seizure for which no specific trigger is identified

EPIDEMIOLOGY

- In the United States, 25,000–40,000 children have a first unprovoked seizure each year
- 1% of children will have an unprovoked seizure by age 14 years
- If normal physical exam, normal EEG, and normal MRI, recurrence risk is 15–30%. If any of these are abnormal, recurrence risk is higher.

DIAGNOSTICS

Laboratory Studies

- CBC, electrolytes, BUN, creatinine, Ca^{2+}, Mg^{2+}, glucose.
- Metabolic screening evaluation if concern for developmental plateau or regression, or other concerning features on history
- Additional studies may be warranted based on clinical circumstances (e.g., vomiting, dehydration, mental status)
- Urine toxicology screen if prolonged post-ictal state or high suspicion
- Lumbar puncture: Required in infants <6 months, for failure to return to mental status baseline, or for meningeal signs
- If increased ICP suspected, obtain head CT before LP

Neuroimaging

- Indications for emergency head CT: Focal deficit on exam; patient does not return to baseline within several hours after the seizure
- Outpatient brain MRI for all children with first unprovoked seizure of unclear etiology.

EEG

- Urgent/inpatient: If patient does not return to baseline
- Outpatient (within 1–2 weeks): Indicated for all children with first unprovoked seizure

MANAGEMENT

- Consider admission if indications for emergency neuroimaging, or if prolonged postictal lethargy for observation.
- Outpatient neurologic consultation within 1–2 weeks

• No evidence that antiepileptic drugs change natural history of seizure disorders. Usually, these drugs are not indicated after a first unprovoked seizure unless there is a risk factor suggesting a high likelihood of recurrence (e.g., abnormal EEG, MRI with structural abnormality, genetic syndrome, etc.).

UNPROVOKED SEIZURE, SECOND

EPIDEMIOLOGY

• Affects 0.4–0.9% of children, 1% of overall population
• Occurs in about 40% of those who had a first unprovoked seizure.

DIAGNOSTICS

• Similar to first unprovoked seizure

MANAGEMENT

• Discuss with neurologic consultant.
• Consider admission if indications for emergency neuroimaging or if prolonged postictal lethargy for observation.
• Initiate anticonvulsant therapy. Common medications, indications, dosing, and adverse effects are outlined in **Table 20-5**. Basic considerations include:
  ✓ Consider if seizure was focal or generalized at onset. Focal seizures may rapidly generalize secondarily.
    ▪ Oxcarbazepine is a good first choice for focal epilepsy, but may worsen generalized epilepsy
    ▪ Levetiracetam is a good first choice for either focal or generalized epilepsy
  ✓ If seizures and clinical picture fit a specific syndrome, treatment should be specific to that syndrome.
  ✓ Age is important. Phenobarbital is typically the first-line therapy for infants <1 year old. Do not use valproic acid in a child <2 years old unless a metabolic disorder has been definitively ruled out.

Nutrition 21

Rosara Bass, MD, MS
Vi L. Goh, MD, MS
Maria R. Mascarenhas, MBBS

ASSESSMENT OF NUTRITIONAL STATUS

Information gathering, growth assessment, estimation of needs, determination of risk factors, identification of goals and provide recommendations and education

ASSESSMENT

- Common causes of impaired weight gain and linear growth are listed in **Table 21-1** and **21-2**.
- Nutrition-focused medical history
  - ✓ Usual intake including types and portion sizes of foods consumed
  - ✓ Fluid intake: Juice, milk, water over 24-hour period
  - ✓ For breast-fed children, assess minutes on each breast and frequency of feeding
  - ✓ Formula: Type, concentration, additives, changes, and response
  - ✓ Oral supplements or tube feedings (delivery method, tolerance, formula, length of time)
  - ✓ Herbal, vitamin, or mineral supplements
  - ✓ Food aversions, allergies, appetite, and religious/ethnic restrictions
  - ✓ Access to food: Food insecurity, use of Women, Infants and Children (WIC) program and food stamps
  - ✓ Note specific conditions that may affect absorption, metabolism, and digestion or increase the caloric needs of the patient (fever, increased respiratory rate and effort, cardiac disease, etc.)
  - ✓ Micronutrient deficiencies from inadequate intake or comorbidities: Vitamin D, iron, zinc
- Gastrointestinal history, including defecation patterns, nausea, vomiting, gastroesophageal reflux (GER) treatment, abdominal surgeries
- Medications and potential food/drug interactions:
  - ✓ Note side effects of drugs that may cause electrolyte wasting, change in stool patterns, or malabsorption.
  - ✓ Note whether the drug's efficacy is reduced by food intake or whether food interferes with absorption or mechanism of action.
- Family history: Food allergies/atopic disease, celiac disease, diabetes, obesity, hypercholesterolemia
- Birth history: Prematurity, intrauterine growth retardation, small for gestational age, necrotizing enterocolitis
- Laboratory values:
  - ✓ Consider evaluating electrolytes, albumin, prealbumin, CBC, and hepatic function and lipid panels if indicated (e.g., in the setting of emesis, diarrhea, poor growth, obesity, supplemental nutrition or when otherwise warranted based on clinical evaluation)
  - ✓ Deficiencies (if diet history indicates): 25-hydroxyvitamin D, zinc, iron profile, vitamin B_{12}, vitamins E and A, fatty-acid panel
- Growth parameters:
  - ✓ Unintentional weight loss: 5–10% loss is moderate, >10% is severe.

TABLE 21-1	Common Causes of Impaired Weight Gain in Childhood (with or without Secondary Impaired Linear Growth)	
Inadequate Intake	**Inadequate Absorption**	**Increased Energy Expenditure**
Food insecurity	Gastroesophageal reflux	Insulin resistance secondary to intra-uterine environment
Poor knowledge of child's nutritional needs	Anatomic obstruction (gastrointestinassl tract)	Congenital infection
Formula dilution	Vomiting	Genetic syndrome
Developmental delay	Cystic fibrosis	Chronic cardiac disease
Breastfeeding difficulty	Celiac disease	Chronic renal disease
Poor oromotor skills	Food protein sensitivity or intolerance	Chronic endocrine disease
Behavioral feeding problem	Chronic diarrhea	Chronic pulmonary disease
Neglect	Malabsorption	Fevers

TABLE 21-2	Common Causes of Impaired Linear Growth in Childhood with Preserved Weight	
Condition	**Distinguishing Features**	**Height Velocity**
Familial short stature	Within range predicted by midparental height	Low-normal
Constitutional delay of growth	Normal height for bone age, but delayed bone age/puberty	Slow in early childhood but prolonged growth in puberty
Small for gestational age infant with catch-up growth	Normal if catch up growth is achieved by 2 years of age	Normal
Hypothyroidism	Sluggishness, cold intolerance, constipation	Slow
Cushing syndrome	Obesity with central fat distribution, buffalo hump	Slow
GH deficiency	Progressive growth failure	Slow
Precocious puberty	Virilization	Initially fast, but early cessation
Genetic disorders	E.g., Turner, Noonan, Silver-Russel syndromes	Slow
Skeletal dysplasias	E.g., Achondroplasia, spondyloepiphyseal dysplasia, osteogenesis imperfecta	Slow

✓ Length/height, weight, head circumference (if <3 years) percentiles
  ▪ Up to 2 years of age—Use 2006 World Health Organization (WHO) growth chart for weight, supine length, and head circumference.
  ▪ 2–20 years of age—Use Centers for Disease Control and Prevention (CDC) 2000 growth charts for weight and standing height. Calculate Body mass index.
  ▪ Plot on all growth measurements including calculated BMI on CDC growth chart or specialty chart (prematurity, disease-specific, etc.) until 20 years of age.
  ▪ Correct for prematurity until 3 years of age.
✓ *Optional:* Obtain triceps skinfold and mid-arm circumference measurements to calculate muscle and fat stores. Measure lower-leg length, knee height, or arm span (when unable to obtain accurate height).

TABLE 21-3	Growth Velocity* (Median Weight Gain in Grams/Day)	
Age	**Boys**	**Girls**
0–4 weeks	34	29
1–6 months	14–40	13–34
6–12 months	8–11	8–11
1–2 years	6–7	7

*For children <2 years of age, review the World Health Organization website for more detailed weight-velocity charts.

✓ Typical growth velocity presented in **Table 21-3**.
✓ Use z-score to express individual anthropometrics in relation to population standard (i.e., 25th percentile weight-for-age = z-score of 1, indicating that weight-for-age is 1 standard deviation from the mean).

Stunting and Wasting

• Wasting is an indicator of acute malnutrition.
• Stunting is an indicator of chronic malnutrition.

Grading Malnutrition

• Acute (<3 months) and chronic (>3 months) malnutrition includes both undernutrition and obesity. Undernutrition can be classified based on a variety of measures, including anthropometrics: weight for length z-score, BMI for age z-score, length/height z-score, mid–upper arm circumference, weight gain velocity, weight loss, deceleration of weight for length or BMI for age as well as nutrient intake.
• Classification based on weight for length and BMI for age z-scores: mild malnutrition z-score, −1.0 to −1.9; moderate malnutrition z-score, −2.0 to −2.9; severe malnutrition z-score, <−3.0 (also including length/height z-score)
• Screen all admitted patients for malnutrition using age-based criteria on admission and assess risk. If more than one risk factor is present, consider involving inpatient nutrition team.

Body Mass Index

• Body mass index (BMI) = Weight (kg)/(Height (cm))^2 × 10,000
• Used for children >2 years of age for assessment of obesity
• BMI percentile 85–95% = overweight and BMI percentile >95% = obese

Estimating Nutrition Needs

There are a variety of methods to estimate energy (calorie) needs.
• The recommended daily allowance (RDA) guideline is recommended for infants and may be used to estimate calorie (**Table 21-4**) and protein (**Table 21-5**) needs for healthy children
• Dietary Reference Intakes: A set of reference values for recommended intake of vitamins, minerals, and nutrients in healthy populations of Americans and Canadians
  ✓ Estimated Average Requirements: Average daily intake of nutrient that will meet nutritional needs of half the individuals in the group
  ✓ Recommended Dietary Allowance (RDA): Amount of nutrition that meets needs of 97–98% of healthy individuals

TABLE 21-4	RDA Requirements for Daily Calories
Age	**Kcal/kg**
0–6 months	108
6–12 months	98
1–3 years	102
4–6 years	90
7–10 years	70
Males	
11–14 years	55
5–18 years	45
Females	
11–14 years	47
15–18 years	40

TABLE 21-5	Daily Recommended Intake for Protein		
Age	**AI (g/kg/day)**	**EAR (g/kg/day)**	**RDA (g/kg/day)**
0–6 months	1.52	—	2.2
7–12 months	—	1.1	1.2
1–3 years	—	0.88	1.05
4–10 years	—	0.76	0.95
11–13 years	—	0.76	0.85
14–18 years			
Males	—	0.73	0.85
Females	—	0.71	0.85

AI = adequate intake (protein intake sufficient if above this level); EAR = estimated average requirement (half of the healthy individuals in this group would meet their protein requirements at this level); RDA = recommended daily allowance (risk of inadequate intake is very small at this level).

✓ Adequate Intake: Expected to meet nutritional need of everyone in the group to give guidance but is not a defined calculation
- The WHO equation (**Table 21-6**) provides a more detailed calculation of energy requirements for children and adolescents to provide the resting energy expenditure (REE). The REE is then modified by activity levels and stress factors, which are important considerations in hospitalized children.
- Once the REE is calculated, an activity or stress factor must be incorporated to account for additional calorie needs under special circumstances. (REE × [Activity or Stress Factor] = estimated caloric needs)
  ✓ REE × 1.3: Well-nourished child on bed rest with mild-to-moderate stress
  ✓ REE × 1.5: Normally active child with mild-to-moderate stress; inactive child with severe stress (trauma, sepsis, cancer) or child with minimal activity and malnutrition requiring catch-up growth
  ✓ REE × 1.7: Active child requiring catch-up growth or active child with severe stress

TABLE 21-6	WHO Equation for Resting Energy Expenditure
Age	**kcal/Day**
Males	
0–3 years	$(60.9 \times Wt) - 54$
>3–10 years	$(22.7 \times Wt) + 495$
>10–18 years	$(17.5 \times Wt) + 651$
>18–30 years	$(15.3 \times Wt) + 679$
Females	
0–3 years	$(61.0 \times Wt) - 51$
>3–10 years	$(22.5 \times Wt) + 499$
>10–18 years	$(12.2 \times Wt) + 746$
>18–30 years	$(14.7 \times Wt) + 495$

Wt = weight in kilograms.

OBESE POPULATION

- Caloric needs vary significantly in the obese population, and equations do not always accurately predict needs. When possible, energy requirements of obese hospitalized children should be assessed using indirect calorimetry
- The Schofield height and weight equation is most accurate for calculating calorie needs.
- When calculating calorie needs for an obese patient, consider using an adjusted body weight (BW) instead of the actual body weight in the WHO equation.
- Adjusted body weight = Ideal body weight + 0.25 × (Actual body weight − Ideal body weight)

CATCH-UP GROWTH

- Calorie requirements for catch-up growth can be calculated using the RDA Guidelines shown in **Table 21-4** and the following equation:

$$\text{Daily Calorie Requirement for Catch-up Growth} = \frac{\text{RDA for Weight Age} \times \text{Ideal Weight for Height}}{\text{Actual Weight}}$$

- Protein requirements for catch-up growth can be calculated using the Dietary Reference Intakes for Protein are shown in **Table 21-5** and the following equation:

$$\frac{(\text{Protein for Weight Age} \times \text{Ideal Weight for Height})}{\text{Actual Weight}}$$

✓ Use weight in kilograms
✓ Weight-age = age at which present weight would be at the 50th percentile on the growth chart

REFEEDING SYNDROME

- Refeeding syndrome (RFS) is an anabolic reaction caused by the introduction of aggressive nutritional therapy in malnourished patients and associated with serum electrolyte

shifts, clinical symptoms, or both, resulting from metabolic changes and a fluid imbalance (e.g., peripheral edema, heart or respiratory failure).

- National Institute for Health and Care Excellence Criteria for patients at highest risk of refeeding syndrome (created for adult patients, no specific criteria for pediatrics):
  ✓ One or more of:
    - BMI <16
    - Unintentional weight loss of >15% in previous 3–6 months
    - Little to no nutritional intake for >10 days
    - Low potassium, phosphorus, or magnesium before refeeding
  ✓ OR Two or more of:
    - BMI <18.5
    - Unintentional weight loss of >10% in previous 3–6 months
    - Little to no nutritional intake for >5 days
    - History of alcohol misuse or use of drugs including insulin, chemotherapy, antacids or diuretics
- Prevention of refeeding syndrome
  ✓ Start feeding at 50 to 75% of measured or predicted REE or 80 to 100% of current caloric intake.
  ✓ Slow advancement of caloric intake (increase by 10–20% per day)
  ✓ Daily electrolyte monitoring with repletion as necessary; can start multivitamin and thiamine prior to initiation of feeding

ENTERAL NUTRITION

TUBE FEEDING

Tube feeding should be considered if the patient has a functional gastrointestinal (GI) tract but is unable/unwilling to consume sufficient calories/protein intake for weight maintenance/growth. Feedings may be intermittent or continuous. Many children benefit from a combination of a daytime bolus and overnight continuous feeding; thus, the regimen should be based on the individual child's needs. Because there is a risk of bacterial contamination, the hang time of formula should not exceed 4 hours for hospitalized patients, especially neonates.

CONTINUOUS FEEDS

- Advantages of continuous feeds:
  ✓ Enhanced tolerance and absorption (especially in patients with a short bowel)
  ✓ Used for nocturnal supplemental feedings (with daytime oral intake)
  ✓ Less likely to cause abdominal distention
  ✓ Physiologic for small-bowel or jejunostomy feeds
- Disadvantages of continuous feeds:
  ✓ Requires a pump and therefore decreases mobility
  ✓ Risk of bacterial contamination if feeds are left at room temperature for a long period
  ✓ May suppress appetite; thus consider limiting to overnight feeds if possible
- Suggested initial regimen and advancement for continuous feeding:
  ✓ For ages 1 month–7 years: Initial regimen, 0.5–2 mL/kg/hr; advance by 0.5–1 mL/kg/hr every 4–24 hours as tolerated
  ✓ For age >7 years: Initial regimen, 10–20 mL/hr; advance by 10–20 mL/hr every 4–8 hours as tolerated
  ✓ Individual tolerance must be closely monitored

INTERMITTENT (BOLUS) FEEDS

- Advantages of bolus feeds:
  - ✓ Easier to administer: Faster and do not always require a pump
  - ✓ Physiologic for gastric feeds: Pattern is similar to mealtimes
  - ✓ Enhances mobility: Not always connected to a pump
- Disadvantages of bolus feeds:
  - ✓ May worsen gastroesophageal reflux
  - ✓ Aspiration risk due to volume of feed in stomach
  - ✓ May impinge on respiratory effort with large bolus feeds
  - ✓ Unable to use it in small-bowel or jejunostomy feeds
  - ✓ Suggested initial regimen and for advancement shown in **Table 21-7**; individual tolerance must be closely monitored

MONITORING WHILE ON ENTERAL FEEDS

- Elevated BUN/creatinine: Check for increased protein content of formula, decreased renal function, or inadequate fluid intake.
- GI tolerance:
  - ✓ Constipation: Evaluate for inadequate fluid and fiber intake, inactivity, and consider evaluating for a fecal impaction.
  - ✓ Diarrhea: Etiologies to consider: hyperosmolar medication or formula, rapid infusion, intolerance to particular component of formula (i.e., carbohydrate and fat content) or modular supplements, tube migration (i.e., from stomach to duodenum with bolus feeds), inadequate fiber intake, low albumin, impaction leading to overflow diarrhea, possible bacterial contamination of formula
  - ✓ Vomiting: Etiologies to consider: delayed gastric emptying; GER; displacement of tube (i.e., in the distal esophagus); gastritis; intolerance of a particular component of formula (i.e., fat content or allergy); rapid infusion rate; also consider a behavioral component.
- Hydration status: Monitor urine specific gravity, input, and output and check whether regimen meets the child's free water requirements.
- Glucose homeostasis: If high blood glucose or glucosuria, consider possible infection or medication side effect (i.e., steroids), check carbohydrate intake
- Anthropometrics: Weight, height, and head circumference (as appropriate for age); adjust calorie/protein intake accordingly.
  - ✓ Consider following weights closely or daily while inpatient to guide adjustments.

TABLE 21-7	Guidelines for Intermittent (Bolus) Enteral Feeding Regimens	
Age	**Initial**	**Advance By**
1 month–7 years	2–5 mL/kg/feed every 3–4 hours Usually full strength	Advance volume by 5–10 mL/feed every 3–12 hours as tolerated OR if hypertonic formula is used, increase caloric density every 8–24 hours as tolerated. Do not advance volume and caloric density at the same time.*
>7 years	90–120 mL/feed every 3–4 hours Usually full strength	Advance volume by 30–60 mL every 4–8 hours as tolerated OR if hypertonic formula is used increase caloric density every 8–24 hours as tolerated. Do not advance volume and caloric density at the same time.*

*Feeding advance should be tailored according to the patient's clinical circumstances and feeding tolerance.

Mechanical problems of gastrostomy and jejunostomy tubes (Table 21-8)
Formulas
A variety of infant and pediatric formulas are available based on the individual child's needs. For infants, maternal breast milk is always the first choice. See **Tables 21-9** and **21-10** for formula choices.

TABLE 21-8	Mechanical Problems of Gastrostomy and Jejunostomy Tubes	
Mechanical Problems	**Prevention**	**Interventions**
Clogged tube	Scheduled water flushes, especially following feeds and instillation of medications	• Attempt to flush with warm water using progressively smaller syringes (e.g., 5, 3, 1 mL). • If the tube does not clear with warm water, consider using an enzymatic solution according to your institutional protocol (e.g., Clog Zapper™) to unclog the tube. • If attempts to clear the clog fail, consider replacement of tube.
Leakage of gastric contents around the gastrostomy site	Prevent leakage by minimizing tube movement (e.g., using a foam [Mepilex®] dressing) and using protective skin care (such as gauze, petroleum jelly, Stomahesive® protective powder).	• Check the amount of water in balloon (refer to manufacturer's instructions) • Ensure the tube size is appropriate. Do not increase the tube size to avoid progressive enlargement of the stoma site. • Consider calling the service that placed device to decide if further action needed.
The tube has fallen out	Secure tube by: • Placing a tape tab around the tube and pin to patient's clothing, or • Tucking tube, extension set into patient's clothing, or • Using ElastiNet, Griplok, or gastrostomy tube protective belt	• Initial tube (review your hospital policy, consider <12 weeks old for tubes placed in by interventional radiologist and 4 weeks old for surgically placed tubes), the patient's parent or guardian should contact the team that placed the tube as soon as possible. • The patient should go to the ED for evaluation and to preserve the stoma site. In the ED, a 10 Fr Foley can be carefully placed (without inflating the balloon) to maintain patency but should not be used for feeding. • Once the appropriate team replaces the tube, consider obtaining a dye study to confirm placement to avoid complications such as peritonitis and death. • If the tube has been changed before and is >12 weeks old (or 4 weeks if surgically placed), the family should replace the tube or place a foley in the stoma to keep it patent until an appropriate tube is available.

(Continued)

TABLE 21-8	Mechanical Problems of Gastrostomy and Jejunostomy Tubes *(Continued)*

| Granulomas at gastrostomy-tube site | Make sure that tube size is appropriate. Ill-fitting tubes are a risk factor for granuloma formation. | • Consider a trial of silver nitrate or triamcinolone cream 1–2 times per day for up to 1–2 weeks. If not improved, contact the service that placed the tube.
• Gastric mucosa prolapse through the stoma is not a granuloma and is a problematic complication that may require temporary removal of tube or surgical revision of site. Surgical consultation is recommended. |

TABLE 21-9	Formula Choices

Infant Feeding

	Human Milk	Formula	Additional Information
Term infants	Human milk (recommended) Donor human milk (DHM)	Standard intact infant formula	19–20 kcal/oz
Premature infants (not yet corrected to term)	Human milk or DHM with fortifier	Preterm formula	24–30 kcal/oz increased protein, Ca, P, Na, and trace elements; formula has 50% Medium chain triglyceride (MCT) oil as primary fat source
Premature infants (corrected to term)	Human milk with fortifier	Transitional formula	22 kcal/oz, fewer trace elements as compared to preterm formula but greater than term formula
Galactosemia	Contraindicated	Soy formula	Formula contains soy protein isolate.
Cow's milk sensitivity	Maternal avoidance of cow's milk and/or soy	Extensively hydrolyzed formula, soy formula if tolerated	Partial protein hydrolysate, amino acid (AA) if not tolerated, 10–30% of patients with cow's-milk sensitivity will also react to soy
IgE-mediated milk protein allergy	Anaphylaxis unlikely with breast milk	Soy formula (if skin test negative), AA-based formula	Anaphylaxis unlikely with breast milk
Gastroesophageal reflux	Consider maternal avoidance of cow's milk.	Term formula thickened with rice cereal or commercially available formula for babies with reflux; consider 2–4 weeks trial of extensively hydrolyzed formula	Avoid cow's milk or hydrolyzed formula trial to exclude symptoms due to cow's-milk sensitivity.

TABLE 21-10	Enteral Formula Selection		
	Infant–1 Year	**1–10 Years**	**>10 Years**
Healthy	Standard intact age appropriate formula	Standard intact age appropriate formula	Standard intact age appropriate formula
Fluid restricted	Concentrate to 22, 24, or 27 kcal/oz	Choose formula with 1.5 or 2.0 kcal/mL	Choose formula with 1.5 or 2.0 kcal/mL
Food allergy	Milk protein allergy: trial of extensively hydrolyzed formula and switch to AA-based if not improved. If IgE mediated, start with AA-based	If IgE-mediated, use a AA-based	If IgE-mediated, use AA-based
Constipation	Not applicable	Fiber-enriched	Fiber-enriched
Malabsorption*	Protein hydrolysate or AA-based or consider MCT-containing formula	Protein hydrolysate or AA-based or consider MCT-containing formula	Protein hydrolysate or AA-based or consider MCT-containing formula
Renal failure	Low protein, concentrate volume, adjust electrolytes	Low protein, concentrate volume, adjust electrolytes	Low protein, concentrate volume, adjust electrolytes
Pancreatitis	Standard formula	Standard formula	Standard formula
Chylothorax	Low-fat, high-MCT formula	Low-fat, high-MCT formula	Low-fat, high-MCT formula

*Use a formula high in MCT in children with cholestasis.

Blenderized Formulas

- Foods can be modified in commercial and noncommercial settings to be provided via a gastrostomy tube.
- Ingredients for recipes might include baby foods; table foods such as meats, fruits, vegetables, milk, and carbohydrates; commercial formula; and vitamin/mineral supplements.
- Examples of when these formulas may be contraindicated can include when a child is ill or has a compromised immune system, before the tube tract has healed from initial placement, if the feeding needs to delivered via a pump, postpyloric feeds, nasogastric route, hang time >2 hours, and small tubes (needs to be at least a size 12 French).
- The need for safe preparation and monitoring of foods for infusion via tube includes the need for monitoring by a registered dietitian/nutritionist with use of both commercial and noncommercial blended mixtures. Reported risks include (but are not limited to) hypernatremia and hyponatremia, tube clogging, dehydration, and nutrient deficiencies.

  Modular Supplements: Can be used to add macronutrients and calories (see **Table 21-11**).

Vitamin D Deficiency

- Etiologies: Exclusive breastfeeding without supplementation, limited sun exposure, limited dietary intake, malabsorptive diseases, renal disease, medications
- Assessment: Deficiency defined as 25-hydroxyvitamin D <12 ng/mL and insufficiency as 12–20 ng/mL; target serum level should be >30 ng/mL; screening recommended for at-risk individuals only (chronic disease, medications known to interfere with vitamin D synthesis)

TABLE 21-11 Modular Supplements			
Modular Type	**Name**	**Components**	**Amount per Serving**
Calorie boosters	Duocal, Super Soluble	Carbohydrate and fat	25 calories per scoop (5 g)
			42 calories per tablespoon (8.5 g)
	BeneCalorie	Fat (91%) and protein (9%) NOT recommended for tube feeding.	330 calories/1.5 oz serving cup
Carbohydrate-based additive	Solcarb	Soluble form of powdered carbohydrate (maltodextrin). Can be added to formula, liquids, and moist foods.	23 calories per tablespoon (6 g)
Fat-based additive	Microlipid	Fat emulsion of both long-chain and medium-chain fatty acids. Used to add calories with minimal increase in total volume and osmolality	4.5 calories/mL
	MCT oil	Medium-chain triglycerides, used in patients with decreased bile flow, defective lymphatic transport.	7.7 calories/mL
	Liquigen	Medium chain triglycerides emulsion (50% MCT, 50% water), indications as above for MCT	4.5 calories/mL
Protein-based additive	ProMod Liquid Protein	Liquid protein and carbohydrate	10 g of protein and 100 calories per 30 mL
	BeneProtein	Whey protein powder, for ages 3 years and up.	6 g protein and 25 calories per scoop or packet (7 g)
	Complete Amino Acid Mix	Essential and nonessential amino acid source, used to add additional protein to formulas.	7.8 g or protein and 31 calories per tablespoon (9.5 g)
	Essential Amino Acid Mix	Essential amino acids, used to add additional protein to formulas.	7.2 g of protein and 28.4 calories per tablespoon (9 g)
	Liquid Protein Fortifier (Infant)	Extensively hydrolyzed protein source for infants, can be added to human milk or formula.	1 g of protein and 4 calories per 6 mL

(continued)

TABLE 21-11	(continued)		
	Human MilkFortifier with Hydrolyzed Protein Concentrated Liquid (Infant)	Extensively hydrolyzed protein source for infants, added to human milk	0.35 g of protein and 7 calories per 5 mL
Fiber additive	BeneFiber Nonflavored Powder	Soluble fiber source: wheat dextrin	1.5 g of fiber and 7.5 calories per teaspoon
	BeneFiber Non-flavored Stick Packs	Soluble fiber source: wheat dextrin, in prepackaged packets.	3 g of fiber and 15 calories per packet or 2 teaspoons (3.5 g)
	NutriSource Fiber (previously, Resource BeneFiber)	Soluble fiber source: partially hydrolyzed guar gum. For ages 3 and up.	3 g of fiber and 15 calories per tablespoon or packet (4 g)

Adapted with permission from the Clinical Nutrition Department, Children's Hospital of Philadelphia, 2015.

- Consequences of deficiency: rickets (defective growth plate mineralization), osteomalacia, (abnormal matrix mineralization of established bone)

PARENTERAL NUTRITION

- Indication: To maintain nutritional status and achieve growth in patients who cannot receive adequate nutrition enterally. Remember that enteral nutrition is the route of choice.
- Peripheral parenteral nutrition (PPN): Used in peripheral veins and therefore is limited to maximum dextrose concentration of 10% (in some circumstances, 12.5%) and osmolality less than 900–1000 mOsm/L. It is intended for nutritional support of <7–10 days' duration.
- Central parenteral nutrition: Used in central veins, which allows for higher dextrose concentrations and osmolality greater than 1000 mOsm/L. It is used when the anticipated duration is >7–10 days.
Parenteral energy intake:
- 10–20% lower than estimated enteral needs due to reduced energy cost for digestion/absorption (see estimating nutritional needs earlier in the chapter)

PARENTERAL NUTRITION (PN) COMPONENTS

- Carbohydrates: Given as dextrose (glucose)
  ✓ Calorie density: 3.4 kcal/g
  ✓ Goal of 40–55% of caloric intake
  ✓ Calculation of glucose-infusion rate (GIR):

$$\text{GIR (mg/kg/min)}: \frac{\% \, \text{Dextrose (g/dL)} \times (\text{Infusion Rate mL/h}) \times 0.167}{\text{Weight (kg)}}$$

TABLE 21-12 Protein and Lipid Requirements for Parenteral Nutrition

Age/Weight	Protein (g/kg/day) Initial	Protein (g/kg/day) Goal	Lipid (g/kg/day) Initial	Lipid (g/kg/day) Goal
Preterm	2	2.5–4.0	2.0	3.5
Term infant	2	2.2–3.5	2.0	3.5
Child 5–20 kg	1.0–2.5	1.0–2.5	1.0	2.0
Child 20–40 kg	1.0–2.0	1.0–2.0	1.0	2.0
Adolescent >40 kg	0.8–2.0*	0.8–2.0*	0.5	1.0

*A maximum of 150 g of protein/day is recommended.

✓ Begin at 10–12.5% and advance daily by 2.5–5.0% to a goal of about 20–25% (GIR: 8–14 mg/kg/min in infants, and 2–5 mg/kg/min in older children and adolescents)
- Protein: Given as amino acids
  ✓ Calorie density: 4 kcal/g
  ✓ Goal of 10–16% of total calories
  ✓ Protein goals as shown in **Table 21-12**. Neonates can start at 2 g/kg/day and advance daily by 1.0 g/kg/day to goal, whereas nonneonates can be started at or near goal.
  ✓ *Exceptions:* Less protein is indicated in the setting of renal or hepatic failure. More protein may be indicated in the setting of trauma, sepsis, or increased protein needs (i.e., ongoing losses, healing from injury or surgery).
- Fat: Given as intravenous lipid
  ✓ Calorie density: 2 kcal/mL of 20% solution (20 g/100 mL)
  ✓ Goal lipid content should account for 25–40% of calories. A minimum of 3–5% total calories is needed to prevent essential fatty acid deficiency. Lipid content should generally not exceed 3.0 g/kg/day or 45–50% of total daily calories.
  ✓ Initial rate of lipid administration: Refer to **Table 21-12**
  ✓ Neonates can advance daily by 1.0 g/kg/day to goal, whereas nonneonates can be started at or near goal. Do not advance beyond 1–1.5 g/kg/day in patients with cholestasis based on prematurity, weight and essential fatty acid status.
  ✓ Volume of lipid solution needed is calculated as follows:

    Weight (kg) × Goal Grams IV Fat/kg/day × 100 mL/20 g IV Fat = mL of 20% IV Fat

  ✓ Triglyceride level should be monitored, with a goal <200 mg/dL in neonates and <400 mg/dL in children and adolescents. Consider reducing lipid dose if the triglyceride level is elevated. Carnitine may be added to improve lipid tolerance (however, data are limited).
  ✓ SMOF lipid (30% soy, 30% MCT, 25% olive oil, 15% fish oil) can be considered as an alternative to low dose intralipid in children with parenteral nutrition-associated liver disease
  ✓ Omegaven (100% fish oil) can be used in patients with soy allergy and if cholestasis is due for PN-related liver disease.
- Minerals and electrolytes: Refer to **Tables 21-13** and **21-14**.

TABLE 21-13	Parenteral Nutrition Mineral Requirements for Children Based on Weight (kg)*			
Element	**<5 kg**	**5–40 kg**	**>40 kg**	**Maximum**
Chromium	0.2 mcg/kg	0.2 mcg/kg	8 mcg	15 mcg
Copper	20 mcg/kg	20 mcg/kg	800 mcg	1500 mcg
Manganese	1 mcg/kg	1 mcg/kg	40 mcg	150 mcg
Selenium	2 mcg/kg	2 mcg/kg	80 mcg	120 mcg
Zinc	400 mcg/kg	125 mcg	5000 mcg	16,000 mcg

*Chromium and manganese are not added separately, as they are contaminants in PPN.

TABLE 21-14	Parenteral Nutrition Electrolyte Requirements			
Electrolyte (mEq/kg/day)	**Infants (0–5 kg)**	**Children (5–20 kg)**	**Children (20–40 kg)**	**Adolescents (>40 kg)***
Acetate[†]	PRN	PRN	PRN	PRN
Ca^{2+}	1.0–4.0	0.5–1.0	10–25	10–20
Cl^-	2.0–5.0	2.0–5.0	2.0–3.0	80–150
Mg	0.3–0.5	0.3–0.5	0.3–0.5	10–30
Phos	2.0–4.0	1.0–2.0	1.0–1.5	30–60
K^+	2.0–4.0	2.0–3.0	1.5–2.5	40–60
Na^+	2.0–5.0	2.0–6.0	2.0–3.0	60–150

*mEq/day for in this age group.
†PRN=- as needed for acidosis. Bicarbonate is not added.
Other considerations:
1. If the patient's serum calcium is low, correct the value based on serum albumin (Corrected Calcium = (0.8 × (Normal Albumin − Patient's Albumin)) + Serum Ca) and obtain an ionized calcium prior to adjusting calcium in total PN (TN).
2. If a patient requires an increase in potassium dose due to hypokalemia, closely monitor for arrhythmia during infusion (in an ICU setting if appropriate).
3. When adjusting sodium content, note the patient's total body sodium status. For example, a patient may have hypervolemic hyponatremia and additional sodium may exacerbate edema. Also, correct sodium for hyperglycemia (e.g., in the setting of diabetic ketoacidosis).
4. In patients with renal failure, magnesium, potassium, and phosphorus should be monitored closely to avoid toxicity due to decreased excretion.
5. Check solubility of your electrolytes (e.g., calcium and phosphorus) with your TPN pharmacy to avoid precipitation.
6. There are currently shortages of several intravenous electrolytes. Consider monitoring electrolytes more frequently if your electrolyte supply is limited and a patient is TPN-dependent. Also consider enteral supplementation if possible.
7. When choosing phosphorus salts for supplementation in premature infants, choose those with minimal aluminum content to avoid toxicity.

- Vitamins:
  ✓ A pediatric multivitamin should be added for children <11 years of age and <40 kg (dose is 5 mL/day for children and 2 mL/kg/day to a maximum of 5 mL/day for neonates). For children >40 kg or >11 years of age, use adult multivitamin (10 mL/day).
  ✓ Vitamin K can also be added separately.

MONITORING LABORATORY STUDIES

- Initial laboratory studies (within 48 hours after PN initiation): CBC, electrolytes, calcium, phosphorus, magnesium, triglycerides, alanine transaminase (ALT), gamma-glutamyl transferase (GGT), total and conjugated bilirubin, albumin, prealbumin. Severe abnormalities in electrolytes should be corrected before initiating PN.
- Daily or every-other-day laboratory studies: Electrolytes, phosphorus, magnesium, and calcium until stable and at full kcal and protein goal. Check a triglyceride level with every increase in IV fat.
- Weekly laboratory studies (once stable): Electrolytes, calcium, phosphorus, magnesium, triglycerides, ALT, GGT, albumin, prealbumin, total and conjugated bilirubin
- Long-term PN and minimal enteral nutrition: Check vitamin, trace elements, cholesterol, iron panel, CBC, reticulocyte count, carnitine (in patients with no enteral intake) and triene to tetraene ratio (in patients receiving a low-fat regimen) and aluminum levels as indicated clinically.

SPECIAL CIRCUMSTANCES: PARENTERAL NUTRITION CYCLE REGIMEN

- Cycling is used in long-term PN to promote normal daily activity and oral intake and to possibly lower the risk of PN-associated steatosis
- The infusion rate of PN solutions with greater than 10% dextrose should be decreased by 50% during the last hour of the infusion to prevent rebound hypoglycemia

Complications of TPN and Central Venous Catheters

- Metabolic and electrolyte imbalances: Follow laboratory monitoring as above.
- Catheter occlusion: May be related to clot, fibrin deposition, or precipitate. Review your hospital policy regarding management.
- Air embolus: Presents with sudden onset of respiratory distress. Clamp the catheter and place the patient left side down in the Trendelenburg position and seek emergency care.
- Catheter breakage, crack, or aneurysm: Stop infusion, clamp catheter, and contact the team that placed the catheter
- Central line-associated bloodstream infection (CLABSI): Obtain cultures in all febrile patients and treat with broad spectrum antibiotics. In patients with recurrent CLABSIs, consider central-line lock therapies (i.e., ethanol locks) according to your hospital policy.
- Malpositioning of a central catheter with extravasation of fluid: Stop infusion, clamp the catheter, and evaluate catheter position.
- Parenteral nutrition-associated liver disease:
  - ✓ Prevent overfeeding
  - ✓ Cycle PN: Decrease the duration of PN (e.g., decrease from 24 hours per day to a goal of 10–12 hours per day) to rest the liver from constant exposure to glucose and other nutrients.
    - Blood sugar should be monitored while cycling TPN.
  - ✓ Decrease IV fat (to a goal of 1–1.5 g/kg/day based on age, gestational age, and fatty acid status)
    - Monitor for essential fatty acid deficiency in this circumstance,

✓ Copper and manganese are both excreted in bile and can accumulate in liver disease. Consider decreasing the copper dosage (generally by 50%) and consider removing manganese if it is in the PN.

✓ Start enteral trophic feeds as soon as possible.

CHAPTER 22

Oncology

Regina Myers, MD
Anne Reilly, MD
Dava Szalda, MD, MSHP

CHEMOTHERAPY

GENERAL PRINCIPLES

- Cancer cells divide rapidly and are, therefore, more susceptible to cytotoxic agents.
- Combination therapy is useful for preventing the development of resistance and overcoming existing resistance by using agents with different mechanisms of action.
  - ✓ Also permits more intensive overall therapy by using agents with nonoverlapping toxicities
- Dose intensification: Effective because most malignancies have a steep dose–response curve
  - ✓ The main approaches are to either increase dose (per cycle or by increasing the total number of chemotherapy cycles) or to decrease the interval between treatment cycles.
- Adjuvant therapy: Administration of systemic chemotherapy in the absence of overt disease
  - ✓ Targeted at micrometastases (see "Solid Tumor" section)
- Toxicities: Myelosuppression, alopecia, and nausea/vomiting are the most common acute toxicities (see "Principles of Supportive Care" sections for management of specific toxicities).
  - ✓ There are also many long-term toxicities (see "Late Effects of Cancer Treatment" section).
  - ✓ See **Table 22-1** for specific toxicities relevant to commonly used agents in pediatric oncology.

RADIATION THERAPY

GENERAL PRINCIPLES

- Delivery of ionizing radiation typically by external beam
- Biologic effect achieved by inducing direct and indirect DNA damage
- Different tumor types have different required doses for efficacy.
  - ✓ Wide range (e.g., 21 Gy for neuroblastoma/lymphoma, up to 60+ Gy for sarcomas)
- Normal tissues have different dose tolerance thresholds before toxicity is seen.
- Effect (and toxicity) can be potentiated by concomitant chemotherapy (e.g., doxorubicin, dactinomycin).
- Radiation recall: Inflammation in previous radiation field after administration of certain chemotherapy (days to years after original treatment)
- Photons versus protons
  - ✓ Photons deliver radiation to all structures in path (i.e., entry and exit doses)
    - ■ Intensity-modulated radiation therapy (IMRT) is used to carve out treatment volume to minimize exposure of normal tissues.
  - ✓ Protons are heavier and deposit radiation more precisely at target.
    - ■ Decreased scatter to normal tissues as protons enter/exit target areas, which may also allow higher doses to be delivered to target

TABLE 22-1	Commonly Used Chemotherapy Agents and Important Agent-Specific Toxicities			
Agent(s)	**Class**	**Mechanism of Action**	**Specific Toxicities**	**Prevention/ Treatment**
Cyclophosphamide Ifosfamide	Alkylators	DNA cross-linking	Hemorrhagic cystitis Fanconi syndrome (ifosfamide) Neurotoxicity (ifosfamide) Infertility	Hydration Mesna Methylene blue (for ifosfamide neurotoxicity)
Cisplatin Carboplatin	Platinums	Plastination/ cross-linking	Ototoxicity Nephrotoxicity (↓CrCl and electrolyte wasting) Infertility	Hydration and electrolyte replacement Audiogram before each cycle to assess if dose reduction required
Doxorubicin, daunorubicin, mitoxantrone, idarubicin	Anthracyclines	DNA intercalation	Cardiac (cardiomyopathy and arrhythmia) Mucositis	Dexrazoxane (cardioprotectant)
Vincristine, vinblastine	Vinca alkaloids	Inhibition of microtubule spindle formation	Constipation Peripheral neuropathy SIADH	Bowel regimen Decreased dose if necessary
Methotrexate	Antimetabolites	DNA precursor analogues	Nephrotoxicity, hepatotoxicity Neurotoxicity (highest risk with intrathecal)	Hydration, urine alkalization, and leucovorin for high dose If nephrotoxicity develops, consider glucarpidase
6-Mercaptopurine Thioguanine	Antimetabolites	DNA precursor analogues	Hepatotoxicity Veno-occlusive disease (thioguanine)	Thiopurine methyltransferase genotyping for slow metabolizers to dose correctly
Etoposide	Epipodophyllotoxin	Topoisomerase inhibitor	Hypotension Anaphylaxis	Slow the infusion rate if hypotension
Asparaginase	Enzyme	Asparagine depletion	Pancreatitis Thrombosis Anaphylaxis	Can switch to another type/hypoallergenic form Consider premedication due to frequent anaphylaxis
Imatinib Sorafenib	Tyrosine kinase inhibitors	Inhibit certain tyrosine kinases	Hypertension Rash Esophagitis/gastritis	Switching to another agent in same class Take medication with lots of fluids

SIADH = syndrome of inappropriate antidiuretic hormone.

INDICATIONS

- Local control: Can be used as sole or complementary way to control disease around primary site of tumor (e.g., in Ewing sarcoma, when margins are positive after resection)
- Metastatic disease: Targeting metastatic sites and bone lesions or total lung radiation for persistent lung metastases (e.g., Ewing sarcoma and Wilms tumor)
- Cranial/craniospinal
  ✓ Brain tumors with metastatic disease or potential
  ✓ Acute lymphoblastic leukemia (ALL) with central nervous system (CNS) involvement
- Total-body irradiation: Conditioning option for Hematopoietic stem cell transplant (HSCT) (particularly in ALL)
- Symptom management: In relapsed disease, can control cancer-related pain, particularly at bony sites
- Emergencies: Occasionally used to manage impending organ-function threats of tumors (e.g., spinal-cord compression, ocular tumors, mediastinal masses)

TOXICITY

- Proportional to dose intensity and radiation field (area exposed). Acute toxicities include
  ✓ Dermatitis
  ✓ Mucositis
  ✓ Cytopenias from marrow damage
  ✓ Fatigue
- There are also many potential late effects of radiation therapy (see "Late Effects of Cancer Treatment" section)

SURGERY

- Typically employed for biopsy of suspected mass to obtain histologic diagnosis and aid with staging a patient via exploration of peritoneal washings and lymph nodes sampling in certain settings (e.g., pelvic masses)
- Depending on the type of tumor, surgery occurs at different points in therapy (typically up front in brain tumors or germ-cell tumors) or after several weeks of therapy as local control in other tumors (some sarcomas and neuroblastoma)
- The goal of surgery may be complete resection, removal of discrete metastatic lesions (e.g., lung metastases in osteosarcoma) or in a palliative setting, debulking the tumor to decrease pressure or symptoms from compression of local structures

BONE MARROW TRANSPLANTATION

TYPES AND INDICATIONS

- Allogeneic: Replace recipient's marrow with hematopoietic stem cells from another individual (allograft)
  ✓ Indications
    - Malignancies: ALL (for patients at very high risk or with relapse), acute myeloid leukemia (AML) (for patients at high risk or with relapse), juvenile myelomonocytic leukemia (JMML), myelodysplastic syndrome (MDS)
    - Bone marrow failure: Aplastic anemia, Fanconi anemia, severe congenital neutropenia, etc.
    - Hemoglobinopathies: β-thalassemia major, sickle cell disease
    - Primary immunodeficiencies: severe combined immunodeficiency syndrome (SCID), hemophagocytic lymphohistiocytosis (HLH), Wiskott-Aldrich syndrome (WAS), chronic granulomatous disease (CGD), etc.
    - Metabolic disorders: Mucopolysaccharidoses, leukodystrophies, osteopetrosis

- Autologous: Infuse patient's previously stored stem cells after delivery of high-dose chemotherapy. Can think of as a rescue after high-dose chemotherapy
  - ✓ Indications: Treatment of certain tumors that are chemosensitive but at high risk for relapse
    - High-risk neuroblastoma and medulloblastoma
    - Relapsed or refractory lymphomas

PRINCIPLES OF ALLOGENEIC TRANSPLANTATION

- Approach depends on goal of transplantation
  - ✓ Hematologic malignancy
    - Treat cancer with high-dose chemotherapy with or without radiation
    - Immunosuppress recipient to accept allogeneic graft
    - Make space in marrow
  - ✓ Defective hematopoietic cell(s)
    - Immunosuppress recipient to accept allogeneic graft
    - Make space in marrow
- Conditioning regimen: Given prior to stem-cell infusion in order to prepare the patient to receive the allograft
  - ✓ Myeloablative: High-dose chemotherapy with or without radiation to completely ablate marrow
  - ✓ Reduced-intensity: Less toxic regimen that is sometimes used for nonmalignant indications or heavily pretreated patients; still highly immunosuppressive
- Donors: Chosen on the basis of the best available human leukocyte antigen (HLA) match, and other factors (sex, CMV status, etc.)
  - ✓ Matched siblings preferred
  - ✓ Alternative donors: Unrelated voluntary donors, umbilical-cord blood, parent (mismatched related, haploidentical)
- Stem-cell sources: Bone marrow, mobilized peripheral-blood stem cells, umbilical-cord blood
  - ✓ Chosen based on availability and type/purpose of transplant
  - ✓ Sources differ by engraftment kinetics, immune reconstitution, risk of graft-versus-host disease (GVHD), etc.
- GVHD: Process by which donor T-cells recognize recipient antigens as foreign and induce tissue damage
  - ✓ Increased risk with increased HLA mismatch
  - ✓ Allograft recipients receive prophylaxis with calcineurin inhibitor with or without steroids or methotrexate or mycophenolate
  - ✓ Acute GVHD: Develops within the first 100 days after transplantation. Skin (erythema and subsequent desquamation), liver (cholestasis), and/or GI tract (diarrhea)
  - ✓ Chronic GVHD: Develops more than 100 days after transplantation; resembles autoimmune diseases like scleroderma
  - ✓ Treatment with immunosuppression (corticosteroids are first line)
- Immune function and opportunistic infections
  - ✓ Patients at very high risk for infection, even after engraftment
  - ✓ Viruses: CMV, adenovirus, HSV, VZV, EBV, HHV-6
  - ✓ Fungus: *Candida, Aspergillus,* mucormycosis
  - ✓ Bacteria: enteric Gram-negative rods, *Streptococcus mitis, Staphylococcus* spp.; bacteremia most common early after transplantation
  - ✓ *Pneumocystis jirovecii* pneumonia: Universal prophylaxis is recommended
- BMT-specific organ toxicities

✓ Veno-occlusive disease: Disorder of vascular damage/thrombosis in small vessels of liver that occurs in first several weeks after transplantation
- Painful hepatomegaly, ascites, weight gain, direct hyperbilirubinemia, portal-vein flow reversal, splenomegaly, refractory thrombocytopenia, kidney injury
- Treated with defibrotide, a fibrinolytic agent. Current studies are evaluating the role of defibrotide as prophylaxis for patients at risk for veno-occlusive disease

✓ TA-TMA: Disorder caused by endothelial injury to the microvasculature, most notably in the kidneys
- Microangiopathic hemolytic anemia, thrombocytopenia, elevated creatinine, neurologic dysfunction, elevated LDH
- Management requires discontinuing calcineurin inhibitors. Eculizumab or plasma exchange may also be used.

✓ Idiopathic pulmonary syndrome: Noninfectious noncardiac respiratory insufficiency occurring in first weeks after transplantation

IMMUNOTHERAPY

GENERAL PRINCIPLES

- Cancer immunotherapies have advanced rapidly in recent years and remain a very active area of cancer research. Currently, a few immunotherapies are used in up-front treatment, but most are used for relapsed or refractory disease. They can be used alone or in combination with conventional chemotherapy, radiation therapy, and/or surgery.
- Immunotherapy treatments work by inducing, enhancing, or suppressing the immune system in order to allow killing of tumor cells.

TYPES AND TOXICITIES OF IMMUNOTHERAPIES

- Monoclonal antibodies: Proteins that are created in the lab that bind to specific antigens on tumor-cell surfaces in order to target the tumor cells for destruction. Examples include the following.
  ✓ Dinutuximab: Used in treatment for newly diagnosed neuroblastoma. Binds to GD2 on neuroblastoma cells, and the complex is destroyed by the immune system.
    - Toxicities: GD2 is also expressed on normal peripheral nerve cells, so the treatment leads to severe pain that is managed with opioid patient controlled analgesia (PCAs) and gabapentin. Infusion reactions can also lead to capillary leak.
  ✓ Blinatumomab: Used for relapsed/refractory B-ALL. Binds to both CD19 on B-ALL cells and CD3 on T cells, to link the cells and activate the T cells to destroy the leukemia cells.
    - Toxicities: Because of immune-system activation, patients can have transient flu-like symptoms or a more toxic cytokine release syndrome.
- Adoptive T cell therapy: Involves collecting and using patients' own immune cells in order to attack their tumor cells. The most successful and well studies adoptive T cells therapies in children are CD19-targeted chimeric antigen receptor (CAR) T-cells.
  ✓ CD19 CAR T-cell therapy: Approved by the FDA to treat B-ALL in children with refractory or second or later relapse of disease. For the procedure, T-cells are collected from the patient, and then genetically engineered with a viral vector to express CAR. Those T-cells are expanded in vivo and then reinfused into the patient. In the patient, there is further proliferation of the T-cells; when the cells come into contact with CD19 (on B-ALL cancer cells), a cytotoxic response attacks the cancer cells.
    - Toxicities: T-cell expansion in the patient can lead to cytokine release syndrome (CRS), which ranges in severity from fevers and myalgias to life-threatening hypotension, coagulopathy and multisystem organ dysfunction. Management involves supportive care (in

the intensive care unit for patients with severe cytokine release syndrome) and cytokine blockade with tocilizumab.

- Checkpoint inhibitors: Substances that block specific mechanisms ("checkpoints") that allow cancers to avoid immune surveillance. Checkpoint inhibitors have been more successful in adult than in childhood cancers, but are currently being studied in early-phase pediatric clinical trials. Some examples follow.
  - ✓ Programmed cell death receptor 1 (PD-1) inhibitors: Restore T-cell cytotoxic function to enhance the immune system's response against the tumor; includes nivolumab and pembrolizumab
  - ✓ Cytotoxic T-lymphocyte–associated protein 4 (CTLA-4) inhibitors: Inhibits CTLA-4's modulation of T-cell responses in order to increase T-cell activation and promote killing of tumor cells. Includes ipilimumab.
  - ✓ Toxicities of checkpoint inhibitors: Common and can affect almost any organ system— infusion reactions (can be life-threatening), colitis, hepatitis, hypopituitarism, pneumonitis, arthritis, etc.
- Other immunotherapies in different stages of development include anticancer vaccines, oncolytic viruses, and cytokines.

ONCOLOGIC EMERGENCIES

FEVER AND NEUTROPENIA

GENERAL PRINCIPLES

- Because of the bone marrow suppression from cancer and its treatment, patients lack a first line of defense against bacterial infections.
- Patients with fever and neutropenia (Absolute neutrophil count (ANC) $<500/mm^3$) deserve critical attention.
- Definitions of fever and neutropenia vary by treating center, but commonly:
  - ✓ Fever: A single temperature taken orally that is greater than 38.3–38.5°C or three temperatures greater than 38.0°C in a 24-hour period
  - ✓ Neutropenia: Different centers have different rules, but a common threshold is an ANC <300 cells/mm^3 or <500 cells/mm^3 and falling

CANCER AND THE IMMUNOCOMPROMISED HOST

- Cancer can increase infectious risk by inherent immunosuppression (leukemia) or by a mass creating obstruction of an organ (bladder, biliary tree, etc.) and subsequent development of infection.
- Therapy disrupts normal barriers against infection, including myelosuppression, disruption of the mucosal epithelium, local tissue breakdown, skin disruption, and the presence of foreign bodies such as a central venous catheter.
- Febrile, neutropenic patients can have an occult infection, but with subtle symptoms due to lack of inflammatory reaction.
- When pathogens are documented, bacteria are the most common (85–90%).
- Infections with mold or fungi are most common in patients exposed to chronic broad-spectrum antibiotics or with prolonged neutropenia.
- High-risk features: Inpatient at the time of diagnosis, uncontrolled cancer, comorbidities (hypotension, tachypnea, hypoxemia, mucositis), prolonged neutropenia (>5 days), higher fever, lower ANC.

APPROACH TO THE HISTORY AND PHYSICAL EXAM

- Key pieces of the history and physical exam:

✓ Determine the date of the most recent chemotherapy to predict the expected direction of the ANC trend, as most agents cause suppression 7–10 days after infusion.

✓ Note any recent blood transfusions (transfusion reaction can cause fever) and history of other infections as this may guide antibiotic choices.

✓ Critical to assess what type of indwelling catheter the child has (none, PICC, Broviac°, Port-A-Cath°), as these carry various risks of infection and antibiotic coverage may differ.

• Perform a thorough physical examination focusing on

✓ The oropharynx—Look for mucositis, gingival involvement.

✓ The central venous line sites—Look for signs of infection such as erythema, tenderness, or discharge at the site of insertion.

✓ Skin—Look for lesions that could indicate opportunistic fungus or molds

✓ Abdominal exam—A neutropenic patient is also at risk for neutropenic colitis (typhlitis), a potentially fatal complication, so perform a thorough abdominal examination and consult with a surgeon if there is any concern.

✓ The perineum—Look for perianal abscesses.

DIAGNOSTICS

• At least one blood culture needs to be drawn from a central line or a peripheral site. (Accessing a central line solely to obtain a blood culture may not be necessary.)

• CT scan (head/sinuses, chest, abdomen) for evaluation of fungal disease with white blood cell (WBC) count recovery in patients who have prolonged febrile neutropenia or in patients on long-standing broad-spectrum IV antibiotics who develop a new fever.

MANAGEMENT

• For reference, may refer to the Children's Hospital of Philadelphia (CHOP) clinical pathway for oncology patients presenting with fever: https://www.chop.edu/pathways ("Oncology Patient with Fever" section).

• Empiric antibiotic therapy

✓ Since gram-positive or gram-negative organisms can cause infection, empiric therapy must be broad spectrum (including antipseudomonal coverage) and bactericidal. Antibiotic choice depends on the individual institutional resistance patterns, and the combinations used are quite varied and are institution-specific. Typical empiric combinations include the following.

  ▪ Monotherapy with cefepime, imipenem, or meropenem

  ▪ Two-drug therapy with a third- or fourth-generation cephalosporin or an antipseudomonal penicillin in addition to an aminoglycoside (usually given for a maximum of 24 hour)

  ▪ Consider addition of vancomycin for gram-positive coverage if

    ▷ High institutional rate of gram-positive organisms leading to severe infection

    ▷ Receipt of intensive chemotherapy known to result in severe mucositis (HSCT, AML)

    ▷ Recent infection sensitive to vancomycin

    ▷ Colonization with vancomycin-sensitive organisms

    ▷ Patients presenting with hypotension

  ▪ Patients with a low risk of bacteremia may be given one dose of IV ceftriaxone and then treated as an outpatient on oral levofloxacin until count recovers.

✓ If there are signs of a specific infection on exam, add appropriate coverage (i.e., gram-positive coverage for skin infection or anaerobic coverage for perirectal or oral infection)

✓ If no organism can be identified, broad coverage (usually with a third- or fourth-generation cephalosporin) should continue until the patient has evidence of bone marrow recovery (e.g., ANC >200 cells/mm^3 and rising)

- Empiric antifungal therapy: Should be started in patients who have persistent febrile neutropenia (>3–5 days) or a new fever while on broad-spectrum empiric antibacterial coverage. Risk is greatest in HSCT and hematologic malignancy patients; patients with solid-organ transplants with expected duration of neutropenia <5 days are at low risk.
- Consider removal of central venous catheters if there is evidence of
  ✓ Subcutaneous tunnel infection
  ✓ Periportal infection
  ✓ Fungemia
  ✓ Atypical mycobacteremia
  ✓ Central line associated bloodstream infection (CLABSI) due to *S. aureus*
  ✓ Persistently positive bacterial blood cultures or in a critically ill patient
- Fever with a true infection may not develop in patients receiving corticosteroids as part of their therapy or for chronic symptom management; empiric antibiotic coverage should be considered in afebrile neutropenic patients taking steroids who have signs or symptoms suggestive of infection.
- Avoid rectal interventions (taking temperature or giving medicines) in a patient with neutropenia, except in an emergency.
- Special considerations for oncology patients with sepsis
  ✓ Consider stress-dose hydrocortisone, especially for patients with recent corticosteroid exposure, as they may not be able to mount an appropriate adrenal response.
  ✓ Consider administration of daily G-CSF or GM-CSF to promote quicker count recovery.

HYPERLEUKOCYTOSIS

DEFINED AS WBC >100,000/MM³ ON PRESENTATION

- Occurs in hematologic malignancies; more often in AML than in ALL or CML
- May be asymptomatic, but symptoms arise from WBC sludging, stasis, and increased blood viscosity and can include
  ✓ CNS: Confusion, headache, focal neurologic symptoms, somnolence
  ✓ Respiratory: Dyspnea, respiratory insufficiency, hypoxemia
  ✓ Renal: From severe tumor burden and associated lysis
- Despite profound anemia, transfusions of packed red cells in patients with hyperleukocytosis have been associated with poor outcomes due to shifts in blood viscosity. If a red-cell transfusion is needed, small-aliquot transfusions should be used initially.
- Symptomatic patients require intervention with leukapheresis; while careful attention should be paid to WBC >200,000/mm³ in AML or 300,000–400,000/mm³ in ALL, there is no WBC value that mandates leukapheresis.
  ✓ May also consider starting corticosteroids or other low-dose cytoreductive therapy in patients with ALL to accelerate tumor-cell lysis
  ✓ Definitive therapy is initiation of cancer-directed treatment.

SPINAL-CORD COMPRESSION

A mass that compromises the integrity of the spinal cord, conus medullaris, or cauda equina

EPIDEMIOLOGY

- Acute compression of the spinal cord develops in 3–5% of children with cancer. This must be differentiated from back pain of other etiologies that develops in 5–10% of patients with cancer.
- Sarcomas (especially Ewing) account for about 50% of cases.
- Other commonly involved tumors include neuroblastoma and lymphoma.

ETIOLOGY

- Tumor in the epidural or subarachnoid space
- Metastatic spread to the cord parenchyma or the vertebrae with secondary cord compression
- Extension of paravertebral tumor through the intervertebral foramina leading to epidural compression
- Subarachnoid spread down the spinal cord from a primary CNS tumor

PATHOPHYSIOLOGY

- Physical compression of the spinal cord, conus, or cauda equina leads to impaired blood flow, which results in venous hypertension and vasogenic cord edema, hemorrhage, ischemia, and eventually, infarction.

CLINICAL MANIFESTATIONS

- Back pain with localized tenderness is the presenting sign in 80% of patients.
- Radicular pain
- Abnormalities of bowel or bladder dysfunction (i.e., incontinence, retention)
- Most have objective motor loss.
- Patient/parent report of weakness, pain, tingling, bowel or bladder dysfunction

DIAGNOSTICS

- Spine radiographs: May be helpful, but are abnormal in less than 50% of cases
- MRI with and without gadolinium: Detects presence and extent of epidural involvement, intraparenchymal spread of tumor, and small lesions compressing nerve roots in the cauda equina
- Cerebrospinal fluid analysis: Important in evaluation of subarachnoid disease and meningeal leukemia or carcinomatosis, but not appropriate before initial imaging

MANAGEMENT

- Perform detailed neurologic exam.
- If patient has focal spinal tenderness or neurologic deficit, determine the nature of the symptoms and whether they are progressive.
- If neurologic symptoms are evolving, discuss initiation of Intravenous corticosteroids and perform MRI with and without gadolinium
- If evidence of spinal-cord compression on imaging, consider urgent chemotherapy, surgery, or local radiation only after careful discussion with all disciplines, as initial management decisions can have a profound effect on future therapy and patient function.
- Dexamethasone: For progressive dysfunction, initiate high-dose dexamethasone to reduce edema and cord compression

- Definitive therapy is initiation of appropriate cancer-directed treatment, so diagnostic biopsy should be pursued emergently; often empiric chemotherapy is initiated to treat most likely diagnosis while awaiting definitive pathology results.

SUPERIOR VENA CAVA SYNDROME AND SUPERIOR MEDIASTINAL SYNDROME

Signs and symptoms that result from compression, obstruction, or thrombosis of the superior vena cava (SVC). Superior mediastinal syndrome (SMS) includes SVC syndrome (SVCS) with associated tracheal compression.

ETIOLOGY

- Malignant (90%): Most commonly seen with non-Hodgkin lymphoma, Hodgkin lymphoma, T-cell ALL, and germ-cell tumors
- Nonmalignant: Vascular thrombosis resulting from the presence of a central venous line, thrombotic complications of cardiovascular surgery for congenital heart disease, infectious masses (i.e., tuberculosis, histoplasmosis, aspergillosis), bronchogenic cyst; hamartoma; ganglioneuroma

PATHOPHYSIOLOGY

- Tumor or infection in the nodes or thymus can compress the SVC, causing venous stasis.
- The trachea and right main stem bronchus in infants and children are smaller than in adults, and minimal compression/swelling can result in obstructive symptoms. Compression, clotting, and edema decrease airflow and reduce venous return from the head, neck, and upper thorax, leading to the signs and symptoms of SVCS and superior mediastinal syndrome.

CLINICAL MANIFESTATIONS

- 75% of children with mediastinal masses have respiratory symptoms that are aggravated when the patient is supine
- Signs: Edema and/or cyanosis of the face, neck, and upper extremities; plethoric appearance; conjunctival suffusion; cervical and thoracic venous distention; wheezing; stridor; pleural/pericardial effusion
- Symptoms: Cough, dyspnea, dysphagia, orthopnea, hoarseness, wheezing, stridor, chest pain, anxiety, headache, confusion secondary to carbon dioxide retention

DIAGNOSTICS

- Chest x-ray demonstrates mass
- Laboratory evaluation
  - ✓ CBC: Pancytopenia, leukocytosis, blasts on smear (leukemia, lymphoma), left shift (infection)
  - ✓ Chemistry panel: Potassium, calcium, phosphorus, creatinine, uric acid, lactic dehydrogenase (LDH) (can be elevated with leukemia, lymphoma)
  - ✓ α-fetoprotein, β-hCG: Elevated in germ-cell tumors
  - ✓ Urine catecholamines: Elevated in neuroblastoma
  - ✓ ESR: Can be elevated with lymphoma
- Assess risk for general anesthesia/surgery
  - ✓ If respiratory distress or orthopnea is present, anesthesia would put patient at high risk.
  - ✓ If patient is asymptomatic or has even minimal symptoms, chest CT and echocardiography are needed prior to undergoing anesthesia.

- Sedation or general anesthesia in patients with a mediastinal mass may be contraindicated because these can decrease respiratory drive and result in respiratory failure, decreased venous return, and circulatory collapse.

MANAGEMENT

- Clinical decision-making
  - ✓ General principle is to establish diagnosis/staging with the least invasive test possible, particularly if high risk for anesthesia
  - ✓ If CBC and other studies confirm diagnosis, begin tumor-specific treatment.
  - ✓ If no diagnosis is made after initial noninvasive studies, continue evaluation and assess anesthesia risk for patient to safely obtain tumor tissue
    - If patient is at low risk for anesthesia, perform diagnostic procedures and then begin tumor-specific treatment.
    - If patient is at high risk for anesthesia, perform necessary procedures while awake or treat empirically with chemotherapy or radiation based on the most likely disease, although this is can complicate the eventual diagnostic procedure.
- General management issues: Respiratory compromise may not be immediately obvious.
- Do not force the patient to lie down or assume another uncomfortable position.
  - ✓ Control the airway, give oxygen, and avoid intubation if possible.
  - ✓ Extreme care in handling the patient: Minimize stress, sedation
  - ✓ If tissue diagnosis is not possible, empiric therapy may be necessary.
  - ✓ Empiric use of steroids, radiation therapy, and chemotherapy can all affect masses and lymph nodes, making subsequent tissue diagnosis and treatment more difficult, but these interventions may be medically indicated.

TUMOR LYSIS SYNDROME

Metabolic abnormalities that result from dying tumor cells and the rapid release of intracellular metabolites into circulation that exceeds the excretory capacity of the kidneys. Tumor lysis syndrome (TLS) can occur at presentation or within 12–72 hours after the start of chemotherapy. The classic triad involves hyperuricemia, hyperkalemia, and hyperphosphatemia.

- Hyperuricemia: Results from the release of nucleic acids from malignant cell breakdown. Uric acid is soluble at physiologic pH but precipitates in the acidic environment of the kidney and can lead to acute renal failure.
- Hyperkalemia: Potassium is the principal intracellular cation, and serum levels can also increase with acute renal failure. High serum potassium can cause fatal dysrhythmias.
- Hyperphosphatemia: Lymphoblasts have four times the content of phosphate as normal lymphocytes; leads to hypocalcemia by decreasing production of calcitriol, decreasing absorption of calcium from the GI tract, and from precipitation; if $Ca^{2+} \times PO_4^{-3}$ product reaches 60, calcium phosphate crystals form and precipitate in the microvasculature, leading to acute renal failure.

ETIOLOGY

- Most common: Burkitt lymphoma, lymphoblastic lymphoma, ALL (T-cell)
- Predisposing factors: Tumors with high growth fraction and sensitivity to chemotherapy, bulky tumors, high pretherapy uric acid or LDH, poor urine output, high WBC count on presentation

CLINICAL MANIFESTATIONS

- Usually no signs or symptoms
- May present with vomiting or diarrhea
- May present with evidence of hypocalcemia: Muscle weakness, spasms, tetany, seizures, renal failure
- Strategies for the prevention and management of tumor lysis syndrome are outlined in **Table 22-2**.

PANCYTOPENIA AND ACUTE LEUKEMIA

GENERAL PRINCIPLES

PRESENTATION

- Manifestations of single or multiple cytopenias
  - ✓ Anemia: Headache, light-headedness, dyspnea on exertion, palpitations, fatigue, pallor, irritability
  - ✓ Thrombocytopenia: Mucosal bleeding, petechiae, purpura, easy bruising
  - ✓ Leukopenia/neutropenia: Fevers, mucosal ulceration, invasive bacterial infections

DIFFERENTIAL DIAGNOSIS

- Broad division between decreased bone marrow production and peripheral destruction (or combination)
  - ✓ Decreased production: Bone marrow failure (inherited or acquired), leukemia, lymphoma, metastatic solid tumor, infection (CMV, EBV, HHV-6, parvovirus, etc.), HLH
  - ✓ Destruction/consumption: Evans syndrome, hypersplenism

EVALUATION

- History: Fever pattern, bone pain, weight loss, night sweats
- Physical examination: Lymphadenopathy, hepatosplenomegaly
- Laboratory evaluation
  - ✓ CBC/differential/reticulocyte count with review of peripheral-blood smear
    - ▪ Smear review critical for blasts and evidence of stressed marrow (nucleated RBCs or teardrop) that may suggest infiltrative process
  - ✓ Electrolytes (with Mg, Ph), BUN/creatinine, hepatic panel
  - ✓ LDH and uric acid to evaluate for tumor lysis syndrome
  - ✓ Prothrombin time/international normalized ratio and partial thromboplastin time; fibrinogen if abnormal
- Other studies
  - ✓ Chest x-ray for mediastinal mass or adenopathy
  - ✓ Bone marrow examination (aspirate and biopsy) for definitive diagnosis
- Features suggestive of a malignancy include prominent constitutional symptoms, bone pain, adenopathy, hepatomegaly, mediastinal mass, or laboratory evidence of tumor lysis syndrome.

ACUTE LEUKEMIA

Accounts for approximately 30% of childhood cancers. Characterized by excessive proliferation of early hematopoietic cells (blasts) whose maturation has been arrested. Lymphoid leukemia (ALL) represents 80% of cases and myeloid leukemia (AML) 20%.

TABLE 22-2	Prevention and Management of Tumor Lysis Syndrome
Diagnosis and monitoring	• CBC, electrolytes, creatinine, uric acid every 4–6 hours • Cardiac monitoring if hyperkalemia or hypocalcemia • Urine output • Chest x-ray to evaluate for mediastinal mass • Abdominal ultrasound if concern about abdominal mass or renal failure
Hydration	• IV fluids without K^+, Ca^+, PO_4 at 1–4 times maintenance fluid rate to maintain urine output at >100 mL/m²/hr • Close monitoring of weight/fluid status • If patient has renal failure and cannot be hydrated appropriately, consider dialysis.
Uric acid reduction	• Allopurinol: xanthine oxidase inhibitor that prevents uric acid synthesis • Urate oxidase (rasburicase): converts uric acid to allantoin, which is much more soluble. Consider in patients at highest risk for developing tumor lysis (WBC >100,000/mm³, uric acid >10 mg/dL, elevated creatinine). As this agent causes significant hemolysis in patients with glucose-6-phosphate dehydrogenase (G6PD) deficiency, use with caution if G6PD status unknown. • Consider alkalinizing fluids for management of hyperuricemia if rasburicase is not available because uric acid is more soluble in an alkaline pH. Maintain urine pH of 7.0–7.5. If alkalinization is used, discontinue prior to starting chemotherapy to reduce the risk of precipitating calcium-phosphorus calculi.
Treatment of metabolic abnormalities	
Hyperkalemia	• Calcium gluconate • Kayexalate • Insulin and 25% glucose to increase cellular uptake of potassium • Consider furosemide or other loop diuretics
Hyperphosphatemia	• Aluminum hydroxide or • Sevelamer • Insulin and glucose as above
Hypocalcemia	Calcium gluconate slow IV infusion *only* if symptomatic
Dialysis indications	• Volume overload: pleural, pericardial effusions • Renal failure • Hyperkalemia • Hyperphosphatemia • Hyperuricemia • Symptomatic hypocalcemia • Uncontrolled hypertension • Oliguria or anuria

CLINICAL MANIFESTATIONS

- Bone marrow replacement: Cytopenias and their associated symptoms
- Uncontrolled proliferation: Bone pain, adenopathy, organomegaly, fever
- Unique presentations: Coagulopathy, acute promyelocytic leukemia (APML), anterior mediastinal mass (T-cell ALL), chloromas (extranodal collections of myeloid blasts), leukemia cutis (cutaneous infiltrates—often bluish), testicular mass (ALL)

INITIAL MANAGEMENT

- Priorities are to obtain a prompt diagnosis and address existing or potential oncologic emergencies
  - ✓ Diagnosis: Unilateral bone marrow aspirate/biopsy and lumbar puncture with intrathecal chemotherapy (if confident about malignancy based on presentation/smear)
  - ✓ Emergencies: TLS, infection, hyperleukocytosis, cytopenias, anterior mediastinal mass, coagulopathy
- Once diagnosis is established, disease-specific therapy (see below) is implemented.

ALL: ACUTE LYMPHOBLASTIC LEUKEMIA

- Divided into two groups based on immunophenotype of blasts: B-cell (80%) and T-cell (20%); T-cell ALL tends to affect older patients and have more extramedullary disease (CNS involvement, lymphadenopathy, mediastinal mass, hepatosplenomegaly).
- Prognosis
  - ✓ The vast majority of children with ALL can be cured of their disease, but there are risk factors that require more intensive or varied therapies. High-risk features include
    - CNS involvement—requires additional CNS-directed therapy
    - Initial total WBC $\geq$50,000/mm³
    - Age $\geq$10 years.
    - Infants $\leq$1 year can have leukemias that are especially difficult to treat).
  - ✓ Cytogenetics abnormalities in the leukemic clone:
    - Favorable: Hyperdiploidy, *ETV6-RUNX1*
    - Unfavorable: Hypodiploidy, t(9;22) (also known as the Philadelphia chromosome), *KMT2A*-rearranged (previously known as *MLL*)
- As molecular testing becomes more sophisticated, additional cytogenetic lesions are being identified and included in risk stratifications.
  - ✓ Response to therapy
    - For B-ALL, failure to achieve an excellent response as defined by >1/10,000 leukemia cells per mononuclear cells in the bone marrow (termed minimal residual disease negative) by the end of the first month of therapy is a poor prognostic factor.
    - For T-ALL, a slower response may be seen. Persistence of minimal residual disease at the end of 2 months of therapy indicates a poor prognosis.
- Treatment
  - ✓ Conventional chemotherapy cures most childhood ALL, is typically delivered over a period of 2–3 years, and is divided into phases, with each having a specific purpose. Exact treatment regimens are based on risk stratification, which is dictated by above prognostic factors.
  - ✓ Standard phases of chemotherapy:
    - Induction: Establish a complete remission
      - ▷ Drugs: Steroid, asparaginase, vincristine with or without daunorubicin
      - ▷ Duration: 1 month

- Consolidation: Increased CNS-targeted therapy and consolidation of systemic remission
  ▷ Drugs: Incorporates different agents than induction; protocol-specific
  ▷ Duration: 1–2 months
- Interim maintenance: Continued CNS treatment; systemic treatment with less myelosuppression
- Delayed intensification: Period of intensive treatment, essentially repeating induction and part of consolidation
  ▷ Duration: 2 months
- Maintenance: Prevent relapse and eradicate residual disease with continuous low-intensity chemotherapy
  ▷ Drugs: Mostly oral chemotherapy (6-MP and methotrexate) with monthly IV vincristine and steroid pulses, and every 3-month LPs with IT-chemotherapy
  ▷ Duration: 1.5–2 years
- CNS treatment: All patients receive CNS-targeted therapy with intrathecal chemotherapy
  ▷ If CNS+ at diagnosis, CNS therapy more intensive +/− cranial radiation
  ▷ T-cell patients more likely to be CNS+ and receive cranial radiation
- Relapsed disease
  ▷ Treatment approach is dictated by risk, which is based on timing and site of relapsed disease
  ▷ Lower risk B-ALL relapse: generally includes later relapses with an excellent response to reinduction; typically, treat with conventional chemotherapy and cranial radiation, if CNS is involved.
  ▷ Higher risk B-ALL relapses: generally includes earlier relapse or late relapses without an optimal response to re-induction; standard of care typically involves HSCT. CD19-targeted CAR T-cell therapy may also be considered.
  ▷ T-cell: HSCT generally recommended regardless of timing or site
  ▷ Second relapse of ALL often indicates chemotherapy-resistant disease, which may be very difficult to cure.
✓ Special groups
- Infants: ALL occurring in children <1 year is a biologically unique disease with frequent *KMT2A* (MLL) rearrangements. It is difficult to cure, with many children dying of relapsed disease. May consider stem-cell transplantation in first remission, but there is no clear evidence of its benefit.
- Trisomy 21: Children with trisomy 21 have a higher risk of ALL. Because of increased sensitivity to chemotherapeutic agents, some decrease in intensity of therapy may be needed for certain patients.
- Ph+ (t(9;22)) ALL: Historically, Ph+ ALL indicated a poor prognosis. However, addition of tyrosine kinase inhibitors (e.g., imatinib, dasatinib) to the backbone of chemotherapy, has improved outcomes substantially.

AML: ACUTE MYELOID LEUKEMIA

- Generally divided into *de novo* AML (occurring in previously well child), secondary AML (occurring in child with history of exposure to certain chemotherapy agents or in child with bone marrow failure syndrome or MDS), and APML.
- Prognostic factors
  ✓ Cytogenetics and molecular features
  - Low risk: includes t(8;21)(q22;q22), inv16, *CEPBPA*, *NPM1*

- High risk: Includes monosomy 7, 5q−, *FLT3* ITD
  - All therapy- or MDS-related AML is considered high risk.
  - Intermediate risk: All others
- As molecular testing becomes more sophisticated and the implications of different cytogenetic features are studied, risk stratifications are being adjusted and additional abnormalities are being assigned to the high- or low-risk groups.
  ✓ Response to therapy
    - Failure to achieve an excellent remission, defined as <1 leukemia cell per 10,000 normal bone marrow cells (minimal residual disease–negative) after first month of therapy is a poor prognostic factor.
- Treatment
  ✓ General approach: Based on combination of cytogenetic features and minimal residual disease status after the first month of therapy, patients can be stratified into low-, intermediate-, or high-risk groups.
    - Patients with low- or intermediate-risk disease can be treated with 4–5 cycles of intensive chemotherapy alone.
    - Patients with high-risk disease are treated with 3 cycles of intensive chemotherapy and then proceed with allogeneic HSCT in first remission
  ✓ CNS disease: Does not alter prognosis of AML, but does require more frequent intrathecal therapy
  ✓ Chloromas: Chloromas in sensitive locations (e.g., orbits) may require emergency up-front radiation.
  ✓ Chemotherapy
    - Intensive chemotherapy cycles include the following agents, given in different combinations
      ▷ Cytarabine (low-dose and high-dose)
      ▷ Anthracyclines (daunorubicin, mitoxantrone)
      ▷ Etoposide
      ▷ Asparaginase
    - Gemtuzumab ozogamicin, an antibody-drug conjugate, is added to several cycles of chemotherapy for patients with CD33+ AML
- Relapse
  ✓ Children with relapsed AML are treated with intensive chemotherapy followed by HSCT if remission can be achieved; prognosis is poor, especially for early relapses.
- Special groups
  ✓ APML: Unique form of AML that has a characteristic cytogenetic abnormality—t(15;17)—making it amenable to targeted therapy with the differentiating agent all trans retinoic acid (ATRA). Arsenic has also been shown to have specific sensitivity for APML blasts. Current APML regimens are using these agents alone or in combination with conventional chemotherapeutic agents.
  ✓ Trisomy 21: Children with trisomy 21 have a higher risk of developing AML, especially a certain subtype called acute megakaryocytic leukemia (AMKL). It is usually diagnosed before age 4 years and associated with a better prognosis than in children without trisomy 21. Generally, AMKL in these children responds to less intensive chemotherapy.
    - *TMD:* Transient myeloproliferative disorder is an escalation of nonmalignant blasts in the first weeks of life without or without organomegaly. Usually responds spontaneously, although sometimes low-dose chemotherapy is needed to control organomegaly or hyperviscosity. Children with TMD have a higher incidence of developing AMKL over the next 4 years of life.

LYMPHADENOPATHY AND LYMPHOMA

GENERAL PRINCIPLES

PRESENTATION

- Features of an enlarged lymph node suggestive of a malignant etiology
  - ✓ Single node >1.5 cm
  - ✓ Generalized or ≥2 nodal regions or any supraclavicular
  - ✓ Firm (rubbery), painless, enlarging, no overlying erythema/cellulitis

DIFFERENTIAL DIAGNOSIS

- Based on pattern (focal/diffuse), characteristics (size, pain, firmness, etc.), associated symptoms, and other physical exam findings. Differential diagnosis includes:
  - ✓ EBV, CMV, toxoplasmosis
  - ✓ Cat-scratch disease
  - ✓ Atypical mycobacterium
  - ✓ Kawasaki disease

EVALUATION

- History and physical exam
- CBC/differential, review of peripheral blood smear, electrolytes, LDH, uric acid, infection testing, ESR (can be elevated in classical Hodgkin lymphoma)
- Chest x-ray important to evaluate for mediastinal mass in a child with worrisome lymphadenopathy
- CT of affected areas (if concern for lymphoma, include neck, chest, abdomen, pelvis)
- Biopsy if concern for malignancy or diagnostic uncertainty in ill child
  - ✓ Should be in consultation with oncologist
  - ✓ Excisional biopsy required as nodal architecture important in lymphoma diagnosis.
- Determining the extent/stage of lymphoma is important:
  - ✓ CT (as above)
  - ✓ Positron-emission tomography (PET) (can be done as PET/CT or PET/MRI)
  - ✓ Bone marrow aspirates and biopsies (bilateral)
  - ✓ Lumbar puncture (if non-Hodgkin lymphoma (NHL))

LYMPHOMA

Generally divided into Hodgkin (40%) and non-Hodgkin (60%) lymphoma based on immunophenotype of malignant cells. Comprises about 10–15% of childhood cancers, and up to 25% in adolescent age group.

HODGKIN LYMPHOMA

- Malignant cell represents the minority of cellular composition of lymph node; remainder is mixed infiltrate of mature lymphocytes, eosinophils, and monocytes/macrophages. In classical Hodgkin lymphoma, the malignant cell is termed the Reed–Sternberg cell and is giant and multinucleated with prominent nucleoli.
- Presentation
  - ✓ Classically present with painless lymphadenopathy. Lymph node enlargement is often more indolent than in NHL.

✓ Cervical and supraclavicular nodes are most frequently involved and anterior mediastinal masses are common (60%).

✓ Constitutional symptoms: Unexplained fevers, drenching night sweats, and unintentional weight loss (>10% of body weight over preceding 6 months) are termed "B" symptoms and are present in 20–30% of patients at diagnosis

✓ Oncologic emergencies in Hodgkin lymphoma are uncommon. Anterior mediastinal masses usually do not enlarge quickly enough to case cardiopulmonary compromise, and the malignant cell does not turn over rapidly enough to cause TLS.

• Classification

✓ Based on histology, can be classified as classical Hodgkin lymphoma (90%) or nodular lymphocyte–predominant Hodgkin lymphoma (10%)

  ▪ Classical Hodgkin lymphoma includes nodular sclerosis, lymphocyte rich, mixed cellularity, and lymphocyte depletion

• Staging and risk stratification

✓ Staging based on site(s) of nodal involvement (Ann Arbor system)

  ▪ Stage I: 1 nodal region
  ▪ Stage II: ≥2 nodal regions on same side of diaphragm
  ▪ Stage III: ≥2 nodal regions on both sides of diaphragm
  ▪ Stage IV: Diffuse disease or bone marrow involvement

✓ Risk stratification: Based on stage, presence of B symptoms, and bulk (specific measurements done by radiology in conjunction with oncologist)

  ▪ Low risk: Stage I or II without B symptoms or bulk
  ▪ High risk:
    ▷ Classical Hodgkin lymphoma: Stage IIB with bulk, III or IV with B symptoms, or IV without B symptoms
    ▷ Nodular lymphocyte predominant Hodgkin lymphoma: Stage III or IV with B symptoms
  ▪ Intermediate risk: All other stages

• Treatment

✓ Multiagent chemotherapy with or without radiation of involved lymph node areas

✓ Since cure of Hodgkin lymphoma is successful in >90% of children, current regimens focus on deintensifying therapy (typically by removal of radiation) in children at lower risk of relapse to avoid late effects.

✓ For low and intermediate risk, if there is a good response to chemotherapy, omission of radiation should be strongly considered.

• Relapse

✓ Many children with relapsed Hodgkin lymphoma can be salvaged. Treatment involves initial chemotherapy to get to as close of a complete remission as possible followed by autologous HSCT with or without radiation

• Late effects

✓ Long-term adverse effects of therapy occur with all childhood cancers, but survivors of Hodgkin lymphoma are among those at highest risk, especially those who received radiation. See "Late Effect of Cancer Treatment" section for more details.

NON-HODGKIN LYMPHOMA (NHL)

• Subtypes

✓ Based on phenotype (B vs. T) and differentiation (mature vs. precursor) of lymphoma cells

  ▪ Mature B-cell: Burkitt lymphoma and diffuse large B-cell lymphoma (DLBCL)
  ▪ Mature T-cell: Anaplastic large cell lymphoma (ALCL)
  ▪ Precursor: Lymphoblastic lymphoma (LL) (This occurs much more commonly with T-cell lymphoblastic lymphoma over B-cell.)

- Presentation
  - ✓ Can present with symptoms similar to Hodgkin lymphoma with a generally more aggressive pattern, or in relatively unique ways based on subtype
  - ✓ Burkitt lymphoma: Presents with rapidly enlarging masses in the nodal regions or in the abdomen that can be mistaken for acute abdomen.
  - ✓ Lymphoblastic lymphoma: Often presents similarly to acute leukemia, but may also see mediastinal mass, effusions, and bulky adenopathy
  - ✓ ALCL: Usually presents with adenopathy, but can also present in other organs and bones.
- Staging
  - ✓ Staging is based on number of nodal areas and sites involved (St. Jude system)
    - Stage I: 1 region (not abdomen or mediastinum)
    - Stage II: ≥2 regions on same side of diaphragm; resectable abdominal tumor
    - Stage III: ≥2 regions on both sides of diaphragm; any chest, paraspinal, or unresectable abdominal tumor
    - Stage IV: CNS or bone marrow involvement
  - ✓ Risk stratification, which guides treatment, is based on a combination of disease histology, stage, and other patient factors.
- Treatment
  - ✓ BL/DLBCL: Short, but intensive, therapy with multiagent systemic and intrathecal chemotherapy
  - ✓ LL: Treated like ALL, with up-front intensive therapy followed by maintenance chemotherapy, over 2–3 years
  - ✓ ALCL: Intermediate intensity and length
- Relapse
  - ✓ Difficult to cure in general; treatment with intensive chemotherapy followed by stem-cell transplantation with or without radiation
- Special groups
  - ✓ Immunocompromised hosts: Children with acquired or inherited immunodeficiencies are at increased risk of developing NHL (particular B-cell)
  - ✓ Recipients of organ transplants: After solid-organ transplantation or HSCT, children are at risk of developing posttransplantation lymphoproliferative disease (PTLD).
    - Encompasses a wide spectrum, ranging from reactive polyclonal B-cell hyperplasia to polyclonal or monoclonal B-cell lymphoma. Most cases are EBV-driven.
    - Can be asymptomatic or present with symptoms such as fever, fatigue, gastrointestinal disturbances, lymph node enlargement, or viral symptoms that resemble an acute infectious mononucleosis.
    - Some patients can present with fulminant PTLD, defined as PTLD with fever, hypotension, and multiorgan involvement.
    - Evaluation includes laboratory tests (CBC, BMP, phosphorous, LDH, uric acid), imaging (CT neck, chest, abdomen and pelvis, PET), site-directed biopsy and bilateral bone marrow biopsies
    - Management: Based on histology and clinical status
      ▷ Polymorphic or monomorphic, non-Burkitt PTLD and clinically stable: First line is to reduce immunosuppression. If unable or unsuccessful, treat with chemotherapy (most commonly cyclophosphamide, prednisone, and rituximab).
      ▷ Fulminant PTLD or Burkitt histology: Treat as de novo Burkitt lymphoma/DLBCL. For other patients, reduce immunosuppression and start chemotherapy right away.
      ▷ Can consider using EBV-directed cytotoxic T lymphocytes for patients with poor response to other therapies or relapsed disease

✓ Primary mediastinal B-cell lymphoma (PMBCL): Biologically unique form of DLBCL that originates from thymic tissue, is locally invasive, and is relatively resistant to conventional chemotherapy.

SOLID TUMORS

ABDOMINAL MASSES

HISTORY

• Duration, pain, vomiting/diarrhea, obstruction, B symptoms (fevers, night sweats, weight loss), age, underlying genetic syndrome

PHYSICAL EXAM

• Location, size, mobility, consistency

EVALUATION

• Labs include CBC, LFTs, uric acid, LDH, urinalysis, tumor markers (α-fetoprotein, β-hCG, urine homovanillic/vanillylmandelic acid)
• Diagnostic imaging (CT/MRI, PET, 123 meta-iodobenzylguanidine (MIBG))

WILMS TUMOR

EPIDEMIOLOGY

• Represents about 5% of childhood cancers
• 90% of cases are diagnosed by age 6 years
• 5–15% of cases can be associated with other congenital anomalies.
  ✓ Cryptorchidism, hypospadias, sporadic hemihypertrophy
  ✓ WAGR (Wilms tumor, aniridia, genitourinary malformation, mental retardation): Germline deletion at 11p
  ✓ Denys–Drash syndrome: Pseudohermaphroditism, renal disease, Wilms tumor—WT1 mutation
  ✓ Beckwith–Wiedemann syndrome (BWS): Macroglossia, omphalocele, visceromegaly, hemihypertrophy
  ✓ Frasier syndrome: Nephropathy, gonadal dysgenesis, gonadoblastoma
  ✓ Simpson–Golabi–Behmel syndrome: Coarse facial features, skeletal and cardiac abnormalities, intellectual impairment

ETIOLOGY/GENETICS

• WT1—Wilms tumor suppressor gene
  ✓ Patients with bilateral disease may have constitutional WT1 mutations
• WT2—Genomic imprinting within the WT2 locus may account for BWS
  ✓ Loss of heterozygosity at 16q and 1p are associated with worse outcomes
• Deregulation of the Wnt pathway also plays a role in Wilms tumor

CLINICAL MANIFESTATIONS

• Painless abdominal swelling or mass, hematuria, fever. Usually, otherwise well-appearing
• Hypertension in 25% of cases on presentation
• Varicoceles can be seen in males with spermatic-vein compression
• Note any signs of syndromes associated with Wilms tumor, including aniridia, facial abnormalities of BWS, hemihypertrophy, or genitourinary anomalies

DIAGNOSIS AND STAGING

- Laboratory evaluation: CBC, urinalysis, electrolytes, BUN/creatinine, LFTs
- Primary tumor imaging: Usually start with an ultrasound and then definitive imaging with CT or MRI
- Metastatic evaluation: Chest CT
- Staging:
  - ✓ Stage I: Tumor confined to the kidney, completely resected
  - ✓ Stage II: Tumor extends beyond the kidney, but is completely resected
  - ✓ Stage III: Gross or microscopic residual tumor remains postoperatively
  - ✓ Stage IV: Distant metastases or lymph node metastases outside the abdomen
  - ✓ Stage V: Bilateral tumors

PROGNOSIS

- Overall, excellent prognosis, but older age, anaplastic histology (especially with stage IV or V disease), loss of heterozygosity at 1p and 16q, and capsular or vascular invasion are associated with worse outcomes.

TREATMENT

- Surgery
  - ✓ When feasible, an up-front nephrectomy is preferred for unilateral tumors. This allows for examination of histology as well as complete staging of lymph nodes.
  - ✓ Unresectable, unilateral tumors may be biopsied, although special consideration should be made for the possibility of "up-staging," should there be intraoperative spillage.
  - ✓ Nephron-sparing surgery is being investigated for patients with bilateral disease.
- Chemotherapy/radiation: Based on risk group, which is based on combination of age, tumor weight, and stage
  - ✓ Very low risk: No chemotherapy or radiation
  - ✓ Low risk: Vincristine and actinomycin, no radiation
  - ✓ Standard-risk: Vincristine, actinomycin, and doxorubicin + radiation (flank, whole abdomen, or whole lung based on local staging)
  - ✓ Higher risk: Same as standard-risk therapy, but add more intensive chemotherapy after 6 weeks if less than optimal response
  - ✓ Bilateral: Chemotherapy based on histology and extent of disease + radiation (flank, whole abdomen or whole lung based on local staging)
  - ✓ Anaplastic: chemotherapy based on local stage and extent of anaplasia (local vs diffuse) + radiation (flank, whole abdomen, or whole lung based on local staging)

NEUROBLASTOMA

A malignant tumor derived from neural crest cells that can be found anywhere along the sympathetic chain, including the adrenal medulla. Variations in location and histologic differentiation result in a wide range of biologic and clinical characteristics.

EPIDEMIOLOGY

- Neuroblastoma is the most common extracranial solid tumor in children.
- Most commonly diagnosed in children <5 years old; median age at diagnosis, 17 months

ETIOLOGY/GENETICS

- *MYCN* amplification is associated with advanced disease and a worse outcome.

- *1p* and *11q* loss of heterozygosity are independently associated with a worse outcome
- Most cases are sporadic, but a small proportion (1–2%) have a family history
  - ✓ *ALK* (anaplastic lymphoma kinase)—the major neuroblastoma predisposition gene. *ALK* activation/amplification is also found in about 10–15% of sporadic cases.

CLINICAL MANIFESTATIONS

- Classic signs and symptoms can include fever, weight loss, limp, periorbital ecchymosis/proptosis ("raccoon eyes"), bone pain, and pancytopenia.
- Tumors can occur anywhere along the sympathetic chain
  - ✓ Abdomen/adrenal—Can be detected as an asymptomatic mass or with abdominal pain; more common in younger children
  - ✓ Thoracic/paraspinal—Can present as an asymptomatic mass or with spinal-cord compression
  - ✓ Cervical—Can present with Horner's syndrome (ptosis, miosis, anhidrosis); more common in infants
- Most common sites of metastases are regional nodes, bone, bone marrow, liver, and skin. Rarely, metastases can occur in lung and brain
- Infants can present with skin involvement (stage 4S) with bluish, non-tender subcutaneous nodules.
- Paraneoplastic manifestations:
  - ✓ Opsoclonus myoclonus ataxia syndrome—Presumed secondary to antineural antibodies
  - ✓ Secretory diarrhea—Associated with vasoactive intestinal peptide secretion

DIAGNOSIS/STAGING/RISK STRATIFICATION

- Biopsy is preferred for histologic confirmation and to have tissue for molecular diagnostic studies
- Laboratory evaluation: CBC with differential, electrolytes, BUN/creatinine, LFTs, urinary homovanillic/vanillylmandelic acid, LDH
- Imaging: CT/MRI of primary tumor including chest/abdomen/pelvis, MIBG scan
- Other evaluation: bilateral bone marrow aspirates and biopsies
- Staging (International Neuroblastoma Staging System)
  - ✓ L1: Localized tumor not involving vital structures as defined by a list of image-defined risk factors and confined to one body compartment
  - ✓ L2: Locoregional tumor with presence of one or more image-defined risk factors
  - ✓ M: Distant metastatic disease (except stage MS)
  - ✓ MS: Metastatic disease in children younger than 18 months with metastases confined to skin, liver, and/or bone marrow
- Risk stratification (low, intermediate, or high): Complex algorithm based on age, stage, *MYCN* status, histology, and ploidy. The majority of patients fall into the high risk category.

PROGNOSIS

- Prognosis dependent on risk group, which is based on age, stage, MYCN status, histology, and ploidy

TREATMENT (RISK-RELATED)

- Neonates with MS disease: Often require urgent treatment secondary to respiratory distress and abdominal competition, especially in those <2 months
  - ✓ Chemotherapy
  - ✓ Radiation therapy—Reserved for cases in which tumor does not respond rapidly enough to chemotherapy

- Low-risk: Surgery alone; very few patients require cytotoxic therapy
- Intermediate-risk:
  ✓ Surgery
  ✓ Chemotherapy—Carboplatin, cyclophosphamide, etoposide, doxorubicin
  ✓ Radiation—Can be considered in cases where tumor bulk precludes surgery and tumor does not respond to chemotherapy
- High-risk: Involves very intensive multimodal therapy delivered over 1–2 years
  ✓ Chemotherapy: Topotecan, cyclophosphamide, vincristine, doxorubicin, cisplatin, etoposide
  ✓ Surgery: Best possible resection of primary tumor
  ✓ Stem cell transplant: Usually, tandem autologous hematopoietic cell transplants
  ✓ Radiation therapy: To primary tumor site and other sites not responding to induction chemotherapy
  ✓ Immunotherapy: Dinutuximab (anti-GD2 immunotherapy) combined with interleukin-2 or GM-CSF. In addition, isotretinoin given with each cycle to promote maturation of any remaining malignant neuroblastoma cells
- Trends in neuroblastoma therapy
  ✓ Biologically favorable disease: reduce or eliminate cytotoxic therapy
  ✓ Biologically unfavorable disease: test more precise therapeutic approaches that target neuroblastoma cells directly (e.g., crizotinib to target *ALK* mutations)
- Relapsed disease
  ✓ Not curable except for local relapses, but treatments are available to slow disease progression
  ✓ Iodine-131 MIBG can be used as a form of target radiation to treat relapsed/refractory disease. Current studies are evaluating MIBG as treatment for newly diagnosed high-risk patients.

BONE TUMORS

Osteosarcoma is a malignant bone tumor arising from mesenchymal cells. It is unique in its production of immature bone (osteoid) by cell stroma. Ewing sarcoma is part of a family of tumors comprising a histologic spectrum ranging from undifferentiated small round blue cells to differentiated cells resembling primitive neuroectodermal tumors (PNETs).

OSTEOSARCOMA

EPIDEMIOLOGY

- Represents approximately 2% of childhood cancers
- The most common age at presentation is adolescence.
  ✓ Likely relationship between rapid bone growth and development of osteosarcoma
- More common in boys than girls
- Usually occurs in metaphyseal portions of long bones (distal femur, proximal tibia, proximal humerus)

ETIOLOGY/GENETICS

- Prior irradiation increases the risk for developing osteosarcoma.
- Associated clinical syndromes:
  ✓ Rothmund–Thomson syndrome (autosomal recessive): Poikiloderma, small stature, and skeletal dysplasia

✓ Hereditary retinoblastoma: germline mutation in *Rb* gene
✓ Li–Fraumeni syndrome: Cancer predisposition syndrome due to *P53* mutation

CLINICAL MANIFESTATIONS

• Pain over involved site with or without associated soft-tissue mass
• Can have erythema, warmth, or swelling that mimics infection
• Can result in pathologic fracture
• Patients usually do not have systemic symptoms.

DIAGNOSIS/STAGING

• Biopsy: Open biopsy should be performed by an experienced orthopedic surgeon (ideally should be the surgeon who will later perform definitive surgery).
• Staging:
  ✓ Imaging of primary tumor: MRI should include both the joint above and the joint below to examine for skip lesions.
  ✓ Metastatic evaluation: Chest CT, PET scan (can be done as PET/CT or PET/MRI)

PROGNOSIS

• Extent of disease at diagnosis (metastatic disease unfavorable)
  ✓ Location of primary tumor
• Axial skeleton is unfavorable, due to difficulty obtaining a full resection
• Tumor size (>15 cm is unfavorable)
• Young age (<10 years is unfavorable)
• Histologic response at the time of local control (<90% tumor necrosis is unfavorable)

TREATMENT

• Presurgical (neoadjuvant) chemotherapy: MAP (methotrexate, doxorubicin, cisplatin)
  ✓ Allows evaluation of tumor responsiveness to chemotherapy in a uniform manner, eradication of micrometastases early instead of waiting until postoperative recovery, and demonstrated improvement in outcome.
• Local control: Surgery
  ✓ Removal of all gross and microscopic tumor is essential to prevent local recurrence. Surgical procedures include either amputation or limb-salvage procedures (allografts, vascularized grafts, endoprostheses, rotationplasty)
  ✓ The type of surgical procedure depends on tumor location, size, presence of metastatic disease, age, skeletal development, lifestyle preference, and desired activities.
• Postsurgical (adjuvant) chemotherapy: Additional MAP chemotherapy
• Radiation therapy is generally not indicated in osteosarcoma therapy as it is not a very radiation-sensitive disease.

EWING SARCOMA

EPIDEMIOLOGY

• Most prevalent in adolescents; median age at diagnosis, 15 years
• More common in boys than in girls
• Usually diaphyseal

ETIOLOGY/GENETICS

• t(11;22) is present in about 85% of tumors.

✓ Results in a chimeric EWS-FLI1 transcription product
✓ Detected by reverse transcriptase–polymerase chain reaction and fluorescence in situ hybridization

CLINICAL MANIFESTATIONS

- Pain over involved site with or without associated soft-tissue mass
- Paraspinal tumors can present with spinal-cord compression
- Can have erythema, warmth, or swelling that mimics infection
- Can result in pathologic fracture
- May also have constitutional symptoms, including fever or weight loss

DIAGNOSIS/STAGING

- Biopsy: Open biopsy should be performed by an experienced orthopedic surgeon (ideally should be the surgeon who will later perform definitive surgery).
- Staging:
  ✓ Imaging of primary tumor—For bone primaries, MRI should include both the joint above and the joint below to examine for skip lesions
  ✓ Metastatic evaluation—Chest CT, PET scan (can be done as PET/CT or PET/MRI), bilateral bone marrow aspirates, and biopsies

PROGNOSIS

- Presence of metastatic disease is the most important adverse prognostic factor
- Primary site (pelvis is unfavorable)
- Larger tumor size is unfavorable
- Poor response to initial therapy is unfavorable
- Older age is unfavorable

TREATMENT

- Presurgical (neoadjuvant) chemotherapy: vincristine, doxorubicin, cyclophosphamide alternating with ifosfamide/etoposide every 2 weeks
  ✓ Every patient is assumed to have micrometastatic disease at diagnosis, and the primary treatment involves combination chemotherapy. The goal is to decrease primary tumor volume for immediate control of micrometastatic disease and for eventual local control.
- Local control: Approach depends on the site and whether radiation would cause significant growth or functional difficulty. Each potential site of disease is associated with varied options for surgery and radiotherapy. Final decision balances the need for complete tumor eradication with the goal of maintaining function.
- Postsurgical (adjuvant) chemotherapy: vincristine, doxorubicin, cyclophosphamide alternating with ifosfamide, etoposide every 2 weeks

RHABDOMYOSARCOMA

Tumor derived from primitive mesenchyme that may develop into muscle, fat, fibrous tissue, bone, or cartilage

EPIDEMIOLOGY

- Represents 2–4% of childhood cancers
- Two-thirds of cases diagnosed in children <6 years (largely embryonal histology)
- Small second peak in adolescence (largely alveolar histology)

- Relationship between age at diagnosis and site of primary tumor/histology:
  ✓ Head and neck tumors most common in children <8 years
  ✓ Extremity tumors more common in adolescents and usually alveolar

ETIOLOGY/GENETICS

- Vast majority of cases are sporadic
- Associated syndromes:
  ✓ Neurofibromatosis type I
  ✓ Li-Fraumeni—*p53* mutation, cancer predisposition
  ✓ Costello syndrome (growth retardation, coarse facies, developmental delay)
  ✓ Alveolar disease usually has characteristic translocation: t(2;13)(q35;q14)
    ▪ Fusion of *PAX3* or *PAX7* with *FOXO1*
  ✓ Embryonal disease usually has loss of heterozygosity at 11p15

CLINICAL MANIFESTATIONS

- Disturbance in normal function due to mass effect:
  ✓ Head/neck: Proptosis, ophthalmoplegia, visual disturbance, chronic sinus obstruction
  ✓ Genitourinary tract: Dysuria, hematuria, pain, urinary obstruction, constipation. Testicular disease often presents with painless unilateral enlargement.
  ✓ Extremity: Pain, tenderness, and erythema of the affected limb
  ✓ Other less common sites: Biliary tract, perineal, intrathoracic, retroperitoneal
- Metastatic disease (present in <25% at diagnosis)
  ✓ Lymph nodes, lung, bone/bone marrow are most common sites

DIAGNOSIS/STAGING

- Biopsy and/or up-front surgical resection: If feasible without excessive morbidity
- Staging evaluation:
  ✓ Imaging of primary tumor: CT or MRI
  ✓ Metastatic evaluation: Chest CT, PET scan (can be done as PET/CT or PET/MRI), bilateral bone marrow aspirates and biopsies
- Based on the initial biopsy/surgery, staging evaluation, and histology/molecular studies, a stage and group are determined, which then leads to stratification into low-, intermediate-, or high-risk disease.
- Group: Depends on extent of initial resection
  ✓ I: Complete resection, negative margins
  ✓ II: Microscopic residual tumor
  ✓ III: Gross residual tumor
  ✓ IV: Metastatic disease
- Stage: Depends on primary site, size of primary tumor, and involvement of nodes
  ✓ 1: Favorable site (orbit, superficial head and neck, biliary tree, paratestis, vagina)
  ✓ 2: Unfavorable site, <5 cm, no nodal involvement
  ✓ 3: Unfavorable site and >5 cm OR <5 cm with nodal involvement
  ✓ 4: Metastatic disease

PROGNOSIS

- Most important factors associated with a worse prognosis are metastatic disease at diagnosis and presence of *PAX3/PAX-7-FOXO1* fusion (usually with alveolar histology, but some embryonal histology can also have the fusion)
- Site of primary disease: Favorable vs. unfavorable

- Size of primary tumor: >5 cm is unfavorable
- Older age is unfavorable.

TREATMENT

- Surgery: Preferred for local control unless impaired function or cosmetic result. Up-front aggressive surgery or wide excision should not be used in the female genital tract, orbit, bladder, or biliary tract.
- Chemotherapy: Combination depends on risk group stratification (low, intermediate or high)
  ✓ Most common agents: Vincristine, actinomycin, cyclophosphamide and vincristine, irinotecan
- Radiation therapy: Dose, fractionation, and therapy for certain tumor locations (orbit/cranial tumors) are variable and controversial. In general, radiation therapy is given for patients with large tumors and for those without surgical options for local control.

CENTRAL NERVOUS SYSTEM TUMORS

Approach to the patient with a suspected brain tumor:
- Patients with brain tumors may be asymptomatic, but diagnosis is commonly made after clinical symptoms such as new-onset seizure, intractable headache, persistent nausea or vomiting (especially in the morning), or new-onset focal neurologic symptoms (visual loss, ataxia, confusion, etc.) lead to imaging studies.
- Tumor location will dictate presenting signs and symptoms. Initial care is directed at emergency management of increased intracranial pressure (ICP), spinal-cord compression, respiratory or cardiovascular compromise, if present.

EPIDEMIOLOGY

- Second most common group of all pediatric malignancies (about 20% of total)
- Most common cause of cancer death
- Age: Incidence peaks in first decade
  ✓ Supratentorial tumors: Most common in patients <1 year and >11 years
  ✓ Infratentorial tumors: More common in patients ages 1–11 years
- Risk factors and predisposing conditions:
  ✓ Genetic disorders (<10% of cases): NF-1, NF-2, tuberous sclerosis, von Hippel–Lindau syndrome, Turcot syndrome, Gorlin syndrome, Li–Fraumeni syndrome, Cowden syndrome, retinoblastoma
  ✓ Ionizing radiation immunosuppression: Higher risk of CNS lymphoma in patients with inherited or acquired T-cell dysfunction (CVID, Wiskott–Aldrich syndrome, ataxia–telangiectasia, acquired immunodeficiency syndrome (AIDS), and solid-organ transplant patients)
  Clinical presentation of tumors based on location (**Table 22-3**).
- Supratentorial (cerebrum, basal ganglia, thalamus/hypothalamus, pituitary pineal, optic): Increased ICP, seizures, visual loss, hemiparesis, headache, emesis; new need for glasses; difficulty in school; behavioral difficulty, personality changes; failure to thrive; change in dominant hand; diencephalic syndrome (failure to thrive with increasing appetite and good mood); endocrinopathies such as diabetes insipidus, short stature; Parinaud's syndrome (poor upward gaze, poor pupillary light reflex but normal to accommodation and convergence nystagmus)

TABLE 22-3 Classification of CNS/Spinal Tumors

Cell Type	Tumors	Most Common Locations	Estimated Incidence[*]	Approach to Treatment[*]
Embryonal	Medulloblastoma	Cerebellum	15–20%	Surgery
	PNET	Supratentorial		Radiation (focal/CSI[†])
	Pineoblastoma	Pineal gland	0.5–2%	Chemotherapy
Glial (gliomas)[‡]	Low-grade astrocytoma (pilocytic, fibrillary)	Any site	15–20%	Surgery with or without radiation and chemotherapy
	High-grade astrocytoma (anaplastic/ glioblastoma)		10–12%	Surgery Radiation (focal) Chemotherapy
	Ependymoma		5–10%	Surgery Radiation (focal)
	Oligodendroglioma		1%	Surgery with or without radiation and chemotherapy
	Diffuse midline glioma	Brainstem	10–20%	Radiation (focal)
Choroid plexus	Papilloma Carcinoma	Ventricles	3%	Surgery with or without radiation and chemotherapy (for carcinoma)
Rathke's pouch	Craniopharyngioma	Suprasellar	3–5%	Surgery with or without radiation (focal)
Germ cell	Germinoma	Suprasellar, pineal	4–5%	Surgery (for mature teratoma)
	Nongerminomatous germ-cell tumors			Radiation with or without chemotherapy

[*]For children >15 kg
[†]Do not use for patients with leukemia or lymphoma, stem-cell transplant patients, or patients receiving steroids as part of their treatment regimen.
[‡]For children >12 years and >40 kg; also requires that concurrent dexamethasone dose be decreased by 50%.
CI = Craniospinal irradiation.

- Infratentorial (cerebellum, brain stem): Ataxia, clumsiness, worsening handwriting, dysarthria; nystagmus; head tilt; cranial nerve palsy; increased ICP from ventricular compression (morning headache and vomiting); extreme vomiting if near area postrema
- Nonspecific signs and symptoms: Change in activity level, change in appetite with associated weight gain or loss, delayed or precocious puberty, macrocephaly in infants, vomiting, complaints consistent with spinal cord involvement such as back pain or bowel/bladder dysfunction (see "Oncologic Emergencies" section)

DIAGNOSTICS

- Initial imaging: CT scan of brain with and without contrast (useful as a quick screen, especially in unstable patients) evaluates ventricular size, midline shift, and hemorrhage; inadequate for anatomic detail and often misses smaller tumors or those in the posterior fossa
- Primary site imaging: Brain MRI with gadolinium
- Biopsy: Surgical biopsy for histologic diagnosis is critical prior to treatment except in cases of diffuse midline gliomas, visual pathway gliomas (in children with NF-1), and tectal gliomas, which are diagnosed from neuroimaging findings and in cases of elevated β-hCG and α-fetoprotein.
- Metastatic evaluation:
  - ✓ Spinal MRI to evaluate for drop metastases/leptomeningeal spread (sometimes seen in PNET, medulloblastoma, germ-cell tumors, ependymoma, GBM)
  - ✓ Lumbar puncture (only after scan and evaluation for increased intracranial pressure) for glucose, protein, culture, cytology, and markers such as α-fetoprotein and β-hCG
  - ✓ Bone marrow aspirate/biopsy for some PNETs
- Note that neuro-oncology is moving away from strict morphologic classification of tumors to molecular subdivision of tumors (e.g., medulloblastomas are divided according to which molecular pathway is activated or mutated).

MANAGEMENT

- Initial management: Increased ICP, respiratory or cardiovascular dysfunction managed with involvement of neurosurgical and critical care services.
- Tumor-directed therapy: Approach is based on biologic potential of tumor and method of spread (see **Table 12–3**). In general, tumors with higher biologic potential require therapy directed at the entire neuroaxis (e.g., craniospinal irradiation/chemotherapy) and those with lower biologic potential or only local invasion may be treated with surgery or local radiation therapy alone.
- Observation: Some benign tumors, such as optic pathway/hypothalamic gliomas can remain stable for years and can be monitored with surveillance imaging, opting for treatment for visual decline or significant tumor progression
- Surgery: Balance preservation of function and maximization of tumor removal. For some tumors (juvenile pilocytic astrocytoma), surgery alone is adequate therapy. Diffuse tumors are not amenable to complete resection, but biopsy and identification of the tumor are often critical and may be achieved using CT- or MRI-guided stereotactic surgical techniques.
- Chemotherapy: Used in combination and specific to tumor type
  - ✓ Presence of the blood–brain barrier is an obstacle to effective therapy, although this may be disrupted in the setting of active neoplasm.
  - ✓ Active agents include alkylating agents (cyclophosphamide, ifosfamide, thiotepa, cisplatin, carboplatin, and temozolomide), antimetabolites (methotrexate), and plant alkaloids (vincristine, etoposide)
  - ✓ For aggressive or recurrent tumors, high-dose chemotherapy with stem-cell rescue has been used
  - ✓ Use of chemotherapy has enabled a decrease in the doses of radiation, reducing late effects to the developing brain.
- Radiation therapy
  - ✓ Aimed at tumor bed and/or craniospinal area for spread or prophylaxis
  - ✓ Proton-beam therapy (versus traditional photon) is being used increasingly in children for its precise targeting and potential for fewer late effects.

✓ Age, comorbidities, and balance of early and late toxicity must be considered.
✓ Radiation is used most commonly in medulloblastoma, PNET, ependymoma, high-grade gliomas, diffuse midline gliomas, and germ-cell tumors.
- Newer methods
  ✓ Antiangiogenic agents are part of many therapies now
  ✓ Other promising agents under investigation include differentiating agents (*cis*-retinoic acid, histone-deacetylase inhibitors), MEK inhibitors, tyrosine kinase inhibitors, other molecular targets (e.g. signal transduction pathways), and immunotherapy (vaccine-based immunotherapy, immune checkpoint modulation),
- Treating most brain tumors requires an experienced, multidisciplinary team, including a pediatric neurosurgeon, oncologist, radiation oncologist, neurocognitive specialist, endocrinologist, and neuro-ophthalmologist.

PRINCIPLES OF SUPPORTIVE CARE

INFECTIOUS PROPHYLAXIS

- Bacterial prophylaxis
  ✓ *P. jirovecii* pneumonia (PCP): Patients receiving chemotherapy or other forms of immunosuppressive therapy are at risk for PCP
  ✓ Most effective prophylactic agent is cotrimoxazole (sulfamethoxazole–trimethoprim), usually given twice a day, 2 days per week
  ✓ Other agents available include dapsone, aerosolized pentamidine (IV for patients <5 years old), and atovaquone, but are not as effective as cotrimoxazole.
  ✓ PCP prophylaxis is typically continued for 3 months after therapy completion or longer (12 months) in stem-cell transplantation patients
  ✓ *Streptococcus mitis:* Patients with a history of *S. mitis* require prophylaxis with future periods of neutropenia, typically with clindamycin, vancomycin, or the narrowest-spectrum antibiotic to which their strain of *S. mitis* was sensitive.
  ✓ Other: Patients with expected periods of profound/prolonged neutropenia (AML, relapsed ALL, stem-cell transplantation) should receive levofloxacin while neutropenic.
- Fungal prophylaxis
  ✓ Increased risk of fungal infection associated with prolonged/profound neutropenia (AML, relapsed ALL, stem-cell transplantation) or profound lymphopenia (transplant patients with GVHD, alemtuzumab exposure, etc.)
  ✓ Patients at high risk for fungal infections should receive an antifungal agent, such as fluconazole or caspofungin, while neutropenic.
- Viral prophylaxis
  ✓ Stem-cell transplantation patients are at risk for viral reactivation and may require CMV, HSV, and/or VZV prophylaxis based on pretransplantation serologies.
- Growth factor support
  ✓ Patients with solid tumors or lymphoma should be given subcutaneous pegfilgrastim (Neulasta) 24–48 hours after completing highly myelosuppressive chemotherapy cycles
  ✓ Daily filgrastim (Neupogen) can be considered in patients with leukemia who are at very high risk for severe sepsis during periods of neutropenia.

MUCOSITIS

Any rapidly dividing cell, like gastrointestinal or oral mucosa, can suffer effects of chemotherapy and break down, become ulcerated or inflamed causing mucositis.

Doxorubicin, daunorubicin, methotrexate, and cytarabine are most commonly associated with mucositis.

SIGNS AND SYMPTOMS

- Pain, drooling, dysphagia, abdominal pain, diarrhea, melena, or hematochezia
- Mucositis can interfere with adequate oral hydration and also create an entry point for infectious agents
  - ✓ Patients receiving high-dose cytarabine or who have undergone HSCT are at particularly high risk for a mucositis-related infection, including S. mitis, which can cause life-threatening sepsis.

TREATMENT

- Debridement with sponges dabbed in sterile saline
- Analgesia with "magic mouthwash" (2% viscous lidocaine, liquid Maalox, and liquid diphenhydramine) every 4 to 6 hours
- Oral mucositis can also be complicated or worsened by oral thrush, so an antifungal agent (nystatin or fluconazole) may be indicated.
- Treatment methods for anal mucositis: Stool softeners, creams applied to the anal verge (nystatin cream, zinc oxide)
- Mucositis can cause significant discomfort and patients may require IV fluids, parenteral nutrition, or IV opioid therapy.

NAUSEA AND VOMITING

GENERAL PRINCIPLES

- Nausea and vomiting can be induced by chemotherapy and radiation.
- Consequences include dehydration, electrolyte imbalance, anorexia, weight loss, and increased susceptibility to infections.
- Chemotherapy-induced nausea and vomiting (CINV) is defined by when it occurs:
  - ✓ Acute: Occurs within the first 24 hours after receiving chemotherapy
  - ✓ Delayed: Occurs >24 hours after administration and can persist up to 1 week after therapy (common with platinum-based chemotherapy)
  - ✓ Breakthrough CINV: Defined as more than three episodes of emesis or retching within 24 hours and occurs despite proper prophylaxis
  - ✓ Anticipatory CINV: A preconditioned emetic response often related to anxiety surrounding treatments due to prior poor control of nausea/emesis; can also be triggered by tastes, odor, or sights

EMETOGENICITY AND TREATMENT GUIDELINES

- Emetogenicity varies among commonly used chemotherapeutic agents (**Table 22-4**).
  - ✓ If multiple chemotherapeutic agents or radiation are given on a single day, the emetogenicity is generally classified based on the most highly emetogenic agent.
  - ✓ If multiple days of chemotherapy are being given consecutively, the emetogenicity is generally classified by the most highly emetogenic agent given each day of therapy.
- For patients receiving emetogenic chemotherapy, scheduled antiemetics are often required as prophylaxis. Additional agents are used as needed for breakthrough nausea or emesis. (**Table 22-5**).
  - ✓ Other agents that can be considered in patients with severe or refractory nausea include cannabinoids (e.g., dronabinol), olanzapine, metoclopramide, and hydroxyzine.

TABLE 22-4	Emetogenic Potential of Each Drug in the Chemotherapy Regimen or by the Site of Radiation		
Minimal	**Low**	**Moderate**	**High**
<10% frequency of emesis in absence of prophylaxis	10–30% frequency of emesis in absence of prophylaxis	30–90% frequency of emesis in absence of prophylaxis	>90% frequency of emesis in absence of prophylaxis
Alemtuzumab	Cytarabine (<200 mg/m2)	Busulfan	Carboplatin
Asparaginase		Carmustine (low dose)	Carmustine
Bevacizumab	Etoposide (oral)	Clofarabine	Cisplatin
Bleomycin	Fludarabine (oral)	Cyclophosphamide (low dose)	Cyclophosphamide (>1 g/m2)
Cladribine	5-Fluorouracil	Daunorubicin	Cytarabine (>3 g/m2)
Dasatinib	Gemcitabime	Doxorubicin	Dactinomycin
Dexrazoxane	Mitoxantrone	Etoposide	Methotrexate (>12 g/m2)
Erlotinib	Nilotinib	Idarubicin	
Gemtuzumab	Paclitaxel	Ifosfamide	Procarbazine
Hydroxyurea	Thiotepa (<300 mg/m2)	Imatinib	Thiotepa
Lenalidomide	Topotecan	Intrathecal therapy	Total body irradiation
Nelarabine		Irinotecan	Brain/Craniospinal radiation
Rituximab		Methotrexate (<12 g/m2)	Abdominopelvic radiaion
Sorafenib		Temozolomide	
Temsirolimus		Vinorelbine	
Thioguanine			
Vinblastine			
Vincristine			
6-Mercaptopurine			

Data from Hesketh PJ: Defining the emetogenicity of cancer chemotherapy regimens: relevance to clinical practice, *Oncologist* 1999;4(3):191–196; and Basch E, Prestrud AA, Hesketh PJ, et al: Antiemetics: American Society of Clinical Oncology clinical practice guideline update, *J Clin Oncol*. 2011 Nov 1;29(31):4189–4198.

- Bone marrow transplantation patients usually receive antiemetics until 24 hours after the last dose of chemotherapy or irradiation.
- Antiemetic regimens are often institution-specific, so consult the formulary at your treating center for dosing guidelines.

NUTRITIONAL SUPPORT

- Malnutrition is common in oncology patients and is often multifactorial. It may consist of
  ✓ Decreased intake, poor absorption, increased caloric losses, and/or increased metabolic demand.
- Malnutrition is associated with increased risk of infection, prolonged hospitalization, and poorer outcomes.
- When supplemental nutrition is required, the enteral route is preferred. May start with oral nutrition supplements, but many children require tube feedings via nasogastric or other routes.

TABLE 22-5	Sample Antiemetic Regimens	
Emetogenicity of Regimen	**Prophylactic Antiemetics (Prescribed "Around the Clock" or Scheduled)**	**Breakthrough Antiemetics (Prescribed to Use as Needed)**
Low (e.g., vincristine)	None	5-hydroxytryptamine antagonist (ondansetron, granisetron)
Moderate (e.g., doxorubicin + vincristine)	5-HT3 antagonist (ondansetron, granisetron) Scopolamine transdermal patch*	Lorazepam Diphenhydramine with or without promethazine
High (e.g., ifosfamide + etoposide)	5-HT3 antagonist (ondansetron, granisetron) Scopolamine transdermal patch* Dexamethasone†	Lorazepam Diphenhydramine with or without promethazine
Very High (e.g. Cisplatin + doxorubicin)	5-HT3 antagonist (ondansetron, granisetron) Scopolamine transdermal patch* Dexamethasone† Aprepitant‡	Lorazepam Diphenhydramine with or without promethazine Consider: dronabinol, olanzapine, metoclopramide, vistaril

*For children >15 kg.
†Do not use for patients with leukemia or lymphoma, stem-cell transplant patients, or patients receiving steroids as part of their treatment regimen.
‡For children >12 years and >40 kg; also requires that concurrent dexamethasone dose be decreased by 50%.
$5\text{-HT}_3 = 5\text{-hydroxytryptamine}$.

✓ Can also consider starting appetite stimulants (e.g., dronabinol, megestrol acetate)
- Placing a gastrostomy tube for nutritional and medication delivery purposes may be beneficial in certain patients (where radiation or severe mucositis may impair eating/taking medications)
- Total parenteral nutrition is less favored, but may be necessary for weight maintenance.
- Being overweight has also been associated with poor outcomes, so maintaining a healthy weight is critical.

PAIN

Somatic or Visceral Pain

- Typically managed with opioid therapy, as antiinflammatory medications like ibuprofen, which can affect platelet function, are contraindicated in patients with actual or expected thrombocytopenia
- Begin with oral regimens and proceed to IV as needed, following the World Health Organization two-step opioid ladder, with some patients requiring a PCA device.
- Proper bowel regimens (stool softeners plus cathartic agents) are required for patients being started on opioid therapy to prevent significant constipation associated with opioid use (which is, of note, the only side effect of opioids to which patients do not become tolerant).

Neuropathic Pain

- Neuropathic pain is a common side effect of several chemotherapy and immunotherapy regimens.

- Gamma-aminobutyric acid analogs like gabapentin and pregabalin are helpful for these symptoms, but require a slow titration to be effective.
- Depending on the length of pain therapy, a slow taper off of the medication may be required.

PSYCHOSOCIAL AND PSYCHIATRIC SUPPORT

- Patients with cancer are at increased risk of psychological distress, including anxiety, adjustment disorder, and depression. They are also more likely to experience sleep disturbances as a result of treatment factors, hospitalizations, medication side effects, and psychosocial stressors.
- Appropriate attention should be paid to addressing these symptoms and their management. Consultation with psychosocial support teams and child life staff is prudent and can be beneficial. Some children and adolescents benefit from pharmacologic intervention (e.g., selective serotonin-reuptake inhibitors)

TRANSFUSION

- There is wide variation in practice, so there may be institutional or disease-specific guidelines available. Patients with clinical indications for blood products (bleeding, anemia, gallops, etc.) should be transfused at the discretion of the treating provider.

Packed Red-Cell Transfusions

- Typically indicated if the patient is symptomatic from anemia or the hemoglobin is <7–8 g/dL
- Ensure that all blood products are irradiated and leuko-reduced;
- For a CMV-negative or pre– or post–bone marrow transplantation patient, blood should also be CMV antibody–negative.

Platelets

- Transfusion of platelets is typically indicated when platelet counts are $<10,000/mm^3$ or there is active bleeding
- In bone marrow transplantation or neuro-oncology patients with residual tumor, or children with bleeding symptoms, higher platelet thresholds are typically followed.
- Platelets should be $>30,000/mm^3$ for lumbar puncture.
- Prior to neurosurgical procedures or other procedures with significant bleeding risk, platelet goal should be over $50,000/mm^3$.
- There is no widely accepted platelet requirement for bone marrow aspirate or biopsy.

Special Situations

- Patients at risk for hyperviscosity syndrome (new diagnosis of leukemia with elevated WBC $>100,000/mm^3$) should be transfused only after discussion with oncologist, given high risk of vascular sludging and sequelae (stroke, pulmonary failure, cardiac dysfunction).
- Patients on concurrent anticoagulation for history of thrombosis are typically maintained at platelet count of at least $20,000$–$50,000/mm^3$.
- Provision of fresh-frozen plasma, cryoprecipitate, or vitamin K may be required for correction of severe coagulopathy in specific cases (e.g., preoperative or in disseminated intravascular coagulation associated with APML) but is not a standard practice in all patients.

VACCINATION

- Aside from the yearly inactivated influenza vaccine, routine immunizations should be deferred in all patients undergoing cancer chemotherapy.

- Revaccination should not begin until at least 6 months after therapy is complete, and longer (at least 8 months) after allogeneic stem-cell transplantation.

VASCULAR ACCESS

- Patients undergoing treatment for chemotherapy usually require indwelling central lines.
- Peripheral IVs should not be used to administer certain chemotherapeutic agents, given concerns for subcutaneous extravasation into skin or joints.
- Peripherally inserted central catheters (PICCs) can provide continuous access but are less favored than subcutaneous ports (Port-a-cath) or tunneled central venous lines (Broviac, Hickman) because of the increased risks for infection and thrombosis.
- The choice of line depends on diagnosis and treatment protocol (based on type and rate of administration of chemotherapy and supportive care requirements), as well as planned future care (stem-cell transplantation, etc.).

OTHER SUPPORTIVE CARE CONSIDERATIONS

Venous Thromboembolism (VTE) Prophylaxis

- Patients receiving cancer therapy are at risk for developing VTEs (including extremity deep-vein thromboses and pulmonary embolisms) because of active malignancy and indwelling central catheters. Other VTE risk factors include mediastinal mass, certain chemotherapeutic agents (e.g., asparaginase), age >12 years, obesity, and altered mobility.
- During hospital admissions, patients should be encouraged to maintain their highest degree of mobility and use mechanical prophylaxis with sequential compression devices while in bed.
- For patients at highest risk for VTE (e.g., adolescent with newly diagnosed T-ALL with mediastinal mass and PICC line in place), pharmacologic prophylaxis should be strongly considered.
  ✓ Enoxaparin is generally used for first-line prophylaxis. Current clinical trials are evaluating the role of direct-acting oral anticoagulants (e.g., apixaban) for VTE prophylaxis in pediatric oncology patients.

Fertility Preservation

- Children, adolescents and young adults receiving cancer treatment are at risk of infertility secondary to therapy (chemotherapy like alkylating agents and radiation therapy).
- At the time of diagnosis, sperm banking should be offered to males who are at least a Tanner stage III, regardless of the gonadotoxicity of their planned treatment.
  ✓ Sperm banking should be done prior to initiating cytotoxic therapies.
- For females, there is a larger risk of premature ovarian failure (though some risk of acute ovarian failure depending on the therapy). Ovarian tissue cryopreservation should be considered, but this does necessitate a delay in initiating therapy.

LATE EFFECTS OF CANCER TREATMENT

- Over 80% of children diagnosed with cancer become long-term survivors. However, childhood cancer survivors are at risk for developing late toxicities of their cancer therapy (**Table 22-6**).
- Late effects are medical conditions that are the direct effects of the cancer diagnosis or treatment. Childhood cancer survivors should receive multidisciplinary, long-term follow-up care in a specialized survivorship program. At entry into a survivorship program, patients should receive the following:

TABLE 22-6	Representative Late Effects According to Cancer Treatment Exposures	
Late Effects by System	**Cancer Treatment Exposure**	**Additional Risk Factors/Other Notes**
Auditory ○ Hearing loss	• Cisplatin	
Cardiac ○ Cardiomyopathy ○ Early atherosclerosis	• Anthracyclines, dose-dependent • Radiation (mediastinal, chest)	• Younger age at diagnosis • Female gender • Other cardiac risk factors: obesity, hypertension, hyperlipidemia
Endocrine ○ Growth hormone deficiency ○ Obesity ○ Luteinizing hormone/follicle-stimulating hormone deficiency ○ Diabetes mellitus ○ Hypothyroidism, hyperthyroidism, thyroid nodules	• Radiation (cranial, thyroid, total body, or abdominal)	
Neurocognitive ○ Decreased IQ ○ Executive functioning	• Radiation (cranial) • Intrathecal therapy	• Important to screen for school performance issues
Psychosocial ○ Anxiety, depression ○ Posttraumatic stress disorder	• Any exposure	
Pulmonary ○ Pulmonary fibrosis	• Bleomycin • Radiation (mediastinal, chest)	• Risk further increased with tobacco use
Reproductive ○ Hypospermia/azoospermia ○ Hypogonadism ○ Premature ovarian failure	• Alkylating agents, dose-dependent • Radiation (testicular, pelvic, total body)	
Renal ○ Chronic kidney disease	• Heavy metals • Alkylating agents • Stem cell transplant	
Subsequent Malignant Neoplasms ○ Leukemia or myelodysplastic syndrome (MDS) ○ Thyroid cancer ○ Osteosarcoma ○ Skin cancers ○ Breast cancer	• Etoposide • Alkylating agents • Radiation	• Chemotherapy induced leukemia (with MDS) usually occurs within 5–10 years after finishing treatment • Therapy induced solid tumors can occur many years of treatment
Visual ○ Cataracts	• Radiation • Corticosteroids	

For additional information and screening recommendations, refer to the Children's Oncology Group Long-Term Follow-Up Guidelines for Survivors of Childhood, Adolescent and Young Adult Cancers, Version 4.0: http://www.survivorshipguidelines.org/

✓ Treatment summary: Lists details of diagnosis and treatments, including medications with doses, surgeries, and radiation with location and doses.

✓ Survivorship care plan: A personalized plan for long-term follow-up care that recommends visits, labs, and other screening tests based on cancer diagnosis and treatment received.

- Customized care plans can be created at the following link: https://smartalacc.onco-link.org/

23 Ophthalmology

Gil Binenbaum, MD, MSCE
Stefanie L. Davidson, MD

OCULAR EXPOSURE

The surface of the eye needs to stay well lubricated or it can lead to vision-threatening complications in the ICU

PATHOPHYSIOLOGY

- Normal ocular surface protective mechanisms include tear production, intact corneal sensation, blinking, and complete eyelid closure.
- Impaired protective mechanisms result in corneal exposure and drying.
- Corneal "dryness" (subclinical epithelial breakdown) may progress to corneal abrasion, ulceration, infection, scarring, thinning, and/or perforation if untreated.

CLINICAL MANIFESTATIONS

- Risk factors for corneal exposure include loss of protective mechanisms due to deep sedation, neurologic impairment, or eyelid abnormality; overhead warmers; and treatments causing air to blow over the eyes.
- Risk increases with poor eyelid closure: Low risk with eyelids that close completely, increasing with white sclera showing, highest with cornea or underlying iris showing.
- Eye exam may reveal conjunctival redness or swelling, corneal haze or opacity, or blunted red reflex.

DIAGNOSTICS

- Slit lamp biomicroscopic exam and fluorescein staining may reveal punctate erosions, corneal abrasion, opacity (ulcer), thinning, or perforation

MANAGEMENT

- Prophylaxis for at-risk patients (e.g., intubated and sedated) is critical:
  - ✓ Lubricating eye ointment (Lacri-lube ointment which consists of mineral oil and white petrolatum); frequency determined according to eyelid position
  - ✓ Closed lids every 12 hours, sclera showing every 6 hours, cornea showing every 2 hours; the frequency of ointment administration may be reduced if the eye and ointment are then covered with a piece of nonsticky plastic wrap (e.g., Saran wrap) to form a "moisture chamber."
  - ✓ Artificial tear drops evaporate quickly and are not useful.
- Prompt ophthalmology consultation for red conjunctiva, corneal haze or opacity, or if the cornea is visible due to incomplete eyelid exposure in an at-risk patient
- Antibiotic ophthalmic ointment (erythromycin, Polysporin) if there is corneal epithelial staining with fluorescein
- Complicated cases may require tarsorrhaphy (suturing of eyelids), bandage contact lens, corneal gluing, or emergent corneal transplantation

CORNEAL CLOUDING AND GLAUCOMA

The cornea should always be clear, with visible iris details and a bright red reflex. Any opacity, whether diffuse or focal, is a sign of serious eye disease. Glaucoma is irreversible optic-nerve damage due to increased intraocular pressure.

DIFFERENTIAL DIAGNOSIS OF CORNEAL CLOUDING IN AN INFANT

- Trauma: Forceps injury, corneal perforation with amniocentesis
- Infection: Syphilis, rubella, herpes simplex virus (HSV), bacterial ulcer
- Infantile glaucoma: Associated with enlarged eye (buphthalmos)
- Corneal or limbal dermoid, associated with Goldenhar syndrome
- Anterior segment dysgenesis: Peters anomaly (central corneal opacity), sclerocornea
- Corneal dystrophy: Congenital hereditary endothelial dystrophy, congenital hereditary stromal dystrophy
- Metabolic: Mucopolysaccharidoses type I. (Hurler syndrome) [MPS -IH]; T type IV, muco-lipidoses), cystinosis, tyrosinemia

EPIDEMIOLOGY AND ETIOLOGY

Primary Glaucoma

- Primary infantile glaucoma (congenital glaucoma): 1 in 10,000 to 1 in 15,000; 90% sporadic
- Caused by developmental defect in the structure of the anterior chamber
- Associated systemic syndromes, including Sturge–Weber, neurofibromatosis type 1, Marfan, Stickler, Lowe, Rubinstein–Taybi, Wolf–Hirschhorn
- Also associated with ocular syndromes such as aniridia, Peters anomaly

Secondary Glaucomas

- Secondary glaucomas of childhood are more common than primary glaucomas
- Traumatic: Acute glaucoma related to a hyphema (see "Hyphema" section) or glaucoma years after trauma secondary to damage of drainage angle in the eye (angle recession)
- Inflammatory: Caused by trabecular meshwork inflammation or clogging with inflamma-tory debris; for example, uveitis associated with juvenile idiopathic arthritis
- Steroid-induced: Can be caused by topical, systemic, or inhaled forms of glucocorticoids, by decreasing aqueous outflow
- Aphakic: Absence of the natural lens usually due to cataract extraction; 8–41% chance of developing glaucoma
- Intraocular neoplasms such as retinoblastoma, juvenile xanthogranuloma

PATHOPHYSIOLOGY

- Intraocular pressure (IOP) is maintained by the balance of aqueous humor production by the ciliary body and drainage by the trabecular meshwork.
- When this drainage system is impaired, IOP increases.
- Elevated IOP causes loss of the nerve fiber layer of the retina, optic nerve damage, and, if left untreated, irreversible blindness.

CLINICAL MANIFESTATIONS

- Children with congenital glaucom <3 years of age present with enlarged eye (buphthal-mos), photophobia, epiphora (tearing), blepharospasm (repetitive involuntary closure of the lids), and cloudy cornea (corneal edema).

- Children >3 years of age may have completely asymptomatic glaucoma until advanced, irreversible visual loss occurs.
- Check ocular size (typically by measuring corneal diameter, see "Diagnostics" section), corneal clarity, and visual acuity.
- Haab's striae: Breaks in Descemet's membrane (basement membrane of the cornea) that occur as the cornea enlarges. Typically seen as horizontal lines in the cornea and develop in children <3 years old.
- Cupping of the optic nerve: Cup:disc ratio >0.4 is suggestive of glaucoma.
- Look for evidence of associated syndromes.

DIAGNOSTICS

- Tonometry: Pressure >21 mmHg in a calm infant is abnormal.
- Gonioscopy: Visually assess the angle anatomy.
- Measure corneal diameter and axial length to follow response to treatment: Normal corneal diameter is 9.5–10.5 mm in newborns and 11–12 mm in adults.

MANAGEMENT

- Ophthalmologist should be consulted on all patients with a clinical suspicion of glaucoma or with any corneal opacity, regardless of concern for glaucoma.

Medical

- Topical Therapy
  - ✓ Beta-blocker (e.g., timolol maleate twice a day) is a common first-line agent.
  - ✓ Initial IOP >30 mmHg or insufficient lowering of IOP to <21 mmHg requires addition of a carbonic anhydrase inhibitor (e.g., dorzolamide or brinzolamide 2–3 times daily) and/or prostaglandin (latanoprost once daily).
- Oral therapy: Acetazolamide for highly or persistently elevated IOP
- Duration of therapy is lifelong unless surgery is performed.

Surgical

- Primary congenital glaucoma is a surgical disease.
- 80% of children can be cured with
  - ✓ Goniotomy: An incision is made in the trabecular meshwork with a blade inserted into the anterior chamber. Improves trabecular outflow and reduces IOP. Can be performed only if the cornea is clear.
  - ✓ Trabeculotomy ab externo: External dissection of Schlemm's canal to increase exit of aqueous fluid. Can be done even if corneal is cloudy (corneal edema).
  - ✓ When primary infantile glaucoma fails above surgeries and other types of glaucomas fail medical management then:
    - ▪ Trabeculectomy: Filtration procedure creating a communication between the anterior chamber and subconjunctival space to allow drainage of aqueous
    - ▪ Glaucoma drainage device: Similar purpose to trabeculectomy but uses an implant
    - ▪ Photocyclocoagulation and cyclocryotherapy: Destroys the ciliary body, thereby reducing production of aqueous fluid; usually a last resort

ABNORMAL RED REFLEX AND LEUKOCORIA

Red reflex testing should be done routinely on all newborns, infants, and young children as part of a complete physical examination. "Leukocoria" is from Greek meaning "white pupil."

EPIDEMIOLOGY

- Congenital cataracts are the most common cause of leukocoria, occurring in 1 in 2500 live births.
- Retinoblastoma occurs in 1 in 15,000 people; extremely rare after 6 years of age.

DIFFERENTIAL DIAGNOSIS

- Cataract (lens opacity) may result in permanent vision loss if not treated early.
- Retinoblastoma is life threatening and the most concerning diagnosis.
- Advanced retinopathy of prematurity and retinal detachment
- Strabismus will cause asymmetric red reflexes.
- High refractive errors cause blunted red reflex.
- Other ocular disorders include retinal dysplasia (developmental anomaly, present at birth), coloboma (missing piece of tissue in the eye, such as a chorioretinal or optic nerve head coloboma), and Coats disease (retinal vascular abnormalities and lipid exudates).

PATHOPHYSIOLOGY

- The vascular choroid behind the retina reflects light, forming the normal "red reflex."
- Light passes through the cornea, aqueous humor, pupil, lens, and vitreous to get to the retina. Interference by any of these structures may lead to a diminished, irregular, absent, white, or asymmetric red reflex.

CLINICAL MANIFESTATIONS

- Red reflex exam: Use a direct ophthalmoscope an arm's length from the infant's eyes in a dark room.
  - ✓ A normal exam shows clear, bilaterally symmetric reflexes with equal color, intensity, and clarity.
  - ✓ Any white spots, opacities, or asymmetry are abnormal and require evaluation.
  - ✓ Darker pigmented children will have reflexes that appear darker.

DIAGNOSTICS

- A patient with abnormal or asymmetric red reflexes or leukocoria urgently requires a full eye exam, including a dilated fundus examination by an ophthalmologist.
- Ocular ultrasound by an ophthalmologist and MRI of the eye provide additional evaluation for retinoblastoma when necessary.

MANAGEMENT

- Depends on etiology
- Congenital cataracts are typically surgically removed by 4–6 weeks of age and require ongoing amblyopia treatment.
- Retinoblastoma treatment is begun immediately because mortality is tied to spread of disease; untreated children will die from extension to the brain.
- Children with bilateral congenital cataracts may require evaluation for congenital infections (toxoplasma, rubella, cytomegalovirus, and herpes simplex virus [TORCH]), metabolic diseases, and chromosomal abnormalities.

UVEITIS

Intraocular inflammation of the uveal tract (iris, ciliary body, choroid)

CAUSES

- Idiopathic
- Systemic inflammatory disorders: Juvenile idiopathic arthritis (JIA) (especially pauciarticular, ANA-positive, rheumatoid factor–negative), sarcoidosis, Behçet's disease, inflammatory bowel disease, HLA-B27 associated disease
- Infection: Lyme disease, HSV, CMV, HIV, TB, toxoplasmosis, *Toxocara*, syphilis
- Tubular interstitial nephritis and uveitis (TINU)
- Trauma
- Neoplasm (masquerade syndrome): Retinoblastoma, leukemia, lymphoma

DIFFERENTIAL DIAGNOSIS

- Conjunctivitis or extraocular inflammation does not affect corneal or red reflex clarity.
- Key warning signs that a red eye is not a simple conjunctivitis: Vision loss, photophobia, eye pain, eye surgery, contact lens use, chronic (>2 weeks), hyperpurulent discharge, corneal opacity, irregular pupil, poor red reflex, vesicles on lids

CLINICAL MANIFESTATIONS

- Symptoms: Photophobia, pain, redness, decrease in vision, floaters
- Children may be completely asymptomatic (no conjunctival redness, no pain), especially with JIA
- Signs: Conjunctival injection, corneal endothelial deposits, anterior chamber cells, hypopyon (grossly visible collection of white cells behind the cornea), irregular pupil from synechiae (scarring between iris and lens behind it), blunted red reflex, inflammatory lesions on fundus exam

DIAGNOSTICS

- Diagnosis is made visually by slit-lamp biomicroscopic and fundus examinations.
- Laboratory and radiographic workup for recurrent, bilateral, or posterior uveitis or suspicion of systemic disease

MANAGEMENT

- Uveitis is a site-threatening condition requiring diagnosis and management by an ophthalmologist, often jointly with a pediatric rheumatologist.
- Aggressive control of intraocular inflammation with topical steroids (e.g., prednisolone acetate 1% every hour until inflammation is controlled)
  - ✓ Systemic steroids if topical steroids do not adequately control the inflammation or if the posterior structures of the eye are involved
  - ✓ Steroid-sparing immunosuppressive agents (e.g., methotrexate, infliximab) if oral steroids cannot be tapered off without recurrence of uveitis
- Cycloplegic eyedrops (e.g., atropine) while active inflammation is present
- Antibiotics as indicated for infectious causes

HYPHEMA

Blood in the anterior chamber of the eye

EPIDEMIOLOGY

- Annual incidence of 17–20 per 100,000; mostly younger than 20 years old

PATHOPHYSIOLOGY

- Blunt or penetrating trauma damages iris blood vessels, causing blood to leak into the anterior chamber with potential to increase IOP
- Bleeding stops when a clot forms.
- Rebleeding risk is highest during first 5 days post-trauma, when the clot weakens, and can result in pressure spike.
- Spontaneous (nontraumatic) hyphema may be caused by intraocular tumors.

CLINICAL MANIFESTATIONS

- Patients present with a history of eye trauma, eye pain, and vision loss.
- Children may be somnolent.
- Some patients have history of bleeding disorders, sickle cell disease, or anticoagulation therapy.
- Blood in the anterior chamber appears as a red or dark meniscus in the aqueous humor behind the cornea and in front of the iris.

DIAGNOSTICS

- Small hyphemas may be seen only with the magnification best provided by a slit-lamp biomicroscope.
- Assess visual acuity and IOP
- Rule out an open-globe injury (see below).
- Sickle cell testing for African Americans, because patients with sickle cell trait or disease are at much greater risk for acute glaucoma with hyphema.

MANAGEMENT

- Ophthalmologist should be consulted for all patients with hyphema.
- Prevent rebleeding with the following measures:
  - ✓ Bed rest
  - ✓ Avoid NSAIDs
  - ✓ Protect the eye with a plastic or metal shield, which covers but does not touch the eye. Do not apply gauze patches, as these touch the eye.
- Admission and/or sedation may be required for young, active children.
- Topical mydriatics (e.g., atropine 1% twice per day) and topical steroids (prednisolone acetate 1% four times per day)
- Glaucoma medications for elevated IOP (see "Glaucoma Management" section, but note that topical and systemic carbonic anhydrase inhibitors are relatively contraindicated in sickle cell or sickle trait–positive patients with hyphema).
- Consider surgical intervention if elevated IOP is unresponsive to medications, in patients with sickle cell disease, and with corneal blood staining.
- Surgical procedures: Anterior chamber washout and clot removal

ORBITAL FRACTURE

Fracture of one or more of the orbital bones due to trauma, including from assault, falls, motor vehicle accidents, and sports

DIFFERENTIAL DIAGNOSIS

- Bruised extraocular muscles, cranial nerve palsy, and orbital edema all present with double vision
- Eye trauma may result in open globe injury, hyphema, retinal detachment, vitreous hemorrhage, lens dislocation or cataract, and/or choroidal rupture.

PATHOPHYSIOLOGY

- The orbit is composed of seven bones: Maxilla, zygoma, lacrimal, ethmoid, palatine, sphenoid, and frontal. The walls are thin; the rims are thick.
- Most fractures occur in the medial wall or posteromedial floor, near the infraorbital groove, which contains the infraorbital nerve (V2), providing sensation to the cheek and upper alveolus/teeth (**Figure 23-1**).
- Extraocular muscle may become entrapped in a fracture, causing oculocardiac reflex (vagal nerve)–induced bradycardia.
- OPEN GLOBE INJURIES (full thickness hole in the wall of the eye) may result from penetrating trauma (laceration) or blunt trauma (ruptured globe), in which increased IOP causes a scleral break and may not be accompanied by an orbital fracture.
- Extensive retrobulbar (orbital) hemorrhage with orbital fracture may cause an orbital compartment syndrome and ischemic injury to the optic nerve and retina; *this is an ocular emergency.*

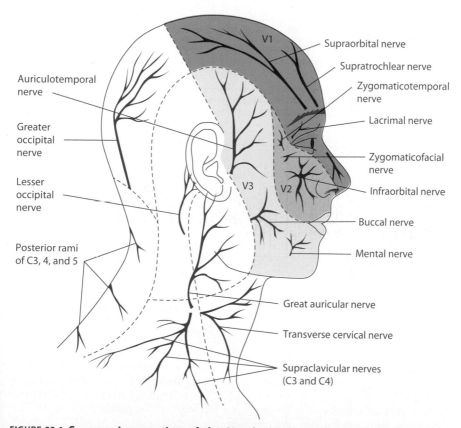

FIGURE 23-1 Sensory Innervation of the Head. The figure shows distribution of the three components of the trigeminal nerve. V1, ophthalmic, sensory; V2, maxillary, sensory; V3, mandibular, sensory, and motor. Adapted with permission from Lalwani AK: *Current Diagnosis & Treatment in Otolaryngology-Head & Neck Surgery*, 3rd ed. New York, NY: McGraw Hill; 2012.

CLINICAL MANIFESTATIONS

- Patients may be asymptomatic ("white-eyed" blow-out fracture) or present with periorbital ecchymosis and swelling, pain on vertical gaze, double vision, and/or decreased sensation in the V2 cranial nerve distribution.
- Check ocular motility, which may be decreased if there is muscle entrapment, and palpate orbital rims for a step off.
- Extraocular muscle entrapment may cause a symptomatic oculocardiac reflex with bradycardia, and presyncopal symptoms, particularly with eye movement.
- Signs of an open globe injury include
  - ✓ Obvious laceration site
  - ✓ Protruding uvea (appears as brown tissue)
  - ✓ Large amount of subconjunctival hemorrhage
  - ✓ Collapsed anterior chamber (cornea and iris come close to one another)
  - ✓ Peaking of the pupil toward wound site
  - ✓ Decreased vision
- Signs of an orbital compartment syndrome include
  - ✓ Decreased vision
  - ✓ Proptosis
  - ✓ Increased eye pressure with an eye that feels hard to palpation

DIAGNOSTICS

- Thin-cut CT in both axial and coronal planes is the study of choice.
- Plain film x-rays are insufficient for ruling out an orbital fracture; MRI depicts bones poorly.

MANAGEMENT

Nonsurgical

- Ice compresses for 48 hours; elevation of head of bed
- Avoid aspirin and NSAID use, minimize coughing and nose blowing.
- The following medications have not clearly been shown to improve outcomes, and some ophthalmologists do not use any of these approaches:
  - ✓ Nasal decongestants to prevent or minimize nose blowing
  - ✓ Oral steroids to reduce edema, particularly if ocular motility is decreased
  - ✓ Antibiotics covering sinus flora (e.g., ampicillin–sulbactam), particularly if there is a concomitant sinus infection

Surgical

- Immediate canthotomy and cantholysis for orbital compartment syndrome with decreased vision
- Urgent surgery for entrapped muscles, particularly if a symptomatic oculocardiac reflex is present
- Otherwise, fracture repair is recommended within 1–3 weeks if patient has diplopia, enophthalmos, soft-tissue herniation into maxillary sinuses, or if >30% of orbital floor is fractured.
- Open-globe injuries should be shielded (not patched) and the patient put on a nothing-by-mouth regimen for urgent surgical repair.

RETINOPATHY OF PREMATURITY (ROP)

A vasoproliferative disease of the developing retinal vasculature in premature infants that can lead to retinal detachment and blindness

EPIDEMIOLOGY

- ROP is a leading cause of childhood blindness worldwide.
- The strongest risk factors for ROP are early gestational age at birth, low birth weight, excessive oxygen administration, and slow postnatal weight gain in the first 6 weeks of life, sepsis, necrotizing enterocolitis, and thrombocytopenia.

PATHOPHYSIOLOGY

- The retinal vasculature normally develops along the surface of the retina anteriorly from the optic nerve, reaching the end of the retina (the ora) by around 40 weeks postmenstrual age.
- Premature birth with or without exogenous oxygen supplemental results in hyperoxia, which causes vaso-obliteration of developing retinal blood vessels and decreased retinal production of the hypoxia-induced vasoproliferative factor, vascular endothelial growth factor (VEGF); and loss of maternal insulin-like growth factor 1 (IGF-1), a key activator of VEGF.
- As retinal development progresses, metabolic demands increase, leading to localized hypoxia and increased retinal VEGF production, but VEGF activity is poor due to low IGF-1 levels.
- Eventually, infant production of IGF-1 begins to rise, activating intraocular VEGF and resulting in pathologic neovascularization into the vitreous and tractional retinal detachment.

CLINICAL MANIFESTATIONS

- ROP is diagnosed on the basis of indirect ophthalmoscopic examination by an ophthalmologist with expertise in the disease and graded with "stage," "zone," and "plus disease," as defined next.
- Stage: 0 = immature retinal vasculature (no ROP); 1 = white demarcation line between vascularized and avascular retina; 2 = elevated ridge; 3 = fibrovascular proliferation onto the ridge and into the vitreous; 4 = partial retinal detachment; 5 = total retinal detachment. Visual prognosis with stage 4 or 5 is very poor.
- Zone: I = most posterior (disease in zone I often more aggressive); II = out to the midperipheral retina; III = most anterior, far peripheral retina. Risk of vision loss is lower once the vessels have reached zone III.
- Plus disease: Increased venous dilatation and arteriolar tortuosity of the vessels directly adjacent to the optic-nerve head
- Plus disease is a major determinant of the decision to treat.
- While stage and zone are judged on the basis of the appearance and location of the most anterior extent of the developing retinal vessels, plus disease is judged posteriorly around the optic-nerve head.

DIAGNOSTICS

- Grading of retinal photographs by an experienced ophthalmologist or a trained nonphysician reader can be used to determine the need for an ophthalmologist's diagnostic examination.

MANAGEMENT

- ROP can progress very rapidly, so careful coordination of ROP examinations is critical to lowering the risk of blindness from late-diagnosed disease.
- ROP screening in the United States: Infants with a gestational age of ≤30 weeks or a body weight of ≤1500 g, or larger infants with an unstable course in the judgment of the neonatologist should receive examinations; criteria are location-specific and older

gestational age, higher body weight infants may develop severe ROP in countries with developing neonatal care systems.

- Diagnostic ROP examinations are initiated at 31 weeks' postmenstrual age or 4 weeks chronologic age, whichever comes later, and continued at 1–3 weeks intervals on the basis of the exam findings.
- Treatment with laser ablation of an avascular retina within 72 hours is recommend for type 1 prethreshold ROP, which is defined as stage 2 or 3 ROP in Zone II with plus disease, any stage ROP in zone 1 with plus disease, or stage 3 in zone 1 without plus disease.
- Intravitreal injection of anti-VEGF agents is an alternative treatment method, especially for infants with posterior disease, but the correct dose and possible long-term systemic effects of these injections are unknown.

PROGNOSIS

- Approximately 85% of ROP regresses spontaneously without treatment
  - ✓ Regressed stage 1 or 2 ROP typically has no long-term visual sequelae.
  - ✓ Regressed stage 3 (and treated ROP) carries a long-term risk of retinal hemorrhage or detachment and requires lifelong ophthalmologic follow-up.
  - ✓ Stages 4 and 5 ROP have very poor visual prognosis.
- Prematurity is associated with increased incidence of high refractive errors, strabismus, and nystagmus, with the risk increasing along with the worst stage of ROP diagnosed in the infant.

WHEN TO CONSIDER AN OPHTHALMOLOGY CONSULTATION

- Discuss exam location and timing with the ophthalmology team. For some conditions, a slit-lamp biomicroscope exam is important and best performed in the ophthalmology clinic. It may be advantageous to wait until the patient is well enough to travel to the office or to arrange an outpatient visit.
- Pupillary dilation with mydriatic eye drops will prevent a reliable pupil exam for 4 or more hours but is necessary for a complete exam.

Symptoms or signs as an inpatient

- Red eye
- Vision loss or blurry vision
- Eye pain
- Diplopia (double vision)
- Risk for corneal exposure
- Corneal opacity
- Irregular pupil
- Abnormal red reflex
- New onset strabismus
- Nystagmus

Based on suspected or confirmed systemic disease (finding)

- Cardiology
  - ✓ Congenital heart disease
  - ✓ CHARGE syndrome
  - ✓ PHACES syndrome
- Child abuse
  - ✓ Intracranial hemorrhage in an infant: Retinal hemorrhages with abusive head trauma
- Craniofacial
  - ✓ Pierre Robin sequence: Stickler syndrome

✓ Hydrocephalus or craniosynostosis: Papilledema
- Dermatology
  ✓ Stevens–Johnson syndrome, toxic epidermal necrolysis
  ✓ Periocular capillary hemangioma
  ✓ PHACES syndrome
  ✓ Incontinentia pigmenti
  ✓ Juvenile xanthogranuloma
  ✓ Oculocutaneous albinism
- Gastroenterology
  ✓ Wilson disease: Kayser–Fleischer ring, cataracts
  ✓ Alagille syndrome: Posterior embryotoxon
- Genetics
  ✓ Marfan syndrome: Lens subluxation
  ✓ Neurofibromatosis: Iris Lisch nodules
  ✓ Tuberous sclerosis
  ✓ Trisomy 21: Nystagmus, strabismus, cataracts, glaucoma, blocked tear ducts, high refractive error
  ✓ 22q11.2 deletion syndrome
- Hematology
  ✓ Hermansky–Pudlak syndrome: Oculocutaneous albinism
- Immunology
  ✓ Chediak–Higashi syndrome: Oculocutaneous albinism
- Infectious disease
  ✓ HIV
  ✓ Preseptal or orbital cellulitis
  ✓ Neonatal conjunctivitis
  ✓ Neonatal herpes simplex virus infection
  ✓ Periocular herpes simplex virus or varicella virus infection
  ✓ Cat-scratch disease: Parinaud's oculoglandular syndrome, neuroretinitis, focal chorioretinitis
  ✓ Lyme disease: Optic neuritis, cranial nerve palsies, uveitis
  ✓ Fungemia: Chorioretinitis, vitritis
  ✓ Endocarditis: Retinal hemorrhages and septic emboli
  ✓ TORCH infections
  ✓ CMV in immunocompromised patient: CMV retinitis
- Metabolism
  ✓ Galactosemia: Cataract
  ✓ Tyrosinemia: Type 2 with corneal deposits causing redness, tearing, photophobia
  ✓ Cystinosis
- Mitochondrial disease
  ✓ MERFF (myoclonic epilepsy with ragged red fibers)
  ✓ MELAS (mitochondrial encephalomyopathy with lactic acidosis and stroke-like episodes)
  ✓ Kearns–Sayre
  ✓ NARP (Neuropathy, ataxia, retinitis pigmentosa)
- Neonatology
  ✓ Neonatal conjunctivitis
  ✓ Extreme prematurity (birth weight ≤1501 g, gestational age ≤30 weeks; guidelines vary for middle income countries)—Retinopathy of prematurity exams
- Nephrology
  ✓ Tubular interstitial nephritis: Uveitis

- Neurology
  - ✓ Seizures, especially infantile spasms
    - Tuberous sclerosis: Retinal hamartomas
    - Aicardi syndrome (X-linked dominant, primarily affecting girls): Retinal lacunae
    - Use of vigabatrin for seizure control
  - ✓ Myasthenia gravis: Ptosis, strabismus, ocular motility deficits
  - ✓ Cranial nerve palsies: 3rd-, 4th-, 6th-, and 7th-nerve palsies
  - ✓ Multiple sclerosis: Optic neuritis, internuclear ophthalmoplegia
- Rheumatology
  - ✓ JIA: Uveitis, slit-lamp exam essential, patients generally asymptomatic
  - ✓ Kawasaki disease: Conjunctivitis and uveitis
  - ✓ Use of hydroxychloroquine: Retinopathy

Brian Vernau, MD
Matthew Grady, MD
Theodore Ganley, MD

BASICS OF PEDIATRIC ORTHOPEDICS

Musculoskeletal complaints and injuries are some of the most commonly encountered problems in pediatrics. In addition, children have immature musculoskeletal systems that pose particular challenges that are quite different from those of adults.

- Children have open growth plates, or physes, located between the epiphysis and the metaphysis.
- Fractures most commonly occur near the metaphysis or physis.
- An open growth plate is cartilaginous, and has not yet calcified, which makes it the weakest part of the immature bone.
- Pediatric bones are less brittle than adults, leading to some distinct fracture patterns.
- In a buckle fracture, compression force leads to partial failure, but the fracture does not traverse the entire bone.
- A greenstick fracture occurs because of tension or torsion force that leaves the cortex and periosteal sleeve intact on one side of the bone.
- Angulated fractures in children have a much greater potential to remodel back to their original shape than do fractures in adults. Remodeling potential is greatest in younger patients, injuries near a growing physis, and those in the plane of motion congruent to an associated joint.
- Open fractures require consultation with orthopedic surgery.
- Consider nonaccidental trauma (child abuse) as a factor in pediatric fractures. Injuries concerning for abuse include bucket-handle (metaphyseal corner) fractures, multiple fractures of different ages, posterior rib or scapular fractures, and long-bone fractures in children who do not walk. Refer to Chapter 7 for details.

FRACTURES

Management of fractures depends on the type, location, and amount of displacement present. Displacement, or loss of normal alignment of the distal fragment, is usually described in terms of translation (repositioning away from but remaining parallel to the long axis), angulation (degrees of bending from a straight line), shortening (overlap) or distraction (increased distance), and rotation (twisting).

FRACTURES OF THE PHYSIS

Physeal fractures are more common than isolated ligament or tendon injuries in skeletally immature patients because the surrounding connective tissues are stronger than the open physis. Injuries involving the physis are described with the Salter–Harris classification as shown in **Figure 24-1** and described in **Table 24-1**.

- Physical exam findings in physeal fractures: Tenderness over long bone physis following an injury, swelling, difficulty bearing weight

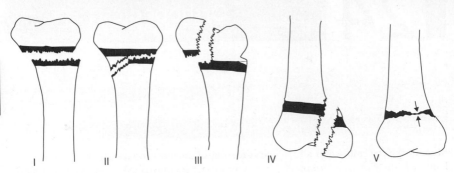

FIGURE 24-1 **Salter–Harris Types I–V.**

TABLE 24-1	Salter–Harris Classification for Fractures Involving the Physis	
Fracture Type	**Characteristics**	**Comments**
SH-I	Shearing injury to the physis without apparent bony fracture	Most common in toddlers; may not be recognized on radiographs
SH-II	Fracture at physis that extends into the metaphysis	Overall the most common pattern
SH-III	Fracture at physis that extends into the epiphysis	Intraarticular extension can lead to joint instability; should be managed by Orthopedic Surgery
SH-IV	Fracture involving the metaphysis, physis, and epiphysis	About 10% of physis fractures. One example is the triplane fracture
SH-V	Crush injury of the physis	Rare, <1% of fractures

DIAGNOSTICS

- Fracture diagnoses are commonly made on plain radiographs.
- Salter–Harris type I fractures may not be visible on initial films. Look for soft-tissue swelling adjacent to the physis in question.
- In equivocal cases, consider imaging the contralateral joint to compare physeal widths.
- Injuries to the physis should be monitored for several months after injury to monitor for growth arrest.
- Injuries that result in some measure of disability, along with tenderness at a physis on exam, should be treated as Salter–Harris type I fractures even if there is no abnormality demonstrated on the radiographs.

UPPER EXTREMITY

Clavicle Fractures

- The most frequently fractured bone in children; most are in the midshaft
- Mechanism of injury: Trauma at birth due to difficult delivery; fall onto shoulder or onto outstretched arm in older children
- Physical exam: Tenderness at clavicle; patient may have visible deformity
- Shoulder range of motion (ROM) likely to be limited, especially forward flexion and abduction
- Assess for associated injuries, especially at the sternoclavicular joint

Diagnostics

- Plain radiographs: True anteroposterior (AP) view of both clavicles, and AP view with beam at 30-degree cephalad angle ("serendipity view")

Management

- Infants: Pin the sleeve to the body of the shirt for comfort; avoid direct pressure on the clavicle.
- Older children: Sling, or figure 8 splint, typically for 3–4 weeks
- A palpable bony callus often remains after healing, but it should not affect function.
- Orthopedic referral required for open fractures, injuries adjacent to the sternoclavicular or acromio-clavicular joint, or when significant skin tenting is present.

Proximal Humerus Fractures

This is a rare injury in children, accounting for <5% of pediatric fractures. Patients with proximal humerus fractures need to be seen by orthopedic surgery service within 24–48 hours.

- Mechanism of injury: Backward fall onto outstretched arm in older children and adolescents
- Children >11 years old usually have Salter–Harris type II pattern
- Assess neurovascular status, especially the axillary nerve by assessing lateral shoulder sensation.

Management

- Consult with orthopedic surgeon
- Infants: Nearly all do well with nonsurgical care.
- Older children and adolescents: Most can be managed with sling and swathe.
- Surgical indications: >50% translation and angulation of >30–40 degrees in adolescents or >60–70 degrees in younger children

FRACTURES AROUND THE ELBOW

All elbow fractures require consultation with orthopedic surgeon. Elbow fractures do not remodel, so alignment for healing fractures needs to be near perfect.

- The lateral epicondyle is the last ossification center to appear, around age 8–11 in girls and 9–13 in boys.
- The medial epicondyle is the last to fuse, at age 14 in girls and 17 in boys.

Supracondylar humerus fracture

- Account for 60–80% of elbow fractures in children.
- Most occur in children <8 years old.
- Up to 15% may be associated with nerve injury, especially the anterior interosseous (Flynn).
- Evaluate by having patient flex thumb interphalangeal joint, and index finger distal interphalangeal joint (making the "OK" sign).

Diagnostics

- In the presence of a posterior fat pad (**Figure 24-2**), there is about a 75% chance of fracture.

Management

- If there is little to no posterior translation of the distal humerus, casting alone may be appropriate.
- Most other fracture patterns require closed reduction and pinning.

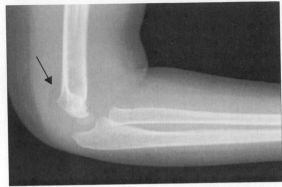

FIGURE 24-2 Presence of the Posterior Fat Pad Indicates High Likelihood of Supra-condylar Humerus Fracture. Reproduced with permission from Rudolph CD, Lister GE, First LR, et al: *Rudolph's Pediatrics*, 22nd ed. New York, NY: McGraw Hill; 2011

Lateral condyle fracture

- Second most common elbow fracture, accounting for about 15% of elbow fractures in children
- Injury often due to varus force to the elbow during a fall

Diagnostics

- Oblique view is of paramount importance to properly assess for displacement.
- Most are treated surgically on the basis of the amount of displacement
- If <2 mm displaced, consider long-arm cast for 4–6 weeks with repeat radiographs in cast at 1 and 2 weeks.
- Fractures displaced >2 mm require surgical treatment.
- Unlike most pediatric fractures, these can show nonunion that may lead to cubitus valgus.

Medical condyle fracture

- More likely in boys (nearly 80%) with peak incidence in early adolescence
- Mechanism is valgus force with associated firing of forearm flexor and pronator muscles
- Association with elbow dislocation in 50% of cases
- Ulnar nerve may be compromised in rare cases.

Management

- Most surgeons accept treatment with cast for displacement 2–5 mm. Internal fixation is advised if displaced >5 mm.
- May be associated with loss of terminal extension, which is more common with dislocation injuries and prolonged immobilization

FOREARM FRACTURES

Forearm fractures account for nearly 50% of fractures in skeletally immature children, and nearly 80% involve the distal third of the forearm. The typical mechanism of injury is a fall onto an outstretched hand.

- Most fractures are buckle, greenstick, or Salter–Harris type II pattern, and displacement is often dorsal.
- Fractures involving both bones (radius and ulna) are more complex, as are diaphyseal and proximal injuries.
- Be sure to evaluate distal vascular status.

Monteggia fractures

- Proximal ulnar fracture with associated dislocation of radial head
- Require management by orthopedic surgery

Diagnostics

- Plain radiographs: AP and lateral views of the forearm to include both the elbow and wrist
- Assess distal and proximal articulations of the radius, ulna, and humerus

Management

- Nondisplaced injuries can be initially managed with volar splint (proximal forearm to metacarpal heads) (**Figure 24-3B**).
- Reduction attempt with sedation is warranted for displaced distal fractures, followed by long-arm splint or cast for 4 weeks.
- Up to 50% translation is likely acceptable if >2 years of growth remains.
- Most metaphyseal fractures are managed successfully in short-arm cast for 4 weeks

HAND FRACTURES

A fall onto an outstretched hand and direct blows are common mechanisms. Overall, the thumb and little finger are most likely to be injured. Tendon and ligament injuries are uncommon until skeletal maturity.

- Distal phalangeal fractures are common.
- Metacarpal fractures most often occur at the neck. Evaluate for rotational displacement by having patient make a fist, which should show all fingers pointing to scaphoid.
- Carpal bone fractures are rare. The scaphoid is the most commonly fractured carpal bone. Patients have snuffbox tenderness, and radiographs may be negative.

Diagnostics

- Consider "scaphoid view" with wrist in ulnar deviation.

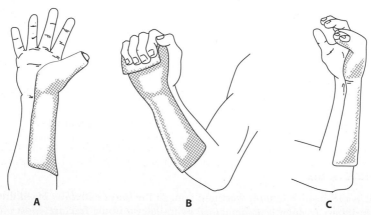

FIGURE 24-3 Splints. A. Thumb spica. B. Volar splint (proximal forearm to metacarpal heads). C. Safe position splint for metacarpal fractures (10 degrees wrist extension, 60–70 degrees flexion at metacarpophalangeal joints, extension at interphalangeal joints).

Management

- Most metacarpal fractures are treated with closed reduction and splint in the "safe position" (10 degrees wrist extension, 60–70 degrees flexion at metacarpophalangeal joints, extension at interphalangeal joints) (**Figure 24–3C**).
- Displaced fractures usually require open reduction and pinning.
- Snuffbox tenderness, even with negative radiographs requires thumb spica (**Figure 24-3A**) immobilization for 2–3 weeks then repeat evaluation with radiographs out of cast. If fracture is present, then total immobilization is usually 6–12 weeks.

LOWER EXTREMITY

Fractures of the lower extremity are more often seen in older children and adolescents.

FEMUR FRACTURES

- Most femur fractures are due to low-energy events in middle childhood (6–10 years) with falls during play being the most common cause (Wells).
- In children <1 year, 80% may be due to abuse.
- In adolescents, most are due to motor vehicle accidents.
- With a femoral shaft fracture, the patient is likely unable to bear weight and may have visible deformity.
- Distal femur physis fractures are most likely Salter–Harris type I or Salter–Harris type II. Knee may be held in flexion due to hamstring spasm. Exam may reveal tenderness at the distal physis, which is just proximal to the joint line near the superior pole of the patella.

Diagnostics

- Plain radiographs: AP, lateral; obtain oblique view for distal injuries. Include the ipsilateral hip and knee.
- For fractures into the joint, consider CT scan to assess displacement in multiple planes.
- Fractures in infants often warrant a skeletal survey to evaluate for child abuse.

Management

- Birth–5 years: Treat with spica cast or Pavlik harness for infants. Most show significant healing in 4 weeks, but may need up to 8 weeks of immobilization.
- 5–10 years: Consider conservative management with inpatient traction then spica casting. Surgical options include intramedullary nails, plates with screws, and external fixation devices.
- >11 years: Surgery is the primary treatment; intramedullary nails are often used and facilitate early weight bearing (Wells).
- There is high risk for growth arrest with distal femur physeal fractures, and treatment of distal physeal injuries depends on fracture pattern.
- Salter–Harris type I injuries may be treated with long-leg or spica cast with knee at 15–20 degrees of flexion.
- Salter–Harris type II fractures may require percutaneous pinning if unstable.
- Salter–Harris type III and Salter–Harris type IV require open reduction and internal fixation (ORIF) with long-leg cast postoperatively.

TIBIA FRACTURES

The tibia is the most commonly fractured bone of the lower extremity in children, and these injuries are frequently accompanied by ipsilateral fibula fracture. Most proximal tibia physeal fractures are Salter–Harris type I or Salter–Harris type II, and if displaced they can compromise the surrounding vascular structures.

- Tibial tubercle avulsion fractures are rare, and occur with a jumping or landing mechanism that typically produces a pop sensation and presents with significant swelling over the tubercle and an inability to do straight leg raise.
- The toddler's fracture is a nondisplaced spiral fracture of the tibial metaphysis in children 1–4 years old. It occurs with an apparently innocuous twist and fall that is often unwitnessed. Child may limp or stop bearing weight.
- The Cozen fracture involves the proximal tibia metaphysis and is seen in children 2–10 years old. It can lead to progressive valgus deformity
- Both Tillaux and triplane fractures are fractures of the distal tibia in adolescents near skeletal maturity. They most often occur because of external rotation of a planted foot and may be mistaken for an ankle sprain.
- The Tillaux fracture is an Salter–Harris type III injury to the anterolateral distal tibial epiphysis.
- A triplane fracture involves coronal, sagittal, and transverse components at the distal tibia. It appears as an Salter–Harris type II fracture on lateral radiographs and as an Salter–Harris type III on AP radiographs.

Diagnostics:

- Plain radiographs: AP, lateral, oblique views to include the ipsilateral knee and ankle
- CT scan may be indicated for Tillaux and triplane fractures to assess the degree of displacement at the joint surface.

Management

- Most tibial shaft fractures are treated with casting; consider closed reduction as needed.
- Nondisplaced tibial tubercle avulsions are managed with casting above the knee; if displaced, they warrant ORIF.
- Cozen fractures are treated with closed reduction and casting.
- Proximal physeal fractures are treated with casting above the knee if nondisplaced. If displaced, they require closed reduction, often under general anesthesia.
- Treat toddler's fracture with above the knee casting, and weight bearing as tolerated, for 3 weeks (Wells).
- Closed reduction may be attempted for Tillaux and triplane fractures, but ORIF is indicated for residual joint step-off greater than 2 mm.

FOOT FRACTURES

Most metatarsal fractures are due to a direct blow. Fractures at the base of the fifth metatarsal require special attention.

- The apophysis at the fifth metatarsal base appears on radiographs as a line parallel to the shaft of the bone. A lucency perpendicular to this is consistent with a fracture.
- Avulsion of the apophysis at the base of the fifth metatarsal occurs with inversion of the foot and ankle with tension from the lateral cord of the plantar aponeurosis pulling on the apophysis.
- Jones fracture is injury at the junction of the metaphysis and diaphysis, distal to the apophysis. It occurs in adolescents, and is often seen as an acute on chronic injury.

Diagnostics

- Plain radiographs: AP, lateral, oblique
- Obtain weight-bearing views, if tolerated.

Management

- Most nondisplaced metatarsal fractures are treated with a short-leg walking cast.
- Immobilization is preferred for avulsion at the base of the fifth metatarsal.
- Nonoperative care can be considered with acute Jones fracture and consists of non–weight-bearing cast for 6–8 weeks. There is a relatively high nonunion rate, and some patients will require internal fixation with a screw.

SIGNIFICANT ORTHOPEDIC ISSUES

COMPARTMENT SYNDROME

Compartment syndrome occurs when increased pressure within an osseofascial compartment leads to impaired blood flow with ischemia of muscle and nerve tissue.

- Most often seen in the lower leg or the forearm
- May result from trauma and hemorrhage or postsurgically; especially likely in the setting of a crush injury
- 75% of cases are associated with a fracture.
- Pain apparently out of proportion to injury and pain with passive stretching are hallmarks that warrant further evaluation.
- Late findings include diminished pulses and pallor.

Diagnostics

- Removal of cast or splint is necessary for proper assessment, which includes visualization, palpation, and ROM.
- Clinical concern can be corroborated with compartment pressure measurement.

Management

- If suspected, immediate surgical consultation is advised.
- Remove any restrictive dressings, including cast material.
- Keep affected limb at the level of the heart. Do not elevate the limb, as this can decrease arterial blood flow.
- Fasciotomy is the definitive intervention.

SLIPPED CAPITAL FEMORAL EPIPHYSIS (SCFE)

Disorder in which the femoral neck slides up and outward along the femoral physis, consistent with an Salter–Harris type I injury. The femoral head remains in place within the acetabulum.

- Typically seen from late childhood (9–10 years) through middle adolescence (15–16 years).
- More likely to occur in obese youth
- May be acute (symptoms <3 weeks), chronic, or a combination thereof
- Symptoms: Unilateral hip, groin, thigh or knee pain. Patients with chronic picture have more vague pain and often a limp.
- Up to 60% can be bilateral
- It is stable if the patient can ambulate either with or without crutches.
- Exam reveals limited internal rotation, abduction, and flexion, with pain upon hip ROM. The affected limb may be held in external rotation, and may appear slightly shortened.

Diagnostics

- Plain radiographs: AP and frog-leg lateral (hips flexed and abducted) views of the pelvis with assessment of both hips
- A line drawn along superior aspect of the femoral neck (Klein's line) should intersect the lateral capital epiphysis. As the femoral neck slips up and outward, the line will intersect

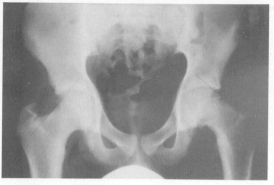

A

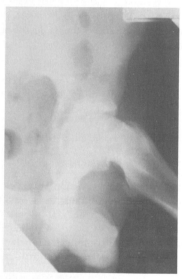

B

FIGURE 24-4 **Left slipped capital femoral epiphysis on plain radiographs (AP and frog-leg lateral).** Klein's line in image A fails to intersect the femoral head on the affected side. Reproduced with permission from Skinner HB, McMahon PJ: *Current Diagnosis & Treatment In Orthopedics*, 5th ed. New York, NY: McGraw Hill; 2014

progressively less of the epiphysis, until it no longer contacts it at all. This is the radiographic finding in SCFE (**Figure 24-4**).

Management

- Upon diagnosis, contact orthopedic surgeon.
- Make patient non–weight-bearing with either crutches or a wheelchair for bilateral involvement.
- Definitive treatment for nondisplaced lesions is in situ fixation using a pin or screw. Surgical intervention for the unaffected hip, whether symptomatic or not, may be considered, but remains controversial.

TRANSIENT SYNOVITIS

- Transient synovitis is the most common cause of hip pain and usually affects children 3–8 years old. It is often associated with recent or current illness, often viral. Children appear nontoxic and are able to bear weight on the affected limb.
- In contrast, the child with septic arthritis may appear more ill and have a higher fever. (See Chapter at for management of septic arthritis.)

Diagnostics

- History and physical exam, along with complete blood count for white blood cells (WBCs), and erythrocyte sedimentation rate (ESR).
- The four primary factors based on the Kocher criteria to consider are: fever, inability to ambulate, WBC count $>12,000/mm^3$, and ESR of 40 mm/hr or higher.
- If all four criteria are met, there is up to a 99% chance that the patient has septic arthritis. The likelihood decreases to 93% if three of four criteria are positive, 40% if two of four are positive, and $<5\%$ if only one of four is positive.
- Joint aspiration is indicated if two or more criteria are met.
- An aspirate is considered indicative of bacterial infection if the fluid has $>50,000$ WBCs/mm^3 or if bacteria are present on Gram stain.

Management

- Most transient synovitis will resolve spontaneously within 2 weeks. Weight bearing is limited for comfort, and nonsteroidal antiinflammatory drugs (NSAIDs) are used as needed.
- Despite its efficacy for pain relief, joint aspiration is reserved for diagnostic purposes as fluid often rapidly reaccumulates.
- The septic joint must be explored surgically and is a relative emergency.

POSTOPERATIVE MANAGEMENT OF SPINAL FUSION

Key elements of postoperative care following spinal fusion surgery include monitoring hemodynamics, managing pain, advancing enteral nutrition, and facilitating early mobility. Hospitalist comanagement is particularly beneficial in patients with multiple comorbidities, neuromuscular or congenital scoliosis and in pediatric patients being cared for by adult spine surgeons. Risk factors for complication include history of renal disease, increased intraoperative blood loss, and prolonged surgical/anesthesia time.

Management

- Pain control and mobility
  - ✓ Regimens vary by surgeon.
  - ✓ Early mobilization and short-term opioid use are key.
  - ✓ Early discontinuation of Patient Controlled Analgesia and demand-only PCA without basal rate are associated with shorter lengths of stay.
  - ✓ Common multimodal regimens include acetaminophen, NSAIDs, gabapentin, and benzodiazepines.
  - ✓ May start sitting up on postoperative day 0 and walking with physical therapist on postoperative day 1.
  - ✓ Goal of 30–60 minutes out of bed three times daily
- Complications
  - ✓ Gastrointestinal and respiratory
    - Postoperative nausea and vomiting and ileus are common.

- Clear liquid diet on postoperative day 0, and advance to bland foods as tolerated on postoperative day 1.
- Manage with ondansetron and antihistamines.
- Aggressive pulmonary toilet, including incentive spirometry or breath-stacking (for those unable to cooperate https://pubmed.ncbi.nlm.nih.gov/26195544/) to treat sedation related respiratory depression and reduce risk of pneumonia.
- Superior mesenteric artery syndrome is rare but well described.
  ▷ Tall and thin, relatively large scoliosis correction
  ▷ Persistent nausea and vomiting a number of days or even weeks after surgery

✓ Neurologic
- Occurs in ~1% of scoliosis surgery.
- Complications include neuropraxia, nerve-root injury, spinal-cord injury and paralysis.
- Due to positioning, direct injury, vascular insult due to either excessive stretch from correction or cord ischemia from hypotension
- Neuropraxia typically recovers spontaneously over time.
- Intraoperative spinal-cord monitoring allows for immediate treatment.
- Delayed neurologic injury (within 48 hours) has been reported.
- Serial neurologic exams recommended throughout the postoperative recovery period: Hip flexion, knee extension, foot dorsiflexion and plantarflexion, great toe extension, sensory nerves to the foot, and foot pulses.

✓ Infection
- In immediate postoperative period, pneumonia is the most frequently encountered infection.
- Perioperative antibiotics within 1 hour of incision and for 24 hours afterward
- Neuromuscular scoliosis patients have higher infection rates, up to 10–20% in some series.
- Most surgical-site infections are delayed (>6 months) and caused by low virulence skin flora (e.g., *Staphylococcus epidermidis, Cutibacterium acnes*).

✓ Hematologic
- Blood transfusion is less common, than previously reported, especially in adolescent idiopathic scoliosis.
- Use of antifibrinolytic therapy (tranexamic acid and aminocaproic acid) has decreased blood loss for this operation.
- Intraoperative blood-cell salvage techniques are frequently utilized.
- Daily CBC for first 2 days
- Transfuse for hemoglobin level <7 g/dL or if symptomatic.
- Venous thromboembolism is rare in pediatric population.
  ▷ Risk factors include surgery done for fracture stabilization, syndromic/congenital scoliosis, or those with hematological risk factors for blood clot.
  ▷ Pharmacologic prophylaxis is not routinely required, especially with early mobilization strategies.

Otolaryngology

25

John Germiller, MD, PhD

ADENOTONSILLAR HYPERTROPHY

Enlargement of palatine tonsils and adenoid lymphoid tissue that contributes to obstruction of the upper airway

- Results in sleep disordered breathing defined as an abnormal respiratory pattern during sleep including snoring, mouth breathing, and pauses in breathing which may be symptoms of obstructive sleep apnea (OSA)

EPIDEMIOLOGY

- Volume of lymphoid tissue increases from 6 months of age to puberty; peak of OSA in preschool years, when tissue makes up greatest proportion of upper airway
- Associated craniofacial and neuromuscular disorders and obesity increase likelihood of symptomatic adenotonsillar hypertrophy..

PATHOPHYSIOLOGY

- The underlying etiology of adenotonsillar hypertrophy is unknown.
- Upper airway obstruction is multifactorial and includes hypertrophied lymphoid tissue, compliance and elasticity of pharyngeal soft tissue, facial morphology, and changes to the pharyngeal musculature during sleep.
- Cyclic airway obstruction during sleep causes hypoxia and hypercapnia, leading to arousals to restore respiration.
- Repeated arousals interrupt rapid eye movement sleep, which can lead to daytime somnolence.

CLINICAL MANIFESTATIONS

- Nighttime: Snoring, apnea, restless sleep, enuresis, nightmares
- Daytime: Somnolence, behavioral changes, learning difficulties, nasal obstruction, mouth breathing, hyponasal speech; in severe cases, dysphagia, failure to thrive
- Degree of tonsillar enlargement: Tonsil within fossa = 0; less than 25% obstruction = 1+; less than 50% obstruction = 2+; less than 75% obstruction = 3+; greater than 75% obstruction = 4+ (Brodsky grading scale) (**Figure 25-1**).

DIAGNOSTICS

- Overnight polysomnography is definitive test for OSA.
- Lateral neck radiograph versus flexible nasopharyngolaryngoscopy (NPL) to assess adenoid size and airway caliber; however, volume of tonsils and adenoids do not always correlate well with severity of OSA.
- ECG and/or echocardiogram in severe, longstanding OSA to rule out cor pulmonale—Right heart strain, right ventricular hypertrophy

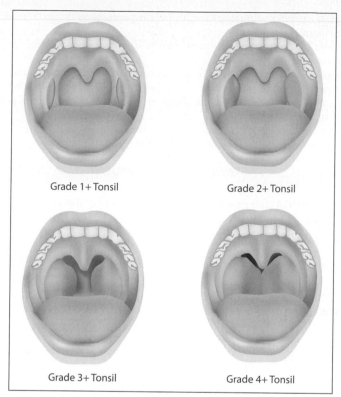

Grade 1+ Tonsil   Grade 2+ Tonsil

Grade 3+ Tonsil   Grade 4+ Tonsil

FIGURE 25-1 **Assessing the Degree of Tonsillar Enlargement Using the Brodsky Grading Scale.** Reproduced with permission from Brodsky L: Modern assessment of tonsils and adenoids, *Pediatr Clin North Am* 1989 Dec;36(6):1551–1569.

MANAGEMENT

Medical

- Nasal corticosteroids decrease nasal turbinate and adenoid hypertrophy and may decrease severity of OSA, improve snoring, and improve nighttime symptoms such an enuresis, though long-term effectiveness is unclear. Dosage—1 spray in each nostril daily (if <2 years, give every other day)
- Noninvasive positive-pressure ventilation (e.g., continuous positive airway pressure)
- Weight loss for obese patients

Surgical

- Indications for adenotonsillectomy
  - ✓ Sleep disordered breathing leading to daytime and nighttime symptoms, and all children with documented OSA
  - ✓ Nasal obstruction causing discomfort in breathing and distortion of speech, or recurrent otitis media (adenoidectomy only)

✓ Dysphagia or speech disturbance (dysarthria or hypernasality) due to large tonsils (tonsillectomy only)

✓ Chronic tonsillitis: Seven episodes in the past year, five episodes per year for 2 years, or three episodes per year for 3 years

✓ Prior complications of tonsillitis (peritonsillar abscess, poststreptococcal glomerulonephritis)

- Risks of surgery include postoperative hemorrhage (0.1–3%), airway obstruction due to edema, prolonged pain and dehydration, anesthesia risks, speech change, and postobstructive pulmonary edema.

- Tracheostomy (temporary or permanent) may be needed in severe, refractory OSA or for children with complex medical/anatomic conditions.

BRANCHIAL CLEFT ANOMALIES

Persistence of branchial cleft resulting in cysts, sinuses, or fistulae of the lateral neck

- Cyst: Persistent lateral neck mass; usually painless unless it is infected
- Sinus: External opening to neck along the anterior border of the sternocleidomastoid muscle (SCM), extending along the tract. May intermittently drain fluid.
- Fistula: Opening both externally in neck and internally in tonsillar fossa or hypopharynx

EPIDEMIOLOGY

- Branchial-cleft anomalies are present from birth but are often not recognized until acute infection, usually in the first decade of life.
- 90% arise from the second branchial cleft.
- Almost always unilateral. Bilateral branchial anomalies may suggest an underlying genetic syndrome (branchio-oto-renal).

ETIOLOGY

- Anomalies develop from ectodermal remnants in the tract of the second branchial cleft, which arises from the anterosuperior border of the SCM, passes between the internal and external carotids and over the 10th and 12th cranial nerves to end at the tonsillar fossa.
  ✓ Third branchial cleft remnants are less common and have a slightly different course, terminating in the hypopharynx. Fourth cleft anomalies are very rare and are almost exclusively on the left side; they also terminate in the hypopharynx.

DIFFERENTIAL DIAGNOSIS

- Differential diagnosis of neck masses is affected by location (**Figure 25-2**).
- Congenital: Hemangioma, cystic hygroma, thyroglossal duct cyst, SCM pseudotumor of infancy (fibromatosis colli), remnant of branchial-arch cartilage, enlarged or ectopic thyroid, epidermoid cyst (usually lateral), neurofibroma (usually lateral), lipoma
- Following trauma: Hematoma, subcutaneous emphysema
- Infectious: Reactive adenopathy, adenitis (see Chapter 15), Kawasaki, infectious mononucleosis syndrome, toxoplasmosis, sarcoid
- Malignant: Leukemia, lymphoma, neuroblastoma, Langerhans-cell histiocytosis, others

CLINICAL MANIFESTATIONS

- Cystic neck mass or opening anterior to midportion of SCM muscle
- May have tenderness, redness, swelling, and/or purulent drainage if infected.
- Internal opening of fistula may be visible near tonsillar fossa.

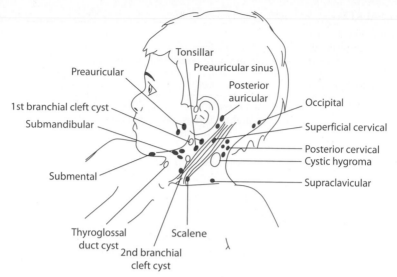

FIGURE 25-2 Typical locations of cystic and solid neck masses. 0 = Cysts/sinuses; ● = lymph nodes.

- Third and fourth branchial anomalies may present with unilateral acute thyroiditis.
- Pertinent negative: Branchial cysts are never midline. A midline mass that moves upward with tongue protrusion or swallowing suggests a thyroglossal duct cyst.

DIAGNOSTICS

- CT or MRI (preferred) usually delineates the mass and any associated tract.
- Ultrasound can distinguish cystic from solid masses.
- Rarely, instillation of radiopaque material is needed to demonstrate the extent of the fistula or sinus.

MANAGEMENT

- Acute infection/abscess is treated with systemic antibiotics (e.g., ampicillin–sulbactam, amoxicillin–clavulanate, or clindamycin) and, if needed, incision and drainage.
- Complete surgical excision is the definitive treatment but is usually deferred until after resolution of acute inflammation.

CLEFT LIP/PALATE

CLEFT LIP

- Complete: Extends into floor of the nose
- Incomplete: Extends part way through the lip

CLEFT PALATE

- Always involves uvula
- Unilateral or bilateral
- Severity depends on degree of soft and hard palate involvement

EPIDEMIOLOGY

- One in 1000 births in whites; 1 in 400 in Japanese; 1 in 3000 in Africans
- Cleft lip: 80% unilateral, 20% bilateral; 75% have associated cleft palate
- Facial clefting associated with approximately 300 syndromes including Van der Woude and Stickler and associated Pierre Robin sequence
- Both genetic and environmental factors have been implicated.

PATHOPHYSIOLOGY

- Embryology: Palatogenesis occurs between 5th and 12th week of gestation.
- Clefting results from incomplete closure of upper lip, with or without incomplete closure of the two halves of the hard palate and the overlying soft palate.
- Feeding difficulties are due to inability to create adequate negative oral pressure with sucking.
- Poor eustachian tube function results from the incomplete sling of palatal musculature. Results in middle-ear effusion and conductive hearing loss. Most children with cleft palate require pressure equalization tubes.
- Speech problems found in most cleft palate patients mostly due to velopharyngeal insufficiency with air escape from nose (hypernasal speech) with associated articulation errors.
- Other congenital abnormalities are common.

MANAGEMENT

- Multidisciplinary approach: Surgeon, dentist, speech pathologist, audiologist, geneticist, social worker, nurse, nutritionist, psychologist

Feeding

- Breastfeeding is possible with cleft lip and palate.
- Bottle feeding with special nipples such as Habermann feeder or Mead–Johnson cleft bottle
- Frequent burping required owing to increased air swallowing
- Nasogastric feeding or gastrostomy tube may be required, more likely with associated syndromes

Surgical

- Cleft lip repair around 10 weeks of age (rule of 10s—10 weeks, 10 lb, 10 g/dL hemoglobin)
- Lip adhesion may be performed as initial procedure to facilitate later definitive closure.
- Presurgical nasoalveolar molding is an orodental appliance that can aid in closure of cleft lip and palate and improve nasal symmetry.
- Cleft palate repair: Goals include separation of nasal from oral cavity, a competent velopharyngeal valve, elongation of the palate, and restoration of palate musculature. All are aimed at yielding improved speech quality. Eustachian tube function also eventually improves.
- Cleft palate repair typically completed by 9–18 months of age

CONGENITAL NASAL PYRIFORM APERTURE STENOSIS

Abnormal narrowing of the anterior nasal vault leading to feeding difficulty, nasal obstruction, and cyclic cyanosis

- The pyriform aperture is a pear-shaped bony opening bordered by the nasal processes and horizontal processes of the maxilla and nasal bones.
- Normal pyriform aperture measures at least 11 mm wide in the full-term neonate.

EPIDEMIOLOGY

- Rare congenital anomaly that may be isolated or may be associated with other congenital "midline defect" anomalies, namely central mega-incisor, holoprosencephaly, absent corpus collosum

ETIOLOGY

- Developmental midline defect believed to be related to overgrowth of the nasal process of the maxilla, or an underdeveloped primary palate
- May accompany other craniofacial anomalies with additional levels of airway obstruction

DIFFERENTIAL DIAGNOSIS

- Very similar presentation as choanal atresia
- Rhinitis (which can be secondary to reflux in neonates), congenital septal dislocation (birth trauma), nasolacrimal duct cyst, hemangioma, encephalocele, glioma, and other midline nasal masses

CLINICAL MANIFESTATIONS

- Classic presentation is cyclic cyanosis relieved by crying. Neonates are obligate nasal breathers.
- Difficulty with feeding due to nasal obstruction. Normally neonates nose-breathe continuously while feeding.
- Can have difficulty passing 6 French suction catheter, feeding tubes; in contrast to choanal atresia, resistance is met right at the entry to the nostrils. Note that passage of catheters does not rule out congenital nasal pyriform aperture stenosis, since the aperture is narrow but never entirely closed.

DIAGNOSTICS

- Anterior rhinoscopy and flexible NPL scope, when possible demonstrates narrowed anterior nasal passage
- Fine-cut CT scan demonstrates pyriform aperture <11 mm and is also useful to evaluate for central mega-incisor, holoprosencephaly, pituitary anomalies, absent corpus collosum
- Pyriform aperture of ≤5.7 mm on CT predicts need for surgical intervention.
- Commonly, stenosis is not limited to the aperture, but involves the entire nasal cavity.

MANAGEMENT

- Most important consideration is that infants will grow out of congenital pyriform aperture stenosis within a few months. Management goals are therefore to ensure a patent nasal airway until growth occurs.
- Initial treatment with nasal steroids and nasal saline to reduce any swelling that may worsen narrowing. Minimizing reflux, if present, can reduce additional nasal edema.

- Oral airway, or orotracheal intubation if airway symptoms are severe
- Surgical if cannot be managed medically
- Mild to moderate cases: Dilation of the pyriform aperture, or of the entire nasal cavity, with or without stenting to maintain the patent airway. This may need to be repeated one or more times until infant grows.
- Moderate to severe cases limited to the pyriform aperture are repaired via the transoral, sublabial approach, with drilling to widen the bony aperture. Most authors advocate stenting postoperatively for up to 6 weeks.

CHOANAL ATRESIA

The choanae are the openings through which the nasal cavity and nasopharynx communicate. They are bound by the vomer, the horizontal plates of the palate, the sphenoid bones, and the medial pterygoid bones.

- Because infants are obligate nasal breathers, bilateral choanal atresia becomes apparent early and is considered a medical emergency.

EPIDEMIOLOGY

- Rare congenital anomaly occurring in approximately 1 in 8000 live births
- Up to 50% present as component of a syndrome, most commonly CHARGE syndrome; therefore, any diagnosis of choanal atresia merits workup for CHARGE syndrome.
- May be unilateral or bilateral
- Atresia may be bony, membranous, or a combination of the two, with bony atresia being most common

ETIOLOGY

- Failure of recanalization of the buccopharyngeal membrane, or incomplete obliteration of the nasobuccal membrane
- Persistent bony and or membranous barrier between the nasal cavity and nasopharynx prevents passage of air and normal mucociliary clearance.

DIFFERENTIAL DIAGNOSIS

- Presentation similar to that for pyriform aperture stenosis, midline nasal mass, and deviated nasal septum.

CLINICAL PRESENTATION

- Bilateral choanal atresia presents at birth with cyclic cyanotic episodes relieved by crying, as well as difficulty feeding, desaturation, and respiratory distress.
- Unilateral choanal atresia typically presents later, with unilateral rhinorrhea and nasal obstruction. Feeding difficulty and respiratory symptoms are not usually present.

DIAGNOSTICS

- Clinical examination shows rhinorrhea in affected side and inability to pass suction catheter.
- No fogging on a mirror held below the nostrils suggests atresia.
- Flexible NPL reveals blind-ended nasal cavity with no evident choanal opening.
- Fine-cut CT of the skull base and facial bones helps determine preoperative degree of bony versus membranous obstruction.

MANAGEMENT

- Bilateral choanal atresia is considered a medical emergency and often requires orotracheal intubation
- May be able to treat patients temporarily with McGovern nipple and oral airway prior to surgery
- Surgical management
  - ✓ Puncture and dilation: A stiff dilator punctures then dilates the atresia plate. Stents made of endotracheal tubes are often placed for several weeks to maintain the opening.
  - ✓ Endoscopic approach uses drill and sinus instruments to remove bony atretic plate and a portion of the bony posterior septum (vomer). This is not always possible in the smallest neonates, who often need puncture and dilation initially, followed by endoscopic repair after interval growth.
  - ✓ Postoperative treatment includes topical steroids.
  - ✓ Restenosis requiring additional surgical intervention is common, especially in children who undergo initial repair within the first several days of life; most infants require two to five procedures.

EPISTAXIS

PATHOPHYSIOLOGY

- Anterior septum (Little's area) is most common site due to vascularity (Kiesselbach's plexus) and exposure (dry air, trauma)
- Epistaxis from trauma (digital or impact), inflammation, dryness, or less often tumor, vascular abnormality, or coagulopathy

CLINICAL MANIFESTATIONS

- Active bleeding or dry blood with or without identifiable source
- Mucosa: Dry, cracked, pale, boggy, prominent vessels
- Localized active bleeding: Anterior, posterior, unilateral, or bilateral. Unilateral epistaxis without obvious source on anterior septum raises suspicion for discrete masses or vascular lesions further posteriorly in nose.
- Check for masses, polyps, and foreign bodies.
- Signs of underlying bleeding disorder: Petechiae, ecchymosis
- Hypertension: Very rarely a factor in children
- History: Bruising, bleeding, or family history of same; use of anticoagulants or platelet inhibitors. Long-term nasal steroid use also predisposes to epistaxis.

DIAGNOSTICS

- None routinely required but clinical situation may warrant the following:
  - ✓ Hematologic/coagulation studies, and/or hematology consultation. Use if no typical, focal bleeding source is identified, or if additional bleeding sites besides epistaxis, or family history of coagulopathy. Initial studies should include prothrombin and partial thromboplastin times and platelet count.
  - ✓ Sinus CT or MRI if neoplasm suspected
  - ✓ Arteriography or MR angiography if vascular anomaly suspected or embolization is considered

MANAGEMENT

Medical

- Hold external direct pressure on soft tissue of nostrils for 5–15 minutes.
- Oxymetazoline (0.05%; Afrin) spray to affected nostril for local vasoconstriction (up to twice daily for maximum of 3 days)
- Anterior nasal packing with absorbable hemostatic agents including Surgicel, MeroGel, or Gelfoam, or with ointment-coated sponges that require removal after 72 hours
- Posterior packing (gauze, nasal tampons/balloons) rarely needed except for severe trauma or tumor bleeding.
- Prophylactic antibiotics (e.g., cephalexin, clindamycin, amoxicillin–clavulanate) while packing in place owing to risk of toxic shock syndrome and sinusitis.
- Treat underlying process (e.g., allergic rhinitis, bleeding diathesis).
- Ear, nose, and throat consult for severe epistaxis, suspicion of occult nasal lesion, or underlying hemorrhagic diathesis
- For chronic recurrent epistaxis from identified source: Petrolatum ointment nightly and humidifier use during dry air seasons; moisten/lubricate with saline spray and gel; keep petrolatum quantity small and avoid long-term use of antibiotic ointments

Surgical

- Chemical cautery (e.g., silver nitrate) of bleeding site; moderately high rate of recurrence
- Electrocautery of bleeding site (avoiding excessive cautery of both sides of nasal septum due to risk of septal ischemia and perforation); lower recurrence rate than chemical cautery but requires general anesthesia
- Limited septoplasty. The mucoperichondrium is simply elevated off the septal cartilage and allowed to heal back into place; the surgical trauma induces enough scarring to reduce the rate of epistaxis.
- Embolization, laser excision, or arterial ligation in severe cases (e.g., tumor, vascular malformation)

FOREIGN-BODY ASPIRATION/INGESTION

EPIDEMIOLOGY

- Highest incidence 1–3 years of age
- Twice as common in boys
- Most common foreign body: Food matter/nuts (aspiration), coins (ingestion)

ETIOLOGY

- Toddlers have less control of swallowing and have immature chewing ability, laryngeal elevation, and glottic closure. They cannot grind foods until molars develop, and dentition ability continues to mature throughout childhood.
- Intellectual disability, autism, and neurologic or seizure disorders increase risk.

CLINICAL MANIFESTATIONS

- History of foreign body in mouth or close to child or unobserved period before appearance of symptoms
- May be asymptomatic for weeks or months before presentation
- Airway foreign body: Wheezing, unexplained coughing spells, significant respiratory distress, pneumonia, decreased breath sounds in obstructed lobe/lung

✓ Upper airway symptoms: Hoarseness, aphonia, stridor, inspiratory wheeze
✓ Lower airway symptoms: Expiratory wheeze, asymmetric aeration of lung fields
✓ Unilateral wheezing or migrating wheeze on physical examination is highly suspicious for foreign body as opposed to reactive airway disease.

- Ingested foreign body: Drooling, throat pain, dysphagia, odynophagia, localizable anterior neck pain, less commonly respiratory distress due to compression of the airway from esophageal foreign body
- Food impaction: Raises suspicion for chronic esophagitis, notably eosinophilic esophagitis, especially if repeat episodes
- Disk-battery ingestion: Full-thickness esophageal wall injury due to electrical discharge and caustic chemical leakage; begins within minutes and rapidly progresses; can result in permanent stricture, perforation

DIAGNOSTICS

- Posteroanterior and lateral chest and neck films together are used to localize radiopaque objects in airway or esophagus
- Chest CT if erosion or extraluminal extension suspected
- Aspiration: Acutely, failure of affected lobe to deflate may be seen on inspiratory/expiratory (hyperinflation on expiratory film) or lateral decubitus (air trapping in dependent lung) chest x-ray. Subacutely or chronically, the chest x-ray may show resorptive postobstructive atelectasis, compensatory emphysema of nonobstructed lobes, pneumonia, pneumothorax, shift of mediastinum during expiration, or abscess
- Ingestion: Most common objects, such as coins, are often radiopaque; esophageal air may delineate tissue-density foreign body on plain film. Barium swallow may identify radiolucent esophageal foreign body. Must rule out presence of disk battery (halo sign on AP view and step-off on lateral view) as this is a true emergency, and delay in removal can be fatal since the battery can burn through vessels and cause severe bleeding.
- Repeated episodes: Consider evaluation of swallowing function (presence of gag reflex, observed feedings, modified barium swallow with speech therapy), or esophageal anatomy (upper endoscopy, biopsy to rule out eosinophilic esophagitis, barium swallow)

MANAGEMENT

- Complete airway obstruction is an absolute emergency. Perform abdominal thrusts on children >1 year of age, and back blows/chest thrusts on children <1 year of age.
- Disk battery/button battery ingestion is an emergency requiring operative endoscopy. Do not delay diagnosis or treatment.
- Endoscopy can be both diagnostic and therapeutic. General anesthesia is required.
- Rigid bronchoscope: Allows visualization of the trachea and bronchi, with removal of the foreign body through the scope; ventilation occurs through the scope
- Rigid esophagoscopy: Allows visualization of the entire esophagus with removal of the foreign body through the scope
- A foreign body that cannot be removed endoscopically may require thoracotomy for direct removal.

HEARING LOSS

Decreased hearing may be present at birth (congenital) or may begin later in childhood (acquired). Hearing loss can be stable or progressive. May be sensorineural (inner ear, nerve, or central source) or conductive (mechanical sound conduction, from outer or middle ear disease).

- Most commonly picked up at newborn hearing screen, school, or well-visit screening tests, or by caregiver concern for hearing or speech delay.

EPIDEMIOLOGY

- Prevalence of congenital or childhood hearing loss is 1 to 2 per 1000.

ETIOLOGY

- Genetic: 50% of congenital loss is genetic. One third of these is associated with a syndrome.
  - ✓ Recessive: Usher (vestibular dysfunction, retinitis pigmentosa), Pendred (thyroid goiter, cochlear dysplasia), Jervell and Lange–Nielsen (prolonged QT, sudden death)
  - ✓ Dominant: Waardenburg (heterochromia, white forelock), branchio-oto-renal (auricular deformity, preauricular pits or tags, branchial cleft anomalies [commonly bilateral], and renal anomalies), Stickler (retinal detachment, cleft palate, arthritis), Treacher Collins (midface hypoplasia, down sloping eyes, conductive hearing loss), neurofibromatosis (café au lait spots, axillary freckling, neurofibromas)
  - ✓ Other syndromes: Fetal alcohol, Down, Goldenhar
  - ✓ Two-thirds of congenital hearing loss is nonsyndromic—that is, there are no other anomalies.
  - ✓ Connexin 26 gap-junction protein mutation: Most common cause of nonsyndromic genetic hearing loss in North America
- Nongenetic
  - ✓ In utero exposure to cytomegalovirus (CMV) most common cause, often otherwise asymptomatic and mother may experience minimal or no symptoms. May account for one third of cases of congenital hearing loss.
  - ✓ Bacterial meningitis, fetal alcohol, congenital rubella, trauma (e.g., temporal bone fracture)
- Other
  - ✓ Cerumen impaction, acute infection, and persistent middle ear fluid (OME) can lead to conductive hearing loss, which is treatable or self-resolving.
  - ✓ Other diseases, such as ear drum retraction, formation of middle ear mass or cholesteatoma

DIFFERENTIAL DIAGNOSIS

- Congenital (present since birth): May be stable or progressive
- External ear causes: Cerumen impaction, foreign body, outer ear infection
- Middle ear causes: AOM, (OME), cholesteatoma (skin cyst, which can be either congenital or more commonly is acquired from repeated infections or retraction) or other middle ear mass, scarring from infection, sclerosis or abnormal formation of the ossicles, trauma
- Inner ear causes—Congenital or progressive sensorineural hearing loss, malformed cochlea or cochlear nerve (cochlear hypoplasia), enlarged vestibular aqueduct, rare mass lesions

CLINICAL MANIFESTATIONS

- Failed screening testing, speech delay, poor school performance, social isolation

DIAGNOSTICS

- Otoscopy: May reveal external or middle ear causes
- Audiogram: Gold standard—distinguishes sensorineural from conductive hearing loss. May be followed over time and with intervention. Different testing available depending on age and ability to cooperate.

- Otoacoustic emissions: Show inner ear hair-cell function. May be used as a screening test, does not require patient participation. Simple, noninvasive; however, not definitive; will miss auditory nerve dysfunction or central hearing loss (auditory neuropathy spectrum)
- Tympanography: Assess movement of ear drum and pressure of middle ear; can determine if there is fluid in middle ear or a perforation
- Auditory brain-stem response: Objective testing on the inner ear and brain stem to assess hearing ability. For children unable to perform standard audiography; often requires sedation after 6 months of age. Used in many centers for newborn screening.
- CT or MRI to assess for middle or inner ear abnormalities in some cases.
- Medical workup for suspected genetic causes may include genetic testing (connexin 26/30 most common), CMV testing in neonates, ECG for bilateral deaf patients (detects long QT abnormalities such as Jervell and Lange–Nielsen syndrome), eye exam

MANAGEMENT

Medical

- Cerumen or foreign body removal, treatment of external or middle ear disease
- Hearing aids standard for permanent hearing loss
- FM systems or wireless assistive hearing devices, preferential classroom seating, early intervention services for all children with hearing loss
- Antivirals can slow progression of hearing loss in symptomatic congenital CMV but are controversial in asymptomatic CMV when hearing loss is the only manifestation.

Surgical

- Ventilating ear tubes for repeated infections or persistent ear fluid (>3 months' duration, associated with hearing loss or in high-risk populations), eustachian tube dysfunction with retraction
- Surgery may be required for cholesteatoma, retraction, ear drum perforation, middle ear mass, or other causes.
- Cochlear implantation for those with bilateral profound hearing loss who do not benefit from hearing aids.

INFECTED PREAURICULAR CYST OR SINUS

Preauricular sinuses or pits, located near the front of the ear, mark the entrance to a sinus tract that travels under the skin near the ear cartilage. These tracts may sequester to produce subcutaneous cysts lined with epithelium or may become infected.

EPIDEMIOLOGY

- Congenital anomalies that may be sporadic or inherited (autosomal dominant with variable penetrance)
  ✓ Inherited cases are more likely bilateral.
- 3–5% occur in association with other syndromes, including deafness and branchio-oto-renal syndrome

PATHOPHYSIOLOGY

- Infection occurs when the opening of the sinus is occluded with bacteria and desquamated skin.
- *Staphylococcus aureus* is most commonly isolated; other pathogens include viridans group streptococci, *Peptostreptococcus* spp., and *Proteus* spp.

CLINICAL MANIFESTATIONS

- Sinus appears as a pinpoint hole anterior to ear, usually just above the tragus.
- Cyst appears as a preauricular mass, often adjacent to an associated sinus.
- Signs of infection include
  - ✓ Preauricular erythema, swelling, and tenderness
  - ✓ Purulent drainage or preauricular granulation tissue may be present.
- Superinfected cyst may manifest as a tender, enlarging preauricular mass.

DIAGNOSTICS

- Clinical diagnosis from symptoms and physical exam
- Imaging rarely needed
- Consider hearing screen and renal ultrasound if dysmorphic features or other congenital abnormalities are also present.

MANAGEMENT

- Oral antibiotics (e.g., amoxicillin–clavulanate, clindamycin) for uncomplicated cases, IV antibiotics if recalcitrant cases or associated with facial cellulitis or high fever
- May require needle aspiration (21-gauge needle); incision and drainage should be avoided, if possible as inflammation may impair wound healing and increases recurrence risk.
- Definitive management is excision of the preauricular sinus and tract once acute infection resolved
  - ✓ 5% to 15% recurrence after surgical excision
  - ✓ Factors associated with recurrence include
    - ▪ Excision performed during active infection or inflammation
    - ▪ Excision under local anesthesia
    - ▪ Poor delineation of sinus tract during surgery

LARYNGOMALACIA

Congenital flaccid larynx

EPIDEMIOLOGY

- Most common laryngeal anomaly in infants
- Accounts for 65–75% of infant stridor

ETIOLOGY

- Exact etiology unknown. Theories include hypotonia or dyscoordination of laryngeal or supralaryngeal structures.
- Gastroesophageal reflux may be contributing factor.

PATHOPHYSIOLOGY

- Prolapse of loose laryngeal tissues into airway on inspiration; causes inspiratory airway noise/obstruction
- Prolapse is caused by excess compliance of the laryngeal cartilages with an omega-shaped epiglottis, short aryepiglottic folds, and possible excess mucosa over the arytenoids.
- Laryngomalacia can be secondary to other airway lesions, from increased work of breathing and negative airway pressures. Examples include cysts of the tongue base or vallecula, glottic or subglottic stenosis, and tracheomalacia (collapse of trachea on inspiration).

- With normal growth, symptoms typically worsen initially and then gradually resolve between 6 and 18 months of age.

CLINICAL MANIFESTATIONS

- Onset of "noisy breathing" or inspiratory stridor within the first few weeks of life, which worsens with agitation and/or supine positioning
- Inspiratory stridor that is typically positional, louder when supine or during sleep; also with agitation or exertion (e.g., feeding, crying, laughing)
- Cry/phonation is typical (expiratory process).
- Evidence of increased work of breathing: Nasal flaring, retractions, pectus excavatum
- Strong association with gastroesophageal reflux

DIAGNOSTICS

- Flexible NPL: Confirms diagnosis and assesses extent of prolapse/obstruction. Allows detection of secondary airway lesions above the vocal cords. Noninvasive, is done in office or at bedside, without sedation.
- Airway fluoroscopy may reveal laryngomalacia but is much less useful than flexible endoscopy.
- For severe cases, rigid laryngoscopy and bronchoscopy under general anesthesia may be warranted.
- Evaluation for additional congenital tracheobronchial anomalies is important in severe or unusual cases. Airway fluoroscopy is useful here, to detect coincident tracheomalacia. Diagnosis of other secondary lesions requires rigid bronchoscopy under anesthesia.

MANAGEMENT

Medical

- Depends on severity of symptoms
  - ✓ Mild: No feeding problems; symptoms not progressive
  - ✓ Moderate: Feeding difficulties but thriving; progressive stridor
  - ✓ Severe: Apnea, cyanosis, failure to thrive
- Mild/moderate: Conservative management with reassurance to family that condition is self-limited, complete resolution may take up to 18 months. Consider proton-pump inhibitor and change in formula. CPR education for caretakers. Home pulse-oximetry monitoring may be indicated.
- Severe: Surgery may be necessary.
- Treatment of gastroesophageal reflux often helps, regardless of severity

Surgical

- Supraglottoplasty: Excision of the obstructive aryepiglottic folds and/or redundant supraglottic tissues
- Rigid laryngoscopy and bronchoscopy is done at time of surgical intervention to detect any secondary lesions.
- Tracheotomy: Rarely indicated, except in most severe cases

TRACHEOSTOMY

Tracheostomy: The actual hole in the trachea following tracheotomy
Tracheotomy: The surgical incision in the trachea used to gain access to the airway

Indications for tracheostomy include ventilator dependency (40%), extrathoracic obstruction (30%), neurologic dysfunction (20%), and intrathoracic obstruction (10%)

TRACHEOSTOMY VERSUS PROLONGED ENDOTRACHEAL INTUBATION

- Risks of prolonged intubation include injury to glottis, subglottis, and trachea due to pressure of tube.
- Endotracheal tube irritation can be minimized by avoiding cuffed tubes and use of nasotracheal placement to minimize tube movements.
- Endotracheal tubes can easily become blocked owing to the small lumen of pediatric tubes.
- Typical recommendation is for tracheostomy after 2–4 weeks of intubation in child, longer in neonates
- Advantages of tracheostomy: Hospital discharge on ventilator support, avoid damage to larynx and subglottis, easier replacement if decannulated, ease of suctioning and pulmonary toilet, improved ability to wean ventilator and associated sedation
- Disadvantages of tracheostomy: Need for frequent cleaning, suctioning, and humidification; surgical risks; risk of general anesthesia; increased requirements for home care

COMPLICATIONS OF TRACHEOSTOMY

- Intraoperative: Hemorrhage, subcutaneous emphysema, pneumomediastinum, pneumothorax
- Early postoperative: Tracheostomy tube plugging, decannulation, tracheitis
- Late: Tracheoesophageal fistula, tracheal granulomas, suprastomal collapse. Rarely, tube can erode anterior tracheal wall, which may lead to tracheoinnominate fistula with life-threatening hemorrhage

TRACHEOSTOMY CARE

- Tracheostomy tube size reflects the inner diameter in millimeters. Outer diameter is variable and depends on manufacturer and/or material.
- Cuffless tubes preferred in young children to minimize pressure on tracheal wall. Cuffless tubes also allow inner diameter to be maximized in these small airways, which maximizes ventilation and minimizes risk of occlusion.
- Humidified air is supplied to prevent drying of tracheal mucosa.
- Trained caregiver, suctioning equipment, and replacement tube should always be available to maintain airway patency.

CHANGING TRACHEOSTOMY TUBES

- Surgeons typically make first change and survey stoma for patency within 1 week after surgery.
- Subsequent changes can be made by other caregivers.
- All tracheostomy changes best made with neck extended, with good lighting and suction available.

SUBGLOTTIC STENOSIS

Pathologic narrowing of the subglottic airway resulting in stridor, increased work of breathing, and respiratory distress.

- The subglottis is the narrowest segment of the infant airway and is housed by the cricoid cartilage. Stenosis of this segment may be congenital, acquired, or idiopathic.

EPIDEMIOLOGY

- Incidence of congenital subglottic stenosis unknown but accounts for roughly 10% of airway malformations
- Incidence of acquired subglottic stenosis in neonates ranges up to 8%, with a downtrend noted in recent decades; now more likely under 4% due to improved intubation practices
- Greatest risk factor for acquired subglottic stenosis is prematurity.

ETIOLOGY

- Congenital subglottic stenosis is due to failure of the recanalization of the laryngeal airway during the 10th week of gestation, or from a developmentally small cricoid cartilage.
- Acquired subglottic stenosis most often results from either direct mechanical trauma or pressure necrosis from an oversized endotracheal tube causing mucosal erosion and exposure of the underlying perichondrium. This may lead to infection, chondritis, and subglottic scarring.
- In older children, subglottic stenosis may result from rheumatologic disorders like granulomatosis with polyangiitis.

DIFFERENTIAL DIAGNOSIS

- Any other cause for stridor and airway narrowing, including croup, tracheal stenosis, laryngeal stenosis, foreign body aspiration, subglottic cyst, hemangioma, tumor (see **Table 25-1**).

CLINICAL MANIFESTATIONS

- Largely dependent on severity of stenosis. Severe congenital subglottic stenosis presents with retractions, stridor, and respiratory distress at birth.
- Infants may present with intermittent stridor and significant fatigue, especially with feeding or agitation.
- Low-grade subglottic stenosis may present as recurrent episodes of croup that are slow to respond to medical therapy. More severe stenosis may present with airway distress, retractions, desaturations, and airway compromise.
- Failure to wean from a ventilator, especially when accompanied by stridor after extubation attempts, or inability to intubate with an age-appropriate endotracheal tube, may be the first signs of subglottic stenosis, especially in the setting of the neonatal ICU.

DIAGNOSTICS

- Rigid microlaryngoscopy and bronchoscopy is the gold standard for diagnosing subglottic stenosis and should be undertaken in any patient suspected of having subglottic stenosis . This allows for airway sizing using endotracheal tubes as well as intervention if warranted.
- Grading of subglottic stenosis typically employs the Cotton–Myer grading system (**Figure 25-3**).
- Airway fluoroscopy provides a dynamic assessment of the airway caliber and can help to identify the level of airway narrowing but is not a substitute for endoscopy.

MANAGEMENT

- Conservative management with observation and close follow-up may be warranted for certain grade 1 subglottic stenosis patients.
- Endoscopic balloon dilation for thin and early, evolving stenosis; often includes injection with steroid

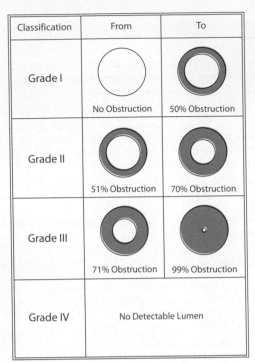

Classification	From	To
Grade I	No Obstruction	50% Obstruction
Grade II	51% Obstruction	70% Obstruction
Grade III	71% Obstruction	99% Obstruction
Grade IV	No Detectable Lumen	

FIGURE 25-3 Cotton–Myer Grading Scale for Subglottic Stenosis. Reproduced with permission from Myer CM, O'Connor DM, Cotton RT: Proposed grading system for subglottic stenosis based on endotracheal tube sizes, Ann Otol Rhinol Laryngol 1994 Apr;103(4 Pt 1): 319-323.

- For infants with low-grade subglottic stenosis, anterior cricoid split widens the subglottis by dividing the cricoid cartilage anteriorly. This may be done endoscopically or as an open procedure and is followed by intubation for several days.
- Laryngotracheal reconstruction involves splitting of the anterior and/or posterior cricoid cartilage followed by cartilage graft augmentation.
- Cricotracheal resection involves surgically resecting the segment of stenotic airway followed by end-to-end reanastomosis.
- Tracheostomy may be needed in moderate to severe subglottic stenosis. Definitive repair can then be deferred until the infant has grown and has improved pulmonary function. This is often necessary in extremely premature infants with chronic lung disease.

TRACHEAL STENOSIS

Narrowing of the tracheal airway secondary to congenital tracheal anomalies, external compression from vascular rings/slings, or acquired from trauma and/or infection

EPIDEMIOLOGY

- Congenital tracheal stenosis is estimated to occur in 1 in 65,000 births.
- The rarity of this entity often leads to delays in diagnosis.

ETIOLOGY

- Abnormal development of the tracheal cartilage resulting in complete rings rather than c-shaped arches
- Compression on the tracheal airway from abnormal vascular anatomy such as double aortic arch, persistent right aortic arch, or prominent distal innominate artery, or left pulmonary artery sling
- Intubation trauma leading to inflammation, scarring, and stenosis

DIFFERENTIAL DIAGNOSIS

- Differential diagnosis for stridor (**Table 25-1**).

CLINICAL MANIFESTATIONS

- Widely variable presentation
- Biphasic stridor which is often wet-sounding, described as "washing machine" stridor
- Recurrent respiratory infections
- Symptoms may be severe but episodic and include apnea, bradycardia, or cyanosis
- Often associated with dysphagia if vascular ring/sling also causes esophageal compression

DIAGNOSTICS

- Chest x-ray
- Microlaryngoscopy with rigid bronchoscopy: Avoid instrumentation of stenotic segment when possible.
- Echocardiography and/or MR angiography to evaluate for cardiac anomalies and aberrant vasculature
- Contrast-enhanced chest CT scan defines anatomy of the tracheobronchial tree and relationship to surrounding vessels.

MANAGEMENT

- Avoid instrumentation of the stenotic segment to prevent edema and further potentially critical narrowing.
- Shallow intubation above the level of stenosis if required
- Segmental resection and reanastomosis has largely been replaced by slide tracheoplasty for complete tracheal rings, tracheal sleeves, and other tracheal stenosis. In this procedure, the stenotic segment of trachea is divided and reattached in a way that makes it shorter yet wider.
- Rerouting of vascular rings/slings via division and reanastomosis when necessary, and aortopexy to suspend innominate artery anteriorly

VOCAL-CORD PARALYSIS

Unilateral or bilateral paralysis of the vocal folds

EPIDEMIOLOGY

- Accounts for 15–20% of cases of stridor in infants
- Rarely an isolated lesion in children
- Unilateral vocal-cord paralysis (VCP) is more common on left side.

TABLE 25-1 Differential Diagnosis for Noisy Breathing

	Laryngomalacia	Subglottic Stenosis	Tracheal stenosis, vascular ring, or sling	Vocal cord paralysis	Neoplasm	Croup	Epiglottitis	Foreign Body
Stridor	Inspiratory especially with agitation, feeding, and when supine	Inspiratory; occasionally biphasic	Biphasic, "washing machine" stridor	Unilateral—usually none but occasionally inspiratory stridor. Bilateral-biphasic	Determined by the location of lesion	Inspiratory with barking cough	Biphasic	Inspiratory or biphasic
Associated Signs and Symptoms	Difficulty feeding, aspiration, poor weight gain, GERD	Recurrent respiratory infections and recurrent severe croup	Dysphagia, Recurrent respiratory infections	Unilateral: Aspiration, hoarseness (weak, breathy cry). Bilateral: severe stridor with normal cry	Widely variable	Fever, cold symptoms, worse breathing at night	Acute onset. fever, dysphagia, drooling, tripod positioning	Witnessed choking event, paroxysmal cough, decreased breath sounds, unilateral wheeze
Age	Weeks to 2 years	Variable	Usually within first few weeks, but may not be discovered until adulthood	Any age for Bilateral, unilateral, or congenital	Any	6 months-3 years	Any	Any

Chronicity	Onset in first few weeks of life	Congenital—may be clinically apparent from birth, or only at times of respiratory infection Acquired—often apparent at time of extubation, but may be delay in clinical manifestation	May be clinically present from birth, or may progress over time	Congenital—present at birth, may resolve within 2 years Acquired—present following inciting incident	Progressive	Acute	Acute	Acute
Diagnosis	Flexible NPL; need fully awake patient	MLB	MLB, Chest CT, MRI, ECHO	Flexible NPL	NPL, MLB, and imaging	Plain Films	Clinical, NPL	CXR, MLB
Management	GERD management, Observation for mild cases, supraglottoplasty if child has poor growth or significant respiratory distress	Observation for some grade 1; Endoscopic dilation; Open or endoscopic Laryngotracheoplasty; Tracheotomy	Slide tracheoplasty, Tracheal resection, Cardiothoracic surgery to repair rings and slings	Observation Tracheostomy Anterior/Posterior Cricoid Cartilage Split Vocal fold injection Recurrent laryngeal nerve reinnervation	Dependent on pathology	Medical management with steroids, humidification	Intubation in the OR, possible tracheostomy	MLB with foreign body removal

CT = computed tomograph; CXR = chest radiograph; ECHO = echocardicgram; GERD = gastroesophageal reflux disease; MLB = microlaryngoscopy and bronchoscopy; MRI = magnetic resonance imaging; NPL = nasopharyngolaryngoscopy

ETIOLOGY

- Bilateral vocal cord paralysis can be idiopathic, or caused by central nervous system immaturity, various lesions, Arnold–Chiari malformation, hydrocephalus, or birth trauma.
- Unilateral paralysis can be caused by birth trauma or by previous intervention; most commonly, cardiothoracic surgery (left recurrent laryngeal nerve recurs around aortic arch and ductus arteriosus)

PATHOPHYSIOLOGY

- Abductors and adductors of vocal cords are controlled by the recurrent laryngeal nerve, a branch of the vagus nerve, which can be damaged anywhere along the path from the brain stem to the larynx.
- Unilateral vocal cord paralysis more commonly due to peripheral-nerve injury
- Bilateral vocal cord paralysis more likely due to central nervous system cause
- Traumatic or prolonged intubation can directly injure or scar glottic tissues and joints. Vocal-cord motion is mechanically restricted, though nerve/muscle function is normal.

CLINICAL MANIFESTATIONS

- Unilateral vocal cord paralysis: Weak vocal cord tends to retract away from the midline and glottis fails to close during swallowing and phonation. Result is weak cry, breathy voice, aspiration, and/or feeding difficulties, ineffective cough, recurrent pneumonia, and/or hoarseness.
- Bilateral vocal cord paralysis: Bilaterally paralyzed vocal cords are often fixed in the midline closed position, causing stridor, and respiratory distress; may have normal cry. Alternatively, weak vocal cords may fall away from the midline and result in aspiration, hoarseness, and/or feeding difficulties, as for unilateral vocal cord paralysis
- Evaluate severity of respiratory impairment: Work of breathing, respiratory rate, oxygen saturation
- Search for associated congenital anomalies, surgical history, hydrocephalus, or predisposing trauma.

DIAGNOSTICS

- Flexible laryngoscopy: Cornerstone of diagnosis; can usually be done at bedside; sedation best avoided to allow full assessment of function
- MRI and/or CT in idiopathic cases to evaluate CNS and course of vagus nerve
- Barium swallow, with or without milk scan, to assess swallowing function and risk of dysphagia or aspiration

MANAGEMENT

Three Goals of Management

1. Safe airway
   - ✓ Tracheostomy: Necessary for 20–50% of bilateral vocal cord paralysis; rarely necessary for unilateral vocal cord paralysis
   - ✓ Spontaneous resolution is common, so period of observation (months in duration) is essential,
   - ✓ Surgical management including posterior cricoid graft, lateralization of vocal cords, or cordotomy, may be needed for unresolved bilateral vocal cord paralysis

2. Intelligible speech
   - ✓ For unilateral vocal cord paralysis, observation for several months is indicated, to allow for spontaneous nerve regeneration. Also, young children often have gradual voice improvement, due to overcompensation by the opposite vocal cord
   - ✓ Surgical medialization of the paralyzed vocal cord, or nerve reimplantation, may be needed for persistent aspiration or poor vocal quality
3. Prevention of aspiration
   - ✓ May require alternative consistency of feedings
   - ✓ May temporarily require G-tube

CHAPTER 26

Procedures 26

Mercedes M. Blackstone, MD
Jeannine Del Pizzo, MD
Sarah Fesnak, MD

BAG VALVE MASK VENTILATION

INDICATIONS

- Apnea, respiratory depression, hypoxia, cardiac, respiratory or neurologic failure

EQUIPMENT

- *Appropriate mask size:* An appropriate mask completely covers the patient's nose and mouth without mask edges hanging off the face or covering eyes
- *Bag:* Self-inflating or anesthesia (flow-inflating) bag

TECHNIQUE

- Position patient's head by either chin lift (stable cervical spine) or jaw thrust (unstable cervical spine) to maximize upper airway diameter.
- Place mask over patient's mouth and nose and hold tight against face using C-E hold (see **Figure 26-1**). The thumb and 2nd finger form a "C" shape over the mask while the 3rd, 4th, and 5th fingers of the same hand form an "E" over the mandible, effectively pulling the patient's jaw up to meet the mask. Be careful not to compress the soft tissues below the mandible
- Squeeze bag to push air into patient's lungs
  - ✓ Self-inflating bag: Simple to use, pop-off valve limits amount of pressure delivered, no air reaches patient unless bag is squeezed, delivers room air unless attached to an oxygen reservoir
  - ✓ Anesthesia bag: Requires experienced operator, requires oxygen reservoir, can deliver blow-by oxygen, continuous positive airway pressure (CPAP), or assisted breaths
- Goal rate of delivered breaths: 8–10 breaths per minute
  - ✓ Unsecure airway during one-person cardiopulmonary resuscitation (CPR): Deliver 2 breaths for every 30 compressions
  - ✓ Unsecure airway during two-person CPR: Deliver 2 breaths for every 15 compressions
  - ✓ Secure airway during CPR: 8–10 breaths per minute
- Chest-wall rise indicates adequate delivery.
- Listen for air leak around mask as each breath is delivered. If an air leak is heard, it can be due to hand position, wrong mask size, or fatigue. Try the following—reposition C-E hold, use two hands for C-E hold with a second provider squeezing the bag, or switch providers.

AIRWAY ADJUNCTS: NASOPHARYNGEAL AIRWAY AND ORAL AIRWAY

NASOPHARYNGEAL (NP) AIRWAY

INDICATIONS

- Upper airway obstruction in a patient with spontaneous respirations
- Used to stent tongue away from posterior pharynx

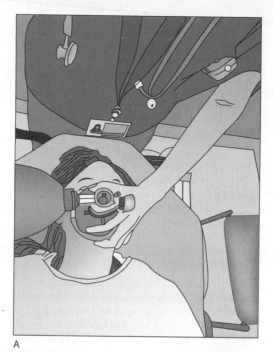

A

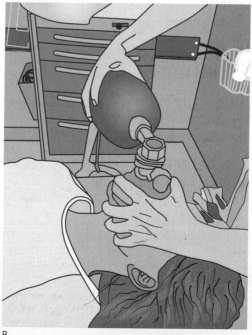

B

FIGURE 26-1 **A and B: C-E Hold for Bag Valve Mask Ventilation.**

- Can be used in conscious patients
- *Do not use* in patients with severe head or facial injuries, or concern for basilar skull fracture

EQUIPMENT

- Appropriately sized NP airway: To estimate appropriate NP airway length, measure the distance from naris to tragus
- Lubrication jelly

TECHNIQUE

- Apply lubrication jelly to insertion end of NP airway.
- Insert NP airway into patient's naris with gentle posterior pressure until the flange rests on the naris edge.
- The NP airway should glide in easily. If resistance is encountered, check NP airway size, lubrication, or patency of nasal passage

ORAL AIRWAY

INDICATIONS

- Upper airway obstruction in an unconscious patient with spontaneous respirations
- Upper airway obstruction in an unconscious patient receiving bag-assisted ventilations
- Used to stent tongue and pharyngeal soft tissues away from posterior pharynx
- *Do not use* in a conscious patient as it may stimulate the gag reflex, emesis, and aspiration

EQUIPMENT

- Appropriately sized oral airway: To estimate appropriate oral airway length, measure the distance from the corner of the mouth to angle of the mandible.
- Wooden tongue depressor

TECHNIQUE

- Using tongue depressor, push tongue away from palate
- Insert the oral airway along the curve of the tongue so that the innermost edge of the oral airway rests just posterior to the tongue
- The flange of the oral airway should rest on the patient's lips
- Be careful not to push tongue back and cause further upper airway obstruction.

ENDOTRACHEAL INTUBATION

INDICATIONS

- Airway protection; existing or impending cardiac, respiratory, or neurologic failure

EQUIPMENT

Mnemonic: "MSOAP"

- Meds: Intubation adjuncts, sedatives, paralytics, resuscitation meds, anticonvulsants
  ✓ See inside back cover for rapid sequence intubation medications
- Monitors: Cardiorespiratory (CR) monitor, pulse oximeter, blood pressure (BP), end-tidal co-oximetry

- Suction: Yankauer (rigid catheter), flexible soft catheter
- Oxygen: Tank or "wall" supply, delivery tubing
- Airway equipment: Endotracheal tubes, stylets, laryngoscope blades, masks, self-inflating bag or anesthesia bag, NP airway, oral airway, laryngeal mask airway, tape, benzoin, syringe for cuff inflation
- Personnel

Choosing an Endotracheal Tube (ETT)

- Beyond the newborn period, cuffed tubes may be safely used
- Formula for uncuffed ETT diameter:

$$\left[\frac{\text{Age (years)}}{4} \right] + 4$$

- Formula for cuffed ETT diameter:

$$\left[\frac{\text{Age (years)}}{4} \right] + 3 \quad \text{or} \quad \left[\frac{\text{Age (years)}}{4} \right] + 3.5$$

Choosing a Laryngoscope Blade

- Straight (Miller) and curved (Macintosh) blades are available. Choose blade based on comfort level of laryngoscopist and size of child. The Miller is more appropriate for someone less experienced and when intubating younger infants and children with a larger and more floppy epiglottis. The Wis-Hipple, modified from the Wisconsin blade, has a length of 1.5 with a slightly wider tip than the Miller.
- Some age-related suggestions:

  ✓ Preemie: Miller 0
  ✓ 0–3 months: Miller 1
  ✓ 3 months–3 years: Miller 1, Miller 2, Wis-Hipple 1.5
  ✓ 3–12 years: Miller 2, Macintosh 2
  ✓ >12 years: Miller 3, Macintosh 3

TECHNIQUE

- Check all equipment and monitors. Preoxygenate with 100% O_2. Administer selected pharmacologic agents (see inside front cover)
- Adjust height of bed to accommodate the person performing the intubation.
- Position patient's head by either chin lift (stable cervical spine) or jaw thrust (unstable cervical spine) to maximize upper airway diameter. Depending on the age of the child, a towel roll under the head or shoulders may help to achieve the "sniffing" position.
- If using stylet, tip should not extend beyond end of ETT.
- Consider having an assistant apply gentle cricoid pressure (Sellick maneuver)
- Open mouth using scissor-finger technique with right hand (thumb on mandibular dental ridge, index or middle finger on maxillary dental ridge)
- Holding the laryngoscope in the left hand, insert blade on the right side of the patient's mouth, and sweep tongue toward the midline. Gently but firmly pull up along the axis of the handle of the laryngoscope maintaining a straight wrist. Do not rock back or lever the laryngoscope on the teeth.

- Suction and reposition as needed until the glottic opening (characteristic inverted V of vocal cords) is visualized.
- While maintaining visualized glottis, introduce ETT with right hand from the right side of mouth and pass tip of tube through the vocal cords.
- Depth of insertion: Internal diameter of the ETT × 3 (length to corner of mouth) or double lines on tube just past vocal cords
- Confirmation of proper placement: Change from purple to yellow on colorimetry, presence of end-tidal CO_2, mist in ETT tube, bilateral chest rise, and equal breath sounds
- Temporarily secure ETT to patient with benzoin and tape. Obtain chest x-ray to confirm placement (ideal tip placement is between clavicles and carina). Definitively secure ETT by splitting tape lengthwise; secure one arm to upper lip and wrap second arm around ETT. Repeat with second piece of tape.

LARYNGEAL MASK AIRWAY (LMA)

INDICATIONS

- Airway protection; cardiac, respiratory, or neurologic failure; difficulty passing endotracheal tube
- Excellent rescue device because fairly easy to use for a variety of providers
- Can serve as a bridge to a more definitive airway

EQUIPMENT

- Appropriately sized LMA: Depends on the patient's weight and the LMA manufacturer. Each LMA will be labeled with a weight range in kilograms that is acceptable for use. Also displayed will be the quantity of air in milliliters that is required to fill the LMA cuff.
- Lubrication jelly
- Equipment as listed in MSOAP pneumonic under "Endotracheal Intubation": Medications, monitors, suction, oxygen, airway equipment, personnel
- See inside back cover for rapid sequence intubation medications.
- If LMA is being placed because of failed intubation, consider calling for additional airway personnel.

TECHNIQUE

- Stand at the head of the bed as if performing intubation
- Check all equipment and monitors. Preoxygenate with 100% O_2. Administer selected pharmacologic agents.
- Apply lubrication jelly to insertion end of LMA.
- Position patient's head by either chin lift (stable cervical spine) or jaw thrust (unstable cervical spine) to maximize upper airway diameter.
- With nondominant hand, grasp the patient's mandible and open the mouth.
- With the dominant hand, hold the LMA as shown in **Figure 26-2** and insert LMA into mouth, skimming along the curve of the tongue into the pharynx until resistance is met.
- Once resistance is met, inflate LMA cuff with appropriate amount of air.
- In younger patients, consider the rotational approach, in which the LMA is first inserted with the opening facing the palate and then rotated 180 degrees into position when resistance is felt.
- Begin ventilating patient. Ensure appropriate LMA placement by checking for presence of end-tidal CO_2, bilateral chest rise, and equal breath sounds.

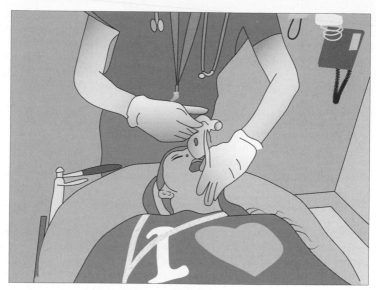

FIGURE 26-2 **Laryngeal Mask Airway Insertion.**

INTRAOSSEOUS LINE PLACEMENT

INDICATIONS

- Immediate vascular access for cardiopulmonary arrest or shock; intravenous access difficult or not possible in critically ill patient
- Can be placed much faster than central venous lines
- May be used to administer fluids, blood products, medications
- Aspirated blood can be sent for diagnostic studies. Values such as WBC count, potassium, calcium, transaminases, and blood oxygen level are less reliable.

EQUIPMENT

- Gloves, gauze; antiseptic solution (povidone-iodine or ChloraPrep); 1% lidocaine; syringe; 22- or 25-gauge needles; saline flush in 10-mL syringe; intraosseous (IO) needle
- If using the battery-powered driver: Device driver, appropriate IO needle, stabilizer dressing, extension tubing, 2% lidocaine
- If no IO needle is available, a bone marrow aspiration needle with trocar or 20-gauge spinal needle can be used.

PLACEMENT SITES

- Proximal tibia: The preferred site is the tibial plateau (anterior, medial flat surface of tibia), 1–2 cm below the tibial tuberosity.
- Distal femur: An alternate site for infants and young children is the midline on the femoral plateau (lower third of femur), approximately 1–2 cm above the superior border of the patella.
- Distal tibia: 1–2 cm above the medial malleolus. Easier to use in children >3 years of age.

- Proximal humerus: Typically requires battery-powered driver device; greater tubercle of humerus appropriate in the older, skeletally mature child. To access the greater tubercle safely, place patient's arm on the abdomen with elbow flexed. The greater tubercle prominence is about 1 cm above the surgical neck of the humerus, or 2 cm below the acromion process.
- Manubrium: The upper part of the sternum has been used more often in adults.

MANUAL INSERTION TECHNIQUE

- In awake patients, inject 1% lidocaine into skin and periosteum.
- Prepare skin with antiseptic solution.
- Stabilize extremity with nondominant hand. (Keep hand away from opposite side of insertion site to avoid injury!) Identify landmarks for insertion, most commonly, the tibial plateau.
- Hold IO needle with hub resting in the palm; stabilize needle with thumb and index finger placed 1–2 cm from the tip.
- Insert needle perpendicular to the bony cortex or slightly angled (10–15 degrees) away from the growth plate. Use steady back-and-forth rotational motion while gradually increasing pressure until a sudden decrease in resistance is felt. Immediately release pressure to prevent piercing opposite end of bone.
- Unscrew the needle cap and remove the trocar. If the needle is secure in the bone, it should stand without support.
- Confirm intramedullary placement with aspiration of blood or bone marrow and/or easy infusion of fluids without extravasation.
  - ✓ Flush the needle quickly with 10 mL of normal saline and connect it to conventional IV tubing.
- Secure needle with a dressing. Avoid bulky dressings that may make infiltration difficult to detect.

BATTERY-POWERED DRIVER TECHNIQUE

- Battery-powered IO needle and driver sets have become more widely available in prehospital and hospital settings (Arrow EZ-IO`, Teleflex Corporation). They are relatively straightforward to use after training and therefore have high success rates.
- Needles come in three sizes:
  - ✓ Small (15 mm) = Pink for patients 3–39 kg
  - ✓ Medium (25 mm) = Blue for patient ≥40 kg
  - ✓ Large (45 mm) = Yellow for patients ≥40 kg with excessive subcutaneous tissues; often needle of choice for humerus site
- Identify appropriate location for insertion and anatomic landmarks. Cleanse insertion site.
- Choose the appropriate needle based on the patient's weight and amount of subcutaneous tissue.

  Note: Weights are rules of thumb; important thing is that one black line is still visible after the needle is through the skin. Because of the amount of subcutaneous tissue, the pink needle often is helpful only in very young patients; the blue needle is the most widely used If in doubt, go with the longer needle to ensure that the marrow is penetrated.

- Remove the safety cap and place the needle into the battery-powered driver
- Position driver with the needle perpendicular to the bone surface and insert needle until you feel bone. Ensure that at least 5 mm of the needle is visible as indicated by the black line (if not, use a longer needle or an alternative site).

- Press trigger to activate the driver, applying gentle downward pressure. Release the trigger when you feel a sudden decrease in resistance.
- Hold the catheter in place and remove the driver by pulling up. Remove the stylet from the catheter by rotating counterclockwise, and safely dispose of the stylet.
- Secure the site with the stabilizer dressing.
- Connect primed connector and draw samples for lab tests, if necessary.
- Flush the catheter quickly with 10 mL of NS (to displace marrow and provide room for infusion).

Note: In an awake or responsive patient, consider infusing 2% lidocaine without epinephrine into IO space prior to this step—infusion into the marrow is quite painful.

LACERATION REPAIR

INDICATION

- Restore integrity and function of injured tissues while minimizing scar formation and infection

EQUIPMENT

- Basics: Light, with or without mask, gloves, povidone-iodine solution
- Irrigation: 20- to 60-mL syringes, sterile saline, splash guard
- Suture tray: Needle holder, nontraumatic tissue forceps, tissue scissors, hemostats, sterile gauze, sterile drapes
- Suture material:
  ✓ Nonabsorbable: Monofilament nylon (Ethilon), polypropylene (Prolene)
  ✓ Absorbable: Vicryl, fast-absorbing gut, chromic gut
    ▪ Nonabsorbable sutures have high tensile strength and are typically used on extremities.
    ▪ Fast-absorbing sutures (Vicryl Rapide, fast-absorbing gut) are frequently used for pediatric facial lacerations and fingertip avulsions.
    ▪ Chromic gut is useful for closure of intraoral lacerations, as well as for nailbed lacerations.
- Size: Face: 6-0 or 5-0; scalp, trunk, extremities: 4-0; sole of foot, over large joints: 4-0 or 3-0

GENERAL TECHNIQUE

- Local anesthesia
  ✓ "LET" gel: Contains lidocaine, epinephrine, and tetracaine. Apply for 15–20 minutes up to three times or until skin blanches. Avoid areas where vasoconstriction is contraindicated (e.g. digits).
  ✓ 1% Lidocaine (10 mg/mL): Infiltrative anesthetic; maximum dose: 4 mg/kg; onset: 2–5 minutes; duration: 30–120 minutes
  ✓ 1% Lidocaine with epinephrine (1:200,000): Infiltrative anesthetic, reduces bleeding; maximum dose: 7 mg/kg; onset: 2–5 minutes; duration: 60–180 minutes; contraindicated in digits, penis, pinna, tip of nose
  ✓ Sodium bicarbonate: Buffers local anesthetic to improve potency and reduce pain. Mix 1 part $NaHCO_3$ to 9 parts lidocaine or lidocaine with epinephrine
- Wound preparation
  ✓ Exploration: Provide hemostasis; explore for foreign body
  ✓ Debridement: Remove devitalized or heavily contaminated tissue
  ✓ Hair: May clip. Alternatively, use petroleum jelly to keep unwanted scalp hair away from wound. Do not shave eyebrows.

✓ Irrigation: Irrigate with NS using 20- to 60-mL syringe and splash-guard. Use 100–200 mL for average 2-cm laceration. Consider cleaning wound periphery using povidone-iodine solution.

- Apply suture using needle holder
  ✓ For better control, hold loaded needle holder near the tip. Do *not* keep fingers in rings of the needle holder while sewing.
  ✓ Enter skin with needle perpendicular to surface. Retrieve needle after each pass with needle holder or forceps.
  ✓ Place just enough sutures so that there are no gaps in the wound.
- Instrument tie
  ✓ Tighten knot so that skin edges just come together, making sure that wound edges are everted to minimize scar formation (**Figure 26-3**).
  ✓ After a double-loop tie, repeat single-loop tie in an over-and-under manner, for a total of four throws. Do not overtighten knots.
  ✓ Cut both ends of suture, allowing adequate length (at least 1 cm) to retrieve suture at time of removal.
  ✓ Suture removal: Neck: 3–4 days; face: 5 days, scalp: 7–10 days; upper extremities, trunk: 7 days; lower extremities: 8–10 days; joint surface: 10–14 days

SUTURE TECHNIQUES

- Simple interrupted sutures: Most common suture used for uncomplicated wounds. Enter skin with needle directed downward or angled slightly away from wound edge (see **Figure 26-3**).
- Inverted ("buried") subcutaneous sutures: Used to counteract tension on wound. Insert needle from within wound at fat–dermal junction (**Figure 26-4**).
- Vertical mattress sutures: Combines a deep and superficial stitch into one suture (**Figure 26-5**). Used in wounds of high tension or where difficult to tie an inverted subcutaneous suture.
- Horizontal mattress sutures: Reinforces subcutaneous tissue and relieves tension from wound edges. Useful as deep layer in relatively shallow lacerations and in areas with minimal subcutaneous tissue (**Figure 26-6**).

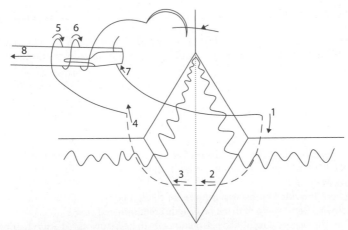

FIGURE 26-3 **Simple Interrupted Suture.**

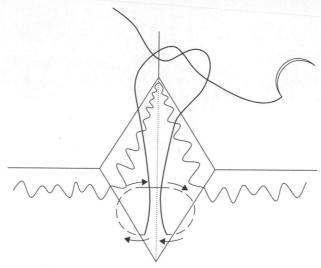

FIGURE 26-4 Inverted Subcutaneous Suture.

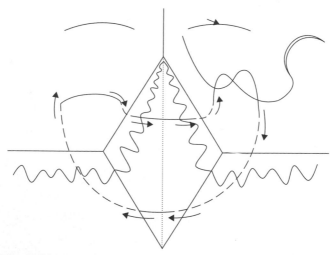

FIGURE 26-5 Vertical Mattress Suture.

- Half-buried or corner suture: Useful in flap closure. Enter skin below and just lateral to the point of V-shaped flap (**Figure 26-7**).
- Simple (continuous) running suture: Limited to linear, clean, low tension wounds. Saves time but breakage unravels entire stitch (**Figure 26-8**).

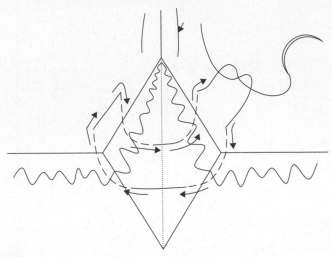

FIGURE 26-6 **Horizontal Mattress Suture.**

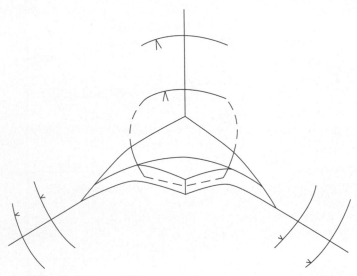

FIGURE 26-7 **Half-Buried (Corner) Suture.**

ALTERNATIVES TO SUTURES

Tape ("Steri-Strips")

- Indications: Linear lacerations under minimal tension; useful for reinforcing or refining other repairs; not useful for wounds requiring meticulous approximation or for moist or hairy areas.

624

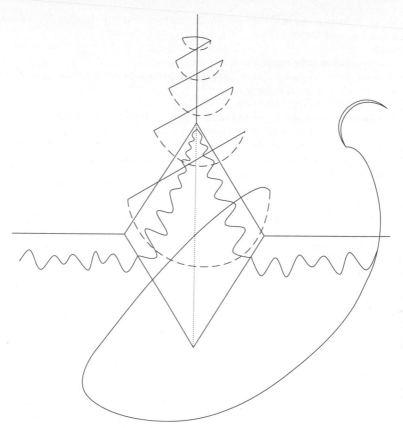

FIGURE 26-8 Simple (Continuous) Running Suture.

• Technique: Clean and dry skin surrounding laceration. Apply adhesive (benzoin) to surrounding skin, and wait 90 seconds for it to become "tacky." Place tape strips perpendicularly across wound, leaving some space for oozing. Place extra tape strips across ends of previous strips and parallel to wound.

Staples

• Best for scalp wounds. Requires staple remover for eventual removal.
• Technique: Prepare wound in same manner as for sutures. Have assistant evert wound edges with tissue forceps or finger pressure. Line up arrow on stapler with center of wound. Place staples by applying steady firm pressure to stapling device. Place staples about 0.5 cm apart.

Tissue Adhesives ("Dermabond")

• Best for linear wounds with minimal tension
• Allows rapid, painless closure of wounds; no removal needed

- Do not use in hairy areas, in the mouth, or near the eyes of young children. Do not use on wounds at high risk for infection.
- Technique
  ✓ Irrigate wound in same manner as for suture repair.
  ✓ Position patient so that adhesive cannot leak into adjacent structures (particularly important for wounds near the eye).
  ✓ The wound must be completely dry.
  ✓ An assistant should hold the wound edges together with forceps or gloved fingers.
  ✓ Activate tissue adhesive applicator (vials often require crushing to start polymerization process and to soak the foam applicator tip).
  ✓ Apply adhesive along surface of wound, creating a thin film.
  ✓ Allow this to dry for a few seconds before applying two to three subsequent layers in concentric ovals around the wound (avoid applying adhesive to inside of wound).
  ✓ Hold wound until dry
- In the event that the tissue adhesive needs to be removed, apply petroleum jelly or antibiotic ointment for about 30 minutes.
- Wears off in 5–10 days

POSTLACERATION REPAIR MANAGEMENT

- In general, cover the wound for the first 24 hours and apply topical antibiotic ointment to wounds. In wounds closed with tissue adhesive, however, no cover is necessary and antibiotic ointments should be avoided.
- Antibiotics are not indicated for the majority of lacerations. Antibiotics may be indicated for high-risk or heavily contaminated wounds. Consider first-generation cephalosporin (e.g., cephalexin). Consider erythromycin if penicillin/cephalosporin allergic. Consider amoxicillin–clavulanic acid for mammalian bites.
- High-risk wounds: Highly contaminated wound, wound with foreign body, bite wounds, wound associated with crush injury, intraoral laceration, wound of hands, feet, or perineum, open fracture, exposed joints and tendons, immunocompromised patient, exposed cartilage, delayed repair, tetanus-prone wounds (**Table 26-1**).

LUMBAR PUNCTURE

INDICATIONS

- Suspicion of CNS infection, suspicion of subarachnoid hemorrhage, measurement of opening pressure, diagnosis and/or treatment of idiopathic intracranial hypertension (pseudotumor cerebri), diagnosis of CNS metastases, suspicion of Guillain–Barré syndrome

TABLE 26-1 Tetanus Prophylaxis		
Prior Tetanus Toxoid Doses	**Clean, Minor Wound**	**Dirty Wounds**
Uncertain or <3 doses	DTaP or Td	DTaP or Td and TIG
3 or more (last >10 years ago)	Td	Td
3 or more (last 5–10 years ago)	None	Td
3 or more (last <5 years ago)	None	None

DTaP, diphtheria, tetanus, acellular pertussis; Td, tetanus, diphtheria; TIG, human tetanus immune globulin.

CONTRAINDICATIONS

- Increased intracranial pressure (unless likely due to idiopathic intracranial hypertension)
- Relative contraindications: Bleeding disorder, cardiopulmonary instability, spinal anomaly, cardiorespiratory instability, overlying rash or skin infection

EQUIPMENT

- Sterile gloves, mask, antiseptic solution (povidone-iodine or chlorhexidine), LP tray, CR monitor and pulse oximeter, topical anesthetic cream (eutectic mixture of local anesthetics, liposomal lidocaine). Resuscitation equipment should also be available.
- LP tray: Typically includes sterile supplies, including drapes, gauze, lidocaine 1%, 3-mL syringe for lidocaine injection, gauze, adhesive bandage strip, collecting tubes, manometer; with or without spinal needle
- Needle size: Usually 22-gauge; infants: 1.5 inch; 1–12 years: 2.5 inch; >12 years/obese patient: 3.5 inch

TECHNIQUE

- Preparing and positioning the patient
  - ✓ Apply topical anesthetic cream to puncture site ≥30 minutes prior to procedure.
  - ✓ Begin monitoring, consider sedation in uncooperative older child.
  - ✓ Two positions commonly used
    - Lateral recumbent: Assistant holds infant in fetal position. In an older child, assistant holds patient in knee–chest position. A firm hold is essential to success. In infants, avoid forcefully flexing the neck, which may lead to respiratory compromise.
    - Sitting position: Patient seated with legs straight out in front over side of bed with neck/upper body flexed forward over pillow on lap or leaning on bedside tray (does not provide accurate measurement of opening pressure).
  - ✓ Locate the puncture site by palpating the superior aspect of the posterior superior iliac crests. A line between the two crests will intersect approximately at top of L4 at midline. The L3–L4 and L4–L5 interspaces are both suitable LP sites.
  - ✓ Prepare the area with antiseptic solution starting at the intended puncture site and swabbing in enlarging circles. Apply sterile drapes; if possible, leave landmarks visible. Anesthetize the interspace with lidocaine 1%. Studies have shown that local anesthetics decrease pain and increase the success rate of LPs.
- Inserting the needle
  - ✓ Ensure that shoulders and hips are perpendicular to the bed.
  - ✓ Slowly insert the bevel-up, styletted needle, aiming slightly cephalad, toward the umbilicus. Infants may require a more acute angle of approach.
  - ✓ After the needle moves through the epidermal and fat layers, some clinicians remove the stylet before advancing further.
  - ✓ Moving beyond the ligamentum flavum/dura into the CSF space, a loss of resistance may be appreciated ("pop"). If the stylet has not been removed, and the "pop" is not appreciated, the physician must remove the stylet every few millimeters to observe for CSF flow.
- Use of manometer
  - ✓ Obtained in the lateral recumbent position.
  - ✓ The manometer should be attached to the needle immediately after CSF flow is seen.
  - ✓ The opening pressure is the highest recorded level that the CSF reaches in the column.
  - ✓ Normal opening pressure is approximately 5–20 cmH$_2$O.
  - ✓ The reading will be falsely high in a struggling patient.

- Collection and completion
  - ✓ Collect approximately 1 mL fluid in each tube. Replace stylet then remove needle. Clean site and apply strip bandage or sterile dressing
  - ✓ Send tubes to lab as follows: Tube 1, Gram stain/culture; tube 2, protein/glucose; tube 3, cell counts; tube 4, any additional studies. If there is concern for subarachnoid hemorrhage, send tubes 1 and 4 for cell count.

PNEUMOTHORAX: NEEDLE DECOMPRESSION

INDICATION

- Tension pneumothorax (which may present with deviated trachea, diminished or asymmetric breath sounds, diminished chest-wall expansion, or sudden cardiopulmonary decompensation)

RISKS

- Can be a lifesaving procedure, so benefit usually outweighs risk
- Very rare complications include lung laceration or air embolism.

EQUIPMENT

- 16- or 18-gauge angiocatheter; 5- to 10-mL syringe; three-way stopcock; antiseptic solution; lidocaine (1%)

TECHNIQUE

- Do not delay for chest x-ray if tension pneumothorax is suspected (absent breath sounds, hypoxia, tracheal deviation hypotension, respiratory distress).
- Place patient in supine position and elevate head of bed to 30 degrees.
- Swab area with antiseptic solution.
- Provide local anesthesia with 1% lidocaine, if time permits.
- Using a 16- or 18-gauge angiocatheter attached to a syringe, insert needle perpendicular to the midclavicular line on the upper edge of the third rib. Gently pull back on the syringe as the needle is advanced into second intercostal space. A loss of resistance in the syringe indicates evacuation of air.
- Advance the catheter over the needle into the pleural space and remove the needle. Attach a one-way drainage device to the catheter or intermittently draw back on a syringe connected to the catheter with a three-way stopcock.
- Immediately obtain chest x-ray.
- Since angiocatheters may not evacuate the whole pneumothorax and can become dislodged or kinked, a chest tube should be placed immediately when there's a large pneumothorax to prevent reaccumulation of air.

UMBILICAL VESSEL CATHETERIZATION

INDICATIONS

- Within the first week of life, frequent arterial or venous blood gases, continuous monitoring of arterial or central venous blood pressures, emergency vascular access, prolonged need for administration of fluids and medications, exchange transfusion

EQUIPMENT

- Umbilical artery catheter (UAC), umbilical vein catheter (UVC), three-way stopcock, radiant warmer, cardiac monitor, pulse oximetry, supplemental oxygen source, antiseptic

solution (povidone-iodine), soft restraints, sterile towels, fenestrated drape, sterile gauze, scalpel: no. 11 or 15, forceps: curved, non-toothed (Iris forceps or vessel dilator), forceps: straight, Crile, hemostats: at least four pairs, scissors, suture: 3.0 or 4.0 silk on curved needle, umbilical tape (approximately 15 inches), 3-mL syringes filled with sterile saline (with heparin 0.5–1 U/mL), sterile gown and gloves, mask, hat
- UAC sizing: Generally 3.5 French, single lumen
- UVC sizing: Infants <1.5 kg: 3.5 French double lumen; infants >1.5 kg: 5 French double lumen

PREPARATION

- Determine appropriate equation for insertion depth.
- Identify appropriate size catheter to be used.
- Gently restrain infant in supine, frog-legged position. Keep infant warm with overhead warmers, and place on cardiac monitor/pulse oximetry with supplemental oxygen available.
- Perform hand hygiene and don hat, mask, sterile gown, and sterile gloves.
- Prepare umbilical lines by connecting a three-way stopcock and 3-mL syringe filled with sterile heparinized saline to each catheter lumen. Flush each lumen with sterile saline and ensure that no air bubbles are present. Turn stopcock so that it is "off to baby."

TECHNIQUE

- Using sterile technique, wash lower 5 cm of umbilical cord and skin surrounding umbilicus with antiseptic solution. Drape with sterile towels.
- Loosely tie umbilical tape at base of cord to prevent bleeding. Use scalpel to cut cord to length of 1–2 cm above the skin surface. Place fenestrated drape (if available) over cut umbilicus, covering patient completely.
- Stabilize cord with forceps or hemostats: Grasp one edge of cord with curved hemostat or grasp opposite sides with two hemostats and evert edges.
- Identify the vessels: One central, cephalad, larger lumen, thin-walled vein; two smaller lumen, thick-walled arteries.
- Hold catheter 1 cm from tip with toothless forceps and insert into vessel lumen with gentle pressure. Blood return at the predetermined depth of insertion signifies proper placement.
  - ✓ Catheterization of the umbilical vein does not require dilation. Insert the umbilical venous catheter to predetermined depth, check for blood return and flush the venous line. Turn stopcock handle toward infant to stop flow ("off to baby").
  - ✓ Catheterization of the umbilical arteries requires gentle dilation with forceps. Dilate arterial lumen using curved, nontoothed, Iris forceps until the arterial opening is large enough to accommodate the umbilical catheter. It is very easy to cause a false track in the Wharton's jelly if this step is skipped. Insert the UAC to predetermined depth, check for blood return, and flush the arterial line. Turn stopcock handle toward infant to stop flow ("off to baby").
- Secure line placement with 3.0 silk suture through Wharton's jelly of umbilical cord. Wrap suture around the catheter two to three times and tie. Do not suture line to skin.
- If able, maintain the sterile field to confirm proper line placement with radiograph of chest and abdomen. Once the sterile field is broken, do not advance the catheter. It may be withdrawn.
- Secure catheters to skin with tape bridge or Tegaderm per unit policy.
- To remove catheter: Place umbilical tape loosely around stump to control bleeding. Remove catheter gradually over 3–4 minutes, allowing vessels to segmentally constrict and/or clot to form.

POSITIONING AND INSERTION LENGTH

- Guidelines vary by institution

"High" UAC

- Catheter tip lies above diaphragm at level of T6–T9.
- Formulas involving body part measurements are more accurate than those using body weight.
- Follow institutional guidelines.
- Common approaches include:
- Shukla and Ferrara method (consistently overestimates length in VLBW infants)
  - ✓ UAC insertion length (cm) = [3 × birthweight (kg)] + 9
- Wright et al formula (superior to Shukla method for VLBW infants)
  - ✓ UAC insertion length (cm) = [4 × birthweight (kg)] + 7
- Gupta et al surface anatomy measurement
  - ✓ (UN − 1cm) + 2 × USp
  - ✓ UN = distance from umbilicus to nipple; USp = distance from umbilicus to symphysis pubis

"Low" UAC

- Catheter tip positioned below diaphragm, just above aortic bifurcation at spinal level L3–L5
- UAC length (cm) = birth weight (kg) + 7 or alternatively, two-thirds the shoulder-to-umbilicus length (cm) distance + length of remaining umbilical cord

UVC

- Normally, catheter tip is placed above diaphragm at the junction of the inferior vena cava and right atrium
- In emergency situations, catheter is passed cephalad for 2–3 cm (preterm) or 4–5 cm (term) until blood return obtained (below portal circulation)
- To estimate normal UVC length: Length (cm) = two-thirds the shoulder-to-umbilicus length (cm) or alternatively (1.5 × birthweight) + 5.5

Risks of procedure

- Bleeding, pericardial effusion/tamponade, air embolus, vessel perforation, arrhythmia, thrombosis, infection

VENTRICULAR SHUNT PUNCTURE

INDICATIONS

- Shunt malfunction, shunt infection. Ideally should be performed by a pediatric neurosurgeon. An indication for a non-neurosurgeon to perform this procedure is life-threatening increased intracranial pressure from suspected shunt malfunction that cannot be managed medically and if no neurosurgeon is immediately available.

CONTRAINDICATIONS

- Overlying skin infection

RISKS

- Introduction of infection (occurs in approximately 1% of procedures)
- Damage to shunt

EQUIPMENT

- 25-gauge butterfly needle (23 gauge may be too large for certain pediatric reservoirs)
- Manometer
- 3-way stopcock
- Syringe
- CSF tubes

- Povidone-iodine or chlorhexidine
- Sterile gloves and drapes

TECHNIQUE

- Important to understand the shunt type and placement location
  - ✓ Proximal catheter (often to the ventricle)
  - ✓ Distal catheter (often to peritoneum, also can be jugular vein, atrium, pleura)
  - ✓ Reservoir (often located near burr hole site)
  - ✓ Valve
  - ✓ Shunt is named for locations of proximal and distal catheter (e.g., venticuloperitoneal shunt, ventriculoatrial shunt)
  - ✓ Multiple shunt types, it is important to know which kind a patient has, if uncertain discuss with neurosurgeon.

PROCEDURE

- Patient should lay supine with shunt located superiorly.
- Identify reservoir, often can be palpated on scalp (small dome), usually can be located on plain film; if uncertain location of reservoir, discuss with neurosurgeon.
- Part hair to reveal reservoir (hair does not need to be shaved or clipped), clean area with povidone-iodine or chlorhexidine.
- Don sterile gloves and place sterile drapes over cleaned area.
- If measuring pressure, attach 3-way stopcock and manometer to tubing of butterfly needle; if not, attach tubing to empty syringe.
- Introduce 25-gauge butterfly needle into reservoir at a slight angle with insertion depth of a few millimeters.
- If there is CSF flow, hold butterfly tubing perpendicular to floor.
- If no immediate flow, apply gentle suction with syringe (avoid vigorous suction, as this can pull choroid plexus into tubing, resulting in obstruction or rupture bridging veins causing hemorrhage).
- Withdraw needle, hold pressure with gauze for several minutes.
- Consider sending sample for CSF studies.
- Interpretation of shunt puncture if there are signs and symptoms of increased ICP and enlarged ventricles on imaging

  - ✓ Rapid flow CSF: Distal catheter obstruction
  - ✓ Slow/absent flow: Proximal catheter obstruction

INTERMITTENT BLADDER CATHETERIZATION

INDICATIONS

- Sterile collection of urine for culture in a child who is not toilet trained
- Relief of urinary retention
- Need for urgent urine testing in child who is unable to void

CONTRAINDICATIONS

- Rarely, due to urologic abnormality, severe phimosis, or labial adhesions, bladder catheterization is not possible or needs to be done by a specialized provider

RISKS

- Microtrauma causing microscopic hematuria
- Iatrogenic infection (extremely rare)

EQUIPMENT

- Antiseptic (e.g., povidone-iodine solution)
- Urinary catheter kit, which typically includes sterile drapes, lubricant, and sterile urine container.
- Appropriate urinary catheter (straight)
- Suggested catheter sizing: 5 French for children ≤6 months; 8 French for those 6 months to adolescence; 10 French for adolescents
- Sterile gloves
- Additional laboratory specimen containers. if required
- Two care providers (one to assist with holding patient)
- Optional: Bladder scanner or ultrasound machine

PROCEDURE

- If unsure of hydration status, consider using a bladder scanner or point-of-care ultrasound to ensure there is adequate urine in the bladder.
- Hold the supine child in the flexed, frog-leg position.
- Open diaper. If soiled, wipe patient with wipes or use wet gauze to clean.
- Open urinary catheter kit then unfold sterile wrapper.
- Unwrap catheter and drop urinary catheter onto sterile field without contaminating.
- Complete hand hygiene and don sterile gloves.
- Squeeze water-soluble lubricant onto sterile field and coat catheter tip.
- Open cleaning agent swab.
- Place sterile drape on genital area.
- Visualize anatomy and identify urethral meatus with nondominant hand. Assistant may need to help with optimal position for visualization.
- Cleanse anterior urethra with antiseptic solution while keeping dominant hand sterile, and allow antiseptic to dry.
- Place distal (unlubricated end) of catheter into sterile urine collection container.
- Advance lubricated catheter into the bladder until urine returns.
- Consider allowing first few drops of urine to be discarded before then filling sterile specimen container for lab.
- Once procedure is complete, remove catheter, clean antiseptic off the skin.

Considerations for boys

- In the uncircumcised male, foreskin should be gently retracted to allow full urethral visualization.
- The nondominant hand should hold the penis upright and perpendicular to the abdomen (to straighten the urethra).
- Resistance may be appreciated at the base of the penis as the catheter touches the external bladder sphincter. Continue to apply gentle upward penile traction while gently advancing the catheter.
- Once procedure is complete, reduce foreskin to prevent a paraphimosis.

Considerations for girls

- Retract labia majora to allow for urethral visualization, which can be challenging (often helps to use gentle traction to pull labia anteriorly, laterally, and inferiorly).
- Utilize first antiseptic swab to locate urethra by wiping in a slow downward motion over anatomical area, looking for pooling of antiseptic in urethral opening..

PITFALL

- Always stop if meeting too much resistance while advancing catheter

27 Psychiatry

Catharyn A. Turner II, MEd, MD
Amy Kim, MD

ACUTE AGITATION/AGGRESSION

Agitation and aggression are nonspecific symptoms that do not necessarily imply a specific etiology.

ETIOLOGY

- Causal or contributing factors
  - ✓ Alcohol and substance intoxication or withdrawal
  - ✓ Infection
  - ✓ Immune-mediated conditions
  - ✓ Primary psychiatric disorders
  - ✓ Psychosis
  - ✓ Severe conduct disorder
  - ✓ Autism spectrum disorders
  - ✓ Intellectual and developmental disabilities
  - ✓ Anxiety
  - ✓ Delirium
  - ✓ Temporal lobe seizures
  - ✓ Other causes (e.g., medication related adverse effects, encephalopathy, cerebritis)
- Risk factors and exacerbating factors

  - ✓ History of prior aggression
  - ✓ History of exposure to aggression/violence
  - ✓ Male gender
  - ✓ Substance abuse/intoxication
  - ✓ Psychiatric disorders or conditions that affect judgement and impulsivity
  - ✓ Pain
  - ✓ Inability to understand treatment plan and/ or their environment (as can be seen in young children, individuals with delirium, autism, or intellectual disability)

CLINICAL MANIFESTATIONS

- Present along a spectrum with verbal and/or physical manifestations. Recognition of early warning signs of agitation or potential for aggression provides opportunity for intervention and prevention of escalation, and to preemptively call for additional help and resources.
- Warning signs and behaviors
  - ✓ Verbal
    - Increased volume of voice, yelling, shouting
    - Use of expletives
    - Threatening statements to harm self or others
    - Verbal refusal to cooperate
  - ✓ Physical
    - Pacing, physical restlessness
    - Violation of typical personal space boundaries
    - Throwing or destroying objects

- Attempts to harm self
- Body contact with other (pushing, hitting, punching, kicking)
- Other clinical manifestations will depend on the underlying cause:
  ✓ Delirium
    - Altered level of alertness and concentration
    - Disorientation
    - Hallucinations or delusions
  ✓ Primary psychiatric disorder
    - Mood/affect lability can be seen in mood disorders, alcohol and drug intoxication or withdrawal
    - Irritability can be seen with mood and anxiety disorders, autism spectrum disorders, disruptive behavior disorders, alcohol and drug intoxication or withdrawal
    - Anxiety can be seen with mood and anxiety disorders, autism spectrum disorders, alcohol and drug intoxication or withdrawal
    - Impulsivity can be seen with attention-deficit/hyperactivity disorder (ADHD), disruptive behavior disorders, as well as other psychiatric, neurologic, medical and developmental conditions
    - Psychotic symptoms can be seen with schizophrenia, mood disorders, delirium, and other neurologic and medical conditions.
    - Suicidal or homicidal ideation may be associated with mood and behavioral disorder, and may contribute to agitation and agression in the inpatient medical setting.
    - Poor insight and impaired judgment are typically present when a patient is agitated or acting in an aggressive manner and can be due to numerous psychiatric, neurologic, medical, and developmental factors.
- Signs of intoxication:
  ✓ Alcohol: Smell of alcohol on breath, dysarthria, incoordination, ataxia
  ✓ Amphetamines: Dilated pupils, altered pulse or blood pressure
  ✓ Marijuana: Tachycardia, dry mouth, conjunctival injection
  ✓ Cocaine: Dilated pupils, hypertension, tachycardia, paranoia
  ✓ Hallucinogens: Dilated pupils, tachycardia, sweating, palpitations, tremors, incoordination
  ✓ Phencyclidine (PCP): Nystagmus, hypertension, tachycardia, ataxia, dysarthria, muscle rigidity, seizures
- Signs of withdrawal:
  ✓ Alcohol: Tremulousness, hypertension, fever, sweating, disorientation, seizures
  ✓ Opiates: Dilated pupils, tachycardia, hypertension, fever, sweating, rhinorrhea,
  ✓ Marijuana: Vomiting, abdominal pain, sweating, fever, chills, headache, restlessness, tremulousness

DIAGNOSTICS

- Urine or serum drug screen
- Consider other studies for altered mental status as clinically indicated (see "Altered Mental Status" section in Chapter 20).

MANAGEMENT

Recognize Early Warning Signs

- Provides opportunity to intervene and prevent escalation and to preemptively call for additional help and resources.

Gather Information

- Interview patient, parents/caregivers, outpatient psychiatrist/therapist
  - ✓ Assess risk factors for agitation or aggression.
  - ✓ Identify warning signs of agitation or aggression specific to the patient.
  - ✓ Identify strategies that have been effective in preventing or successfully managing agitation or aggression in the past.
- Mental status exam and physical exam may help to identify underlying cause/etiology.
- Diagnostic tests to identify potential underlying causes (altered mental status workup)
- Identify and treat the underlying cause of the agitated behavior.

Prevention/De-escalation Strategies (Table 27-1)

- Provide a safe and nonthreatening environment
  - ✓ Remove objects/equipment that could potentially cause injury.
  - ✓ Use developmentally appropriate language, directions, an explanations.
  - ✓ Decrease sensory stimulation (dim lights, speak softly, lower volume on TV/music, etc.).

TABLE 27-1	Prevention/De-escalation Strategies
Environmental Controls	Dim lights
	Play low music
	Put on a favorite TV show
	Minimize noise and unnecessary activity, people in the room
	Remove any object/equipment that could potentially cause injury
Psychological Interventions	Provide verbal support
	Involve family for support or limit family visitation (as appropriate)
	Implement 1:1 staff observation, explaining safety and support aspects of this intervention
	Make uninterrupted time to listen to the patient
	Remain neutral and calm
Behavioral Interventions	Child life interventions (as applicable)
	Use simple age-appropriate directions and explanations
	Try verbal redirection
	Consider distraction techniques
	Set reasonable limits
	Explain consequences of behavior in simple concrete terms
Other	Assess patient for any physical/medical causes for behavior
	Assess for the need for as-needed medication
	Consultation for medication alternatives
	Initiate a safety observation level
	Explain safety and support aspects of observation level

Adapted with permission from Lavelle, J. et al. ED Pathway for Evaluation/Treatment of Children with Behavioral Health Issues. The Children's Hospital of Philadelphia Clinical Pathways. 2021. https://www.chop.edu/clinical-pathway/behavioral-health-issues-clinical-pathway

✓ Limit the number of people in the room.
- If patient is becoming verbally agitated
  ✓ Remain neutral and calm.
  ✓ Listen to patient and allow them to vent, as long as the physical behavior remains safe.
  ✓ Attempt to verbally redirect patient.
  ✓ Offer alternative strategy.
  ✓ Consider distraction techniques.
  ✓ Set reasonable limits.
  ✓ Explain consequences of behavior.
- Remove any family members/caregivers contributing to patient's agitation or who are the target of the patient's aggression.
- Consider use of oral medication as needed for anxiety or agitation, if appropriate.
- Consider 1:1 staff for support and monitoring for safety.

Restraints

- Start with least restrictive and coercive methods (i.e., behavioral/environmental interventions).
  ✓ Level of agitation, potential for violence, and developmental level influence approach.
  ✓ Chemical or physical restraints should be used only after less restrictive means have failed and the aggression or behavior is so severe that it places the patient or others in imminent danger.
  ✓ Safety of patient and staff are both priorities.
  ✓ Minimize staff physical intervention, as this contributes to catecholamine surge.
  ✓ Ideally use personnel with training in nonviolent crisis intervention methods to ensure safety of patient and staff.
- Chemical restraints
  ✓ Refers to the use of medication to achieve behavioral control or sedation (Table 27-2)
  ✓ Consider previous medications used that yielded a positive or negative response.
  ✓ Consider current home medications and potential interactions.
  ✓ Ensure that current prescribed medications are given; consider an extra dose or an early dose.
  ✓ Always attempt to offer oral medications first.
  ✓ Be mindful of onset of action and give medications time to take effect.
  ✓ If inadequate results achieved with multiple doses of a medication, consider addition of another therapeutic class of medication.
  ✓ Confer with psychiatry whenever possible
  ✓ Monitor the patient
    ▪ Once patient has responded to interventions, reassess mental status.
    ▪ Monitor heart rate, respiratory rate and effort, and oxygen saturation. Continuous cardio-respiratory monitor and pulse oximetry are optimal.
    ▪ Consider obtaining a baseline ECG.
    ▪ All accredited facilities should have a formal policy that adheres to Joint Commission guidelines regarding the ordering and use of chemical restraints, related patient assessment and documentation requirements. Become familiar with it.
- Physical/mechanical restraints
  ✓ Any manual method/hold, physical or mechanical device that reduces mobility of the patient's body, arms, legs, or head
  ✓ Should be used only when a patient's behavior becomes so violent or aggressive that it endangers his/her own safety or that of others

TABLE 27-2 Medications for Acutely Agitated Patients

Class	Drug	Route	Dose	Relative Contra Indications	Side Effects/Adverse Effects	Comments
Antihistamines	Diphenhydramine	PO IM IV	1 mg/kg (maximum, 25 mg for children <12 years; 50 mg for children ≥12 years)	Prior paradoxical reaction to diphenhydramine, developmental delay, or current anticholinergic/TCA use	Anticholinergic effects, disinhibition	May be ineffective for acute delirium
Benzodiazepine	Lorazepam	PO IM IV	0.02–0.05 mg/kg (maximum, 1 mg for children <12 years; 2 mg for children ≥12 years) May repeat IV/IM after 20 min or PO after 30 min	Disinhibition, respiratory instability, acute angle-narrow glaucoma	Respiratory depression, disinhibition	May be ineffective for acute delirium If inadequate effect achieved after 2 doses or disinhibition occurs, then consider addition of an antipsychotic
Antipsychotic	Olanzapine	ODT	5 mg for weight 30–60 kg; 10 mg for >60 kg: 10 mg	QT prolongation, anticholinergic intoxication, active seizure disorder	QT prolongation, orthostatic hypotension	
	Risperidone	ODT	0.25 mg for weight 20–45 kg; 0.5 mg for >45 k	QT prolongation, anticholinergic intoxication, active seizure disorder	QT prolongation, tachycardia, hypertension, extrapyramidal symptoms	
	Haloperidol	PO IM	0.01 mg/kg (maximum, 2.5 mg for children <12 years; 5 mg for children ≥12 years) May repeat once in 30 min	QT prolongation, anticholinergic intoxication, active seizure disorder, withdrawal syndrome	QT prolongation, dystonic reaction, extrapyramidal symptoms, neuroleptic malignant syndrome	Full effect may take 30 minutes. If patient did not receive any benzodiazepine, then consider giving dose of lorazepam

IM = intramuscular; IV = intravenous; ODT = orally disintegrating tablet; PO = per os (orally).

Note: If muscle stiffness/dystonia or movement problems develop after use of an antipsychotic, give diphenhydramine 1 mg/kg/dose PO/IM/IV (maximum, 50 mg). If symptoms persist, consider administering second dose of diphenhydramine or adding benztropine 0.02–0.05 mg/kg/dose for children >3 years of age (not recommended for children <3 because of serious adverse events).

Adapted with permission from Lavelle, J. et al. ED Pathway for Evaluation/Treatment of Children with Behavioral Health Issues. The Children's Hospital of Philadelphia Clinical Pathways. 2021. https://www.chop.edu/clinical-pathway/behavioral-health-issues-clinical-pathway.

- Examples include four-point restraints, papoose board, manual physical holds by trained staff or security
✓ Patients in physical restraints may be at increased risk for injury, suffocation, and aspiration.
  - Continuously monitor patient while in restraints (vital signs, extremity range of motion, skin integrity, circulation).
  - Attend to nutrition, hydration, and elimination needs.
  - Check restraint device for proper application and fit.
✓ Inform parents or guardians.
✓ Discontinue restraints as soon as behavior is controlled and patient no longer poses threat to self or others.
✓ Debrief the patient regarding why restraints were used and future alternative strategies, and provide opportunity for patient to apologize or make amends.
✓ All accredited facilities should have a formal policy that adheres to Joint Commission guidelines regarding the ordering and use of physical and mechanical restraints, related patient assessment and documentation requirements.

Special Considerations for Children with Autism, Intellectual, Developmental Disabilities

- Inpatient medical hospitalization can be a very stressful experience for children with autism and their parents/caregivers because of
  ✓ Communication challenges
  ✓ Sensory issues
  ✓ Increased anxiety due to unfamiliar surroundings
  ✓ Frequent interactions with unfamiliar people
  ✓ Disruption in routine
  ✓ Difficulty understanding or tolerating aspects of the diagnostic or treatment plan (such as hunger due to nothing-by-mouth status for scheduled procedure)
  ✓ Dietary restrictions/food aversions
- Stressors may contribute to behavioral changes, including increased frequency of self-stimulating or repetitive stereotypical motor movements ("stimming"), irritability and/or agitation
- Obtain and incorporate the following information from the caregiver(s) in terms of which measures are most helpful (**Table 27-3**):
  ✓ Environmental interventions
    - Maintaining a quiet, calm environment (single-occupancy room)
    - Muting or turning the volume down on equipment monitors and alarms
    - Avoiding use of fluorescent lights (patient room with windows and access to natural light)
  ✓ Providing access to preferred sensory or calming items from home or to a sensory room (if available)
- Use simple language.
- Provide instructions about what behavior you would like to see (rather than what not to do).
- Tell the patient what you are going to do, even if the patient does not appear to understand or be paying attention.
- Allow extra time for the patient to process what has been said/asked and to respond.
- Allow self-calming repetitive behaviors such as hand flapping, pacing, rocking, etc.
- Minimize the number of different staff people working with the child and the number of people in the patient room at any given time.

TABLE 27-3	Questions to Ask Parent/Caregiver to inform Patient-Specific Agitation Prevention and Intervention Strategies.
How does your child communicate?	Verbal, nonverbal
	Assisted communication device
	Communication board
	Sign language/baby sign
Are there any triggers that may upset or aggravate your child?	Too many people in the room at one time
	Loud noises
	Other
Are there any interventions that help when your child becomes upset or aggravated?	Light-up toys
	Music or other sounds
	Weighted blanket
	Other sensory items
	Being alone
	Favorite or calming items
What are your child's favorite things?	Allow favorite or calming items to be brought from home
Does your child have a daily routine schedule?	Incorporate aspects of daily routine during the hospital stay
What is the best way to prepare your child for upcoming tests/procedures/ transitions?	Verbal information
	Visual information
	Picture books, social stories
	Providing a lot versus a little information
	Explaining before the procedure happens or while it's happening
Is there anything else that would be helpful for us to know?	Special dietary needs
	Specific sensory issues
	Other

Adapted with permission from Lavelle, J. et al. ED Pathway for Evaluation/Treatment of Children with Behavioral Health Issues. The Children's Hospital of Philadelphia Clinical Pathways. 2021. https://www.chop.edu/clinical-pathway/behavioral-health-issues-clinical-pathway.

- Incorporate aspects of the daily home routine during the hospitalization.
- Consider medications for anxiety or agitation
  - ✓ Which previous medications yielded a positive or negative response?
  - ✓ Consider current home medications and potential interactions.
  - ✓ Ensure that prescribed outpatient medications are given during the hospitalization.
    - ▪ Consider an extra dose of a medication routinely prescribed for baseline irritability.
    - ▪ Consider giving a dose earlier than scheduled.
  - ✓ Offer oral medications first.
  - ✓ Children with autistic spectrum disorder and developmental disabilities may be more sensitive to medication effects and side effects, so start at lower-range doses and monitor closely for adverse effects.

PSYCHOSIS

Psychotic symptoms include

- Positive symptoms: Auditory, visual, tactile, olfactory, or gustatory hallucinations, delusions
- Negative symptoms: Flattened affect, alogia, avolition, anhedonia, social withdrawal, decreased emotional expression
- Formal thought disorder: Disorganized or incoherent speech, illogical thought, loose associations

DIFFERENTIAL DIAGNOSIS

- Mood disorders (depression, bipolar affective disorder)
- Substance-induced
  ✓ Intoxicants: Alcohol, amphetamine, D-lysergic acid diethylamide (often known as LSD), PCP, marijuana, 3,4-methylenedioxymethamphetamine (ecstasy)
  ✓ Medications: Stimulants, steroids, opiates, benzodiazepines, anticholinergics
- "Organic" causes
  ✓ Delirium
  ✓ Brain tumor
  ✓ Congenital malformation
  ✓ Head trauma
  ✓ Seizure disorder (e.g., temporal lobe epilepsy)
  ✓ Neurodegenerative disorder
  ✓ Metabolic disorder
  ✓ Toxins (heavy metals)
  ✓ Infections (Herpes simplex virus [HSV] encephalitis, human immunodeficiency virus [HIV])
  ✓ Thyroid disease
  ✓ Immune-mediated (anti-N-methyl-D-aspartate receptor encephalitis, lupus cerebritis, paraneoplastic syndromes)
- Schizophrenia
- Autistic spectrum disorders
- Intellectual disability
- Posttraumatic stress disorder
- Anxiety disorders

PATHOPHYSIOLOGY

- Altered neurotransmission in the dopamine and glutamate pathways of the hippocampus, midbrain, corpus striatum, and prefrontal cortex

CLINICAL MANIFESTATIONS

- Agitation or disruption
- Younger children's delusions tend to be less complex and less fixed.
- Adolescent's delusions may be paranoid, grandiose, or bizarre.
- Signs of intoxication may be present (see "Acute Agitation/Aggression" section).
- Mental status exam: Presence of psychotic symptoms (auditory/visual/tactile hallucinations, delusions), alteration of mood and affect (depression, anxiety, irritability, and lability), presence of suicidal or homicidal ideation, impaired judgment

DIAGNOSTICS

- Urine or serum drug screen
- Comprehensive metabolic panel (electrolytes, liver function, renal function)
- Thyroid studies
- Consider evaluation for altered mental status, including electroencephalography, lumbar puncture, head computed tomography or magnetic resonance image

MANAGEMENT

Gather Information

- Interview patient, parents/caregivers, outpatient providers
  - ✓ Assess risk factors: Genetic predisposition, substance use- particularly cannabinoids and synthetic cannabinoids.
- Physical exam
- Mental status exam

Evaluate for Safety

- Impaired judgment risks injury of self/others.
- Disruptive behavior/agitation risks injury to self/others.
- Admit patient if there are safety concerns.

If Patient Requires Admission

- Admit to appropriate level of care until medically stable.
- Consider 1:1 supervision of patient for monitoring of safety.
- Consult child psychiatrist.
- Consider antipsychotic medication.
- Evaluate for inpatient psychiatric care.

Antipsychotic Medications

- Atypical antipsychotic drugs (risperidone, olanzapine, aripiprazole, quetiapine)
  - ✓ Associated with lower incidence of extrapyramidal symptoms and tardive dyskinesia than typical antipsychotics
  - ✓ Increase risk of elevated blood glucose, risk of developing diabetes, risk of elevated triglycerides and cholesterol, and significant weight gain.
  - ✓ Lower the seizure threshold in children with known epilepsy
- Typical antipsychotic drugs (haloperidol, chlorpromazine)
  - ✓ Common side effects: Sedation, orthostatic hypotension
  - ✓ Extrapyramidal symptoms: Acute dystonic reaction (treat with diphenhydramine, benztropine), neuroleptic-induced parkinsonism, akathisia (treat with beta-blocker, benzodiazepine)
  - ✓ Neuroleptic malignant syndrome: Life-threatening condition characterized by hyperthermia, muscle rigidity, altered mental status, choreoathetosis, tremors, and autonomic dysfunction (arrhythmias, hypertension, sweating)
  - ✓ Anticholinergic effects (confusion, agitation, constipation, blurred vision, urinary retention)

SUICIDALITY

Thoughts, threats, events, actions or behaviors characterized by the desire to cause death or harm to oneself

- Suicidal ideation (SI): Thinking about, considering or planning for suicide. Suicidal ideation may be characterized as passive (wishing to be dead, not alive anymore, to fall asleep and not wake up) or active (wanting to end one's life or desire to kill oneself.) Suicidal ideation may be a precursor to suicide.
- Suicidal intent: Thoughts of killing oneself with some intent to act on such thoughts. Suicidal intent can be present with or without having a method conceptualized or a plan worked out.
- Suicide Attempt: Any self-directed potentially injurious behavior with any intent to die as a result of the behavior. A suicide attempt may or may not result in injury.
- Suicide: Death caused by self-directed injurious behavior purposefully performed with any intent to die as a result of the behavior.
- Nonsuicidal self-injury (NSSI): Any self-directed potentially injurious behavior without any intent to die as a result of the behavior. Often, youth report engaging in NSSI in an attempt to feel better or to relieve emotional/psychological distress.

EPIDEMIOLOGY

- Among youth in grades 9–12
  - ✓ 17% seriously considered suicide during prior 12 months
  - ✓ 13% had made a suicide plan
  - ✓ 7% had attempted suicide one or more times
- Suicide is the second leading cause of death among persons 10–24 years of age.
- Suicide rates among youth have been increasing every year since 2007. Isolation and distancing during the COVID-19 pandemic may have exacerbated this trend.
- Females attempt suicide more often than males.
- Males complete suicide more often than females because they use more lethal methods.
  - ✓ Firearms are the most commonly used method of suicide among males.
  - ✓ Poisoning is the most common method of suicide for females.

ETIOLOGY/RISK FACTORS

- Current suicidal ideation, self-injurious behaviors, or recent suicide attempt
- Prior history of suicidal or self-injurious behaviors
- Availability and access to lethal means, which can include firearms, weapons, ropes, sharp objects (razors and knives), cleaning supplies, medications, intoxicating beverages, illegal substances
- Presence of a mental health diagnosis: mood disorders (depression, bipolar disorder), Post-traumatic stress disorder (PTSD), psychosis, conduct disorder, ADHD, eating disorders
- Alcohol and substance use and/or intoxication
- Family history of psychiatric illness, suicidal behavior, substance abuse
- Psychological factors: Hopelessness, anhedonia (loss of enjoyment/pleasure), impulsivity, aggression, emotional dysregulation, limited problem-solving and coping skills, social skills deficits
- Medical Conditions: Central nervous system disorders (epilepsy, traumatic brain injury/concussion), pain/chronic pain conditions, chronic medical condition, sleep disruption
- Stressful life events: Exposure to violence or trauma, physical abuse, sexual abuse, interpersonal conflict with family and friends, recent significant negative life event or loss, engaging in bullying or being a victim of bullying, triggering events that lead to feelings of humiliation, shame, or despair (bullying, victimization, pending legal charges, academic failure)
- Sexual orientation: Lesbian, gay, bisexual, transgender, and queer or questioning youth may be at higher risk for suicidality due to increased psychosocial stressors (shame, stigma, bullying/victimization, lack of family or community support)

• Suicide contagion effect: Knowing or hearing about someone who recently completed suicide, including news media coverage of an adolescent who completed suicide

DIFFERENTIAL DIAGNOSIS

• Accidental versus intentional injury
• High versus low risk of injury or lethality

PATHOPHYSIOLOGY

• Associated findings include altered serotonergic function, lower cerebrospinal fluid serotonin levels, alterations in hypothalamic–pituitary function, disturbed sleep

CLINICAL MANIFESTATIONS

• Clinical presentation of suicidality may include:
  ✓ Expressing a wish to die or a wish to kill oneself
  ✓ Looking for a way to kill oneself, such as searching online or attempting to buy a gum
  ✓ Talking about feeling hopeless or having no reason to live
  ✓ Feeling trapped or in unbearable pain
  ✓ Feeling like a burden to others
  ✓ Showing rage or talking about seeking revenge
• Clinical presentation after a suicide attempt depends on the method used: Drug ingestions/overdose, shooting, hanging, suffocation, stabbing, drowning, burning, running into traffic, intentional motor vehicle accidents
• Mental status exam: Assess current suicidal ideation/intent/plan, presence of delusions or psychotic symptoms, mood and affect (depression, anxiety, irritability, and lability), level of insight and judgment

MANAGEMENT

Gather Information

• Interview patient, parents, and outpatient psychiatrist/therapist to assess overall suicide risk.
• Assess past and current suicidal ideation:
  ✓ Have you ever thought you would be better off dead?
  ✓ Do you have thoughts of wanting to kill yourself?
  ✓ Have you thought about what you could do to end your life?
  ✓ How many times have you had these thoughts? How long do the thoughts last?
  ✓ When was the last time you had thoughts like these?
• Assess current suicide intent:
  ✓ Do you think that this is something you might actually do?
  ✓ How likely are you to carry it out?
• Assess past and current suicidal behaviors:
  ✓ Have you ever tried to hurt yourself on purpose? Why did you do that?
  ✓ Have you ever done anything to try to kill yourself or make yourself not alive anymore?
  ✓ Has there ever been a time when you started to do something to kill yourself but you changed your mind and stopped yourself before you actually did anything?
  ✓ Has there ever been a time when you started to do something to kill yourself but someone or something stopped you before you actually did anything?
  ✓ Have you done anything to get ready to end your life or kill yourself, like giving things away, writing a goodbye note, or gathering things you needed to kill yourself?

- Assess access to means and potential for lethality
  - ✓ To what components of your plan do you have access? (e.g., firearms, medications for overdose, rope for hanging)
  - ✓ If you attempted your plan, how likely is it that you would truly die?
- Assess precipitants/stressors that preceded the attempt.
  - ✓ What were the events that led up to the suicide attempt?
  - ✓ What has happened recently that caused you to decide to make an attempt now?
- Assess reasons for living
  - ✓ What is keeping you from acting on your suicidal thoughts or urges?
  - ✓ What are some reasons to keep on living? Is there any way we can make that stronger?
  - ✓ To what extent are you hopeful that treatment can help you?
  - ✓ To what extent do you regret having attempted suicide?
- Assess protective factors: Restricted access to lethal means, family/social support, responsibility to family or pets, positive therapeutic relationships, consistent mental health care utilization, antidepressant treatment, religious beliefs, ability to cope with stress, healthy problem solving skills, good impulse control and frustration tolerance, absence of psychosis

Evaluate Suicide Threat/Attempt

- Degree of suicidal intent
- Amount of planning
- Method used
- Assessing potential for lethality
- Desire for death as an outcome
- Awareness of death as a likely outcome
- Likelihood of discovery
- Motivation for the attempt

If Patient Requires Admission

- Admit to appropriate level of medical care until patient is stable.
- If patient is admitted for medical hospitalization, consider the following:
  - ✓ 1:1 supervision of patient for monitoring of safety.
  - ✓ If available, placement in a room that has been modified to reduce ligature and self-injury risk.
  - ✓ Remove items from the patient room that could be used for self-injury (sharp objects; medical tubing, extra linens, electric cords, shower and privacy curtains that could be used for hanging or strangulation; plastic trash/linen bags that could be used for suffocation, etc.).
  - ✓ Order meals delivered on modified trays that reduces access to objects that could be used for self-harm (removal of knife and fork from tray, replacing ceramic plates with paper plates).
  - ✓ Search patient's belongings for items that could be used for self-harm.
- Periodic repeated assessment of level of suicidality
- Consult child and adolescent mental health specialist. Depending on resources available at your institution, this may be a child and adolescent psychiatrist, general psychiatrist, child psychologist, or social worker.
- Evaluate for indications for transfer to inpatient psychiatric care.
- Consider starting psychiatric medication to treat primary psychiatric condition(s).
- Use of medication as needed if patient becomes agitated or aggressive or there is concern for imminent harm to self or others.

If Stable for Discharge Home

- Develop a safety plan
  - ✓ Identify warning signs of increased emotional distress/suicidality.
  - ✓ Identify effective coping strategies to manage distress/suicidal ideation.
  - ✓ Identify social supports, family and friends to contact for support or when in crisis.
  - ✓ Provide information about crisis resources.
    - Contact information for local mental health crisis services (psychiatric emergency services, mobile crisis service
    - National Suicide Prevention Lifeline 1-800-273-8255
    - Indications to call 911 and/or when to go to the local emergency room
- Identifying ways to make the environment more safe
  - Reduce access to lethal means by locking or removing guns, firearms, ammunition, ropes, sharp objects (knives, scissors, razors), medications (over-the-counter, prescribed, supplements), cleaning supplies, alcohol and drugs
  - Increase adult observation and supervision of patient, particularly during periods of distress.
  - Supervise medication administration.
  - Monitor online and social media activity and communication.
- Provide information on accessing outpatient mental health treatment services,
- If patient is already engaged in mental health care, contact the outpatient psychiatrist, therapist, and/or pediatrician to coordinate the discharge plan,

AVOIDANT/RESTRICTIVE FOOD INTAKE DISORDER (ARFID)

Diagnostic and Statistical Manual of Mental Disorders, 5th ed., Criteria

- An eating or feeding disturbance (e.g., apparent lack of interest in eating or food; avoidance based on the sensory characteristics of food; concern about aversive consequences of eating) as manifested by persistent failure to meet appropriate nutritional and/or energy needs associated with at least one of the following:
  - ✓ Significant weight loss or failure to achieve expected weight gain or faltering growth in children
  - ✓ Significant nutritional deficiency
  - ✓ Dependence on enteral feeding or oral nutritional supplements
  - ✓ Marked interference with psychosocial functioning
- Disturbance not better explained by lack of available food or by associated culturally sanctioned practice.
- Eating disturbance does not occur exclusively during the course of anorexia nervosa or bulimia nervosa, and there is no evidence for a disturbance in the way one's body weight or shape is experienced
- Eating disturbance is not attributable to a concurrent medical condition or not better explained by another mental disorder.

EPIDEMIOLOGY

- Occur at any age, though generally at younger ages; more likely to be male; and more likely to have a comorbid physical or psychiatric illness than children with anorexia nervosa
- Occurs in a heterogeneous group of children who come to the hospital with malnutrition or acute food refusal that fall into different categories depending on what drives the maladaptive eating behavior

✓ Anxiety: Acute food refusal due to generalized anxiety, chronic but diffuse gastrointestinal symptoms with no apparent biologic cause but anxiety around nausea/vomiting/abdominal pain, obsessive–compulsive disorder–like behaviors targeting food and eating rituals, and various phobias like choking or vomiting.

✓ Autism spectrum disorder, intellectual disability, or developmental delay: Perseverative behaviors surrounding eating that have become more selective over time (due to aspects of food such as, smell, color, texture or other preference that has narrowed)

✓ Oppositional type or volitional behaviors: Withholding eating serves as a means for secondary gain (control in family system)

✓ In all three of these categories, children do not tend to have body image concerns and are not preoccupied with gaining or losing weight

DIFFERENTIAL DIAGNOSIS

- Anorexia nervosa
- Gastroenteritis
- Gastroesophageal reflux
- Celiac disease
- Choking phobia
- Parasitosis
- Malignancy

CLINICAL MANIFESTATIONS

- History of selective (picky) eating or history of very restricted eating, choosing certain foods secondary to texture, color, smell, or other sensory factors.
  ✓ ARFID represents a chronic problem.
  ✓ Often present after an illness in which resumption of limited food intake is markedly impaired
- Acute in onset and may come as a result of a gastrointestinal illness, persistent abdominal pain, gastroesophageal reflux disease, an episode of choking, a fear of vomiting (often associated with an illness), or an allergic reaction to a food
  ✓ Phobic reaction can develop, and children may be afraid to eat and even to drink for fear of choking, or vomiting.
  ✓ Fear may lead to limited intake of food that are "safe" or perceived to not cause vomiting to choking, or soft foods, or foods that require little chewing.
- Usually comes to clinical attention after a child has lost weight or failed to grow in a typical manner.
- May present with dehydration, weight loss, and, occasionally, electrolyte derangements secondary to malnutrition
  ✓ ARFID has a more indolent course and usually lacks the initial electrolyte and vital sign derangements characteristic of the rapid weight loss in anorexia nervosa.
  ✓ Severe malnutrition may require enteral feeding, which puts patient at risk for refeeding syndrome.
  ✓ No issue of body image
    - These children do not think of themselves as fat and typically want to gain weight but often have fear or anxiety that limits their intake.
    - Consider an alternative eating disorder diagnosis if the child has a fear of gaining weight or has other body image issues.

DIAGNOSTICS

- History
  - ✓ Avoidance based on the sensory characteristics of food
  - ✓ Concern about aversive consequences of eating (choking, vomiting)
  - ✓ Dependence on enteral feeding or oral nutritional supplements
  - ✓ Behavioral factors will inform treatment decisions and support correction of weight loss.
- Physical examination:
  - ✓ Signs and sequelae of malnutrition
  - ✓ Signs that support other medical or psychiatric causes in the differential diagnosis
    - Self-induced vomiting may cause inflamed gums or tooth decay, mouth sores, swollen glands in the neck, broken blood vessels in the eyes, teeth marks on the back of the hands or calluses on the knuckles.
  - ✓ Check vital signs (hypothermia, bradycardia, hypotension) and orthostatic blood pressure
- Studies relate to assessing degree of malnutrition and for evaluating other potential causes of weight loss

  - ✓ ECG (disturbances associated with electrolyte abnormalities)
  - ✓ Complete blood count (anemia, leukopenia)
  - ✓ Serum electrolytes, blood urea nitrogen, creatine (hypokalemia, hypoglycemia)
  - ✓ ↓Calcium, ↓magnesium, ↓phosphorus
  - ✓ Amylase, lipase
  - ✓ Thyroid function studies
  - ✓ Celiac panel (alternate cause of symptoms)
  - ✓ Urinalysis
  - ✓ Ferritin
  - ✓ ↓Vitamin D, 25-hydroxycalciferol
  - ✓ ↓Vitamin B12
  - ✓ ↓Zinc

MANAGEMENT

Goal is to support patient and family to be able to resume normal age-appropriate functioning around feeding and eating during meals, with the child able to eat enough food to support daily nutritional needs, metabolic function, and physical growth expectations.

- Nutrition
  - ✓ Schedule meals and snacks throughout the day to meet required daily nutritional and caloric needs.
    - Oral nutritional supplements or nasogastric feeds if patient cannot meet daily calorie goals
    - Nasogastric feeds are generally not required for mild malnourishment, as this may interfere with resumption of age appropriate feeding/eating.
  - ✓ Monitor meals and snacks, initially by staff with later transfer to parent.
  - ✓ Monitor intake and output
  - ✓ Obtain daily weights in a consistent manner (after emptying bladder, wearing same clothing, using the same scale)
  - ✓ Monitor vital signs
  - ✓ Cardiac monitoring if concern for potential cardiac instability
  - ✓ Monitoring for refeeding syndrome may be indicated (see "Anorexia Nervosa" section in Chapter 1).

- Behavioral needs
  - ✓ Consultation with a therapist experienced in both behavioral management and refeeding strategies when feasible
  - ✓ Behavioral interventions may include:
    - Relaxation strategies to reduce anxiety associated with eating/meal times
    - Diaphragmatic (deep) breathing
    - Progressive muscle relaxation
    - Visualization/imagery
    - Graded exposures to the stimuli that contribute to anxiety with eating/avoidance of foods
    - Positive reinforcement (praise, rewards, token economy) for achieving specific tasks related to the treatment plan
  - ✓ Consider consultations
    - Nutritionist
    - Psychology for cognitive behavioral therapy-based strategies for children who are particularly anxious or phobic
    - Psychiatry may be consulted to identify and treat other comorbid psychiatric conditions, and to assess for indications/recommendations for anxiolytic medication.

Pi Chun Cheng, MD, MS
Julie Fierro, MD, MPH
Howard B. Panitch, MD

MECHANICAL VENTILATION AND PULMONARY ASSESSMENT

BLOOD GAS INTERPRETATION

Step 1: Acidemia or Alkalemia?

- Normal pH 7.35–7.45
  - ✓ Alkalemia: pH above normal range
  - ✓ Acidemia: pH below normal range

Step 2: Metabolic or Respiratory?

- Primary respiratory alkalosis: pH above normal range and $PaCO_2$ <40
- Primary metabolic alkalosis: pH above normal range and $PaCO_2$ >40
- Primary respiratory acidosis: pH below normal range and $PaCO_2$ >40
- Primary metabolic acidosis: pH below normal range and $PaCO_2$ <40

Step 3: Is the problem acute or chronic?

- For respiratory acidosis/alkalosis, a 10 mmHg change in $PaCO_2$ causes a 0.08 change in pH in the acute setting or a 0.03 change in the chronic setting.
- For metabolic acidosis/alkalosis, a 10 mEq/L change in HCO_3^- causes a 0.15 change in pH.
- For *acute* respiratory acidosis, expect an increase in HCO_3^- of 1 mEq/L for every increase in $PaCO_2$ of 10 mmHg.
- For *acute* respiratory alkalosis, expect a decrease in HCO_3^- of 1–3 mEq/L for every decrease in $PaCO_2$ of 10 mmHg.
- For *chronic* respiratory acidosis, expect an increase in HCO_3^- of 4 mEq/L for every increase in $PaCO_2$ of 10 mmHg.
- For *chronic* respiratory alkalosis, expect a decrease in HCO_3^- of 2–5 mEq/L for every decrease in $PaCO_2$ of 10 mmHg.

Step 4: Is there a second primary problem?

- In other words, are changes in pH greater than expected from the primary disorder alone?
  - ✓ *Example:* An infant with bronchopulmonary dysplasia is receiving diuretics and is hypochloremic, with pH 7.42, $PaCO_2$ 75, and HCO_3^- 34. The blood gas values reflect not only the patient's chronic respiratory acidosis but also a second primary problem (i.e., hypochloremic metabolic alkalosis).
  - ✓ A compensatory process alone *never* restores pH completely back to normal.
  - ✓ For metabolic acidosis, expect a decrease in $PaCO_2$ of 1–1.5 mmHg for every decrease in HCO_3^- of 1 mEq/L.
  - ✓ For metabolic alkalosis, expect an increase in $PaCO_2$ of 0.5–1 mmHg for every increase in HCO_3^- of 1 mEq/L.

Step 5: In metabolic acidosis, calculate the anion gap.

$$\text{Anion Gap} = Na - (Cl + HCO_3^-)$$

- The normal anion gap is less than 12 mEq/L.
- In normal gap metabolic acidosis, hyperchloremic acidosis results from the loss of HCO_3^- in the gut or kidneys.
- Anion-gap acidosis results from the addition of nontitratable acid to the system. Causes include MUDPILES (methanol, uremia, diabetic ketoacidosis, paraldehyde/propylene glycol, isoniazid/iron/infections, lactic acidosis, ethanol, salicylates).

Step 6: If there is an anion-gap metabolic acidosis, consider the possibility of a second metabolic abnormality.

- This is done by calculating the delta–delta gap (where AG = anion gap):

$$\Delta - \Delta\,Gap = (Measured\ AG - Normal\ AG) / (Normal[HCO_3^-] - Measured[HCO_3^-])$$

- If there is a Δ–Δ gap:
  - ✓ <1 = concurrent non–anion-gap acidosis
  - ✓ = 1 = pure anion-gap acidosis
  - ✓ >1 = concurrent metabolic alkalosis
  - ✓ *Example:* A 12-year-old with diabetic ketoacidosis has an anion gap of 22, a pH of 7.2, and an HCO_3^- of 17.
  - ✓ Calculate the Δ–Δ gap: $(22 - 12)/(24 - 17) = 1.4$. This tells you that there is a metabolic acidosis with a concurrent metabolic alkalosis (e.g., from vomiting) present.

HYPOXEMIA

PULMONARY CAUSES OF HYPOXEMIA

- Ventilation/perfusion(V'/Q') mismatch
- Hypoventilation
- Shunt
- Diffusion block
- Low FiO_2

ALVEOLAR–ARTERIAL GRADIENT (A-a GRADIENT)

- A measure of the difference between the alveolar and arterial concentration of oxygen. It is useful in determining the cause of hypoxemia (**Table 28-1**).

$$A\text{-}a\ gradient = PAO_2 - PaO_2$$

$$PAO_2 = FiO_2(P_{atm} - P_{H_2O}) - (PaCO_2 / R)$$

where

TABLE 28-1	Determining the Cause of Hypoxemia		
	$PaCO_2$	**Corrected with 100% O_2?**	**A-a Gradient**
Hypoventilation	↑	Y	N
V/Q mismatch	↑, Normal or ↓	Y	↑
Shunt	Normal or ↓	N	↑
Diffusion block	Normal or ↓	Y	↑
Low FiO_2	Normal or ↓	Y	N

- PAO_2 = partial pressure of oxygen in alveoli.
- PaO_2 = partial pressure of O_2 measured in arterial blood. Normally 80–100 mmHg.
- $PaCO_2$ = partial pressure of CO2 measured in arterial blood. Normally 35–45 mmHg.
- P_{atm} = atmospheric pressure: at sea level; approximately equal to 760 mmHg, but will vary with altitude

$$P_{H_2O} = \text{water vapor pressure at } 37°C = 47\,mmHg$$

- R = respiratory quotient; 0.8 under normal circumstances
- Normal A-a gradient: <10 mmHg
- *Example:* A patient presents to the emergency department for asthma exacerbation. He is breathing room air. An arterial blood gas is obtained and has a $PaCO_2$ of 60 mmHg and a PaO_2 of 50 mmHg.
- You calculate the A-a gradient: PAO_2 = 0.21 (760 − 47) − (60/0.8) = 75. The A-a gradient = 75− 50 = 25. This tells you there is an increased A-a gradient consistent with likely V'/Q' mismatch.

MECHANICAL VENTILATION

A method to support/assist or replace spontaneous breathing mechanically

- Common indications for initiating mechanical ventilation are to improve alveolar ventilation, improve arterial oxygenation, prevent or reverse atelectasis, reverse hypoxemic or hypercarbic respiratory failure, and prevent or reverse respiratory muscle fatigue.
- Most ventilators use positive pressure to augment the work of the respiratory muscles, although negative pressure devices are still occasionally used.
- A ventilator can use either pressure control (PC) or volume control (VC) to assist breathing.
- Pressure control: The clinician sets the desired pressure to be delivered by the ventilator. The tidal volume varies from breath to breath depending on respiratory system compliance and resistance. The inspiratory flow depends on the pressure being delivered and how quickly the peak pressure is set to be achieved (rise time, or slope). The resulting flow pattern is one of decelerating flow. Because you are able to deliver a uniform pressure over a set inspiratory time, this mode is useful in children with a large leak around a tracheostomy tube or noninvasive interface.
- Volume control: The clinician sets the volume of the breath to be delivered. The flow is delivered with a square wave pattern (e.g., flow is constant) to a set tidal volume (V_T), allowing the pressure to vary as the compliance and resistance of the system change.
- Breaths are classified according to what triggers (starts) and/or cycles (stops) inspiration. These events can be either patient or ventilator initiated. Trigger variables include time, pressure, and flow. A few ventilators can also use abdominal movement or diaphragm electromyography (EMG) as trigger variables. Cycle variables can include pressure, volume, flow, or time.
- If a positive pressure breath is triggered by the patient and cycled by the patient (or by the inherent mechanical characteristics of the patient's respiratory system as with pressure support), the breath is considered to be spontaneous.
- If the ventilator triggers OR cycles a breath independently of the patient's effort or mechanics, the breath is considered to be mandatory.

THREE BASIC BREATH SEQUENCES OF A VENTILATOR

- Intermittent mandatory ventilation: Mandatory breaths are interspersed with breaths that are spontaneous. This would include modes that are commonly referred to as intermittent

mandatory ventilation (IMV), synchronized IMV (SIMV), SIMV with pressure support, or airway pressure release ventilation (APRV).

- Continuous spontaneous ventilation (CSV): All breaths are spontaneous. This would include modes like continuous positive airway pressure (CPAP) or CPAP with pressure support. Pressure support is considered to be a pressure-limited, flow- or pressure-triggered, or flow-cycled spontaneous breath. The breath is supported to a preset pressure by the ventilator and terminated based on characteristics of the patient's respiratory system. This mode enhances the patient's native respiratory drive, reducing respiratory work while allowing the patient to determine respiratory rate as well as the length and depth of breaths. Pressure support is often used in conjunction with mandatory ventilation as a tool for weaning.
- Continuous mandatory ventilation: No breaths are spontaneous. This would include modes that are commonly referred to as control ventilation and assist/control ventilation.

TYPES OF SUPPORTED VENTILATION (ALL BREATHS ARE SPONTANEOUS)

- CPAP: Supplies a constant airway pressure above atmospheric pressure during both inspiratory and expiratory phases of spontaneous ventilation. It is often used to overcome upper airway obstruction or to maintain functional residual capacity (FRC)
- Bilevel positive airway pressure (BLPAP): Supplies both inspiratory positive airway pressure (IPAP) and expiratory positive airway pressure (EPAP). The patient triggers inspiration, and cycle variables are set to end inspiration and allow exhalation. BLPAP can also be a form of assisted ventilation if a respiratory rate is set. It is often used to improve ventilation

TYPES OF MANDATORY VENTILATION (NO SPONTANEOUS BREATHS)

- High-frequency ventilation (high-frequency oscillatory ventilation [HFOV]): Delivers low tidal volume breaths (1–3 mL/kg) at very high rates (3–15 Hz = 180–900 breaths per minute). HFOV settings are mean airway pressure, frequency (in Hz), and amplitude or power. Indications include severe neonatal respiratory distress syndrome (RDS), acute RDS (ARDS), and severe air leak syndromes

TYPES OF ASSISTED VENTILATION (MIXTURE OF MANDATORY AND SPONTANEOUS BREATHS)

- SIMV: The most frequently used mode of ventilation in most pediatric institutions, SIMV allows spontaneous breathing between ventilator breaths that are delivered in either PC or VC mode. Mechanical breaths can be programmed to trigger with patient-initiated breaths or independently of the patient's respiratory effort and are synchronized so as not to occur while the patient is exhaling.
- Pressure-regulated volume control (PRVC): The delivered tidal volume is set by the practitioner, but the ventilator monitors both the volume delivered and the pressure used to deliver the breath. The pressure is adjusted from breath to breath to meet the targeted tidal volume. Flow is delivered with a decelerating wave form. This allows the ventilator to respond to changes in compliance and resistance in the system, thereby limiting volutrauma and barotrauma.
- APRV: Allows spontaneous ventilation while maintaining mean airway pressure (MAP) with a high level of CPAP for a preset time (T high) and a "release" that intermittently drops the mean airway pressure to a lower CPAP level for a shorter period of time (T low). This is designed to open and maintain collapsed alveoli and enhance ventilation of lungs with poor compliance without excessive peak inspiratory pressure (PIP).

INITIAL VENTILATOR SETTINGS

The following should be used as a general guide: Evaluation of the patient's response and care by physicians experienced with managing the mechanically ventilated child are critical

to ensure that the settings provide an appropriate level of support. Initial settings depend on the age and indication.

- In patients with decreased lung or chest wall compliance, a short inspiratory time and higher pressure would be recommended to deliver a set V_T. Examples would include premature infants with RDS or a child with severe interstitial lung disease.
- In obstructive lung patterns for which the time constant of the respiratory system (the product of resistance and compliance) is long, a larger tidal volume and a slow mandatory rate with a longer inspiratory time and longer expiratory time are recommended to allow adequate time for the lungs to fill and to empty. Examples would include a child with asthma or patient with severe bronchopulmonary dysplasia (BPD).

Conventional Ventilation

- Mode: In order to pick one of the five main modes listed here, you will need to decide whether breaths will be mandated, spontaneous, or a combination of the two.
  - ✓ Continuous mandatory ventilation in pressure control (PC-continuous mandatory ventilation) or volume control (VC-continuous mandatory ventilation) mode
  - ✓ Intermittent mandatory ventilation in pressure control (PC-IMV) or volume control (VC-IMV) mode
  - ✓ Continuous spontaneous ventilation in pressure control (PC-CSV) mode
- Mandated respiratory rate (per minute): Typical starting ventilator rates assuming minimal spontaneous respiratory rates of 30–40 for neonates, 20–30 for infants, and 15–20 for children. If allowing for the patient to take some spontaneous breaths, begin supporting at one-half to two-thirds of the normal respiratory rate for age.
- FiO_2: Set at 1.0 (or last known effective FiO_2) and wean to desired oxygen saturation as measured by pulse oximetry (SpO_2).
- Positive end-expiratory pressure (PEEP): 3–5 cm H_2O is considered "physiologic" and helps to maintain FRC. Neonates with severe lung disease may require much higher levels of PEEP to treat parenchymal disease or to support collapsible airways. Older children with ARDS may require a PEEP of 12–15 cm H_2O to recruit surfactant-deficient lung units and prevent injury from recruitment–de-recruitment cycling.
- V_T: Set to 8–12 mL/kg; if low tidal volume strategy is desired, begin with 4–6 mL/kg as tolerated.
- T_i (inspiratory time): Neonates, 0.3–0.4 second; infants, 0.4–0.7 second; children, 0.5–1.0 second.
- Inspiratory:expiratory ratio: 1:2, with longer expiratory times in obstructive disease to prevent breath stacking and the development of dynamic hyperinflation.
- Positive inspiratory pressure: In PC mode, set PC to achieve adequate chest wall movement and desired V_T.

High-Frequency Ventilation

- Frequency: Set at 10–15 Hz in neonates; may need 5–7 Hz with severe ARDS.
- Mean airway pressure: Set 1–4 cm H_2O higher than that needed on conventional ventilation. Wean slowly once recruitment established.
- Amplitude: Set to level with best chest-wall movement.

ADJUSTING VENTILATOR SETTINGS

Ventilator settings are manipulated in order to minimize iatrogenic injury while providing adequate ventilation and oxygenation to support cellular function (**Table 28-2**).

TABLE 28-2	Some Possible Effects of Ventilator Changes	
Change	**PaCO$_2$**	**PaO$_2$**
↑ RR	↓	No change or ↑
↑ PIP	↓	↑
↑ PEEP	↑, No change, or ↓	↑, No change, or ↓
↑ I time	↓	↑, No change, or ↓
↑ FiO$_2$	No change	↑
↑ Amp	↓	No change
↑ Hz	↑	No change
↑ MAP	↓	↑

- Conventional ventilation: To increase CO$_2$ exchange, increase either respiratory rate (RR) or V$_T$. To increase oxygenation, increase mean airway pressure or FiO$_2$. mean airway pressure increase can be achieved by increasing PEEP, PIP, or inspiratory time.
- High-frequency ventilation: To increase CO$_2$ exchange, increase amplitude or decrease frequency. Increase oxygenation by increasing FiO$_2$ or mean airway pressure.

WEANING VENTILATION

The most common weaning modes are SIMV, pressure support ventilation, and T-piece trials.

- Weaning with SIMV: Gradually wean rate of ventilator as the rate of spontaneous breaths increases. Once all breaths are spontaneous, consider supporting each breath to allow adequate oxygenation and ventilation. This method may increase the metabolic cost of breathing for the patient during the weaning process.
- Weaning with PSV (two options):
  - ✓ Using SIMV mode with PSV, initiate short trials of only PSV, gradually lengthening the time off SIMV until the patient is maintained on only minimal PSV.
  - ✓ Place patient on full PSV mode to produce a fully supported tidal volume. Gradually wean down the PSV until the patient is minimally supported. If tolerated, wean off support.

INDICATORS OF READINESS TO WEAN

Negative inspiratory force (NIF): Measures maximum negative deflection during inspiration after occlusion of airway. Used to assess adequacy of spontaneous breaths. A NIF less than −15 cmH$_2$O in an adult has 97% sensitivity for weaning failure. However, there is poor positive predictive value for this test in children.

- Measured vital capacity: Adequate vital capacity is 10–15 mL/kg
- Spontaneous tidal volume: At least 4 mL/kg
- Able to maintain PaO$_2$ >60 mmHg in FiO$_2$ <0.35
- Respiratory rate: Physiologic (lack of rapid shallow breathing); in adults, a respiratory frequency/tidal volume (in liters) ratio of <105 during a spontaneous breathing (T-piece) trial is associated with weaning success (rapid shallow breathing index).
- Rapid shallow breathing index (RSBI): RSBI adapted for children (see formula below) of ≥8 has both a sensitivity and a specificity of 74% in predicting successful extubation in some studies. In children, RSBI occasionally used in clinical practice.

$$RSBI = RR(breaths \ / \ min) \ / \ V_T(mL \ / \ kg)$$

PULMONARY FUNCTION TESTS

Pulmonary function tests (PFTs) are used to diagnose, assess severity, and assess response to therapy in pulmonary disease. To assess reversible airway obstruction or bronchodilator responsiveness, an inhaled bronchodilator is administered and the test is repeated. Histamine, methacholine, exercise, isocapnic cold dry air, and hypertonic or hypotonic aerosol challenges can also help assess airway reactivity.

SPIROMETRY

Lung volumes are shown in **Figure 28-1**.

- Forced vital capacity (FVC): Volume that can be maximally forcefully exhaled after a complete inspiration
- FEV_1: Volume of air that is forcefully exhaled in the first second following a complete inspiration
- FEV_1/FVC: Ratio expressed as a percentage
- FEF_{25-75}: Average forced expiratory flow over the midportion of the FVC
- Peak expiratory flow (PEF) rate during forced exhalation

A volume is the amount that describes a compartment of the lung; when two or more volumes are added together, the new amount is called a capacity. All volumes except the residual volume (RV) can be measured by spirometry; any capacity that includes the RV requires specialized equipment for its measurement.

- Expiratory reserve volume (ERV): Volume that can still be exhaled following normal exhalation
- FRC: Volume remaining in the lungs at the end of normal exhalation (RV + ERV)
- Inspiratory capacity (IC): Volume in the lungs at full inspiration (IRV + V_T)
- Inspiratory reserve volume (IRV): Volume that can still be inhaled after normal inspiration
- Residual volume (RV): Volume remaining in the lungs after maximal expiration (FRC-ERV, or TLC-VC)

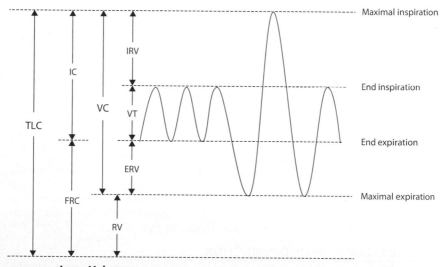

FIGURE 28-1 Lung Volumes.
ERV = expiratory reserve volume; FRC = functional residual capacity; IC = inspiratory capacity; IRV = inspiratory residual volume; RV = residual volume; TLC = total lung capacity; VC = vital capacity; VT = tidal volume.

- V_T: Volume inhaled and exhaled during normal breathing
- Total lung capacity (TLC): Total volume of gas in the lungs at full inspiration (VC + RV, or IC + FRC, or IRV + V_T + ERV + RV)
- Vital capacity (VC): Maximal volume that can be exhaled from a full inspiration (IRV + TV + ERV; TLC-RV)

EQUIPMENT COMMONLY USED TO MEASURE LUNG FUNCTION

- Body plethysmograph: Apparatus for measurement of FRC, RV, TLC, and airway resistance. Fractional lung volumes can also be measured with dilution techniques using helium or nitrogen.
- Spirometer: Apparatus for measuring lung volumes (except RV) and flow rates. Spirometry is used to plot a volume–time curve and a flow–volume loop.

ANTHROPOMETRIC MEASUREMENTS AFFECTING LUNG FUNCTION

- Height: Taller individuals have larger lung volumes and airways, so flow rates are higher.
- Age: Lung volumes change with increasing age in the pediatric population; RV and FRC increase, ERV decreases.
- Sex: Males have larger lung volumes than females.
- Ethnicity: TLC is generally lower in African Americans as compared with Caucasians because African Americans have smaller ratios of upper to lower body segments.

OBSTRUCTIVE LUNG DISEASE

Obstruction to airflow during expiration leads to decreased flow rates, gas trapping, increased RV, decreased, increased, or normal VC, and increased to normal TLC (**Figure 28-1**). Common causes include asthma, bronchiolitis, chronic bronchitis, cystic fibrosis, and bronchiectasis. Spirometry demonstrates a low FEV_1 (<80% predicted), variable FVC, low FEV_1/FVC (<75% predicted), decreased FEF_{25-75}, and an expiratory flow–volume curve that is concave to the volume axis, reflecting lung units that empty at different rates (**Figure 28-2B**).

- Small-airway obstruction is represented by low a FEV_{25-75}.
- A significant response to bronchodilators is defined as a >12% increase in the FEV_1 and/or FVC.
- A methacholine challenge that results in a decrease in FEV_1 of ≥20% from baseline at a dose of <16 mg/dL, or exercise or cold dry air challenge that results in a ≥15% decrease in FEV_1 from baseline are used to diagnose airway hyperreactivity.

RESTRICTIVE LUNG DISEASE

Restrictive lung diseases cause reductions in lung volumes due to decreased lung compliance, decreased chest-wall compliance, or muscle weakness. Causes include interstitial lung disease, neuromuscular diseases, and chest-wall or spine abnormalities. TLC is decreased, whereas flow rates are proportionally normal or slightly increased. Spirometry reveals a low FEV_1 (<80% predicted), low FVC (<80% predicted), normal FEV_1/FVC ratio, and "miniaturized" appearance of the flow–volume curve (**Figure 28-2C**).

VARIABLE EXTRATHORACIC OBSTRUCTION

During inhalation, narrowing of the extrathoracic airway accentuates any obstruction, and airflow through the narrowed portion of the extrathoracic airway decreases. This results in flattening of the inspiratory flow–volume loop (**Figure 28-2D**). If the narrowing is not present during exhalation, the expiratory flow–volume curve is normal. Spirometry

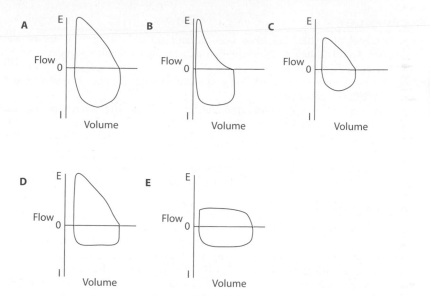

FIGURE 28-2   FLOW–VOLUME LOOPS. A. Normal flow–volume loop. During expiration (E), the normal loop can be straight or slightly convex to the volume (x) axis. B. Obstructive flow–volume curve. During expiration, the expiratory loop is concave toward the volume axis. A normal peak flow (as in this case) does not preclude an obstructive process. C. Restrictive flow–volume curve. The flows are normal when corrected for low lung volumes. D. Variable extrathoracic obstruction. The expiratory loop remains normal, but there is flattening of the inspiratory (I) loop. E. Fixed obstruction. Both the expiratory and inspiratory loops reach a plateau at low flow.

reveals normal FVC and FEV$_1$, but the ratio of forced expiratory to inspiratory flow at 50% of vital capacity (FEF$_{50}$/FIF$_{50}$) is usually >1. Causes include vocal-cord dysfunction and vocal-cord paralysis

FIXED AIRWAY OBSTRUCTION

There is no change in the caliber of the airway with a fixed intrathoracic or extrathoracic obstruction during the entire respiratory cycle. As a result, airflow limitation through the obstruction is independent of the phase of respiration and results in flattening of both inspiratory and expiratory flow–volume loops (**Figure 28-2E**). Etiologies include tumors, tracheal or subglottic stenosis, and foreign bodies in the trachea.

PULMONARY DISEASES AND SYNDROMES

PEDIATRIC ACUTE RESPIRATORY DISTRESS SYNDROME (PARDS)

Pediatric Acute Lung Injury Consensus Conference definition of PARDS: Acute respiratory failure not fully explained by cardiac failure or fluid overload, that occurs within 7 days of a known clinical insult resulting in hypoxemia and new infiltrates on chest imaging consistent with acute pulmonary parenchymal disease. It excludes causes of respiratory failure secondary to perinatal-related lung disease. Severity of disease is determined by the oxygenation index (OI) or the oxygen saturation index (OSI).

EPIDEMIOLOGY

• The incidence of PARDS has likely been underdiagnosed owing to a lack of specific guidelines. Approximately 1–4% of children undergoing mechanical ventilation in North America have ARDS.
• Incidence in children varies greatly, but in the United States, it ranges between 2.9 and 9.5 cases in 100,000 children per year.
• Mortality depends on age, etiology, pre-morbid conditions, and severity of oxygenation deficit: Mortality rate for PARDS is 22–40%.

ETIOLOGY

• The most common cause is infections, including sepsis and pneumonia.
• Other causes include aspiration, near-drowning, and concomitant cardiac disease.

PATHOPHYSIOLOGY

• ARDS follows a predictable progression of histologic and clinical stages:
  ✓ Inflammatory stage: Release of proinflammatory cytokines and influx of neutrophils lead to epithelial and endothelial injury, noncardiogenic pulmonary edema, impaired gas exchange, surfactant deficiency/deactivation, and diffuse alveolar damage.
  ✓ Proliferative stage: Proliferation of type II alveolar cells, squamous metaplasia, interstitial infiltration by myofibroblasts, and early deposition of collagen
  ✓ Fibrotic stage: Obliteration of normal lung architecture, diffuse fibrosis, collagen deposition

CLINICAL MANIFESTATIONS

• The initial presentation can include cyanosis, dyspnea, tachypnea, and diffuse crackles.

DIAGNOSTICS

• Arterial blood gas: Profound hypoxemia, usually refractory to supplemental oxygen administration; elevated A-a gradient. Calculate the oxygenation index ($[FiO_2 \times MAP \times 100]/PaO_2$) or the oxygen saturation index ($[FiO_2 \times MAP \times 100]/SpO_2$) to determine the severity of ARDS. Initially, the $PaCO_2$ is low because of hyperventilation, but later there is CO_2 retention.
• Indicators of end-organ damage and multiorgan failure: Follow liver enzyme levels, coagulation studies, and cardiac enzyme and creatinine levels.
• Chest radiograph: New alveolar infiltrates
• Chest computed tomography (CT) scan: New patchy airspace opacities in dependent areas of lung
• Expected changes in lung function and mechanics: Decreased TLC, decreased FRC, large intrapulmonary shunt fraction, decreased pulmonary compliance

MANAGEMENT

Management involves supportive ventilation and correction of underlying causes while treating comorbidities and limiting complications.

• Ventilation: Goal is to achieve adequate (not necessarily normal) alveolar gas exchange while limiting complications by using low V_T to avoid alveolar overdistention, low FiO_2 to reduce oxidant injury, and high PEEP to limit barotrauma and maximize lung recruitment:
  ✓ Minimize tidal volume: Goal 5–8 mL/kg of predicted body weight
  ✓ Permissive hypercapnia: Smaller tidal volumes to minimize ventilator-induced lung injury result in an elevation of $PaCO_2$

✓ PEEP: 10–15 cmH$_2$O to prevent or reverse atelectasis at end expiration
✓ Limit inflating (plateau) pressure (e.g., after an inspiratory hold) to 28 cmH$_2$O allowing for slightly higher pressures (29–32 cmH$_2$O) for patients with reduced chest-wall compliance
✓ Goal SpO$_2$ for mild PARDS with PEEP <10 cmH$_2$O is 92–97%. For severe PARDS with PEEP >10 cm H$_2$O, an SpO$_2$ goal of 88–92% should be considered.
✓ Goal pH 7.15–7.30

- Adjunctive therapies have not been proven to reduce mortality but include high-frequency oscillation, inverse inspiratory-to-expiratory ratio ventilation, PRVC ventilation, APRV, prone positioning, systemic steroids, inhaled nitric oxide, exogenous surfactant administration, extracorporeal membrane oxygenation, and neuromuscular blockade.
- Supportive treatment:
  ✓ Limited fluid resuscitation ensures adequate tissue perfusion while limiting alveolar edema. Measures to decrease oxygen demand are helpful.
  ✓ Inotropic support; blood transfusion, if necessary; diuretics; sedation; antipyretics
- Experimental therapies: Liquid ventilation, dietary antioxidant therapy, granulocyte macrophage colony-stimulating factor, statins, macrolide antibiotics, beta-agonists
- Manage comorbidities: Renal failure, cardiac failure, hepatic failure, central nervous system failure, disordered coagulation
- Manage complications: Ventilator-associated pneumonia, barotrauma, bacterial tracheitis, sepsis, systemic inflammatory response syndrome (SIRS), chronic respiratory failure, generalized deconditioning, critical illness neuropathy, central line infections, central-line thrombosis, decubitus ulcer formation, nosocomial infection, delirium

CYSTIC FIBROSIS (CF)

An autosomal recessive defect in the cystic fibrosis transmembrane conductance regulator (*CFTR*) gene, located on the long arm of chromosome 7. Abnormal transport of chloride and sodium across epithelium results in viscid mucous secretions and elevated sweat chloride levels. Progressive chronic pulmonary disease and exocrine pancreatic insufficiency are the primary clinical manifestations.

EPIDEMIOLOGY

- Carrier frequency in certain white populations as high as 1 in 25
- >2000 mutations of the *CFTR* gene identified to date
- *Phe508del-CFTR* is the most common mutation in the Northern European white population and accounts for approximately 70% of *CFTR* mutations in the United States.

PATHOPHYSIOLOGY

- Failure of epithelial cells to conduct chloride and the associated water transport abnormalities results in tenacious secretions in the respiratory tract, pancreas, small and large intestines, liver/gallbladder, and genitourinary tract.
- Decreased clearance of viscid secretions causes obstruction of progressively larger airways, starting with bronchioles.
- Chronic airway inflammation and bacterial colonization damage airways. This injury progresses to bronchiectasis, bronchiectatic cysts, and emphysematous bullae. Loss of normal airway architecture causes secondary obstructive changes with air trapping and hyperinflation.
- Long-term treatment goals aim to minimize lung damage and to maintain normal lung function as long as possible.

✓ Treatment of acute pulmonary exacerbations is directed at restoring lung function to pre-illness baseline.

✓ Maintain good nutrition by eating a high-calorie, high-fat diet with vitamins, mineral supplements, and pancreatic enzymes, if needed.

✓ Stay fit, with regular physical activities and exercise.

CLINICAL MANIFESTATIONS

Respiratory Tract

- Cough is the most consistent symptom.
- Infants and young children: Tachypnea, chronic or recurrent episodes of wheezing, respiratory distress with crackles and wheeze, and/or nonproductive cough; recurrent lower respiratory tract infections; respiratory cultures grow *Escherichia coli*, *Klebsiella pneumoniae*, *Staphylococcus aureus*, or *Haemophilus influenzae*.
- Older children and adolescents: Progressive respiratory symptoms including mucopurulent cough worse in the morning and with activity, exercise intolerance, recurrent wheezing, and hemoptysis (occasionally massive). Physical exam findings include increased anteroposterior chest diameter, thoracic hyperresonance, persistent crackles, wheezing, and digital clubbing. Respiratory cultures usually grow *Pseudomonas aeruginosa*.
- Progressive lung pathology includes bronchiectasis, atelectasis, fibrosis, and occasionally pneumothorax. Right heart failure is usually a late consequence of chronic hypoxemia but can present secondary to acute respiratory failure.
- Pansinusitis is common and chronic; acute sinusitis is less common.
- Nasal polyps can be a presenting finding.
- Colonization with select genomovars of *Burkholderia cepacia* and nontuberculous mycobacteria correlate with more rapid disease progression.
- Allergic bronchopulmonary aspergillosis (ABPA) can occur:

  ✓ Obstructive symptoms and fall in lung function tests that do not respond to aggressive antibiotic and airway clearance therapies. Major diagnostic features include:
  - Immediate skin test reactivity to *Aspergillus* antigens
  - Precipitating serum antibodies to *Aspergillus fumigatus*
  - Elevated serum total IgE concentration (>1000 ng/mL)
  - Peripheral blood eosinophilia >500/mm^3
  - Elevated specific serum IgE and IgG to *A. fumigatus*
  - Chest radiograph demonstrates fleeting pulmonary infiltrates, while chest CT imaging usually demonstrates central bronchiectasis

  ✓ Treatment for ABPA consists of a prolonged course of systemic corticosteroids and an antifungal agent.

Gastrointestinal Tract

- Obstructive symptoms due to paucity of intestinal water and large malabsorptive stools: 15% of CF newborns present with no passage of stool in the first 24–48 hours of life, abdominal distention, bilious emesis, and meconium ileus. Infants can present with rectal prolapse in association with straining. Children and adolescents can present with constipation, emesis, abdominal distention, and abdominal pain; the constellation of symptoms is referred to as distal intestinal obstruction syndrome.
- Pancreatic insufficiency: Most patients with CF (90%) have pancreatic insufficiency and suffer from intestinal malabsorption with associated fat-soluble vitamin (A, D, E, and K) deficiencies. Recurrent pancreatitis can occur.

- About 20% of adolescents and 40–50% of adults patients develop CF-related diabetes, which shares features of both types 1 and 2 diabetes.
- Biliary tract: Persistent neonatal direct hyperbilirubinemia, cholelithiasis, and biliary sludge
- Failure to thrive
- Physical exam: Rectal prolapse, protuberant abdomen, decreased muscle mass, delayed Tanner staging, right-lower-quadrant stool mass, hepatosplenomegaly

Genitourinary

- Average delay in sexual maturity of 2 years
- Increased risk of nephrolithiasis
- Males: Atretic epididymis, vas deferens, and seminal vesicles secondary to failure of Wolffian development and inspissation of secretions; obstructive azoospermia and infertility; normal sexual function; higher incidence of anatomic defects including hernia and undescended testes
- Females: Increased rate of secondary amenorrhea with pulmonary exacerbations; tenacious cervical mucus leads to increased risk of cervicitis but does not reduce fertility; pregnancy tolerance is correlated with lung function; increased risk of *Candida* vaginitis in the setting of frequent antibiotic therapy; stress incontinence (experienced by 1 in 4 women with CF) due to weak pelvic floor due to chronic coughing.

Metabolic Abnormalities

- Higher risk for acute salt and volume depletion with gastroenteritis or dehydration (hyponatremic dehydration) and chronic hypochloremic metabolic alkalosis due to increased losses of sodium and chloride in sweat
- History of "tasting salty" or salt crystallization on forehead

DIAGNOSTICS

Both history/physical findings AND laboratory confirmation are required to make the diagnosis of CF (**Table 28-3**).

- Tests for abnormal *CFTR* are used to confirm a diagnosis in a patient with one or more clinical features consistent with the CF phenotype, a history of CF in a sibling, and/or a positive newborn screen.
  - ✓ Sweat test (by pilocarpine iontophoresis): Sweat chloride concentration of >60 mmol/L on two separate occasions with adequate amounts (>100 mg) of sweat collected; values of 30–60 mmol/L are considered borderline and the test must be repeated.
  - ✓ Identification of two *CFTR* mutations: Finding two *CFTR* mutations in association with clinical symptoms is diagnostic, but negative results on genotype analyses do not exclude the diagnosis.
- Tests suggesting CF (these supporting findings need confirmation with a diagnostic test)
  - ✓ Positive newborn screen: Blood test for immunoreactive trypsinogen
  - ✓ Elevated fat content in 72-hour stool collection
  - ✓ Low vitamin D, A, and E levels
  - ✓ Prolonged prothrombin time (PT)
  - ✓ Semen analysis: Obstructive azoospermia
  - ✓ Ultrasound finding of congenital bilateral absence of the vasa deferentia
  - ✓ Bronchoalveolar lavage fluid positive for *P. aeruginosa*
  - ✓ Sputum microbiology positive for *S. aureus* or *P. aeruginosa*, especially the mucoid form

TABLE 28-3	Diagnostic Criteria for Cystic Fibrosis (Patient must have at least one finding from each column)
Patient History	**Evidence of *CFTR* Gene Dysfunction**
1. One or more characteristic phenotypic features	1. Elevated sweat chloride
2. Sibling or parent with cystic fibrosis	2. Identification of mutation in each *CFTR* gene known to cause cystic fibrosis
3. Positive newborn screen	3. Characteristic abnormalities in ion transport across nasal epithelium

- Data used to follow clinical course
  - ✓ Chest radiograph: Hyperinflation, atelectasis, and peribronchial thickening are initial findings. Advanced findings include bowed sternum, cyst or nodule formation, extensive bronchiectasis, dilated pulmonary artery, pneumothorax, and scarring.
  - ✓ Chest CT: Not recommended for routine monitoring of disease status and progression, but can be considered if patient is not responding to appropriate therapy
  - ✓ Sinus CT: Panopacification + failure of frontal sinus development
  - ✓ Pulmonary function testing: Initially can be normal. Early changes indicate an obstructive pattern, whereas advanced disease displays a combined obstructive and restrictive pattern due to fibrosis or marked air trapping. A decrease of 10% or more from baseline FEV_1 may prompt hospital admission.
- Laboratory evaluation during an acute exacerbation:
  - ✓ Fluid balance, renal function, liver enzymes, glucose, magnesium (especially in patients with a history of frequent intravenous aminoglycoside use)
  - ✓ Complete blood cell count with differential
  - ✓ PT/international normalized ratio
  - ✓ Aminoglycoside levels (after institution of therapy)
  - ✓ Serum total IgE level if history of or concern for ABPA
  - ✓ Consider vitamin and mineral levels (A, E, zinc, 25-hydroxyvitamin D)
  - ✓ Hemoglobin A_{1c} if signs or history of diabetes mellitus
  - ✓ Obtain sputum culture, cough swab, or deep throat culture before starting antibiotics. Repeat sputum cultures on day 7 after admission.
  - ✓ Urinalysis to look for glucosuria, hematuria, proteinuria, and hypercalciuria

Miscellaneous Diagnostics

- Dual-energy x-ray absorptiometry (DEXA) scan (bone density scan). All patients over 18 years of age should have a DEXA scan and it should be repeated every 1–5 years depending on results
  - ✓ Obtain a DEXA if patient is >8 years of age and has any of the following:
    - Ideal body weight <90%
    - Body-mass index <50%
    - FEV_1 <50% predicted
    - Glucocorticoid use of ≥5 mg/day for ≥90 days/year
    - Delayed puberty
- Audiology exam (especially in those exposed frequently to aminoglycosides)

MANAGEMENT

Respiratory Management of Pulmonary Exacerbation

- Antibiotics: Empiric parenteral administration of two antipseudomonal antibiotics for 14–21 days (e.g., aminoglycoside and beta-lactam antibiotic such as tobramycin + imipenem, ticarcillin–clavulanate, or piperacillin–tazobactam). Specific therapy should be based on the identification and susceptibility testing of bacteria isolated from sputum.
  - ✓ Administration of long-term aerosolized antibiotics (e.g., tobramycin, aztreonam, colistin) delivers high concentrations of medication directly to the site of infection and can reduce exacerbations and improve lung function and quality of life.
  - ✓ Ideally, sputum culture should be obtained at every visit, but at least quarterly, along with pulmonary function tests when the patient is able to perform them.
- Nonpharmacologic secretion clearance alternatives
  - ✓ Chest physiotherapy with postural drainage
  - ✓ High-frequency chest-wall compression with an inflatable vest
  - ✓ Intrapulmonary percussive ventilation
  - ✓ Positive expiratory pressure device
  - ✓ Autogenic drainage, directed breathing techniques
- Pharmacologic secretion clearance
  - ✓ Inhaled hypertonic saline can reduce the viscoelasticity of sputum
  - ✓ Inhaled human recombinant DNase can reduce the viscoelasticity of infected sputum
  - ✓ Bronchodilator therapy (beta-2-agonist) can increase ciliary beat frequency, and is also used if there is a history of airway hyperreactivity
- Antiinflammatory therapy
  - ✓ Azithromycin is used for the long term for its antiinflammatory effects to improve lung function and reduce the number of exacerbations.
  - ✓ Inhaled corticosteroids are added only when there is a concomitant history of asthma.
  - ✓ Ibuprofen can be used as a long-term antiinflammatory agent in children 6–17 years of age with $FEV_1 \geq 60\%$ of predicted, and serum levels should be maintained 50–100 mg/mL.
- *CFTR* modulators: Small-molecule pharmacologic agents that target defects in *CFTR* gating, processing, and synthesis

  - ✓ Potentiators: Increase flow of chloride through *CFTR* proteins at the cell surface by "holding the gate open," thus regulating the amount of water at the surface of the cell. Ivacaftor is a potentiator. It is recommended for individuals with at least one G551D *CFTR* mutation, or a gating mutation. Ivacaftor is found to improve lung function and quality of life and reduce exacerbations. It also reduces sweat chloride concentrations to near normal levels
  - ✓ Correctors: Repair defective *CFTR* processing by facilitating proper folding and delivery of *CFTR* to the cell surface. Lumacaftor and tezacaftor are correctors. They are recommended for individuals with two copies of Phe508del mutation
  - ✓ Combination therapy with ivacaftor–lumacaftor and tezacaftor–ivacaftor are approved for all patients who are homozygous for the Phe508del mutation, which constitutes nearly half the CF population in the United States. The combination therapy has been shown to improve FEV_1 by up to 4% and, more impressively, to reduce the rate of pulmonary exacerbations by nearly 40%.
  - ✓ Combination therapy with elexacaftor-tezacaftor-ivacaftor is approved for all patients 12 years and older with at least one copy of the Phe508del mutation, which is present in nearly 90% of patients. This triple combination therapy was shown to improve FEV1 by 14%, reduce pulmonary exacerbations by 63%, and significantly reduce sweat chloride concentrations.

Nutritional Management

- Diet: Most patients have increased caloric needs. Children and adolescents require a high-calorie, high-protein, and extra-salt diet
  - ✓ Oral glucose-tolerance test should be done annually after 8 years of age to screen for CF-related diabetes.
- Pancreatic exocrine enzyme replacement
  - ✓ Doses should not exceed 2500 lipase units/kg/meal or 10,000 lipase units/kg/day to avoid fibrosing colonopathy and colonic strictures.
- Vitamins A, D, E, and K in doses used for malabsorption

HEMOPTYSIS

The expectoration of blood or blood-tinged sputum from the lower respiratory tract. The immediate danger is from suffocation, not from exsanguination.

- Massive or major: >200 mL in 24 hours or >100 mL per day for several days
- Minor: Smaller volumes
- Life-threatening: >8 mL/kg/24 hour

PATHOGENESIS

The lung contains two separate blood supplies

- The pulmonary arterial circulation: High-volume, low-pressure system. Its branches accompany the bronchi down to the level of the terminal bronchioles. Pulmonary vessels branch to supply the capillary bed in the walls of the alveoli and then return to the left atrium via the pulmonary veins.
- The bronchial circulation: Small volume, systemic pressures. Typically there are three bronchial arteries, two that supply the left lung and one that supplies the right. These arteries usually originate from the aorta or the intercostal arteries and perfuse conducting airways approximately to the level of the terminal bronchioles.

ETIOLOGY

- Minor hemoptysis: Direct mucosal injury (e.g., shearing forces dislodging mucus from airway wall, direct trauma from suction catheters)
- Massive hemoptysis: Usually from bronchial artery (high-pressure system) to pulmonary artery anastomosis
- Infection is the most common cause of hemoptysis in children.
- Bleeding from tracheostomy
- Foreign-body aspiration, especially long-standing
- Congenital heart disease with pulmonary vascular obstruction or enlarged collateral bronchial circulation
- Cystic fibrosis (areas of bronchiectasis and inflammation)
- Bronchiectasis
- Tuberculosis
- Nasopharyngeal bleeding (nonpulmonary source of bleeding—not true hemoptysis)
- Immune-mediated: Henoch–Schönlein purpura, granulomatosis with polyangiitis, polyarteritis nodosa, Goodpasture syndrome, systemic lupus erythematosus, Heiner syndrome (reversible non–IgE-mediated hypersensitivity to cow's milk resulting in pulmonary disease in young infants)

- Less frequent: An infected pulmonary sequestration, pulmonary embolism, tumor, neoplasm, pulmonary arteriovenous malformation, idiopathic pulmonary hemosiderosis, coagulopathy, iatrogenic from procedures including lung biopsy

DIAGNOSTICS

- Assess adequacy of ventilation
- Orthostatic pulse and blood pressure to estimate blood loss
- Chest radiograph
- Complete blood count, PT, partial thromboplastin time
- If indicated: serum chemistries, blood urea nitrogen, creatinine, tuberculin skin test (purified protein derivative) or interferon-γ release assay (QuantiFERON Gold), rheumatologic markers including antinuclear antibody, double-stranded DNA, erythrocyte sedimentation rate, C-reactive protein, complement levels, antineutrophil cytoplasmic antibodies, anti–basement membrane antibodies, IgG levels
- Urinalysis
- Sputum Gram stain and culture
- Chest CT: Can help define structural abnormalities, including arteriovenous malformations and masses
- Angiography in cases of severe refractory hemoptysis
- Fiberoptic bronchoscopy: Performed when bleeding is not acute to identify a source of bleeding and obtain a lavage
  ✓ The presence of hemosiderin-laden macrophages from bronchoalveolar lavage confirms pulmonary bleeding; they typically appear 72 hours after the event and last for several weeks.
- Rigid bronchoscopy is best for acute bleeding to suction large volumes and control the airway if necessary. Allows better visualization of the airway and removal of a foreign body.
- Cardiac evaluation including echocardiography with visualization of pulmonary veins

MANAGEMENT

- Management is typically supportive, except in the case of massive hemoptysis, and is directed at treating the underlying cause of bleeding.
- Secure the airway and ensure adequacy of ventilation; deliver increased PEEP.
- Support circulating volume with crystalloid until red-cell transfusion is possible.
- In the case of life-threatening massive hemoptysis, emergency bronchoscopy may be required. Sites of bleeding can be slowed by either balloon catheter tamponade or with the use of topical oxymetazoline, epinephrine, or cold saline.
- If bleeding cannot be controlled, emergency arteriography may help to localize the area of bleeding and can allow selective embolization

OBSTRUCTIVE APNEA (OSA)

Disorder of breathing during sleep characterized by prolonged partial upper airway obstruction and/or intermittent complete obstruction (obstructive apnea) that disrupts normal ventilation during sleep and normal sleep patterns

EPIDEMIOLOGY

- Occurs at all ages, although may be more common in preschoolers
- Prevalence in school-age children from 2 to 12%

ETIOLOGY

- Risk factors: Adenotonsillar hypertrophy, obesity, craniofacial anomalies, neuromuscular disorders, trisomy 21, chronic lung disease, sickle cell disease, hypotonia

CLINICAL MANIFESTATIONS

- The most common symptom of clinically significant OSA is snoring.
- Other common manifestations: Labored breathing, restless sleep, apnea while asleep, enuresis, morning headaches, daytime sleepiness, sleeping with neck hyperextended, learning problems, attention-deficit/hyperactivity disorder
- Severe presentations: Cor pulmonale, failure to thrive, cognitive impairment
- Possible exam findings: Adenotonsillar hypertrophy, adenoidal facies, micrognathia/retrognathia, hypertension, loud pulmonary component of S2, underweight or overweight

DIAGNOSTICS

- Polysomnography requires overnight admission to a sleep laboratory. It is the only method that quantifies ventilatory and sleep abnormalities, therefore, it is the gold standard.
  - ✓ Apnea–hypopnea index: Normal, <1.5 events/hour; severe, >10 events/hour. Severe OSA is not an acute emergency.
- If full polysomnography is not available: Nocturnal pulse oximetry, oximetry with capnography, and abbreviated polysomnography or nap sleep study can be done. These all have weaker positive and negative predictive values than full nocturnal polysomnography, so a normal study does not rule out sleep disordered breathing

DEFINITIONS (BASED ON POLYSOMNOGRAPHIC FINDINGS)

Obstructive Apnea

- Drop in the peak signal excursion by ≥90% of the pre-event baseline using an oronasal thermal sensor
  - ✓ Lasts at least two breaths during baseline breathing
  - ✓ Respiratory effort as evidenced by chest-wall and abdominal motion present throughout the entire period of absent airflow

Hypopnea

- Peak signal excursions drop by ≥30% of pre-events baseline using nasal pressure
- Duration of the ≥30% drop lasts for at least two breaths
- Associated with ≥3% desaturation from pre-event baseline or with an arousal

Central Apnea

- Drop in the peak signal excursion by ≥90% of the pre-event baseline using an oronasal thermal sensor with cessation of breathing effort and one of the following conditions:
  - ✓ The event lasts 20 seconds or longer
  - ✓ The event lasts at least the duration of two breaths during baseline breathing and is associated with an arousal or ≥3% oxygen desaturation
  - ✓ For infants <1 year of age, the event lasts at least the duration of two breaths during baseline breathing and is associated with a decrease in heart rate to <50 beats per minute for at least 5 seconds or <60 beats per minute for 15 seconds
- Adjunctive tests: Electrocardiography to evaluate for right ventricular hypertrophy; elevated serum bicarbonate reflects chronic hypoventilation

MANAGEMENT

Acute

- Positioning: Upright, side lying, or sniffing position. In the case of hypotonia or tracheomalacia, prone positioning may relieve obstruction
- Nasal airway: Use preformed nasal trumpet or trimmed down endotracheal tube (ETT). Positive pressure can be delivered through a nasopharyngeal ETT
- Antibiotics: If acute infection
- Antiinflammatory agents: May acutely help reduce swelling, consider dexamethasone.
- Intranasal corticosteroids can be used as treatment for mild OSA.
- Oxymetazoline nasal spray or nebulized racemic epinephrine can diminish intranasal or extrathoracic airway obstruction.
- Tracheal intubation/tracheostomy placement: Reserved for severe refractory cases

Chronic

- Adenotonsillectomy: First line of treatment for pediatric OSA
  ✓ Reassess OSA signs and symptoms 6–8 weeks after surgery to determine if repeat polysomnography is indicated.
- CPAP: Used in patients with specific contraindications to adenotonsillectomy, minimal adenotonsillar tissue, persistent OSA after adenotonsillectomy or for those who prefer nonsurgical alternatives
- Weight loss: Improves OSA if patient is obese

BRONCHOPULMONARY DYSPLASIA (BPD)

Most commonly, chronic lung disease of prematurity in infants born at <32 weeks of gestational age with a supplemental oxygen requirement at 28 days of life. Severity of disease is categorized on the basis of respiratory support needs at 36 weeks of postmenstrual age (Table 28-4).

EPIDMIOLOGY

- BPD affects approximately 10,000 to 15,000 preterm infants per year in the United States (**Table 28-4**).
- Despite advances in neonatal care translating into improved survival of extremely premature infants, the prevalence of BPD has not changed or it has increased slightly.
- The incidence of severe BPD is inversely correlated with gestational age.

ETIOLOGY

- Primary risk factor: Prematurity
- The exact pathogenic mechanisms underlying the development of the disease are unknown. However, prematurity leading to disruption of alveolar growth and pulmonary vascular development contribute to the development of BPD. Other factors, including oxygen toxicity, mechanical ventilation, infection, inflammation, and nutritional deficits further contribute to compromised development of the lung in an infant with BPD.
- Genetic and environmental factors leading to the development of BPD are still being elucidated. Demographic factors associated with the development of BPD include male sex, patent ductus arteriosus, sepsis, and surgical necrotizing enterocolitis.

TABLE 28-4	BPD Definition with Severity		
BPD Severity	Definition (Modified from Jobe and Bancalari)	Relative incidence (Data from Ehrenkranz et al)	Postdischarge mortality (Data from Ehrenkranz et al)
None	O_2 treatment <28 d and breathing room air at 36 wk PMA or discharge home, whichever comes first	23.1%	1.8%
Mild	O_2 treatment at least 28 d and breathing room air at 36 wk PMA or discharge home, whichever comes first	30.3%	1.5%
Moderate	O_2 treatment at least 28 d and receiving <30% O_2 at 36 wk PMA or discharge home, whichever comes first	30.2%	2.0%
Severe (type 1)	O_2 treatment at least 28 d and receiving ≥30% O_2 or nasal CPAP/HFNC at ≥36 wks	16.4%	4.0%
Severe (type 2)	O_2 treatment at least 28 d and receiving mechanical ventilation at ≥36 wks		

HFNC, high flow nasal cannula; O_2, Oxygen.
Reproduced with permission from Abman SH, Collaco JM, Shepherd EG, et al: Interdisciplinary Care of Children with Severe Bronchopulmonary Dysplasia, *J Pediatr* 2017 Feb;181:12-28.

PATHOPHYSIOLOGY

- The histologic features of classical BPD feature interstitial fibrosis, alveolar overdistention alternating with areas of atelectasis, smooth-muscle hyperplasia, and airway abnormalities.
- The "new BPD," seen in the postsurfactant era, is characterized by an arrest in alveolar development leading to alveolar simplification. There is a reduction in the number of alveoli, and those alveoli that are present are larger.
- Characteristics of both "classic" and "new" BPD can be seen in those infants with severe ventilator-dependent BPD.

DIAGNOSTICS

- Diagnosis is dependent on patients who meet historical and clinical factors as described in the clinical definition. There is no specific test that has been established for the diagnosis of BPD.
- Chest radiography can be relatively insensitive and nonspecific in BPD ,with findings including hyperexpansion, hyperlucency, and linear opacities.

- A high-resolution CT scan is more sensitive at detecting abnormalities that can include areas of hyperaeration, linear opacities, cystic lesions, and subpleural opacities.
- A flexible bronchoscopy may be useful to assess for tracheomalacia or bronchomalacia.

MANAGEMENT

- Management of comorbidities requires an interdisciplinary team approach. These conditions include neurodevelopmental impairment, pulmonary hypertension, gastroesophageal reflux, retinopathy of prematurity, and feeding difficulties.
- The goal of BPD management is to support the breathing of the patient while promoting growth and development.
- The use of supplemental oxygen or noninvasive ventilation may be necessary to support the long-term respiratory needs of the infant; however, some patients go on to require long-term mechanical ventilation via a tracheostomy.
- Ventilator strategies for long-term mechanical ventilation of patients with established BPD reflect the abnormal airway mechanics of the disease, which include high airway resistance, air trapping, and heterogeneous aeration of the lung. Ventilation strategies are characterized by larger tidal volumes and prolonged inspiratory times. A higher PEEP may be needed to overcome dynamic airway collapse and optimize gas exchange.
- Medications
  ✓ Bronchodilators (albuterol and levalbuterol) can lower airway resistance with improved short term outcomes, but no studies have assessed long-term, sustained benefits of bronchodilators in infants with BPD.
  ✓ Inhaled steroids may decrease airway inflammation; however, long-term effects of these medications is not known.
  ✓ Diuretics, including furosemide, chlorothiazide, and spironolactone, treat and prevent pulmonary edema. Short-term use improves lung compliance; however, there are no data to support long-term use and improved outcomes.
- Immunizations are important in infants with BPD owing to an increased risk of recurrent respiratory infections and hospitalizations. Prophylaxis with palivizumab, a monoclonal antibody against RSV, and an annual influenza vaccine are recommended for infants with BPD.
- Patients with BPD are at an increased risk for developing pulmonary hypertension (PH) because of dysmorphic pulmonary vasculature and compromised angiogenesis. PH is present in approximately 25% of infants with severe BPD.

  ✓ Echocardiography is the best noninvasive screening tool for assessing for PH, although some cases of PH can be missed. Findings on echocardiography include an increased tricuspid regurgitant jet velocity, septal-wall flattening, and right ventricular dilation.
  ✓ Cardiac catheterization can be used for diagnosis or guidance of therapy; however, the availability of this procedure, as well as the potential risks and benefits, would need to be considered.
  ✓ Management of the underlying lung disease is essential in management of BPD-associated PH.
  ✓ Pulmonary vasodilator therapy is the mainstay of treatment for pulmonary hypertension. Current therapies include supplemental oxygen, inhaled nitric oxide, phosphodiesterase type 5 inhibitors (sildenafil and tadalafil), endothelin receptor antagonists (bosentan and ambrisentan), prostacyclin analogs (treprostenil), and calcium-channel blockers

NEUROMUSCULAR DISORDERS (NMD)

NMD is a general term that refers to diseases that affect any component of nerve and muscle function. Weakness involving inspiratory, bulbar, or expiratory muscles leads to impaired airway clearance and progressive ventilatory failure.

EPIDEMIOLOGY

- These disorders vary greatly in pattern of inheritance, genetic mutation, presentation, degree of respiratory impairment, and therefore, prognosis.

ETIOLOGY

- Duchenne muscular dystrophy (DMD) and spinal muscular atrophy (SMA) are two of the most common and severe forms of neuromuscular disease. Other muscular dystrophies and myopathies make up a variety of NMDs, each with different disease presentation and progression.
- DMD is the most common muscular dystrophy; it is inherited as an X-linked recessive trait. DMD presents in boys with proximal muscle weakness at 3–5 years of age. Respiratory impairment and failure develop, with progressive respiratory muscle weakness, usually in the second decade of life.
- SMAs are a group of autosomal recessive neurodegenerative disorders including type I (Werdnig–Hoffman disease), type II, type III (Kugelberg–Welander disease), and type IV, based on the age of onset of muscle weakness and clinical severity

  ✓ SMA type I: Symptom onset is at birth or by the age of 6 months, with respiratory failure by the age of 18 months. Infants never sit independently.
  ✓ SMA type II: Symptom onset between the ages of 7 and 18 months. Toddlers never ambulate.
  ✓ SMA type III: Symptom onset after 18 months
  ✓ SMA type IV: Symptom onset in adulthood

PATHOPHYSIOLOGY

- Children with progressive neuromuscular weakness undergo a stereotypical progression of respiratory involvement, beginning with impaired airway clearance, which predisposes patients with NMD to chronic atelectasis and recurrent pneumonia. This in turn can reduce lung compliance, increase airway resistance, and increase ventilatory demands. Over time, this leads to nocturnal and then diurnal ventilatory failure.

CLINICAL MANIFESTATIONS

- Secretion retention and lower airway infection: Reduction in inspiratory, glottic, and expiratory muscle strength results in reduction of cough effectiveness, which leads to inability to expectorate secretions. This predisposes individuals to atelectasis and lower-airway infections.
- Sleep disordered breathing:
  ✓ Upper airway obstruction and obstructive apnea: Due to bulbar musculature weakness, macroglossia (DMD), and malar flattening
  ✓ Hypoventilation: Initially NMD patients develop nocturnal hypoventilation due to their weakness and low tidal volume breathing; worse during rapid-eye-movement sleep.
  ✓ Both hypoxemia and hypercapnia result from above breathing derangements during sleep, causing frequent arousals, reduced sleep efficiency, and eventually sleep deprivation. As the severity of neuromuscular weakness progresses, patients can develop diurnal hypercapnia.

- Aspiration lung disease: Swallowing dysfunction occurs owing to loss of control of the larynx and pharynx. Ineffective cough also contributes to increased risk for aspiration. Aspiration causes inflammation within the lungs, leading to worsening obstructive and restrictive lung disease in the form of bronchiectasis and pulmonary fibrosis.
- Mechanical effects of progressive scoliosis: Scoliosis results in reduced vital capacity by causing asymmetric inspiration, diaphragm dysfunction, and a reduction in chest wall compliance.

DIAGNOSTICS

- Clinical assessment of respiratory health should be directed toward identifying progressive muscle weakness, ability to cope with respiratory infection, aspiration, progression of scoliosis and sleep-disordered breathing.
- Pulmonary function testing in NMD patients typically shows a restrictive pattern with diminished vital capacity, total lung capacity, and functional residual capacity, and with a relative preservation of the FEV_1/FVC ratio.
- Standing height cannot be reliably measured in patients with scoliosis or ankle contractures or in those unable to stand independently owing to weakness. Ulnar length or arm span should be used to predict lung function in children with NMD whose height cannot be accurately measured.
  - ✓ VC should be measured in all patients with NMD who are capable of performing spirometry. A $\geq 25\%$ fall in VC between seated and supine maneuvers reflects significant diaphragm weakness.
  - ✓ FEV_1, maximal inspiratory pressure (MIP), maximal expiratory pressure (MEP), cough peak flow, peak expiratory flow rate, and sniff nasal inspiratory pressure should be used to monitor respiratory status.
  - ✓ Cough peak flow can be used as part of the assessment of effective secretion clearance in children with NMD over the age of 12 years.
- Sleep disordered breathing can be assessed with formal overnight polysomnography.
- Video fluoroscopic swallow assessment for risk of aspiration

MANAGEMENT

- In general, airway clearance should be considered in patients with recurrent pneumonia, qualitative assessment of a weak cough, and clinical loss of respiratory functions.
  - ✓ Mechanical insufflation/exsufflation applies a positive pressure to the airway (insufflation) then rapidly shifts to negative pressure (exsufflation). The rapid pressure shift produces a high expiratory flow, simulating a natural cough.
  - ✓ Various mucus-mobilization techniques such as high-frequency chest-wall compressions and intrapulmonary percussive ventilation may be considered in children who have difficulty mobilizing secretions and with persistent atelectasis, despite use of other airway clearance techniques.
- Nebulized normal saline may be considered in children who have continued tenacious secretions.
- The goal of assisted ventilation is to reverse or ameliorate the cause of respiratory compromise (daytime or nocturnal hypoventilation), improve physiologic function as well as quality of life, and reduce morbidity and mortality. It also serves to promote physical and developmental growth of an individual.
  - ✓ Noninvasive ventilation (NIV) should be the first-line treatment for children with NMD and chronic respiratory failure unless there are contraindications, which include poor glottic function, inability to achieve adequate ventilation noninvasively, unstable airway, or lack of caregiver expertise.

✓ Invasive ventilation via tracheostomy is used in young children who require continuous mechanical ventilation, those with severe craniofacial malformations (upper airway or central airway obstruction), those with severe bulbar dysfunction, and hypoventilation that cannot be corrected by NIV.

✓ The decision to advance from noninvasive to invasive ventilation must be individualized, considering both the child's overall health state and the caregivers' ability to perform and preference for care.

- Multidisciplinary care should consist of a primary pulmonologist, respiratory therapist, nutritionist, nurse, and social worker to provide overall wellness in conjunction with subspecialty care.

- Subspecialty care

  ✓ Neurology: Evaluation and management of progressive neuromuscular weakness. Novel gene therapies are now available for DMD and SMA, among other NMDs, to stop or slow the progression of muscle weakness and improve quality of life.

  ✓ Cardiology: Referral for treatment of disease related cardiomyopathy, dysrhythmias, hypertension, pulmonary hypertension, and congenital cardiac disease

  ✓ Gastroenterology: Evaluation of gastroesophageal reflux disease and aspiration, need for gastrostomy tube with fundoplication for chronic aspiration. Other common GI disorders include dysmotility, aerophagia from NIV, and constipation.

  ✓ Rehabilitation/physiatry: Referral for strengthening exercises as treatment of neuromuscular weakness; Botox injections and baclofen pump for contractures.

  ✓ Orthopedic surgery: Evaluation and surgical treatment of thoracic insufficiency syndrome with scoliosis and rib deformities ("collapsing parasol")

  ✓ Transition to adult care coordination: Dedicated transition planning to help young adults develop age-appropriate medical knowledge and self-management skills. Efforts should be made to allow for a smooth transition from pediatric to adult providers by providing information and support for patients and families, in addition to identifying an adult provider with NMD expertise and providing adequate medical summary to the receiving adult medical team,

  ✓ Palliative care team: Provide multidimensional health-related quality of life management, and assist patients and families to make informed choices that are consistent with their own values and preferences.

Emily Liebling, MD
Rosemary Peterson, MD
Jay Mehta, MD

DERMATOMYOSITIS/JUVENILE DERMATOMYOSITIS (JDM)

Most common pediatric inflammatory myopathy; Bohan and Peter diagnostic criteria (definite JDM: heliotrope rash or Gottron papules plus at least three criteria; probable JDM: heliotrope rash or Gottron papules plus two criteria)

- Heliotrope rash (eyelids) or Gottron papules (extensor surfaces)
- Progressive symmetric proximal muscle weakness
- Elevated skeletal muscle enzymes (creatine phosphokinase, aspartate aminotransferase [AST], aldolase, lactate dehydrogenase [LDH])
- Electromyogram (EMG) consistent with myopathy
- Biopsy evidence of myositis
- Updated criteria will likely include muscle abnormalities on MRI short T1 inversion recovery (STIR) or T2 sequence

EPIDEMIOLOGY

- Incidence: About 2–3 cases in 1 million children
- Peaks at 4 to 9 years of age
- Girls > boys (2:1)
- Unlike in adults, JDM has no definite associations with malignancy in children.

ETIOLOGY

- Potential infectious triggers: Group A beta-hemolytic *Streptococcus*, coxsackievirus B, parvovirus, Epstein–Barr virus (EBV), others
- HLA and tumor necrosis factor α (TNF-α) alleles may predispose a child to JDM.
- Molecular mimicry is suspected.
- Sun exposure may trigger onset of rash.

DIFFERENTIAL DIAGNOSIS

- Rheumatologic
  ✓ Juvenile polymyositis is rare in children (2–8% of inflammatory myopathies) and has a higher age at onset and a more severe disease presentation, includes proximal and distal weakness and muscle atrophy, and lacks skin abnormalities; calcinosis is rare.
  ✓ Systemic lupus erythematosus (SLE) and related conditions (e.g., mixed connective tissue disease, Sjögren syndrome)
  ✓ Systemic Sclerosis
  ✓ Juvenile idiopathic arthritis; polyarticular or systemic
  ✓ Polyarteritis nodosa
  ✓ Eosinophilic fasciitis
- Infectious
  ✓ Viral myopathies: Influenza, coxsackievirus, echovirus, parvovirus, EBV, herpes simplex virus, parainfluenza virus, adenovirus, enterovirus
  ✓ Bacterial and parasitic myopathies: *Staphylococcus*, *Streptococcus*, *Toxoplasma*, *Trichinella*

- Metabolic/genetic
  - ✓ Muscular dystrophies
  - ✓ Congenital myopathies
  - ✓ Myotonic disorders
  - ✓ Glycogen storage diseases
  - ✓ Periodic paralysis
  - ✓ Endocrinopathies
- Other
  - ✓ Trauma
  - ✓ Toxins
  - ✓ Drug-induced myopathies
  - ✓ Disorders of neuromuscular transmission

PATHOPHYSIOLOGY

- Autoimmune angiopathy
- Perivascular inflammation, mostly mononuclear cells
- Swelling and blockage of capillaries, tissue infarction, perifascicular atrophy
- Chronic inflammation ensues, with fibrosis and microscopic calcification

CLINICAL MANIFESTATIONS

- Proximal muscle weakness (neck flexors, shoulders, abdomen, thighs): Gower sign, difficulty climbing stairs or combing hair
- Skin: Heliotrope rash (violaceous rash of eyelids); facial erythema, possibly in malar distribution (with involvement of nasolabial folds in contrast to SLE); papulosquamous eruption on extensor surfaces (Gottron rash), particularly over interphalangeal joints; shawl sign (erythematous rash in a shawl distribution); cutaneous calcinosis and ulceration
- Nailfolds: Capillary drop-out, capillary dilation, cuticular hypertrophy
- Arthritis: Can be transient or persistent, with or without tenosynovitis, flexor nodules; flexion contractures due to myofascial inflammation
- Mucocutaneous: Oral ulcers, gingival inflammation
- Pulmonary: Shortness of breath, cough, crackles can be consistent with interstitial lung disease or aspiration pneumonia.
- Gastrointestinal (GI): Dysphagia, enteric ulceration with or without perforation, bleeding, constipation, diarrhea, abdominal pain
- Other manifestations: Lipodystrophy, polyneuropathy, retinal exudates, and cotton wool patches
- Other complications: Calcinotic lesions may spontaneously drain, causing local inflammatory response and superinfection; can form exoskeleton; vasculitic ulcers; rare arrhythmias and cardiomyopathy; complications of chronic corticosteroid exposure (growth failure, hypertension, vertebral compression fractures, striae, avascular necrosis, cataracts, glaucoma)

DIAGNOSTICS

- Complete blood count (CBC): Lymphopenia, anemia of chronic inflammation; iron deficiency anemia should raise concern for GI blood loss.
- Erythrocyte sedimentation rate (ESR): Normal or elevated; CRP: usually normal
- Elevated muscle enzymes: Creatine phosphokinase, aldolase, AST, alanine aminotransferase (ALT), lactate dehydrogenase (LDH)
- Antinuclear antibody (ANA): Positive in 41–72% of cases

- Neopterin and von Willebrand factor antigen: Elevations correlate with disease activity (not widely used)
- Myositis-specific autoantibodies: associated with certain disease phenotypes; anti-Mi2 (mild JDM with classic skin rashes), anti-Jo1 (interstitial lung disease and high mortality), anti-p155/140 (severe cutaneous involvement, lipodystrophy), anti-MJ (more severe disease, joint contractures, calcinosis, GI ulceration)
- Myositis-associated antibodies: 18% of patients, associated with myositis overlap syndromes; anti-U1–anti-ribonuclear protein RNP (myositis + mixed connective tissue disease) and PM-Scl (myositis + scleroderma)
- Urinalysis to rule out renal involvement (may indicate SLE overlap)
- MRI pelvis with T2- or STIR-weighted images of muscles: Localizes active disease sites
- High-resolution chest computed tomography: Evaluate for interstitial lung disease if clinical concern from abnormal pulmonary function tests
- Modified barium swallow: Detect palato-esophageal dysfunction due to hypopharyngeal muscle weakness
- X-ray: Detect calcinosis and soft-tissue and muscle edema
- Electrocardiography (ECG): May detect arrhythmias
- Echocardiography: May detect cardiomyopathy (rare)
- Muscle biopsy: If diagnosis uncertain; myositis, perifascicular atrophy with degenerating and regenerating fibers
- Electromyography (EMG): Only if necessary to confirm diagnosis or guide biopsy; fibrillations, insertional irritability
- Pulmonary function tests: Can see restrictive pattern due to respiratory muscle weakness or interstitial lung disease

MANAGEMENT

- Mild disease: Corticosteroids (2 mg/kg/day then taper), methotrexate, hydroxychloroquine (especially for cutaneous disease)
- Moderate-to-severe disease: Add pulse corticosteroids (IV methylprednisolone 30 mg/kg/day, up to 1000 mg) × 3 then oral (2 mg/kg/day then taper), IVIG (2 g/kg every 3–4 weeks)
- Refractory disease: If active disease persists on a maximal regimen including methotrexate, IVIG, and hydroxychloroquine, other agents such as cyclophosphamide, mycophenolate mofetil, rituximab, calcineurin inhibitors (cyclosporine, tacrolimus), intermittent pulse methylprednisolone, tumor necrosis factor inhibitors, and abatacept can be considered
- Interstitial lung disease: Cyclophosphamide, tacrolimus, pulse corticosteroids, tofacitinib
- Sunscreen: Minimum Sun protection factor (SPF) 30 with ultraviolet (UV) A and UVB protection
- Nutritional supplements: Vitamin D and calcium
- Calcinosis: Decreased with early aggressive therapy, case reports of successful therapy with a variety of agents including bisphosphonates
- Physical and occupational therapy
- Immunizations
  - ✓ No live vaccines for individuals on high-dose systemic corticosteroids or other immunosuppressive agents
  - ✓ Administer inactivated influenza (annually) and pneumococcal vaccines.
  - ✓ Delay measles, mumps, rubella (MMR) vaccination until 11 months after last IVIG treatment if not otherwise contraindicated (e.g., on other immunosuppressants).

HENOCH–SCHÖNLEIN PURPURA (HSP)

Small-vessel vasculitis affecting the skin, joints, GI tract, and kidneys. EULAR/PRINTO/ PRES 2010 criteria: Purpura or petechiae (mandatory) with lower-limb predominance not due to thrombocytopenia and at least one of the four following criteria: abdominal pain, leukocytoclastic vasculitis with immunoglobulin (Ig) A deposits or proliferative glomerulonephritis with IgA deposits on histopathology, arthritis or arthralgia, or renal involvement.

EPIDEMIOLOGY

- Most common childhood vasculitis in the United States
- Age range: 3–15 years; peak: 7 years
- Boys > girls (1.5:1)
- Incidence: 3 in 100,000 to 17 in 100,000
- Some seasonal variation (less common in summer), often preceded by upper respiratory tract infection

DIFFERENTIAL DIAGNOSIS

- Rheumatologic
  - ✓ SLE and related conditions
  - ✓ Antineutrophil cytoplasmic antibody (ANCA)–associated vasculitis
  - ✓ Hypersensitivity vasculitis
  - ✓ Cryoglobulinemia
  - ✓ Urticarial vasculitis
  - ✓ Polyarteritis nodosa
- Hematologic/oncologic
  - ✓ Immune thrombocytopenic purpura
  - ✓ Infantile acute hemorrhagic edema
  - ✓ Leukemia/lymphoma
- Infectious/postinfectious
  - ✓ Sepsis
  - ✓ Viral and bacterial enterocolitis
  - ✓ Poststreptococcal glomerulonephritis
  - ✓ Hemolytic–uremic syndrome
- GI:
  - ✓ Crohn disease
  - ✓ Ulcerative colitis

PATHOPHYSIOLOGY

- Small-vessel vasculitis affecting capillaries and precapillary and postcapillary vessels
- Mediated by immune complexes (typically IgA, can see IgG and activated complement C3), which are deposited in end organs, causing inflammation
- May be associated with antecedent infection (group A beta-hemolytic *Streptococcus*, mycoplasma, parvovirus, other viral pathogens)

CLINICAL MANIFESTATIONS

- Classic presentation includes nonthrombocytopenic purpuric rash, musculoskeletal pain, and colicky abdominal pain.
- Rash: Most common presenting symptom
  - ✓ Nonblanching, purpuric lesions developing in gravity- or pressure-dependent areas, usually distal to the elbows and below the waist

✓ Early lesions may appear erythematous, petechial, or urticarial, evolving into hemorrhagic or ecchymotic lesions. Lesions may take other forms, such as bullous.

✓ Lesions may ulcerate.

✓ Koebner phenomenon may occur (lesions appear at sites of skin injury).

- Musculoskeletal pain: Second most common manifestation; symptoms may be persistent or intermittent

  ✓ Periarticular or articular pain with impaired mobility and minimal joint warmth and effusion, typically affecting the ankles, knees, elbows, wrists, digits

- GI manifestations: Occurs in two-thirds of children within a week of rash onset, but can precede other manifestations; colicky abdominal pain, vomiting, hematemesis, melena; massive GI hemorrhage, bowel perforation, or intussusception in 5% of children

- Renal involvement: Occurs in one-third of patients and usually develops within the first 4–6 weeks; may lead to end-stage renal disease; poorest prognosis in children with nephritic/nephrotic syndrome at onset

  ✓ Manifestations include microscopic or macroscopic hematuria with or without proteinuria, hypertension, glomerulonephritis, ureteritis, urethritis, and cystitis.

- Rare manifestations:

  ✓ Genitourinary: Scrotal swelling/hemorrhage mimicking testicular torsion, testicular torsion (rare)

  ✓ Central nervous system (CNS): Headache, seizures, hemorrhage, cerebrovascular thrombosis, focal deficits, and peripheral neuropathies

  ✓ Pulmonary: Interstitial disease, alveolar hemorrhage, and respiratory failure

  ✓ Cardiovascular: Carditis, myocardial infarction

- Vital signs: Low-grade fevers; hypertension due to renal disease; tachycardia due to anemia or pain

- Duration of symptoms: Average 4 weeks if untreated, chronic HSP is unusual.

- Recurrence: Up to 33%, usually within the first year after diagnosis, with each episode briefer and milder than previous one

DIAGNOSTICS

- CBC: Moderate leukocytosis in some children; normocytic anemia may be due to GI blood loss, platelet count normal to mildly elevated.

- Coagulation studies: Normal

- ESR and CRP: Normal to mildly elevated

- BUN and creatinine: Normal or possibly elevated with renal disease or volume depletion

- Albumin: Decreased with proteinuria and gastrointestinal losses, malnutrition, and inflammation

- Urinalysis: Proteinuria and/or hematuria; red-cell casts

- Stool: May be hemoccult-positive

- Immunologic

  ✓ ANCA should be negative in HSP. If ANCA is positive, consider granulomatosis with polyangiitis (c-ANCA, positive antiproteinase 3), microscopic polyangiitis, or rarely, eosinophilic granulomatosis with polyangiitis (EGPA) (p-ANCA, positive antimyeloperoxidase)

  ✓ Elevated IgA levels in 50% (not routinely sent)

  ✓ Cryoglobulins should be negative (not routinely sent)

- Abdominal x-ray, barium studies, ultrasound, and CT may be useful for assessment of abdominal obstruction and intussusception.

- Skin biopsy: May aid diagnosis in nonclassic presentations; light microscopy demonstrates leukocytoclastic vasculitis and IgA deposition on immunofluorescence.

- Renal biopsy: Useful if proteinuria/hematuria is significant or does not resolve; crescentic glomerulonephritis with IgA deposition may be seen.

MANAGEMENT

- Ibuprofen for analgesia; avoid nonsteroidal antiinflammatory drugs (NSAIDs) if GI or renal involvement
- Monitor for renal involvement with routine blood pressure checks and urinalyses; almost all cases present in first 6 months after illness onset (weekly for the first month, every other week until 3 months, then at 6 months and 1 year after presentation).
- Corticosteroids: Beneficial for significant abdominal manifestations, or significant musculoskeletal pain. Benefit for renal disease is controversial.
  - ✓ For mild or moderate disease, consider prednisone or methylprednisolone 2 mg/kg/day up to 60 mg/day for 1 week with 2–3 weeks taper.
  - ✓ For severe disease, consider pulse methylprednisolone up to 30 mg/kg/day (maximum, 1000 mg/day) up to 3 days then prednisone 2 mg/kg/day up to 60 mg/day for 1 week with a 2–3-week taper
- Immunosuppressive therapy (cyclosporine, cyclophosphamide, azathioprine, methotrexate, rituximab) should be considered in patients with complicated nephritis, pulmonary, cutaneous, and/or CNS manifestations.
- Supportive care: Severe pain may require narcotics. Severe GI involvement may require nothing-by-mouth status, nasogastric suction, and total parenteral nutrition, though response to corticosteroids is often dramatic with prompt initiation of therapy.

JUVENILE IDIOPATHIC ARTHRITIS (JIA)

Chronic, noninfectious, synovial inflammation of unknown cause with onset prior to 16 years of age and leading to arthritis in one or more joints for at least 6 weeks. The 2001 International League of Associations for Rheumatology classification criteria for JIA include seven specific subtypes, as described next.

- Oligoarthritis: Arthritis involving one to four joints during the first 6 months of disease
- Polyarthritis (rheumatoid factor negative): Involvement of five or more joints during the first 6 months of disease; rheumatoid factor test negative
- Polyarthritis (rheumatoid factor positive): Involvement of five or more joints during the first 6 months of disease; two rheumatoid factor tests positive at least 3 months apart during first 6 months of disease
- Enthesitis-related arthritis: Arthritis and enthesitis (tenderness at the site of tendon insertion on bone); or arthritis or enthesitis with at least two of the following: sacroiliac tenderness or inflammatory lumbosacral pain, HLA-B27 positive, onset of arthritis in a male >6 years old, acute (symptomatic) anterior uveitis, first-degree relative with a history of ankylosing spondylitis, enthesitis-related arthritis, sacroiliitis with inflammatory bowel disease, reactive arthritis, or acute anterior uveitis
- Psoriatic arthritis: Arthritis and psoriasis, or arthritis with two of the following: dactylitis, nail pitting, onycholysis, or psoriasis in a first-degree relative
- Systemic arthritis: Arthritis in one or more joints with or preceded by a fever of 2 weeks' duration with a quotidian fever for at least 3 days plus at least one of the following: evanescent (nonfixed) erythematous rash, generalized lymphadenopathy, hepatomegaly and/or splenomegaly, or serositis
- Undifferentiated arthritis: Arthritis that does not fulfill the above criteria based on subtype-specific exclusion criteria or fulfills criteria in two or more of the above categories

EPIDEMIOLOGY

- Most common chronic childhood rheumatologic disease
- Sex distribution is subtype-specific

- Incidence: 1 in 100,000 to 20 in 100,000 in children <16 years old
- Proportion of arthritis subtypes: Oligoarthritis (50%), polyarthritis (20%, of which 85% are rheumatoid factor negative), enthesitis-related arthritis (8–19%), psoriatic arthritis (1–11%), systemic arthritis (5–15%)

ETIOLOGY

- Genetic and environmental factors suspected
- HLA associations exist
- Associated with immunodeficiencies: IgA deficiency, 22q11 deletion
- Link between infectious triggers and arthritis is not fully established.

DIFFERENTIAL DIAGNOSIS OF CHRONIC ARTHRITIS

- Critical to distinguish acute from chronic arthritis as a first step.
- Other rheumatic and inflammatory diseases such as inflammatory bowel disease, sarcoidosis, SLE, and vasculitis can present with an acute or chronic oligoarthritis or polyarthritis with or without fever
- Oligoarthritis: Trauma, reactive arthritis, septic arthritis, hemarthrosis, Lyme disease, foreign body, leukemia, bone or synovial tumor, Legg–Calve–Perthes disease, slipped capital femoral epiphysis, pigmented villonodular synovitis, cystic fibrosis arthropathy, metabolic disorders (e.g., gout)
- Polyarthritis: Serum sickness, reactive arthritis, septic arthritis (*Neisseria* spp.), parvovirus B19 infection, sickle cell disease, scleroderma, congenital arthropathies, mucopolysaccharidosis
- Systemic arthritis: Kawasaki disease, leukemia, lymphoma, primary or secondary hemophagocytic lymphohistiocytosis, septic arthritis, Lyme disease, EBV, parvovirus B19, *Bartonella henselae*, mycoplasma, acute rheumatic fever, periodic fever syndromes and other autoinflammatory syndromes, Langerhans-cell histiocytosis, chronic recurrent multifocal osteomyelitis, Castleman disease

PATHOPHYSIOLOGY

- Synovitis with villous hypertrophy and hyperplasia
- T-cell activation and recruitment into joint synovium leads to release of proinflammatory cytokines by multiple cell types
- Pannus formation in late disease, causing progressive erosion of cartilage and bone
- Systemic arthritis is an autoinflammatory condition and has a unique pathophysiology compared to other subtypes with prominence of innate immune activation resulting in elevated levels of several inflammatory cytokines.

CLINICAL MANIFESTATIONS

- General: Limp, joint swelling with morning stiffness (25% of children may have painless swelling), pain with inactivity. Systemic symptoms of significant fatigue, weight loss, and anorexia only with severe polyarticular disease, systemic arthritis, and/or associated condition such as inflammatory bowel disease or celiac disease; should prompt suspicion for malignancy.
- Oligoarthritis: Usually involves knees, ankles, fingers, wrists, elbows
- Polyarthritis: May involve large and small joints, spares distal interphalangeal joints
- Systemic arthritis: High fevers 1–2 times/day for at least 2 weeks, temperature often returns to normal or subnormal, with fever accompanied by erythematous macular rash on trunk and proximal limbs; hepatosplenomegaly and generalized lymphadenopathy; serositis (pericarditis and/or pleuritis); pericardial tamponade may ensue.

- Musculoskeletal: Swelling/effusion; limited range of motion (including decreased cervical-spine motion); warmth; contracture/deformity; with or without limb-length discrepancies and wasting of surrounding muscles (gastrocnemius or quadriceps); joint erythema not a common finding
- Arthritis of temporomandibular joint may cause failure to thrive secondary to pain with chewing. Micrognathia or jaw deviation may ensue.
- Anterior uveitis: Asymptomatic in oligoarthritis and polyarthritis; can be symptomatic in enthesitis-related arthritis and psoriatic arthritis; not associated with systemic arthritis. Pupil irregularities, synechiae, band keratopathy on exam; may lead to visual loss, cataract, glaucoma; most common in ANA-positive young females.
- Macrophage activation syndrome/secondary hemophagocytic lymphohistiocytosis is a potentially life-threatening complication seen with systemic arthritis.
  - ✓ Symptoms may include unremitting fever, hepatosplenomegaly, lymphadenopathy, coagulopathy with bruising and mucosal bleeding, liver dysfunction, respiratory distress, encephalopathy, and renal involvement progressing to multi-system organ failure
- Other complications: Fractures, pseudoporphyria with NSAID use. Untreated arthritis can lead to contractures and limb-length discrepancy.

DIAGNOSTICS

- No laboratory test can confirm the diagnosis of chronic arthritis.
- ESR and CRP: High with systemic arthritis; usually normal in other subtypes, but can be elevated in severe oligoarthritis or polyarthritis, sacroiliitis, or overlapping inflammatory bowel disease
- CBC: Leukocyte count normal or high; platelets may be elevated.
- ANA: Highest frequency in younger girls, rarely positive in systemic arthritis; positive ANA associated with increased risk of developing uveitis in subtypes other than systemic arthritis
- Rheumatoid factor: Positive in minority of patients with polyarthritis, useful for prognostic purposes only (predictive of more severe and protracted disease course)
- Anticitrullinated peptide antibodies: Most common in rheumatoid factor-positive polyarthritis, predictive of more severe disease course
- HLA-B27: Positive in 90% of children with juvenile ankylosing spondylitis and 60–80% of enthesitis-related arthritis; not diagnostic without other disease features (present in 8% of healthy population)
- Joint fluid aspirate: Usually 2000–50,000 WBCs/mm^3 (but may be higher); neutrophil predominance (see **Table 15–8 in Chapter 15** for reference values)
- Imaging: Radiographs can be used to establish baseline for evaluation of joint erosions, MRI in atypical presentations to evaluate for malignancy and pigmented villonodular synovitis, ultrasonography to confirm joint effusion and/or assess for synovial proliferation
- If cervical-spine range of motion limited, order cervical lateral flexion and extension spinal films to assess for atlantoaxial instability and subaxial ankylosis prior to surgery, intubation, sports participation
- Macrophage activation syndrome/secondary hemophagocytic lymphohistiocytosis: Fall in WBCs, hemoglobin and platelets, elevated liver enzymes, low ESR due to hypofibrinogenemia, elevated D-dimer, elevated LDH, prolonged prothrombin time and partial thromboplastin time (PTT), hypertriglyceridemia, hyperferritinemia, elevated soluble interleukin (IL)-2 receptor, evidence of macrophage hemophagocytosis on bone marrow biopsy

MANAGEMENT

- Oligoarthritis: Treatment of choice is intraarticular corticosteroid injections; NSAIDs (e.g., naproxen 20 mg/kg/day, divided twice per day) for symptomatic relief; if no response to intraarticular corticosteroid injections or manifestations are severe, then use methotrexate and/or biologic therapy.
- Polyarthritis: Intraarticular corticosteroids, methotrexate, TNF-α inhibitors (e.g., etanercept, adalimumab, infliximab), CTLA-4 Ig fusion protein (abatacept), IL-6 receptor antagonist (tocilizumab), B-cell depletion (rituximab). Rheumatoid factor and/or anticitrullinated-antibody positive has poor prognosis and necessitates aggressive therapy.
- Systemic arthritis: Corticosteroids, IL-1 inhibitors (anakinra or canakinumab), IL-6–receptor Antagonist (tocilizumab), cyclosporine (particularly with refractory macrophage activation syndrome), tacrolimus, intraarticular corticosteroids; cyclophosphamide for refractory disease or interstitial lung disease
- Regular ophthalmology exams: Slit-lamp exam to diagnose asymptomatic uveitis
  ✓ Frequency is every 3–6 months initially, depending on age at onset and ANA status, except in systemic arthritis, in which every 12-month screening is adequate.
- Dietary evaluation: Ensure adequate calcium, vitamin D.
- Physical and occupational therapy: To maintain and improve joint function and motion
- Immunizations
  ✓ Avoid live vaccines (varicella, MMR, intranasal influenza) for individuals on high-dose systemic corticosteroids or immunosuppressants.
  ✓ Administer inactivated influenza (annually) and pneumococcal vaccines.

REACTIVE ARTHRITIS

Self-limiting, predominantly lower-extremity, asymmetric arthritis with demonstration of a preceding enteric or genitourinary infection with "arthritogenic" gastrointestinal and genitourinary pathogens

EPIDEMIOLOGY

- Accounts for 4.1–8.6% of rheumatology clinic visits
- Boys (peak age, 6–8 years) > girls, but age and sex distribution vary by causative organism
- Chlamydial infections are more common in adolescents and adults.

ETIOLOGY AND PATHOGENESIS

- Preceding infections: Yersinia, Salmonella, Shigella, Campylobacter (GI), Chlamydia (genitourinary)
- Strong association with HLA-B27, role still unknown; probable CD8+ T-cell cross reactivity with bacterial epitopes

DIFFERENTIAL DIAGNOSIS

- Postviral/transient synovitis
- Septic arthritis
- Acute rheumatic fever/poststreptococcal arthritis
- Serum sickness
- Inflammatory bowel disease–related arthritis
- Early JIA
- Behçet disease
- Kawasaki disease

CLINICAL MANIFESTATIONS

- Vary by causative organism
- Most children have a monophasic course, but HLA-B27–positive patients often have recurrent episodes, with more joints involved, more severe symptoms, and the triad of arthritis, conjunctivitis, and urethritis, which may also later evolve into enthesitis-related arthritis or juvenile spondyloarthropathy.
- Acute oligoarthritis with or without enthesitis; infrequently polyarthritis
  - ✓ Polyarthralgia is common.
  - ✓ Painful, often with overlying erythema
  - ✓ Usually knees and ankles, but sometimes small joints of the hands and feet
  - ✓ Follows enteric infection (varies by organism) within 7–30 days
- Fever, weight loss, fatigue
- Abdominal pain, diarrhea
- Dysuria, asymptomatic urethral/vaginal discharge
- Purulent conjunctivitis with or without uveitis; occurs in two-thirds of children, usually severe
- Painless oral ulcers
- Skin lesions, particularly erythema nodosum

DIAGNOSTICS

- Requires documentation of preceding infection
  - ✓ Stool cultures
  - ✓ Urethral cultures
- Supportive labs and imaging:
  - ✓ ESR/CRP: Usually elevated; supportive, but nonspecific
  - ✓ CBC: Anemia in severe disease, thrombocytosis, leukocytosis; supportive, but nonspecific. May see marrow suppression in the setting of a viral or postviral arthritis.
  - ✓ Urinalysis: May show sterile pyuria
  - ✓ X-ray: May show nonspecific soft-tissue swelling, periarticular osteopenia, or slight periosteal irregularity at entheses
  - ✓ Ultrasound: Useful to evaluate for hip effusions or if physical exam is equivocal. May show joint effusions, synovial and tendon-sheath thickening, bursal fluid accumulation
  - ✓ MRI: Not usually necessary if other signs present to support diagnosis; may show marrow edema, synovitis with or without tenosynovitis.

MANAGEMENT

- Supportive; there is no evidence that medication alters disease course
- NSAIDs; indomethacin particularly effective
- Sulfasalazine; particularly useful for HLA-B27–positive patients
- Corticosteroids; for severe, widespread disease. Start at 2 mg/kg/day with short taper for rapid disease control
- Intraarticular corticosteroid injection; consider for monoarthritis, provides rapid relief

KAWASAKI DISEASE

An acute, febrile vasculitis of childhood defined by ≥5 days of fever and ≥4 of the following: Conjunctivitis, mucous membrane changes, peripheral-extremity changes, polymorphous rash, or cervical adenopathy (>1.5 cm). Incomplete Kawasaki disease may

present with fewer than 4 criteria with supplemental laboratory criteria and/or coronary artery caliber changes. It is more common in infants <6 months old.

EPIDEMIOLOGY

- Incidence: United States: about 12 in 100,000; Japan: about 112 in 100,000
- Median age, 2 years; 80% of cases occur before 5 years of age and 95% before 10 years
- Recurrence <1% in the United States but 3% in Japan
- Children <1 year have increased likelihood of developing coronary artery aneurysms

DIFFERENTIAL DIAGNOSIS

- Viral:
  - ✓ Measles
  - ✓ EBV
  - ✓ Adenovirus
  - ✓ Enterovirus
  - ✓ Parvovirus B19
- Bacterial:
  - ✓ Scarlet fever
  - ✓ Staphylococcal scalded skin syndrome
  - ✓ Toxic shock syndrome
  - ✓ *Yersinia pseudotuberculosis*
  - ✓ Typhoid fever
  - ✓ Leptospirosis
  - ✓ Rocky Mountain Spotted fever
  - ✓ Rat bite fever
- Allergic:
  - ✓ Drug reaction
  - ✓ Serum sickness
  - ✓ Stevens–Johnson syndrome
- Rheumatologic:
  - ✓ Systemic arthritis
  - ✓ Polyarteritis nodosa
  - ✓ Reactive arthritis
- Toxic:
  - ✓ Mercury poisoning
- Multisystem inflammatory syndrome in children (MIS-C)
  - ✓ Follows infection with severe acute respiratory syndrome coronavirus 2 (SARS-CoV-2), the causative virus of coronavirus disease 2019 (COVID-19)
  - ✓ Given the rapidly evolving state of knowledge, check https://www.cdc.gov/mis-c/hcp/ for updates to diagnosis and treatment.
  - ✓ Diagnostic criteria evolving, but include
    - Age <21 years with fever, laboratory evidence of inflammation (elevated CRP, ESR, fibrinogen, procalcitonin, D-dimer, ferritin, LDH, or IL-10/TNFa, or reduced lymphocytes, elevated neutrophils, and low albumin), and clinically severe illness requiring hospitalization with two or more organ systems involved (cardiac, renal, respiratory, hematologic, gastrointestinal, dermatologic, or neurological) AND
    - No alternative plausible diagnosis AND
    - Positive for current or recent SARS-CoV-2 by PCR, serology, or antigen test or exposure to a person with suspected or confirmed COVID-19 within prior 4 weeks

✓ Common manifestations include persistent fever, abdominal pain, vomiting, diarrhea, skin rash, mucocutaneous lesions, and, occasionally, hypotension. Most patients have evidence of damage to the heart (e.g., elevated troponin, B-type natriuretic peptide). Some patients develop cardiac dysfunction and acute kidney injury.

PATHOPHYSIOLOGY

- Vasculitis of medium-sized arteries
- Edema of endothelial and smooth muscle cells; inflammatory infiltration of vascular wall
- The etiology is unknown, multiple environmental factors have been hypothesized
- Up to one-third have an identified coexisting infection

CLINICAL MANIFESTATIONS

- Three phases: Acute febrile phase (7–14 days), subacute phase (14–24 days), and convalescent phase (>24 days)
- Fever: High (can be >40°C) and persistent
- Conjunctival injection: Bilateral, bulbar (limbic-sparing), generally nonpurulent and painless
- Peripheral-extremity changes: Edema ("sausage-like" digits), erythema; desquamation 2–3 weeks after fever onset
- Mucous membrane changes: Injected oropharynx, dry fissured, peeling, cracking lips, "strawberry" tongue
- Polymorphous rash: May be maculopapular, urticarial, morbilliform, scarlatiniform, or targetoid; prominence in groin area and groin desquamation may occur by end of first week
- Cervical adenopathy: ≥1.5 cm, generally unilateral and may be tender
- Coronary artery aneurysms: Develop in up to 25% of patients not treated within 10 days of onset, but in fewer than 5% of treated patients
- Other manifestations: Extreme irritability, aseptic meningitis, cranial-nerve palsy, transient sensorineural hearing loss, myocarditis, valvular disease, MAS, shock-like syndrome, pleural effusions, gallbladder hydrops, hepatitis, jaundice, hepatosplenomegaly, abdominal pain, vomiting, diarrhea, arthralgias, arthritis of small and large joints, urethritis, uveitis, testicular swelling

DIAGNOSTICS

- Elevated ESR and CRP
- CBC: WBC normal or leukocytosis (>15,000/mm³ in 50%); normocytic anemia; thrombocytosis (platelet count ≤1,000,000/mm³) after first week
- Mildly elevated ALT, AST, gamma glutamyl transferase, bilirubin, alkaline phosphatase, but low albumin (<3 g/dL)
- Urinalysis: Sterile pyuria in 70% (>10 leukocytes per high-power filed), catheter sample may miss urethritis.
- CSF: Pleocytosis with lymphocyte predominance in 25–50% of patients who undergo lumbar puncture
- Chest x-ray: May show pneumonitis, pleural effusion, cardiomegaly
- ECG: May show arrhythmia, ischemia, low voltages or ST-segment or T-wave changes
- Echocardiography: Perform at time of diagnosis; may reveal coronary artery ectasia or aneurysms, pericardial effusion, valvular abnormalities, or diminished ventricular function
- Slit-lamp exam: Not routinely done; anterior uveitis is common (>85% of patients) but usually self-resolving without sequelae
- Arthrocentesis: Synovial fluid WBC 50–300,000/mm³, normal glucose, negative Gram stain and culture

MANAGEMENT

- Initial treatment (based on coronary artery change risk stratification):
  - ✓ Age >6 months: IVIG 2 g/kg, high-dose aspirin (80–100 mg/kg/day) for 24 hours then low-dose aspirin (3–5 mg/kg/day)
  - ✓ Age <6 months: IVIG 2 g/kg, corticosteroids 2 mg/kg/day, low-dose aspirin (3–5 mg/kg/day)
  - ✓ Abnormal echocardiogram (ALL patients): IVIG 2 g/kg, corticosteroids 2 mg/kg/day, low-dose aspirin (3–5 mg/kg/day)
- Fever OR lingering clinic symptoms >24–36 hours after completion of IVIG
  - ✓ Re-treat with IVIG 2 g/kg
- Unresponsive to second dose of IVIG
  - ✓ Start corticosteroids 2 mg/kg/day (if not already started in case of abnormal echocardiogram)
  - ✓ Consult Rheumatology and consider infliximab 5 mg/kg (may repeat dose if symptoms/fever persist after 24 hours)
- Anticoagulants: Dipyridamole, clopidogrel, warfarin, or low-molecular-weight heparin, and abciximab can be used for the treatment of coronary aneurysms.
- Other: Current ongoing clinical trial of anakinra (IL-1 receptor antagonist) in Kawasaki disease with early coronary artery abnormalities; few cases of effective use of cyclosporine in IVIG-resistant Kawasaki disease
- Disposition: Close follow-up with pediatric cardiologist. Repeat echocardiography is routinely performed 6–8 weeks after treatment and depending on the presence of coronary aneurysms. Follow-up with pediatric rheumatologist if steroids are necessary (to exclude other mimicking diagnoses after steroids are withdrawn)
- Immunizations: Defer MMR and varicella vaccinations for 11 months following IVIG. Those on long-term salicylate therapy should have an annual influenza vaccination.

RHEUMATIC FEVER

Postinfectious manifestation of group A streptococcal (GAS) pharyngitis. The diagnosis is based on the Jones criteria (Table 29-1).

- Should be distinguished from poststreptococcal reactive arthritis, a GAS-associated reactive arthritis that does not fulfill Jones criteria and is less likely to cause cardiac disease

TABLE 29-1	Jones Criteria of Rheumatic Fever*	
Two Major or One Major and Two Minor PLUS Evidence of Prior GABHS Infection		
Major	**Minor**	**Evidence of Prior GABHS Infection**
Carditis	Arthralgias	Throat culture
Erythema marginatum	Elevated acute phase reactants (ESR and CRP)	Antistreptolysin O[†]
Polyarthritis[‡]	Fever	Antideoxyribonuclease B
Subcutaneous nodules	Prolonged PR interval	
Sydenham chorea		

*Exceptions: Chorea as sole manifestation, indolent carditis; if recurrent need one major or greater than one minor criterion.
[†]Peaks at 2–3 weeks.
[‡]Can by migratory.
GABHS = group A beta-hemolytic streptococcal.

EPIDEMIOLOGY

- Most common in children 5–15 years old
- Annual incidence in the United States is less than 1 in 100,000, but up to 51 in 100,000 in developing countries such as India. Outbreaks are common in overcrowded areas,
- Carditis more common in young children,
- Arthritis more common and severe in teenagers and young adults,

ETIOLOGY

- Usually develops 2–3 weeks following untreated GAS pharyngitis

DIFFERENTIAL DIAGNOSIS

- Bacterial
  - ✓ Septic arthritis
  - ✓ Lyme arthritis
  - ✓ Reactive arthritis (including poststreptococcal)
  - ✓ Osteomyelitis
  - ✓ Endocarditis
  - ✓ Mycoplasma pneumonia
- Viral
  - ✓ Parvovirus
  - ✓ EBV
- Rheumatologic
  - ✓ Systemic arthritis
  - ✓ Kawasaki disease
  - ✓ SLE
  - ✓ Antiphospholipid syndrome (primary or secondary)
  - ✓ Behçet disease
  - ✓ Polyarteritis nodosa
- Immunologic:
  - ✓ Serum sickness
- Neurologic
  - ✓ Hereditary disorders such as juvenile Huntington disease
  - ✓ Wilson disease
  - ✓ Benign hereditary chorea
  - ✓ Inborn errors of metabolism
  - ✓ Nutritional or electrolyte disturbance
  - ✓ Arteriovenous malformation
- Oncologic
  - ✓ Leukemia
  - ✓ Lymphoma
- Hematologic
  - ✓ Sickle cell arthropathy

PATHOPHYSIOLOGY

- Potential role of antigenic mimicry: Antibodies formed against streptococcal antigens (components of M protein) cross-react with the corresponding tissues that share antigenic determinants and lead to inflammation in the heart, joints, and brain.
- Chorea may result from protein kinase activation by ANAs, leading to elevation of tyrosine hydroxylase and subsequent dopamine release in the basal ganglia.

CLINICAL MANIFESTATIONS

- Arthritis: Migratory and/or additive, typically affects knees, ankles, elbows; joints may be swollen, warm, tender, limited range of motion; joint involvement is more severe and common in teenagers.
- Subcutaneous nodules: Previously more common in severe disease with progression to chronic rheumatic heart disease, but now very rare; firm and painless; found over extensor surfaces of joints, occipital region, thoracic or lumbar spinous processes
- Erythema marginatum: <5% of patients; pink/red blanching rash with raised borders, central clearing, not pruritic or indurated; may worsen with fever
- Carditis: Affects mitral valve and aortic valve most commonly. It is a pancarditis that can involve the endocardium, myocardium, and pericardium, but congestive heart failure, if present, is most commonly due to valvular dysfunction.
- Chorea: Involuntary, purposeless movements; associated with muscle weakness and emotional lability that usually disappears over weeks to months; rarely recurs. "Milkmaid sign"; irregular contractions of hand muscles when trying to squeeze examiner's fingers

DIAGNOSTICS

- Evidence of prior infection: Increased antistreptolysin O, anti-DNase B, positive throat culture, recent history of scarlet fever; Streptozyme test not recommended as it is neither sensitive nor specific
- ESR and CRP: Usually very elevated acutely
- CBC: Normocytic, normochromic anemia
- Blood culture: Should be negative
- Joint fluid: Sterile, WBC count may be in septic range (>50,000/mm^3)
- X-rays of affected joints: Normal or effusion present
- Chest x-ray: May see cardiomegaly
- ECG: May see heart block (usually 1st degree)
- Echocardiography: May see mitral- and/or aortic-valve thickening and regurgitation. Stenotic lesions are associated with chronic valve disease in rheumatic fever

MANAGEMENT

- GAS infection treatment (10 days' duration)
  - ✓ Penicillin
  - ✓ Erythromycin or other macrolide antibiotic
  - ✓ Clindamycin
  - ✓ Cephalexin
- GAS prophylaxis
  - ✓ Penicillin G benzathine every 4 weeks: preferred over oral penicillin if carditis present
    - <27 kg: 600,000 units
    - ≥27 kg: 1.2 million units
  - ✓ Penicillin V 250 mg twice per day
  - ✓ Sulfadiazine or sulfisoxazole
    - ≤27 kg: 0.5 g daily
    - >27 kg: 1 g daily
  - ✓ Macrolide if allergic to penicillin and sulfonamide
  - ✓ Duration
    - Without carditis: Treat for 5 years after last episode or until age 21, whichever is longer.
    - With carditis: Treat for 10 years after last episode or until age 21, whichever is longer.

- With carditis and valvular disease: Treat for 10 years after last episode or until age 40, whichever is longer. Lifelong prophylaxis may be needed if risk of exposure is high.
- Aspirin: 80–100 mg/kg/day divided four times per day for arthritis and carditis (4–8 weeks depending on clinical response). Naproxen may be used for isolated joint disease.
- Corticosteroid therapy may be used in cases of severe, acute carditis and congestive heart failure to avoid solute load of aspirin (prednisone 2 mg/kg/day divided twice per day with 2–3-week taper)
- Chorea: Diazepam, haloperidol, valproic acid, corticosteroids

SYSTEMIC LUPUS ERYTHEMATOSUS (SLE)

Multisystem autoimmune disease caused by pathologic production of autoantibodies with tissue deposition of immune complexes, and characterized by global immune dysregulation

EPIDEMIOLOGY

- 15–25% of all patients present in first two decades of life, often after puberty.
- Female > male in all age groups; 5:1 in children, 9:1 in adults
- Overall increased incidence and disease severity in African Americans and Hispanics, as compared to Caucasians (varying by location)

ETIOLOGY

- Genetic predisposition (HLA haplotype associations)
- Complement deficiencies
- Innate and adaptive immune system dysregulation
- Environmental stimuli (UV light, drugs, EBV/CMV infections, smoking)
- Hormonal factors (particularly estrogens)
- Abnormal regulation of apoptosis

DIFFERENTIAL DIAGNOSIS

- Rheumatologic
  - ✓ Drug-induced lupus
  - ✓ Cutaneous lupus
  - ✓ Mixed connective-tissue disease
  - ✓ Sjögren syndrome
  - ✓ Juvenile dermatomyositis
  - ✓ Systemic sclerosis
  - ✓ JIA (systemic arthritis, polyarthritis)
  - ✓ Henoch–Schönlein purpura
  - ✓ ANCA-associated vasculitis
  - ✓ Hypersensitivity vasculitis
  - ✓ Cryoglobulinemia
  - ✓ Polyarteritis nodosa
  - ✓ Takayasu arteritis
  - ✓ Sarcoidosis
  - ✓ Primary antiphospholipid syndrome
  - ✓ IgG4-related disease
  - ✓ Castleman disease
  - ✓ Acute rheumatic fever

- Hematologic
  - ✓ Thrombotic thrombocytopenic purpura
  - ✓ Idiopathic thrombocytopenic purpura
  - ✓ Autoimmune hemolytic anemia
  - ✓ Evan syndrome
  - ✓ Aplastic anemia
- Immunologic
  - ✓ Common variable immunodeficiency
  - ✓ Autoimmune lymphoproliferative syndrome
- Oncologic
  - ✓ Leukemia
  - ✓ Lymphoma
  - ✓ Other malignancies causing marrow infiltration and/or serositis
- Cardiac
  - ✓ Infectious pericarditis
  - ✓ Autoinflammatory syndromes (e.g., idiopathic recurrent pericarditis and periodic fever syndromes)
- Renal
  - ✓ Membranoproliferative glomerulonephritis
  - ✓ Minimal change disease
  - ✓ Focal segmental glomerulosclerosis
  - ✓ Tubulointerstitial nephritis
- Gastrointestinal
  - ✓ Autoimmune hepatitis
  - ✓ Inflammatory bowel disease
  - ✓ Celiac disease
- Endocrine
  - ✓ Autoimmune thyroiditis
- Viral
  - ✓ EBV
  - ✓ Cytomegalovirus
  - ✓ Enteroviruses
  - ✓ Parvovirus B19
  - ✓ Viral hepatitis
  - ✓ Viral encephalitis
- Bacterial:
  - ✓ Lyme disease
  - ✓ Ehrlichiosis
  - ✓ Rocky Mountain Spotted Fever
  - ✓ *B. henselae*

PATHOPHYSIOLOGY

- Autoantibodies are directed against nuclear and cytoplasmic antigens. Organ-specific antibodies to cell-surface antigens are also present
- Disease can be secondary to pathogenic autoantibodies (renal disease, thrombocytopenia, antiphospholipid antibody syndrome, neonatal lupus and fetal loss, CNS disease), pathogenic immune complexes (secondary to quantity and size, and tissue tropism), and T-lymphocyte dysregulation (skin disease)

CLINICAL MANIFESTATIONS

- Many children have nonspecific symptoms months before diagnosis, often presenting with fatigue, fever, malaise, weight loss, lymphadenopathy, arthritis and rash before other organ manifestations.
- Mucocutaneous: Photosensitivity, malar "butterfly" rash, discoid rash, alopecia, painless palatal ulceration, Raynaud phenomenon with or without digital ulceration, vasculitic rash
- Musculoskeletal: Arthralgia and arthritis are frequent at presentation; often polyarticular and nonerosive. Myositis can be seen in overlap syndromes and mixed connective-tissue disease.
- Pleuropulmonary: Pleural effusion, pneumonitis, interstitial lung disease, shrinking lung syndrome, pulmonary hemorrhage, pulmonary embolus. Consider infection as a cause of pulmonary infiltrates in patients with SLE.
- Cardiovascular: Pericarditis, Libman–Sacks endocarditis, valvulitis, myocarditis, atherosclerotic vessel disease leading to myocardial infarction
- Gastrointestinal: Hepatosplenomegaly, hepatitis, mesenteric vasculitis, pancreatitis, enterocolitis. Esophageal dysmotility and reflux may be part of mixed connective-tissue disease.
- Renal: Can present on a spectrum of nephritic or nephrotic syndromes (e.g., hypertension, proteinuria) varying by histopathologic classification; can also be associated with interstitial nephritis and renal-vein thrombosis
- Neurologic: Headaches, mood changes, "brain fog," psychosis, seizures, headaches, catatonia, chorea, ataxia, stroke (ischemic or hemorrhagic), cranial-nerve palsy, peripheral neuropathy, transverse myelitis. Neuropsychiatric testing is helpful in evaluating for cognitive impairment.
- Hematologic: Anemia of chronic inflammation, autoimmune hemolytic anemia, thrombocytopenia, and leukopenia (usually lymphopenia), secondary hemophagocytic lymphohistiocytosis, thrombosis (due to secondary antiphospholipid syndrome)
- Ocular: Retinal vasculitis, episcleritis, central retinal vein thrombosis (due to secondary antiphospholipid syndrome), optic neuritis (with neuromyelitis optica overlap or secondary Sjögren syndrome)
- Endocrine: Autoimmune thyroid disease, short stature, delayed puberty, bone fragility

DIAGNOSTICS (TABLE 29-2)

Initial Evaluation

- CBC: Leukopenia ($<4,000/mm^3$), lymphopenia ($<1,500/mm^3$), thrombocytopenia ($<100,000/mm^3$), and autoimmune hemolytic anemia (AIHA). Work up AIHA as follows:
  - ✓ Peripheral smear; schistocytes are suggestive of thrombotic microangiopathy instead of antibody-mediated hemolysis
  - ✓ Reticulocyte count
  - ✓ Direct antiglobulin test (Coomb's test)
  - ✓ LDH
  - ✓ Indirect bilirubin
- Metabolic panel: Elevated creatinine, hypoalbuminemia suggests renal disease with proteinuria, may see elevated transaminases due to either liver disease or myositis
- Urinalysis: Proteinuria (first morning protein:creatinine ratio >0.2) and/or cellular casts suggests nephritis, gross hematuria suggests renal vein thrombosis.
- Amylase/lipase: Can be elevated both in lupus pancreatitis and chronic kidney disease
- Complement: Low C3 and C4; very low CH50 suggests complement deficiency.
- ANA profile: ANA is rarely negative in SLE.
  - ✓ Anti–double-stranded DNA is specific for SLE and is associated with renal disease.

TABLE 29-2	American College of Rheumatology Criteria for the Diagnosis of Systemic Lupus Erythematosus

Need 4 of 11 Criteria for the Diagnosis (at once or sequentially)

Malar rash

Discoid rash

Oral or nasopharyngeal ulceration (usually painless)

Photosensitivity

Nonerosive arthritis

Serositis (pleuritis or pericarditis)

Renal disorder (persistent proteinuria >0.5 g/day or cellular casts)

Neurologic disorder (seizures or psychosis)

Hematologic disorder (hemolytic anemia with reticulocytosis, leukopenia less than 4000/mm³, lymphopenia less than 1500/mm³, thrombocytopenia less than 100,000/m³)

Immunologic disorder (presence of anti-double stranded DNA, anti-Smith, anti-cardiolipin antibody [IgM or IgG], lupus anticoagulant, false positive rapid plasm reagin test)

Antinuclear antibody

✓ Anti-Smith is specific for SLE.
✓ RNP is seen in SLE and in mixed connective tissue disease (high titer)
✓ Anti-Scl-70 is seen in scleroderma and overlap syndromes.
✓ Anti-SS-A and SS-B are seen in either Sjögren syndrome or SLE.
✓ Anti-Jo1 raises suspicion for interstitial lung disease in juvenile dermatomyositis/polymyositis and overlap syndromes.
- Antiphospholipid antibody syndrome laboratory evaluation
  ✓ Can be primary or secondary to SLE
  ✓ Requires at least one laboratory and one clinical criterion:
  ✓ Laboratory: Elevated functional lupus anticoagulant (PTT or dilute Russell viper venom time), anticardiolipin IgM and/or IgG, or anti-β_2-glycoprotein-I IgM and/or IgG on one or more occasions, at least 12 weeks apart
  ✓ Clinical: Vascular thrombosis (clinical or biopsy evidence) or recurrent fetal loss
- Potential further workup
  ✓ Renal biopsy if significant proteinuria (>200 mg/24 hours or a first morning urine protein:creatinine of ≥0.2), hematuria, cellular casts, hypertension, or renal-function impairment
  ✓ Allows for characterization of nephritis and choice of therapy based on WHO classification
  ✓ Biopsy of skin rash if diagnosis unclear
  ✓ Arthrocentesis and culture if concerned about septic arthritis
  ✓ Low threshold for blood culture if febrile, given functional immunosuppression from hypocomplementemia and medications
  ✓ Chest x-ray and pulmonary function tests if clinical concerns for cardiopulmonary compromise (e.g., serositis, interstitial lung disease)
  ✓ ECG and echocardiography for baseline evaluation and if subsequently indicated
  ✓ Brain/spine imaging, electroencephalography, and/or lumbar puncture may be required for focal neurologic exam, severe headaches, or psychiatric symptoms to evaluate for neuropsychiatric lupus (e.g., cerebritis, CNS vasculitis, transverse myelitis).

✓ CSF studies: cell count, protein, glucose, Gram stain, oligoclonal bands, IgG, IgG synthesis rate, and neuromyelitis optica antibodies are useful (with varying sensitivity and specificity). IgG synthesis rate can be measured with the IgG index: CSF IgG/serum IgG)/(CSF albumin/serum albumin

MANAGEMENT

Pharmacologic Management

- Tailor to symptoms and balance benefits of therapy with adverse effects
  Systemic immune suppression
- Corticosteroids: To capture disease control at diagnosis and/or ongoing disease activity
  ✓ Initial oral dose depends on disease severity. Can range from 0.5–2 mg/kg/day up to 60 mg/day with a taper over 3–6 months. Eventual discontinuation is the goal, but a few patients require a low maintenance dose indefinitely.
  ✓ Life- or organ-threatening disease: IV pulse methylprednisolone 30 mg/kg/day up to 1000 mg daily for 3 days
- Cyclophosphamide: For severe organ-specific complications (e.g., pulmonary hemorrhage, neuropsychiatric disease, proliferative glomerulonephritis)
- Mycophenolate mofetil: For induction and maintenance of lupus nephritis and as maintenance steroid-sparing therapy
- Azathioprine, cyclosporine, or sirolimus: For maintenance as steroid-sparing therapy
- Rituximab: For refractory disease or immune-mediated cytopenias
- Belimumab: May be helpful in combination with standard therapy, particularly for mucocutaneous manifestations; use cautiously in patients with comorbid psychiatric illness given possible increased risk of suicidal ideation
- Methotrexate: For mild-to-moderate disease; beneficial for mucocutaneous manifestations and arthritis
- IVIG: For immune-mediated cytopenias or as Ig replacement
- Therapeutic apheresis: For severe, life-threatening disease such as thrombotic thrombocytopenic purpura, pulmonary hemorrhage, or neuropsychiatric disease

Adjunctive therapy

- NSAIDs: For symptomatic relief of musculoskeletal symptoms. Use with care in individuals with renal disease
- Hydroxychloroquine: Reduces rates of disease flare in general; specifically useful for musculoskeletal symptoms, rash, and alopecia
- Topical or intralesional steroids: For skin lesions
- Angiotensin-converting–enzyme inhibitor or angiotensin-receptor blocker: For hypertension and/or proteinuria
- Low-dose aspirin: For lupus anticoagulant or presence of antiphospholipid antibodies. Hydroxychloroquine may suffice as anticoagulation in some patients.
- Anticoagulation: For thrombotic event (deep-vein thrombosis, pulmonary embolus, arterial thrombus, recurrent fetal loss)

Health Maintenance

- Monitor serum cholesterol, low- and high-density lipoproteins, and triglycerides
- Encourage regular exercise, weight loss, smoking cessation, and low-fat diet
- Calcium and vitamin D supplementation for patients on chronic corticosteroids. Regular dual-energy x-ray absorptiometry scans to monitor bone density

- Yearly ophthalmologic exams for monitoring of hydroxychloroquine toxicity, xerophthalmia in secondary Sjögren syndrome, and cataracts as steroid side effect
- Avoid estrogen-containing oral contraceptives, particularly if antiphospholipid antibodies are present.
- Counseling about risk of neonatal SLE risk in patients positive for anti-Ro/SSA and anti-La/SSB antibodies
- Sun avoidance and protection (minimum SPF-30 with UVA/B protection), as sun exposure can induce lupus flares
- Avoid live vaccines if taking immunosuppressive medications.
- Influenza and pneumococcal (PCV13, PPSV23) vaccination are recommended, as is meningococcal vaccination in the appropriate age group.
- Specialized nursing, social work, physical and occupational therapy, psychology, and nutritional counseling as needed.

Surgery

Erin G. Brown, MD
Peter Mattei, MD

NEONATAL SURGERY

CONGENITAL DIAPHRAGMATIC HERNIA

Failure of complete formation of the diaphragm characterized by pulmonary hypoplasia due to intrauterine compression of the developing lungs by herniated viscera

EPIDEMIOLOGY

- Incidence is 1000 per year (1 in 2000 to 1 in 5000 live births); female:male = 2:1
- 7–10% gestations end in fetal death
- Defects more common on left side (about 80%)
- Associated anomalies (10–35%) include central nervous system (CNS) lesions, tracheobronchial abnormalities, omphalocele, cardiovascular (CV) lesions, skeletal malformations and syndromes (trisomy 13, 18, 21, Beckwith–Wiedemann, Brachmann–de Lange, and Pallister–Killian, among others)

ETIOLOGY

- Unknown currently, though several pharmacologic and environmental factors have been implicated, including a possible role for vitamin A deficiency and/or retinoid-regulated gene defects
- Embryologic theory: Lack of closure of the posterolateral pleuroperitoneal canals in the 8th week of gestation fails to separate the thoracic and abdominal cavities.
- Portions of the diaphragm and pulmonary parenchyma arise from thoracic mesenchyme; if disrupted, this may lead to absence of part of hemidiaphragm and pulmonary hypoplasia.
- Most cases are sporadic; familial cases occur (2%)

DIFFERENTIAL DIAGNOSIS

- Cystic adenomatoid malformation, cystic teratoma, pulmonary sequestration, bronchogenic cyst, neurogenic tumors, primary lung sarcoma, diaphragmatic eventration

PATHOPHYSIOLOGY

- Herniation of abdominal contents into thoracic cavity through posterolateral foramen of Bochdalek
- The diaphragmatic defect may be small or may include entire hemidiaphragm (diaphragmatic agenesis).
- The pulmonary vasculature has increased muscularization of pulmonary arterioles and decreased branching of vessels resulting in pulmonary hypertension
- The lungs are hypoplastic owing to chronic compression, with decreased numbers of bronchial branches on both the ipsilateral and contralateral sides.

CLINICAL MANIFESTATIONS

- Most patients present with respiratory distress within the first hours of life secondary to severe pulmonary hypoplasia and associated pulmonary hypertension.

- 10–20% may have a delayed presentation characterized by less severe pulmonary hypoplasia and pulmonary hypertension, as well as gastrointestinal (GI) symptoms (e.g., vomiting, abdominal pain, constipation)
- Pneumothorax
- On exam: Absence of breath sounds; bowel sounds in chest; scaphoid abdomen; increased anteroposterior diameter of chest; shifted heart sounds

DIAGNOSTICS

- Prenatal ultrasound able to detect defect as early as 11th week, mean gestational age at diagnosis is 24 weeks; accuracy has been reported to be between 40 and 90%.
- Antenatal diagnosis is associated with more severe defects and a worse prognosis; if diagnosed by ultrasound, fetal magnetic resonance imaging (MRI) should be performed.
- During the fetal period, a lung–head ratio (area of contralateral lung to fetal head circumference on ultrasonography) of <1 indicates severe disease.
- Observed-to-expected lung–head ratio (O/E LHR) accounts for changes in LHR with gestational age, and O/E LHR <25% suggests severe CDH
- Echocardiography and amniocentesis to detect other anomalies

MANAGEMENT

Initial Medical Management

- Initial resuscitation includes correction of hypoxia, hypercarbia, acidosis, and hypothermia, as they increase pulmonary vascular resistance and worsen pulmonary hypertension.
- Intubate early to avoid inflation of the stomach with bag-mask ventilation.
- Nasogastric decompression to decrease bowel distension
- Umbilical arterial and venous lines should be placed in severe cases.
- Peripheral oxygen saturations and/or blood gases should be obtained to determine adequacy of gas exchange.
- Echocardiography to determine cardiac anomalies and determine severity of pulmonary hypertension and shunting
- Permissive hypercapnia and gentle ventilation may improve survival and decrease need for extracorporeal membrane oxygenation (ECMO); avoid paralysis.
- Surfactant has not been clearly shown to improve outcomes.
- Response to nitric oxide is inconsistent.
- Persistent right-to-left shunting may require ECMO.

Surgical Management

- Repair typically performed electively (age 3–15 days) when clinically stable.
- Abdominal surgical approach most common. Large defects may require the use of a synthetic patch or muscle flap. Minimally invasive approaches (both laparoscopic and thoracoscopic) have been utilized successfully in selected candidates.
- In utero reduction and repair have been successfully performed but have not consistently shown a benefit to survival. Trials of fetoscopic tracheal occlusion are underway.

Prognosis

- Poor prognosis seen with "liver up" CDH, associated major anomaly, symptoms prior to 24 hours, distress requiring ECMO, delivery in nontertiary center and bilateral defects
- Survival 60–97% with initial stabilization, then surgical repair
- Long-term sequelae may include neurodevelopmental problems, gastroesophageal reflux, nutritional deficiencies, skeletal anomalies, and bronchopulmonary dysplasia

- CDH lungs never reach normal alveolar number or structure, leading to persistent risk of emphysema, pneumonia, bronchiolitis, and pulmonary hypertension

CONGENITAL LUNG LESIONS

Developmental anomalies of the respiratory tree resulting in abnormal lung tissue

EPIDEMIOLOGY

- Congenital lung lesions are seen in 1 in 30,000 live births.
- Large lesions can be associated with pulmonary hypoplasia.
- Includes congenital cystic airway malformation, congenital lobar emphysema, bronchopleural sequestration, and bronchial atresia

PATHOPHYSIOLOGY

- Congenital cystic airway malformation (CCAM): Typically associated with abnormal alveolar tissue and excessive respiratory bronchioles; can be microcystic or macrocystic based on nature of the cysts
- Congenital lobar emphysema: Defective bronchial cartilage leading to air trapping and progressive overinflation of one or more lobes
- Bronchopleural sequestration: Lack of communication between a portion of the lung and the tracheobronchial tree; characterized as extralobar (lesion has own pleura) or intralobar (lesion within pleura of normal lung)
- Bronchial atresia: obstruction of the airway leading to accumulation of lung fluid within the lung segment in utero

CLINICAL MANIFESTATIONS

- Large lesions may be associated with fetal hydrops in up to 40% of cases and pulmonary hypoplasia.
- May present shortly after birth with respiratory distress
- May present with recurrent infections, cough, fever, dyspnea, failure to thrive
- Can present with pneumothorax

DIAGNOSTICS

- Typically diagnosed on prenatal ultrasonography; CCAM volume ratio (CVR) can be calculated to predict severity; CVR >1.6 predicts high risk lesion.
- Chest x-ray at birth may demonstrate lung lesion with or without mass effect.
- CT angiography of the chest can be used to characterize the mass as well as any aberrant blood supply

MANAGEMENT

- Prenatal steroids may be used to decrease the size of the lesion, especially for large and/or macrocystic lesions.
- Large lesions at risk for hydrops may be candidates for fetal intervention such as shunt placement or thoracentesis.
- Ex utero intrapartum treatment (EXIT) or thoracotomy with lobectomy immediately after birth may be indicated for large and/or symptomatic lesions.
- Asymptomatic lesions can undergo elective resection via open thoracotomy or thoracoscopic approach as early as 6 weeks of age.

- Complications: Prematurity due to polyhydramnios, respiratory distress, recurrent pneumonia, pneumothorax, hemothorax, risk of malignancy, death (either in utero due to hydrops or postnatally due to pulmonary hypoplasia)
- Morbidity and mortality in neonates are related to cardiopulmonary comorbidity; development of fetal hydrops is a poor prognostic sign.

ESOPHAGEAL ATRESIA AND TRACHEOESOPHAGEAL FISTULA

Anatomic lesions that may be congenital or acquired and involve a blind pouch of the esophagus; often associated with a fistula to the trachea

EPIDEMIOLOGY

- Esophageal atresia seen in 1 in 2500 to 1 in 4500 live births.
- 90% of infants with esophageal atresia have an associated tracheoesophageal fistula (TEF)
- Associated with trisomy 18 or 21, 22q11.2 deletion syndrome, Feingold syndrome, Pierre Robin syndrome, and Potter syndrome, among others
- 30% of affected infants born prematurely
- Associated anomalies in >50%: Musculoskeletal (rib and vertebral anomalies), cardiovascular, GI (duodenal atresia, intestinal malrotation), genitourinary (choanal atresia):
  ✓ VACTERL association (vertebral, anal, cardiac, tracheal, esophageal, renal, limb)
  ✓ CHARGE association (coloboma, heart disease, choanal atresia, retarded growth and development, genital hypoplasia, and ear anomalies)

PATHOPHYSIOLOGY

- Esophageal atresia with distal TEF: Most common type (>85% cases). Proximal esophagus is dilated and thickened and ends around level of third thoracic vertebra. Fistula at distal esophageal segment enters back wall of lower trachea (**Figure 30-1**).
- Pure esophageal atresia (without TEF): 3–5% of cases. Proximal esophageal pouch ends around third thoracic vertebrae and distal pouch is usually short.
- Isolated TEF without atresia: 3–6% of cases. H-type fistula; level of thoracic inlet. Majority of fistulas are single.
- Esophageal atresia with proximal fistula: 2% of cases; narrow and short fistula
- Esophageal atresia with fistulas to upper and lower tracheal segment: 3–5% of cases. Similar to most common type with additional short, narrow fistula from proximal pouch to trachea

CLINICAL MANIFESTATIONS

- Association with polyhydramnios, though uncommon to be diagnosed prenatally
- May present shortly after birth with excessive secretions and need for frequent suctioning because infant is unable to swallow secretions
- May have aspiration events
- Feeding leads to immediate regurgitation with choking, coughing, and sometimes cyanosis
- Detection of H-type fistula may be delayed

DIAGNOSTICS

- Typically noted by the inability to pass a nasogastric/orogastric tube to the level of the stomach
- Chest x-ray will show coiled catheter in upper esophageal pouch

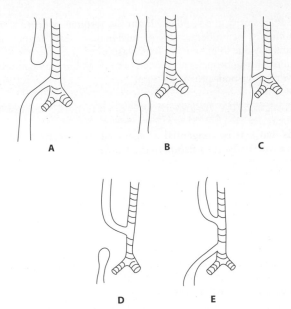

FIGURE 30-1 Types of Tracheoesophageal Fistulas (TEFs). A. Esophageal atresia with distal TEF (>85%). B. Pure esophageal atresia (without TEF) (3–5%). C. Isolated TEF without atresia (3–6%). D. Esophageal atresia with proximal fistula (2%). E. Esophageal atresia with fistulas to upper and lower tracheal segment (3–5%). Reproduced with permission from Lalwani AK: *Current Diagnosis & Treatment in Otolaryngology-Head & Neck Surgery*, 3rd ed. New York, NY: McGraw Hill; 2012.

- Gasless abdomen is evidence of esophageal atresia without distal fistula; air in abdomen on x-ray confirms a distal TEF
- Contrast studies of upper esophagus are not routinely necessary, except to diagnose H-type
- H-type is more difficult to diagnose and often presents beyond the newborn period with history of recurrent pneumonia
- Rigid bronchoscopy provides definitive diagnosis
- Echocardiography and renal ultrasonography to evaluate for associated abnormalities

MANAGEMENT

- Avoid pneumonia from aspiration of upper pouch secretions. Use double-lumen Replogle tube and position patient to maximize drainage.
- Surgical repair is either primary or staged.
  - ✓ Staged repair is usually reserved for critically ill or very-low-birth-weight neonates and involves initial ligation of fistula and placement of gastrostomy tube for feeding followed by future esophageal anastomosis.
- Surgical correction of pure esophageal atresia involves placement of a gastrostomy tube followed by serial calibration until ready for repair.
- Contrast swallow should be done 4–7 days after anastomosis to evaluate for anastomotic leak. Oral feedings are then initiated.

- Complications: Dysphagia, anastomotic stricture, tracheomalacia, airway obstruction, vascular compression, reflex apnea
- Morbidity and mortality in neonates are related to cardiopulmonary comorbidity.

GASTROSCHISIS

Derived from Greek word meaning "belly cleft," a defect in the abdominal wall lateral to the intact umbilical cord

EPIDEMIOLOGY

- Incidence: 2 in 10,000 to 5 in 10,000; male > female
- Associated with young maternal age, low socioeconomic status, maternal smoking, alcohol use, medications (aspirin, ibuprofen, acetaminophen, pseudoephedrine)
- Occasionally associated with intestinal atresia, volvulus, and/or perforation; worse prognosis for "complicated gastroschisis"

ETIOLOGY

- Postulated to be result of vascular accident during embryogenesis
- Studies suggest a possible inherited tendency

PATHOPHYSIOLOGY

- In utero, abdominal viscera herniate through abdominal defect lateral to the umbilicus (usually to the right) and float in the amnion
- Contains midgut and may contain stomach and/or gonad
- Normal bowel rotation and fixation do not occur.

CLINICAL MANIFESTATIONS

- Herniation of viscera through lateral abdominal wall, with or without a skin bridge between the cord and the defect
- Intact umbilical cord
- Absence of peritoneal sac covering bowel

MANAGEMENT

- Delivery may be vaginal or cesarean section; preterm delivery has not been shown to improve outcomes.
- Protect exposed viscera with saline-moistened sterile wraps or plastic bag immediately.
- May need fluids 2.5–3.0 times above maintenance rate because of increased losses.
- Up to 75% may be candidates for primary surgical closure (either in operating room or with sutureless technique at bedside).
- Remaining 25% have prosthetic, extraabdominal compartment or "silo," which allows for gradual manual reduction.
- Postoperative complications include prolonged ileus, parenteral nutrition–related cholestatic liver disease, sepsis, and necrotizing enterocolitis.

PROGNOSIS

- Survival ≥90%

INTESTINAL ATRESIAS

Most common cause for neonatal intestinal obstruction, including complete discontinuity of the small bowel, severe stenoses, and webs

EPIDEMIOLOGY

- Duodenal atresia incidence: 1 in 6000 to 1 in 10,000 births
- Jejunoileal atresia incidence: 1 in 10,000 to 2 in 10,000 births
- Up to 50% of affected infants with duodenal atresias may have another congenital anomaly, compared with 25–35% of those with jejunoileal atresias.
- Often associated with trisomy 21, annular pancreas, malrotation, congenital heart disease, esophageal atresia, and anorectal malformations.

ETIOLOGY

- Duodenal atresia thought to result from failure of recanalization following obliteration of the intestinal lumen after the 6th week of gestation—85% occur in second part of duodenum (**Table 30-1**).
- Jejunoileal atresias likely reflect mesenteric vascular compromise in later gestation (**Table 30-1**).

TABLE 30-1	Types of Duodenal and Jejunoileal Atresias	
Type	**Relative Prevalence (%)**	**Description**
Duodenal atresia		
Type I	92	Obstructing septum/web without muscular defect with intact mesentery
Type II	1	Two blind ends of duodenum connected by a fibrous cord without mesenteric defect
Type III	7	No connection between two blind ends with V-shaped mesenteric defect.
Jejunoileal atresia		
Type I	23	Obstructing septum without mesenteric defect
Type II	27	Two blind ends connected by a fibrous cord without mesenteric defect
Type IIIa	18	No connection between two blind ends with V-shaped mesenteric defect
Type IIIb	7	"Apple peel" or "Christmas tree"—distal small bowel spirals around vascular supply with large mesenteric defect and significant bowel shortening
Type IV	24	Multiple atresias

CLINICAL MANIFESTATIONS

- Presentation may be variable, depending on level of obstruction; polyhydramnios/emesis more common with proximal obstruction, abdominal distention more common with distal obstruction.
- Most prenatally diagnosed atresias are duodenal.

DIAGNOSTICS

- Plain abdominal x-ray findings for duodenal atresia include "double bubble" appearance.
- Jejunoileal atresias often show dilated proximal loops of bowel with air/fluid levels.
- In duodenal atresia, echocardiography and renal ultrasonography should be performed to evaluate for other midline defects.

MANAGEMENT

- Gastric decompression to minimize bowel distention is imperative; note presence of bile in aspirate.
- Intravenous fluid resuscitation should be provided and basic laboratory tests obtained.
- Operative repair should be undertaken as soon as safely possible; duodenoduodenostomy is routinely performed for duodenal atresia, and treatment of jejunoileal atresia may vary depending on the nature of the bowel defect.
- All patients should be evaluated for malrotation and volvulus, and Ladd's procedure should be performed if it is present. If malrotation cannot be excluded, laparotomy should be pursued.
- Tapering enteroplasty may be necessary in the setting of significant size mismatch between proximal and distal limbs.
- Evaluate for multiple atresias.

OMPHALOCELE

A central defect of the umbilical ring through which bowel and abdominal viscera herniate. The abdominal contents are covered with a membrane composed of the inner layer of peritoneum fused to the outer layer of amnion.

EPIDEMIOLOGY

- Occurs in 1 in 2500 to 1 in 5000 live births
- Up to 30–50% of affected infants have associated karyotypic anomaly (e.g., trisomy 13 or 18)
- Can be associated with Beckwith–Wiedemann syndrome and pentalogy of Cantrell (combination of severe defects of the sternum, heart, diaphragm, and abdominal wall)
- >50% have other malformations: Cardiovascular anomalies most common; also renal, skeletal, neural tube, sternum, diaphragm, and bladder
- 10% have "giant" omphalocele, where liver and intestine herniate through an 8- to 10-cm defect

PATHOPHYSIOLOGY

- Failure of migration and fusion of embryonic folds
- Most are lateral fold defects, and all involve the umbilicus
- Failure of the gut to migrate from the yolk sac to the abdomen
- Extruded abdominal contents (may contain midgut, liver, spleen, and/or gonad) are covered by a two-layered membrane; umbilical cord inserts into membrane
- Size >4 cm and contents distinguish omphalocele from umbilical-cord hernia

DIAGNOSTICS

- Detected in second-trimester ultrasound
- Associated with increased α-fetoprotein (AFP) and acetylcholinsesterase in maternal serum and amniotic fluid
- Amniocentesis: To evaluate for associated chromosomal abnormalities

MANAGEMENT

- May be delivered vaginally or via cesarean section
- Cover exposed membranous sac with sterile saline-soaked dressings to prevent heat and fluid losses
- Correct fluid and electrolytes preoperatively
- Extrauterine echocardiography before surgical repair to evaluate for cardiac defect
- Surgical primary repair when possible; staged closure for large defects
- Nonoperative techniques include placement of a "silo" for sequential reduction or use of eschar-producing agents ("paint and wait") when primary repair is not possible owing to loss of abdominal domain

PROGNOSIS

- Survival 70–95%
- Mortality is generally related to comorbidities.

GENERAL SURGERY

APPENDICITIS

Inflammation of the appendix caused by obstruction of the appendiceal lumen. Classically difficult to diagnose in children, because typical signs and symptoms may be absent in more than half of the patients presenting to the ED.

EPIDEMIOLOGY

- Approximately 1 in 12 people will have appendicitis in their lifetime, occurs in 1 in 1000 children per year.
- Peak incidence in adolescence, uncommon in children <5 years of age
- Slight male predominance

DIFFERENTIAL DIAGNOSIS

- Mesenteric adenitis, bacterial enterocolitis (especially with *Yersinia enterocolitica* and *Campylobacter jejuni*), intussusception, Meckel diverticulitis, inflammatory bowel disease, urinary-tract infection, right lower lobe pneumonia, testicular torsion, and gynecologic etiologies such as ectopic pregnancy, ovarian torsion, and pelvic inflammatory disease

PATHOPHYSIOLOGY

- The appendix is a blind pouch that can be obstructed by fecaliths, hypertrophied lymphoid follicles, parasites, or foreign bodies.
- Can also have bacterial invasion without previous obstruction
- This closed-loop obstruction causes edema, inflammation, and vasocongestion, which lead to necrosis and perforation.
- Once this process starts, children are more prone to earlier perforation and development of peritonitis than adults.

CLINICAL MANIFESTATIONS

- Classically, pain begins in periumbilical region and moves to right lower quadrant (RLQ); presentation can be variable, especially in younger children.
- May be associated with nausea, vomiting, anorexia, fever, and dysuria.
- In children, particularly those <2 years, clinical signs can be more vague and misleading and can include irritability, upper respiratory infection symptoms, lethargy, abdominal rigidity, or refusal to walk.
- Perforation usually occurs 36–48 hours after symptom onset and should be considered in context of patient with persistent symptoms, high fevers, and peritoneal signs
- Bowel sounds usually normal or hyperactive, occasionally hypoactive but are unreliable
- Abdominal tenderness: Typically in the RLQ; can also be diffuse
- Coughing, driving over a bump, or standing on the toes and dropping the heels may worsen the pain; this is indicative of peritonitis.
- Presence of one or more of the following may suggest appendicitis:
  - ✓ Rovsing's sign: Palpation of left lower quadrant (LLQ) causes pain in RLQ
  - ✓ Psoas sign: Patient flexes right hip against resistance. Increased abdominal pain indicates positive sign.
  - ✓ Obturator sign: Raise patient's right leg with the knee flexed. Rotate the leg internally at the hip. Increased abdominal pain indicates a positive sign.
- Rectal exam can show rectal masses, abdominal abscesses, or right-sided rectal tenderness, but is often nonspecific and not necessary in most cases.
- Guarding and rebound are more likely with perforation.

DIAGNOSTICS

- Difficult to diagnose, particularly in young children
- 3–6% overall negative appendectomy rate, though rates are considerably higher in children <5 (15–25%) and somewhat higher in females (5–10%) than in males (1–5%)
- Can be diagnosed on basis of history and physical exam alone, but adjunctive radiologic studies often helpful
  - ✓ Abdominal flat plate films have limited utility. Findings include fecalith, localized ileus, soft-tissue mass, splinting, loss of peritoneal fat stripe, or free air
  - ✓ Ultrasound can be diagnostic; sensitivity and specificity vary among studies. Findings include increased appendiceal diameter or thickened wall, target sign, echogenicity surrounding the appendix, appendicolith, pericecal or perivesical free fluid.
  - ✓ CT has sensitivity of 87–100% (increased with oral and rectal contrast) and specificity of 83–97%. Findings include fat streaking, increased appendiceal diameter, and cecal apical thickening.
  - ✓ MRI has sensitivity and specificity of 96%. Findings include focal periappendiceal inflammation. MRI is a suitable alternative to CT for evaluation of appendicitis in children and avoids unnecessary exposure to ionizing radiation.
- Studies suggest that children evaluated at nonpediatric specialty centers are more likely to undergo CT scans during workup.
- Obtain urine pregnancy test in females of reproductive age
- Complete blood count (CBC), urinalysis, C-reactive protein frequently ordered
- Often see leukocytosis and high percentage of neutrophils on CBC with differential; one of these is elevated in 90–96% of cases, but no laboratory studies are sensitive and specific for appendicitis. Some children with early appendicitis may be offered antibiotics only as a form of therapy, avoiding appendectomy altogether in some cases (roughly one third will have recurrent appendicitis within 1–2 years)

MANAGEMENT

- Patient should have nothing by mouth.
- Fluid resuscitation as needed for dehydration or sepsis
- Broad-spectrum IV antibiotics that cover enteric aerobes and anaerobes in cases of perforation or sepsis (e.g., ampicillin–sulbactam with or without aminoglycoside, ticarcillin–clavulanate, ampicillin plus gentamycin plus metronidazole, or ciprofloxacin plus metronidazole)
- Standard of care is urgent appendectomy in uncomplicated appendicitis.
- Surgical intervention is often indicated in perforated appendicitis; in cases of longstanding perforation or well-formed abscess, nonoperative management may be preferred.
- Following appendectomy, children with uncomplicated appendicitis do not require further antibiotic therapy; children with evidence of perforation should receive additional antibiotic therapy; length of administration should be determined by clinical criteria (fever, pain, bowel function, white blood cell count) in nonoperative management of perforation

EXTRACORPOREAL MEMBRANE OXYGENATION (ECMO)

Extracorporeal life support may include venoarterial cardiorespiratory support or venovenous access for respiratory support with or without less severe secondary cardiac failure.

EPIDEMIOLOGY

- Survival is approximately 85% in neonates with respiratory indications and 57–68% for all other indications and age groups.

MECHANICS

- Circuit comprised of a pump, a membrane oxygenator, and a heat exchanger, along with invasive monitoring devices.
- Venoarterial cannulation generally achieved via jugular vein and carotid arteries and/or femoral vein and artery, though when ECMO is employed in patients unable to wean from cardiorespiratory bypass intraoperatively, chest cannulation may be performed.
- Venovenous access may be achieved via cannulation of two different veins or using a double-lumen venous cannula.
- Venovenous configuration preferable (less morbidity) in the absence of cardiac disease.
- In children, cannula size to achieve adequate flow may compromise entire vessel lumen, leading to distal ischemia; a distal reperfusion catheter may be indicated to preserve distal blood flow.

INDICATIONS

- Oxygenation index (OI) = [(Mean airway pressure $\times$ FiO$_2$)/Postductal PaO$_2$] $\times$ 100
- ECMO may be considered for OI >20, and it is routinely indicated for OI >40.
- Clinical signs of decreased perfusion, including end-organ damage, shock, and cardiac arrest
- Primary diagnoses may include CDH, meconium aspiration syndrome, acute respiratory distress syndrome, sepsis, congenital cardiac defect, cardiomyopathy, trauma, or cardiac arrest, among others.

CONTRAINDICATIONS

- Prematurity—ECMO should not be used in newborns <30 weeks' gestation or weighing <1.5 kg owing to a high risk of intracranial bleeding.
- Existing intracranial hemorrhage grade >2
- Profound neurologic impairment, multiple congenital anomalies, or other condition with poor prognosis

- Relative contraindications include prolonged mechanical ventilation (due to high incidence of bronchopulmonary dysplasia and irreversible fibroproliferative pulmonary disease), CDH with severe pulmonary hypoplasia, multiorgan system failure, severe burns, immunodeficiency, and active bleeding.

MANAGEMENT

- Heparin should be titrated to maintain therapeutic anticoagulation during extracorporeal life support.
- Generally, activated clotting time should be maintained at 50–60% above normal levels.
- Management of the ECMO patient requires a coordinated care team, including surgical/ neonatal intensivists, intensive care unit nurses, and ECMO perfusionists.
- During ECMO perfusion, ventilator settings should be maintained at low levels to provide lung rest; recruitment maneuvers will generally be required to transition from extracorporeal support.
- Blood volume should be titrated to a right atrial pressure of 5–10 mm Hg; fluid management should be aimed at achieving and maintaining dry weight.
- Cannula sites should be meticulously cleaned and maintained in accordance with institutional protocols.

COMPLICATIONS

- Bleeding associated with heparinization
- Technical failure (15%) includes circuit thrombus (26%), cannula issues (10%), oxygenator failure (10%), pump malfunction (2%), and air embolus (4%).
- Neurologic sequelae: Ischemic or embolic stroke, seizures (10–13%)
- Pneumothorax (5–15%)
- Hemolytic anemia (6–12%)
- Chronic pulmonary disease (60%)
- Growth delay (40%)
- Neurologic abnormalities in up to 50% with detailed testing
- Infection

HIRSCHSPRUNG DISEASE

Congenital aganglionic megacolon; abnormal innervation of the bowel beginning in the internal anal sphincter and extending proximally

EPIDEMIOLOGY

- Incidence 1 in 5000 live births; male:female = 4:1
- Most common cause of lower intestinal obstruction in neonates
- Associated with Down syndrome, Laurence–Moon–Bardet–Biedl syndrome, Waardenburg syndrome, and cardiovascular abnormalities (especially defects in cardiac septation or tetralogy of Fallot)

ETIOLOGY

- Multifactorial genesis and complex pattern of inheritance (up to 25% familial)

PATHOPHYSIOLOGY

- Absence of ganglion cells in the bowel wall, which extends proximally from the anus for variable distance

- Arrest of neuroblast migration from proximal to distal bowel
- Limited to the rectosigmoid colon in 75% of patients and involves the entire colon in 10% of patients
- Histologically, absence of Meissner and Auerbach plexus and hypertrophied nerve bundles. Increased nerve endings in aganglionic bowel results in increased acetylcholinesterase.

CLINICAL MANIFESTATIONS

- Often presents with delayed passage of meconium; 99% of normal full-term infants pass meconium within 48 hours of birth.
- Constipation is presenting symptom later in life.
- Bowel dilatation proximal to transition zone leading to increased intraluminal pressure, resultant decreased blood flow and deterioration of the mucosal barrier may lead to stasis and proliferation of bacteria with subsequent enterocolitis.
- Patients with enterocolitis (about 10%) may present with fever, abdominal distention and diarrhea, confusing the diagnosis.
- On exam: Palpable fecal mass in left lower abdomen but absence of stool in rectum
- Rectal exam reveals normal anal tone but is often followed by massive release of gas and feces.

DIAGNOSTICS

Roentgenographic (Barium Contrast Enema)

- Use water-soluble contrast for neonates
- Transitional zone seen after 1–2 weeks of age as a funnel-shaped area of intestine by barium contrast enema

Rectal Biopsy

- Gold standard for diagnosing Hirschsprung's disease
- Obtained no closer than 2 cm to dentate line because there is a normal area of hypoganglionosis at anal verge.
- Early rectal biopsy should be avoided in premature infants owing to physiologic immaturity of normal ganglion cells.
- Need submucosa to accurately evaluate
- Specimen is stained for acetylcholinesterase, which should reveal a characteristic pattern of expression throughout the mucosa and submucosa.
- Hematoxylin and eosin staining shows aganglionosis and hypertrophied nerve bundles.
- Positive specimens rarely, if ever, stain for calcitonin.

MANAGEMENT

- Initially, decompression with nasogastric tube; repeated emptying of rectum using rectal tubes and irrigations
- Resuscitation should include IV fluids and broad-spectrum antibiotics to cover multiple enteric pathogens when presenting with signs of enterocolitis.
- Associated anomalies should be addressed prior to operative repair.
- Definitive treatment is surgical resection: Swenson's technique, Duhamel–Grob technique, Soave-endorectal pull-through and may be staged or primary.
- Postoperative complications: Recurrent enterocolitis (about 25%), constipation (about 20%), stricture (about 6%), prolapse (2%), fecal soiling (about 5%)

INGUINAL HERNIA

A protrusion into the groin of contents of the abdominal cavity, most commonly small bowel, into a persistently patent processus vaginalis. There are three types: indirect,

direct, and femoral. Indirect hernias enter the inguinal canal through the internal inguinal ring and are by far the most common in children (>95%). Femoral hernias are rare in children.

EPIDEMIOLOGY

- Incidence of approximately 1–5% in children; male:female = 3:1–10:1
- More common in premature infants (16–25% incidence); typically present in infancy
- Approximately 10% of inguinal hernias are complicated by incarceration.
- Likelihood of incarceration decreases sharply with time; the risk is greatest during the first 6 months of life.
- More often right-sided (60%) but bilateral in approximately 10%
- Patients with abdominal-wall defects, connective-tissue disorders, chronic respiratory disease, or undescended testes are at higher risk. Processes causing increased intraabdominal pressure such as ascites, ventriculoperitoneal shunting, or peritoneal dialysis can lead to high incidence of previously unrecognized inguinal hernias.

DIFFERENTIAL DIAGNOSIS

- Lymphadenopathy, lymphoma, undescended or retractile testes, hydrocele, testicular torsion
- May be difficult to differentiate hydrocele from inguinal hernia. Hydroceles typically transilluminate, but hernias may as well. Unlike hydroceles, neck of hernia can often be felt at the inguinal ring. Also, hydroceles cannot be fully reduced and do not fluctuate in size.

PATHOPHYSIOLOGY

- Embryologically, the processus vaginalis is a diverticular portion of the peritoneum, which herniates through the abdominal wall and into the inguinal canal. The testes descend into the scrotum external to the processus vaginalis by the 29th week of gestation. The processus vaginalis usually fuses and is obliterated by the time a pregnancy reaches term or shortly thereafter. Partial or complete failure to obliterate results in a range of inguinal anomalies from hydroceles to hernias.
- With increased intraabdominal pressure, bowel (or ovary in females) can slip into this communication with risk for possible incarceration (being unable to reduce the hernia), strangulation (compromised blood supply), and subsequent necrosis.

CLINICAL MANIFESTATIONS

- Most children are asymptomatic unless incarceration and/or strangulation occurs.
- Characterized by intermittent groin, scrotal, or labial swelling that spontaneously reduces; more prominent with Valsalva maneuver
- Examine testes first because retractile testes can be mistaken for hernias.
- Classically, an inguinal bulge is noted at the inguinal ring or a scrotal/labial swelling that is reducible or changes in size
- Causing an infant to cry or having an older child stand can increase intraabdominal pressure, making diagnosis easier.
- Evidence indicates that digital photos taken by family members may be useful to document the diagnosis in equivocal cases.
- Incarcerated hernia may present with signs of obstruction (emesis, poor feeds, abdominal distention, lack of bowel movements)
- With time, area surrounding an incarcerated hernia will become indurated, tender, and erythematous.

MANAGEMENT

- Once an asymptomatic inguinal hernia is diagnosed, the patient should be scheduled for an elective operative repair; data suggest that repair within 2 weeks may decrease the rate of incarceration.
- An incarcerated hernia must be immediately reduced to avoid strangulation, necrosis, and perforation. Manual reduction is done by placing a calm child in Trendelenburg position and applying gentle upward pressure while trying to milk herniated tissues back into the peritoneal cavity.
- Consider analgesia and sedation for difficult or painful reductions. Unsuccessful reductions require immediate surgical repair.
- In cases of successful manual reduction, prompt surgical repair can be electively scheduled as outpatient with strict instructions to return to ED in case of reincarceration.
- In cases where intestinal obstruction is present, patient needs nasogastric tube, laboratory studies, fluid resuscitation, and immediate surgical consultation.
- Current data supports the use of transinguinal laparoscopic evaluation of the contralateral side in younger patients with a preoperative diagnosis of unilateral inguinal hernia.
- Laparoscopic and open hernia repair demonstrate equivalent recurrence rates (<5%).

INTUSSUSCEPTION

An invagination of a proximal portion of the bowel and its mesentery (the intussusceptum) into an adjacent distal bowel segment (the intussuscipiens)

EPIDEMIOLOGY

- Incidence: 1 in 2000 to 4 in 2000
- Male:female = 2:1
- Majority of cases occur between 3 months and 2 years, with peak incidence between 3 and 9 months of age
- Seasonal incidence, with peaks in winter and summer
- More common in underweight children
- Occurs in neonates, older children, and adults but usually secondary to a pathologic lead point

ETIOLOGY

- Cause is unknown in approximately 90% of cases
- Incidence follows peak seasons of viral gastroenteritis. Postulated theory is that Peyer's patches become inflamed secondary to viral infection and serve as a lead point.
- Pathologic lead points occur in 1.5–12% of cases. Causes include Meckel diverticulum, intestinal polyps, B-cell lymphoma, submucosal hemangioma, carcinoid tumor, and *Ascaris lumbricoides* infestation.
- Certain conditions, such as cystic fibrosis, Henoch–Schoenlein purpura, Peutz–Jeghers syndrome, and hemolytic–uremic syndrome predispose to lead points.
- Can also occur as a postoperative complication following a laparotomy

DIFFERENTIAL DIAGNOSIS

- Gastroenteritis, incarcerated hernia, Meckel diverticulum, malrotation with midgut volvulus
- For patients who present with lethargy, consider vast differential for change in mental status.

PATHOPHYSIOLOGY

- Proximal portion of bowel and its mesentery telescopes into distal portion—usually ileocolic, but can be ileoileal or colocolic as well

- Constriction of the mesentery causes engorgement of the intussusceptum and venous congestion with eventual bowel necrosis.

CLINICAL MANIFESTATIONS

- Classic triad is intermittent colicky abdominal pain, vomiting, and "currant jelly" stools (due to mucosal sloughing).
- However, this triad is present in less than half of cases and grossly bloody stool is often a late finding.
- Pain typically occurs in screaming spells every 20–30 minutes, during which the child draws up his/her legs. Children often look healthy and even playful between these episodes.
- Emesis becomes bilious as obstruction progresses.
- Up to 10% of patients present with only lethargy or hypotonia.
- Child can be febrile and have other abnormal vital signs.
- Even in infants without grossly bloody stools, stools will be guaiac-positive in approximately 75% of cases.
- Sausage-shaped mass in the right upper quadrant (Dance sign)
- Abdomen often distended; bowel sounds high-pitched or normal
- Up to 20% may reduce spontaneously

DIAGNOSTICS

- Plain abdominal x-ray: Can see paucity of intestinal gas, minimal stool in the colon, small bowel obstruction, and right upper quadrant soft-tissue mass; however, plain films may be normal.
- Upright or decubitus film: Rule out intraperitoneal air.
- Ultrasound has been shown to be an effective and cost-efficient first test aimed at decreasing the number of negative studies involving radiation; may see pseudokidney sign, target sign, or complex hyperechoic mass.
- Barium or water-soluble contrast enemas: Gold standard study for diagnosis and treatment of intussusception, which classically has a "coiled spring" appearance. Air contrast enemas have been shown to be as effective as barium enemas in diagnosis and treatment and can decrease the risks associated with a potential perforation.
  - ✓ Obtain surgical consultation before attempted reduction because (1) there is a risk of intestinal perforation during reduction and (2) a failed reduction attempt requires surgical correction.
  - ✓ Barium contraindicated if clinical peritonitis or free air on abdominal x-ray
- May see nonspecific lymphocytosis and electrolyte abnormalities consistent with dehydration.

MANAGEMENT

- Patient should have nothing by mouth.
- Begin antibiotics (e.g., ampicillin–sulbactam, cefazolin) and fluid resuscitation in preparation for barium or air enema.
- Surgery and anesthesiology staff should be standing by in case radiologic reduction is unsuccessful. In this event, laparotomy is performed with manual reduction and appendectomy.
- Enemas are successful in 60–90% of patients, but are less successful in patients <1 year, those who have had symptoms for >48 hours, when bowel obstruction is obvious on plain films, or when multiple ultrasound findings are present.
- Recurrence of intussusception after barium or air reduction can occur in up to 10% of cases, usually within the first 24 hours.
- If the intussusception recurs, repeated radiologic reduction may be attempted once before surgical reduction. Recurrence is rare following surgical resection (about 2%).

MALROTATION AND MIDGUT VOLVULUS

Malrotation, an abnormal midgut development, results in anomalous positioning of the small intestine, cecum, and ascending colon. Abnormal bands of tissue are present (Ladd bands) from attempts at colonic fixation. A midgut volvulus occurs when the malrotated intestine twists on the axis of the superior mesenteric artery, compromising intestinal blood flow.

EPIDEMIOLOGY

- Detected in 0.2% of live births, 1–2% of autopsy studies
- Approximately 30% of cases detected by 1 week of age, 60% by 1 month, and 90% by 1 year. Remaining 10% may present at any age.
- Up to 70% of patients have associated anomalies that include abdominal heterotaxia, omphalocele, gastroschisis, congenital diaphragmatic hernia, intestinal atresia, mesenteric cysts, Hirschsprung disease, anorectal anomalies, situs inversus, atrial septal detect, ventricular septal detect, transposition of the great vessels, dextrocardia, anomalous systemic or pulmonary venous return, asplenia, and polysplenia.

DIFFERENTIAL DIAGNOSIS

- Bilious (green or yellow) emesis in a neonate is a midgut volvulus until proven otherwise.
- Malrotation may be considered when patients present with failure to thrive, cyclic vomiting, chronic abdominal pain, intermittent apnea, testicular torsion, and incarcerated hernia.

PATHOPHYSIOLOGY

- Normally, in the 5th–6th week of development, intestinal size exceeds the space of the abdominal cavity causing them to protrude into the umbilical cord. As the embryo grows, the midgut structures (duodenum, jejunum, ileum, ascending colon, and half the transverse colon) reposition in the abdominal cavity, rotating 270 degrees around the superior mesenteric artery in a counterclockwise direction.
- Malrotation occurs when the normal counterclockwise rotation of the midgut is incomplete; great variation in degree of abnormality in rotation.

CLINICAL MANIFESTATIONS

- Varies from acute intestinal obstruction to chronic, intermittent abdominal pain
- Delayed presentation of a midgut volvulus and significant intestinal necrosis includes shock with hematochezia or melena and abdominal distention.
- With a midgut intestinal obstruction, the abdomen should be flat or scaphoid. Abdominal distention suggests a more distal small bowel or colonic obstruction.
- Abdominal-wall distention, edema, erythema, and crepitus suggest gangrenous or necrotic bowel. *Bowel viability is time-dependent.*

DIAGNOSTICS

- Plain abdominal x-ray: Gastric and duodenal dilation with a paucity of distal gas suggests a midgut obstruction. However, a normal film does not exclude the possibility of malrotation with or without volvulus.
- An upper GI series is the best test to diagnose intestinal malrotation:
  - ✓ To exclude malrotation, the duodenum should be in the retroperitoneal position on lateral projections, the ligament of Treitz should cross the midline to the left of the spine and rise to a level of the pylorus

• Ultrasound and CT scan may be used. A midgut volvulus on ultrasound has a "barber pole" or "whirlwind" appearance of the small intestine wrapping clockwise around the axis of the superior mesenteric artery.

MANAGEMENT

• Given the potential for volvulus and obstruction, with rare exception, a patient with a diagnosis of malrotation requires operative intervention.
• Ladd procedure: Counterclockwise volvulus reduction, lysis of adhesive bands, conservative (necrotic) bowel resection, appendix removal, and repositioning of small intestine to RLQ and cecum to LLQ
• May need repeat operations to assess bowel viability 24–48 hours later if ischemia present at initial operation
• Postoperative course may be complicated by wound infection, shock, sepsis, intraabdominal abscess, small-bowel obstruction, recurrent volvulus, bowel necrosis, intussusception, short gut syndrome, strictures, and dysmotility.

PERIRECTAL ABSCESS

Infection of the perirectal area via spread from the anal crypts to the anal ducts and glands

EPIDEMIOLOGY

• 68–90% of affected children are male
• May be related to androgen levels in infants <12 months of age; in later childhood/adolescence often occur in the setting of inflammatory bowel disease

ETIOLOGY

• Small tears in the anal mucosa may lead to infection, or infection may arise from the anal glands and extend into the anal crypts.
• When cultured, abscesses usually are polymicrobial. Most frequent organisms isolated are *Escherichia coli*, *Klebsiella pneumoniae*, *Staphylococcus aureus*, and anaerobes (e.g., *Bacteroides* species).

CLINICAL MANIFESTATIONS

• 42% of children <2 years of age have history of diarrhea
• Fever (81%), rectal pain (69%), rectal mass (40%), pain on sitting (27%), pain with defecation (21%), abnormal gait (19%)
• On exam, there is erythematous, painful swelling in the perirectal area with or without fluctuance or drainage.

MANAGEMENT

• Most patients require surgical drainage or needle aspiration followed by oral antibiotic therapy (e.g., cephalexin, amoxicillin–clavulanate, clindamycin) and sitz baths
• 10–20% may progress to fistula-in-ano, for which first-line treatment involves identification and either excision or incisional drainage of the fistulous tract
• MRI may be of use in the setting of Crohn's disease to delineate complex fistulae
• IV antibiotic therapy (e.g., cefazolin, ampicillin-sulbactam) may be required for nonimmunosuppressed patients with extensive abscesses or evidence of systemic disease

PNEUMOTHORAX

Collection of extrapulmonary air within the chest

ETIOLOGY

- Often due to penetrating or blunt thoracic trauma
- Can result from disruption of pulmonary parenchyma, injury to tracheobronchial tree, bleb, or esophageal rupture
- Occurs in 5% of children hospitalized for asthma
- Occurs in 10–25% of patients >10 years old with CF
- Spontaneous pneumothorax far more common among males (18 in 100,000 to 28 in 100,000/year, vs. 1.2 in 100,000 to 6 in 100,000 in females)
- Iatrogenic: Tracheotomy, subclavian line placement, thoracentesis, and transbronchial biopsy
- Bilateral pneumothoraxes are rare beyond neonatal period.
- Tension pneumothorax will develop in up to 20% of patients with simple pneumothorax.
- Other causes: Lymphoma or other malignancies, staphylococcal pneumonia

DIFFERENTIAL DIAGNOSIS

- Localized/generalized emphysema, extensive emphysematous bleb, congenital cystic adenomatoid malformation, diaphragmatic hernia, gaseous distention of stomach

PATHOPHYSIOLOGY

- Primary spontaneous pneumothorax: Occurs in patients without trauma or underlying lung disease (e.g., Ehlers–Danlos disease, Marfan syndrome)
- Secondary spontaneous pneumothorax: Arises secondary to underlying lung disorder but without trauma. Examples include pneumonia with empyema, pulmonary abscess, gangrene, infarct, rupture of cyst, rupture of emphysematous bleb, foreign body
- Tension pneumothorax: A one-way entry of air into the pleural space. This collection of air causes collapse of the ipsilateral lung and compression of the contralateral lung. Mediastinal structures may shift, and there may be a decrease in venous return to the heart and cardiovascular compromise.

CLINICAL MANIFESTATIONS

- Onset may be abrupt; may be asymptomatic; severity of symptoms depends on extent of lung collapse.
- Pain, dyspnea with respiratory distress, cyanosis, splinting on involved side, agitation, increased pulse rate
- Respiratory distress: Retractions, tachypnea, cyanosis
- Crepitus over neck and chest, may be indicative of subcutaneous emphysema.
- Decreased breath sounds on auscultation of affected lung
- Percussion of area involved is tympanitic
- Larynx, trachea, and/or heart may be shifted to unaffected side.

DIAGNOSTICS

- Chest x-ray: Expiratory views emphasize the contrast between lung markings and area of pneumothorax. Tension pneumothorax limits expansion of contralateral lung.
- Chest CT scan: May be obtained after reexpansion of the lung to detect predisposing anatomic abnormalities (e.g., bleb).

MANAGEMENT

Medical

- Small (<15%) or moderate-sized pneumothorax in healthy child may spontaneously resolve within 1 week without intervention.
- Because a small pneumothorax can quickly progress to a tension pneumothorax, even asymptomatic trauma patients with pneumothorax should be admitted for observation.
- Data suggest that blunt trauma patients with occult pneumothorax (visible on CT scan but not on chest x-ray) may be safely observed without intervention despite requirement for positive-pressure ventilation.
- Administration of 100% oxygen may increase nitrogen pressure gradient between pleural air and blood and shorten time to resolution.
- Analgesia: If needed, but consider respiratory depressant effects of opioids

Surgical

- Tube thoracostomy: Indicated for symptomatic patients and, generally, those receiving positive-pressure ventilation. Tube is placed at the midaxillary line at the level of the fifth intercostal space (approximately nipple level) over the top of the rib to avoid the intercostal neurovascular bundle.
- Needle decompression for tension pneumothorax: Needle is placed in midclavicular, second intercostal space of the ipsilateral side; an immediate release of air is noted, and tube thoracostomy must be performed (see "Pneumothorax: Needle Decompression" section in Chapter 26).
- Recurrent pneumothorax: May use sclerosing agent that induces an adhesion between the lung and chest wall (tetracycline, talc, silver nitrate), or induce mechanical adhesions via laparoscopic or open approaches
- Video-Assisted thoracoscopic surgery allows for plication of blebs, closure of fistula, stripping of pleura, and basilar pleural abrasion and has largely replaced open thoracotomy in the surgical treatment of recurrent pneumothorax.

PYLORIC STENOSIS

Enlarged pylorus with increased muscular thickness, which generally leads to gastric-outlet obstruction and projectile emesis

EPIDEMIOLOGY

- Occurs in approximately 3 in 1000 to 6 in 1000 infants
- Male:female = 4:1; more common in white infants
- 10–20% of infants of mother with history of pyloric stenosis

ETIOLOGY

- Hereditary and environmental factors thought to be involved
- Other factors: Abnormal muscle innervation, erythromycin therapy during first 2 weeks of life, maternal stress in third trimester, and B and O blood groups
- Underlying defect is thickened pyloric musculature, leading to a gradual obstruction.

CLINICAL MANIFESTATIONS

- Typically presents between 2 and 8 weeks of age (most common 3–5 weeks)

- Nonbilious vomiting is initial symptom, often described as projectile
- Weight loss and dehydration
- Patients are often hungry and eager to feed.
- "Olive-shaped" mass may be palpated in the midepigastrium beneath the liver edge
- Gastric peristaltic wave may be visible in a distended stomach
- Jaundice occasionally present

DIAGNOSTICS

- Clinical diagnosis possible in 60–80% of patients
- Electrolyte panel: Hypokalemic, hypochloremic metabolic alkalosis due to loss of gastric HCl; however, may be acidotic if severe dehydration present
- Plain abdominal x-ray: Dilated stomach bubble
- Abdominal ultrasound: Radiologic study of choice (sensitivity around 90%); positive ultrasound characterized muscle thickness ≥4 mm and/or channel length ≥18 mm, lack of fluid emptying from stomach
- Upper GI series: Sensitive and specific, but risk for aspiration. Barium studies may show elongated pyloric channel, bulge of pylorus into antrum, and parallel streaks of barium in the channel.

MANAGEMENT

Medical

- Initial IV fluids: 5% dextrose with normal saline
  ✓ Risk of hyponatremia if hypotonic saline is used
- Potassium chloride can be added to IV fluids when urine output is established.
- Correction of alkalosis to bicarbonate >30 is essential to prevent postoperative apnea.

Surgical

- Delay surgery until adequate rehydration and electrolyte correction are established.
- Ramstedt pyloromyotomy is procedure of choice. This involves splitting the pyloric muscle without violating the mucosa.
- Can be performed laparoscopically or through small incision
- Families should be counseled preoperatively to expect vomiting after the procedure; in most cases, feeds can begin within a few hours after the procedure and patients should continue to be fed despite vomiting to improve oral tolerance.

UROLOGIC SURGERY

OVARIAN TORSION

Twisting of the ovary or adnexa resulting in venous and lymphatic congestion and eventual loss of arterial perfusion with resulting ovarian necrosis

EPIDEMIOLOGY

- Incidence: 4.9 in 100,000 in girls 1–20 years old
- Rare in children; occurs predominantly in neonates and early adolescence

ETIOLOGY

- Torsion typically occurs in the setting of enlarged ovaries containing either follicular cysts or tumors; however, normal ovaries can also undergo torsion.

- Torsion is the most common complication of ovarian tumors in children, occurring in 3–16% of patients. Ovarian tumors that undergo torsion are more commonly benign.

DIFFERENTIAL DIAGNOSIS

- Appendicitis, gastroenteritis, ruptured ovarian cyst, ectopic pregnancy, pelvic inflammatory disease, tubo-ovarian abscess, nephrolithiasis

PATHOPHYSIOLOGY

- Ovarian mass (follicle, cyst, tumor) acts as a "weight" to promote twisting of the ovary on its vascular pedicle
- Right ovarian torsion is more common than left (3:2)
- Initially, venous and lymphatic drainage are compromised, leading to an enlarged ovary. If prolonged (>8 hours), arterial supply is affected and necrosis, gangrene, and peritonitis can result.
- Neonatal ovarian torsion typically occurs in ovaries with large (>5 cm) follicular cysts that are believed to develop in response to exposure to maternal hormones. Torsion can occur either in utero or postnatally.

CLINICAL MANIFESTATIONS

- Presentation is highly variable: Abdominal pain (90–100%); nausea/vomiting (70–80%); fever (5–20%); leukocytosis (20%); palpable abdominal mass (20%); dysuria (14%)
- Patients note pain on abdominal (RLQ, LLQ) and pelvic exam

DIAGNOSTICS

- Pelvic ultrasound with Doppler: The preferred imaging modality. Can show complex echogenic pelvic mass and absence of blood flow. Normal ultrasound US and Doppler flow does not exclude ovarian torsion. If clinical suspicion is high, prompt surgical evaluation is indicated.
- Pelvic CT scan: Helpful if ultrasound unavailable and can help to rule out other abdominal processes
- Beta human chorionic gonadotropin: Quantitative to rule out ectopic pregnancy and germ cell tumors
- AFP: Order if tumor diagnosed; abnormal with teratoma or endodermal sinus tumors

MANAGEMENT

- Prompt laparoscopy (preferably by 8 hours from onset of symptoms) with detorsion
- Management of a normal ovary under torsion should be as conservative as possible; detorsion and careful observation is recommended to preserve fertility in the ovary; literature suggests that up to 70% of adnexae can be salvaged following torsion.

TESTICULAR TORSION

Surgical emergency of males in which testis and spermatic cord twist, leading to acute ischemia of testis

EPIDEMIOLOGY

- Incidence 1 in 4000 males <25 years old; not common in newborns
- Peaks at 1 year of age and onset of puberty

ETIOLOGY

- Most common in individuals with "bell-clapper deformity," in which the tunica vaginalis extends up to the spermatic cord, suspending the testes freely within the tunica cavity.
- Deformity is frequently bilateral and can be detected by examining testes for a horizontal lie.
- Undescended testes are ten times more likely to undergo torsion.
- Intravaginal torsion (associated with bell-clapper deformity) is typically seen in adolescents.
- Extravaginal torsion (torsion of the cord and coverings) tends to occur in neonates secondary to highly mobile testes.
- Can result from contraction of cremasteric muscle after sex, trauma, cold, or exercise; can occur at rest.

DIFFERENTIAL DIAGNOSIS

- Torsion of appendix testis, epididymitis, orchitis, scrotal trauma, incarcerated inguinal hernia, Henoch–Schönlein purpura, idiopathic scrotal edema, varicocele

PATHOPHYSIOLOGY

- Spermatic cord twists within the tunica vaginalis
- Arterial blood flow interrupted: Leads to ischemia
- Prolonged torsion: Leads to infarction and necrosis
- Recurrent episodes if spontaneously untwists before significant damage done; one-third of patients have had past transient episodes.
- Can result in abnormal spermatogenesis and infertility

CLINICAL MANIFESTATIONS

- Acute-onset testicular pain (89%); vomiting (39%), dysuria or frequency (5%), history of similar pain or swelling (36%)
- Scrotal pain can radiate to the abdomen, thigh, flank
- Usually afebrile, no dysuria or penile discharge
- On exam: Swollen and tender testis, scrotal edema and erythema, high-riding testicle (twisted cord) with horizontal lie, thickened tender spermatic cord, absent cremasteric reflex, palpable secondary hydrocele
- Fever and erythema are late signs.

DIAGNOSTICS

- Doppler ultrasonography is study of choice, but very operator-dependent. Blood flow on Doppler does not rule out torsion.
- 99m-Technetium radioisotope scan (rarely available)

MANAGEMENT

- Surgical emergency: Obtain immediate consultation.
- Detorsion: Cord is untwisted and the testis wrapped in warm saline-soaked gauze while reperfusion is assessed. Necrotic testes are removed, orchiopexy (attach testes to tunica vaginalis) viable testicle. Orchidopexy of the contralateral testis is present.
- Testis removed if not viable because of the risk of infertility secondary to the development of antisperm antibodies.

Madeline H. Renny, MD
Diane P. Calello, MD

GENERAL APPROACH TO THE POISONED PATIENT

- See **Table 31-1**.

TOXIDROMES

- See **Table 31-2**.
- Describe the combination of signs and symptoms that are seen with certain toxins
- When approaching a poisoned patient, use toxidromes for proper assessment and development of a differential diagnosis; though actual clinical manifestations may vary.

DECONTAMINATION AND ENHANCED ELIMINATION

ACTIVATED CHARCOAL

- Decreases absorption of some drugs in the stomach; however, not routinely recommended unless a potentially toxic amount of poison has been ingested
- Should be used soon as soon as possible after ingestion
- Technique: Activated charcoal given orally or by nasogastric (NG) tube at dose of 1 g/kg (maximum, 100 g); repeat dose 0.5–1 g/kg every 4–6 hours, if necessary (see entry for multiple-dose activated charcoal)
  ✓ Ideally should achieve ratio of at least 10 g charcoal per gram of drug ingested
- Does not bind metals (iron, lithium, lead) or common electrolytes, mineral acids or bases, alcohols, cyanide, solvents, and water-insoluble compounds such as hydrocarbon
- Poses aspiration risk, especially among patients who vomit or receive charcoal via NG tube
- Contraindicated in caustic or hydrocarbon ingestion and in patients without protected airway (altered mental status or unconscious)

GASTRIC LAVAGE/GASTRIC EMPTYING

- Gastric lavage still performed, but exceedingly difficult in young children owing to size of tube required
- Efficacy not proven, but most effective if done within 1 hour after ingestion
- Technique: Place patient on left side with head lower than rest of body. Use large-bore orogastric tube.
  ✓ Aspirate gastric contents prior to lavage.
  ✓ Lavage with normal saline until return of fluid is clear. Fifty to 100 mL per cycle should be used, and up to 200 mL in adolescents.
- May delay administration of charcoal
- Contraindicated in patients with altered mental status (inability to protect airway), hydrocarbon or caustic ingestion, cardiac arrhythmia, or possibility of foreign-body ingestion
- Syrup of ipecac is no longer recommended.

TABLE 31-1	General Approach to the Poisoned Patient

History

- Exposure, timing, amount, formulation, symptoms
- Intent of exposure: often related to age of the patient
  - Young children: Unintentional, exploratory exposures; rarely child abuse by poisoning
  - Adolescents: Self-harm by intentional overdose; illicit drug use

Assess vital signs and perform complete physical exam

- Key components: Mental status, pupils, mucous membranes, skin, bowel sounds, bladder size
- Identify the presence of a toxidrome (see Table 30–2).

Diagnostics

- Bedside blood glucose testing, electrocardiography; exposure-specific testing based on history and clinical presentation
- Determine acetaminophen concentration in all patients with intentional overdose.

Management

- Airway, breathing, circulation
- Exposure-specific; consider decontamination and antidote therapy.
- Consult the Poison Control Center (1-800-222-1222)
- Psychiatric evaluation for all intentional ingestions

EXTRACORPOREAL REMOVAL

- Includes methods such as hemodialysis, plasmapheresis, and exchange transfusion
- Reserved for life-threatening poisonings or renal failure; consult pediatric nephrologist
- Hemodialysis is most commonly used. Blood is pumped through dialysis machine and toxins diffuse passively from blood into dialysate solution.
- Unstable patients may undergo continuous renal replacement therapy (such as continuous veno-venous hemofiltration) but the efficacy for poisoning is much less than hemodialysis
- Plasmapheresis and exchange transfusion are seldom necessary but may be useful in neonates or infants.

ENHANCED ELIMINATION

- Urinary alkalinization enhances clearance of certain agents, such as salicylates, phenobarbital, and chlorpropamide, via "ion trapping."
  - ✓ Alkaline environment favors generation of ionized drug species, which cannot readily cross the renal tubular membrane, thus preventing reabsorption.
  - ✓ Performed with sodium bicarbonate at 1–2 mEq/kg over 1–2 hours with careful monitoring for electrolyte abnormalities
- Whole-bowel irrigation (WBI)
  - ✓ Uses: Iron ingestions, massive ingestions, ingestion of sustained-release or enteric-coated preparations, ingestion of packets of illicit drugs, lead poisoning if radiographic evidence of lead in the gastrointestinal tract, late presentations when gastric emptying and charcoal will be unlikely to be effective, and when charcoal cannot be used, such as in lithium ingestion.
  - ✓ Technique: Give preparation via NG tube until stool is clear.

TABLE 31-2 Common Toxidromes

Drug Class	Vital Signs: HR/BP/RR/T	Mental status	Pupils	Skin	Bowel sounds	Comments
Anticholinergics (i.e., antihistamines)	Increased HR, BP, T; RR variable	Delirium	Dilated	Dry/flushed	Decreased	"Blind as a bat, mad as a hatter, red as a beet, hot as Hades, full as a flask, dry as a bone, and the heart runs alone."
Cholinergics (i.e., organophosphates)	Variable	Depressed	Constricted	Diaphoresis	Increased	Salivation, lacrimation, urination, defecation, bronchorrhea, bronchospasm, fasciculations, paralysis
Sedative-hypnotics (i.e., benzodiazepines) or ethanol	Normal or decreased	Depressed	Variable	Normal	Decreased	
Opioids (i.e., heroin)	Decreased	Depressed	Constricted	Normal	Decreased	
Sympathomimetics (i.e., amphetamines, cocaine)	Increased	Agitated	Dilated	Diaphoresis	Normal/ increased	Seizures

BP = blood pressure; HR = heart rate; RR = respiratory rate; T = temperature

✓ Use polyethylene glycol solution, such as GoLYTELY at 500 mL/hr in children and 2 L/hr in adolescents.
✓ Contraindicated in patients with ileus or intestinal obstruction, caustic ingestions, as well as in patients who are unable to protect airway (may require intubation)
✓ Charcoal may be less effective when used together with WBI.
• Multiple-dose activated charcoal (MDAC):
✓ Some recommend repeat doses after large ingestion (listed in "Management" sections for specific drugs).
✓ May improve results by decreasing enterohepatic recirculation
✓ Requires effective peristalsis
✓ Use caution with sorbitol: May result in electrolyte abnormalities (sorbitol should not be administered more than every third dose)

SPECIFIC POISONINGS

• See **Table 31-3**.

ACETAMINOPHEN

Over-the-counter (OTC) analgesics (e.g., Tylenol), OTC cold remedies, prescription combination medications (e.g., Percocet)

TOXICOLOGY/PHARMACOLOGY

• Most common pharmaceutical poisoning exposure
• May be occult: 1 in 500 suicidal overdose patients will have a significant acetaminophen concentration without history of exposure
• Hepatic metabolism, including cytochrome P450
• Toxicity via metabolite, *N*-acetyl-*p*-benzoquinone imine, which is normally detoxified by glutathione; in overdose, glutathione is depleted and metabolite causes direct hepatic-cell injury and death
• Toxic dose is 150 mg/kg in children and 6–7 g in adults.
• Fulminant liver failure develops in 3–4% of children with hepatotoxicity.

CLINICAL MANIFESTATIONS

• Early (first 24 hours): Asymptomatic or nausea, vomiting, malaise
• Initial symptoms may resolve 1–4 days after ingestion despite ongoing hepatotoxicity
✓ Symptoms may include right upper quadrant abdominal pain and jaundice
• Three to 5 days after ingestion, those with severe toxicity may develop symptoms or signs of fulminant hepatic failure with encephalopathy or coma; coagulopathy; renal failure; death from liver failure possible

DIAGNOSTICS

• Measure acetaminophen level 4 hours after ingestion (also at 8 and 12 hours if extended-release form or if ingested with medications that delay gastric emptying) (**Figure 31-1**).
• *Labs:* Aspartate aminotransferase, alanine aminotransferase, glucose, prothrombin time, bilirubin, electrolytes, creatinine (elevated creatinine associated with higher mortality), venous blood gas, lactate, urinalysis (proteinuria and hematuria suggest acute tubular necrosis)
• Single doses of <200 mg/kg are unlikely to cause serious harm; however, accuracy of ingestion amount and timing may be unreliable in intentional overdose.

TABLE 31-3	Specific Poisonings and their Antidotes	
Toxin	**Antidotes**	**Comments**
Acetaminophen	N-acetylcysteine	
Anticholinergics	Physostigmine	Can lead to seizures, cholinergic crisis
Anticholinesterases/carbamates	Atropine	
Organophosphate	Pralidoxime	
Benzodiazepines	Flumazenil	Seldom used due to seizure risk
Beta-blockers	Glucagon	Causes vomiting
Calcium-channel blockers	Calcium chloride/calcium gluconate	Use caution with peripheral IV
Cyanide	Amyl nitrite + thiosulfate or hydroxocobalamin	Caution with nitrites: methemoglobinemia
Digitalis	Digibind	
Lead	BAL, EDTA, DMSA	
Iron	Deferoxamine	
Methanol/ethylene glycol	Fomepizole	
Opioids	Naloxone	
Tricyclics	Sodium bicarbonate	
Local anesthetics	Intralipids	

BAL = bronchoalveolar lavage; EDTA = ethylenediamine tetraacetic acid; DMSA = dimercaptosuccinic acid.

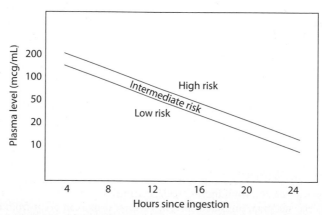

FIGURE 31-1 **Nomogram for estimating severity of acute acetaminophen poisoning.** Modified with permission from Rumack BH, Matthew H. Acetaminophen poisoning and toxicity, *Pediatrics* 1975 Jun;55(6):871–876.

MANAGEMENT

- Gastric lavage is controversial; give charcoal if within 4 hours.
- For acute ingestions, base need for subsequent treatment on nomogram (see **Figure 31-1**).
- N-acetylcysteine (Mucomyst, Acetadote) has greatest benefit in preventing liver toxicity if given within 8 hours after ingestion, but is still beneficial even if initiated many hours to days later.
- If 4-hour level is above the nomogram, administer N-acetylcysteine.
  - ✓ If patient presents 6–8 hours following ingestion, administer N-acetylcysteine while obtaining a blood level measurement.
  - ✓ If patient presents 8–24 hours following ingestion, administer N-acetylcysteine while obtaining a blood level measurement; if >24 hours after ingestion, administer N-acetylcysteine if acetaminophen is detectable or there is evidence of hepatotoxicity.
- N-acetylcysteine dose
  - ✓ Oral dose: Loading dose, 140 mg/kg orally; maintenance dose, 70 mg/kg orally every 4 hours for 17 doses
  - ✓ IV dose: Loading dose, 150 mg/kg given over 1 hour; second dose, 50 mg/kg given over 4 hours; third dose, 100 mg/kg given over 16 hours
  - ✓ Amount of diluent is based on patient age; consider consultation with a pharmacist.
  - ✓ Orally N-acetylcysteine can be difficult to tolerate; this problem is avoided by giving the IV form; the greatest risk of IV N-acetylcysteine is anaphylactoid reactions.
- Cannot use nomogram to determine need for treatment in chronic ingestions; decision to treat in these cases is based on amount ingested (150–200/kg in 24-hour period) or evidence of hepatotoxicity.
- Criteria for admission: Admit all patients who require treatment with N-acetylcysteine. All intentional ingestions warrant psychiatric evaluation.

AMPHETAMINES

Prescribed for narcolepsy, attention-deficit/hyperactivity disorder, fatigue, and weight loss; found in OTC diet pills and some nasal decongestants; includes illicit agents such as methamphetamine, which is the most commonly abused amphetamine, and hallucinogenic amphetamine derivatives such as MDMA (3,4-methylenedioxymethamphetamine, "ecstasy")

TOXICOLOGY/PHARMACOLOGY

- Increase synaptic concentrations of catecholamines causing central nervous system (CNS) stimulation
- Toxic effects are due to excess sympathetic stimulation as well as dopaminergic effects causing psychosis.
- Toxicity through various routes: Ingestion, inhalation, or injection
- Tolerance develops with chronic use; low therapeutic index

CLINICAL MANIFESTATIONS

- Gastrointestinal: Nausea, vomiting, anorexia, diarrhea
- CNS: Euphoria, agitation, pressured speech, seizures; stroke can occur from either hypertension or vasculitis.
- Cardiac: Palpitations, chest pain, hypertensive crises, arrhythmias, myocardial infarction, and circulatory collapse

- Psychiatric: Psychotic state with hallucinations and paranoia, which can be confused with schizophrenia. Hallucinations and altered perception may result with hallucinogenic amphetamine derivatives.
- Other: Hyperthermia, sweating, tremor, difficulty urinating, dilated pupils, rhabdomyolysis, hyponatremia
- With chronic use may see: Cardiomyopathy, cerebral vasculitis, and weight loss. Psychiatric disturbances may be permanent.

DIAGNOSTICS

- Based on history of ingestion and clinical presentation
- Urine toxicologic screen (may not detect all compounds)
- Laboratory studies: Electrolytes, glucose, blood urea nitrogen (BUN), creatinine, creatine phosphokinase (to detect rhabdomyolysis), urinalysis (positive "blood" on dipstick in absence of red blood cells suggests rhabdomyolysis)
- Electrocardiography (ECG), computed tomography (CT) of head if concern for cerebrovascular accident

MANAGEMENT

- Decontamination: Activated charcoal; do not induce emesis
- Symptomatic care: Hydration; treat seizures or agitation with benzodiazepines; if seizures or altered mental status due to severe hyponatremia, give hypertonic saline; treat hypertension with peripheral vasodilator (nitroprusside, phentolamine); treat hyperthermi0
- Treat hyperthermia with active cooling (ice water immersion)
- Treat arrhythmias and rhabdomyolysis if they occur.
- Criteria for hospitalization: Monitor for at least 6 hours; if symptomatic, admit for observation.

ANTIHISTAMINES

OTC and prescription allergy medicines, cold and cough medicines, sleep aids, motion sickness medications

TOXICOLOGY/PHARMACOLOGY

- Antihistamines block H1 receptors.
- Can cause CNS stimulation or depression
- In overdose, can result in anticholinergic symptoms
- Elimination half-lives are variable, ranging from hours to days, depending on the specific drug
- The toxic dose is around three to five times the therapeutic dose.

CLINICAL MANIFESTATIONS

- Lower doses: CNS depression–sedative effect
- Higher doses: CNS stimulation–agitation, confusion, hallucinations, excitement, tremors
- Neurologic: Seizures (diphenhydramine only)
- Cardiac: QRS widening with diphenhydramine (Benadryl)
- Anticholinergic toxidrome: Delirium, flushed skin, dry mouth, fever, tachycardia, hypertension, dilated pupils

DIAGNOSTICS

- Diagnosis based on history and presence of anticholinergic syndrome
- Can be detected on comprehensive urine toxicologic screen
- Laboratory studies: Electrolytes, glucose, blood gas; ECG

MANAGEMENT

- Charcoal and/or gastric emptying; WBI may be helpful when antihistamine is in sustained-release form
- Manage hyperthermia with external cooling.
- Manage agitation or seizures with benzodiazepines.
- If presence of anticholinergic symptoms and no contraindications, then consider use of physostigmine.
  - ✓ Physostigmine dose: 0.02 mg/kg (to a maximum dose of 0.5 mg) given over 5 minutes; dose can be repeated in 15 minutes if there is no response and no adverse effects.
    - Contraindications: QRS widening on ECG, history of asthma/reactive airway disease or current wheezing, bradycardia, and/or tricyclic overdose
  - ✓ Perform ECG before giving physostigmine to rule out conduction delays.
  - ✓ Give slowly: Rapid administration can precipitate seizures or asystole.
    - Stop administration if patient develops any cholinergic effects, including tearing or sweating.
  - ✓ Have atropine ready if needed for cholinergic cardiac effects (bradycardia and hypotension)
  - ✓ Atropine dose is half the amount of physostigmine given

BETA-BLOCKERS

Most common use is for cardiac disorders, such as hypertension, angina, and arrhythmia; noncardiac uses include migraines, essential tremor, thyrotoxicosis, glaucoma, and anxiety.

TOXICOLOGY/PHARMACOLOGY

- In treatment doses, drugs are beta-receptor–specific; in overdose, this specificity is lost.
- Sustained-release preparations exist.
- Can be fatal in doses of only two to three times the therapeutic dose

CLINICAL MANIFESTATIONS

- Cardiac: Bradycardia, hypotension, atrioventricular block; asystole can occur but rare
- CNS: Coma
- Bronchospasm: Mostly seen in patients who have asthma
- Labs may show hypoglycemia in young children; children require serial glucose checks to assess for fasting hypoglycemia.
- ECG may show prolonged PR interval or wide QRS if severe; sotalol ingestion can result in a prolonged QT interval and torsade de pointes.

DIAGNOSTICS

- Diagnosis based on history and vital signs.
- Laboratory studies: Electrolytes, glucose, BUN, creatinine, blood gas
- ECG

MANAGEMENT

- Decontamination: Gastric lavage if large ingestion or immediate presentation; activated charcoal; consider WBI for sustained-release preparations
- Hypotension/bradycardia: Treat with fluids; glucagon; vasoactive pressor infusions may be needed.
- Glucagon dose: 50 µg/kg (maximum, 5 mg) over 5–10 minutes; can repeat dose, if necessary; if heart rate and blood pressure respond, then consider IV infusion. Side effects can include nausea and vomiting .
- Magnesium for torsade de pointes
- Bronchodilators for bronchospasm
- Cardiac pacing or extracorporeal membrane oxygenation (ECMO) is reserved for patients who do not respond to medical management.
- Criteria for hospitalization: For asymptomatic patients, observe and perform ECG monitoring for 6 hours after ingestion; all symptomatic patients, pediatric ingestions, and ingestions with sustained-release preparation should be admitted.

CALCIUM-CHANNEL BLOCKERS

Medication for treatment of hypertension, atrial fibrillation, angina, migraines

TOXICOLOGY/PHARMACOLOGY

- Toxicity due to vasodilatory effects on both coronary and peripheral vessels, decreased myocardial contractility, slowing of the conduction system both at sinus node and through the atrioventricular (AV) node
- Toxicity can occur from therapeutic use or an overdose.
- Can be fatal in small doses
- Most severe toxicity seen with verapamil or diltiazem
- Sustained-release preparations available

CLINICAL MANIFESTATIONS

- May be asymptomatic for hours after ingestion with sustained-release preparations
- Cardiac: Hypotension, bradycardia (verapamil, diltiazem), reflex tachycardia followed by bradycardia as poisoning worsens (amlodipine, nifedipine)
- Neurologic compromise (altered mental status, convulsions, coma) may result from impaired cerebral perfusion, but late in clinical picture. Mental status usually preserved at initial presentation.
- Other symptoms: Hyperglycemia, metabolic acidosis; serum calcium may be normal.

DIAGNOSTICS

- Based on history and clinical presentation
- Laboratory studies: Electrolytes, BUN, creatinine, glucose (risk for hyperglycemia, hypokalemia, metabolic acidosis), blood gas
- ECG shows prolonged PR interval with normal QRS.
- Troponin or other cardiac biomarkers may help differentiate drug-induced from ischemic causes of bradycardia.
- Urine toxicology screen (to detect co-ingested drugs)

MANAGEMENT

- Decontamination:
  - ✓ Gastric lavage: Only if within 1 hour and will not delay charcoal administration
  - ✓ Activated charcoal
  - ✓ WBI for sustained-release preparations
- Treating hypotension:
  - ✓ IV fluids (normal saline bolus)
  - ✓ Calcium gluconate (60 mg/kg IV to maximum of 3 g) or calcium chloride (20 mg/kg IV; only if central access)
  - ✓ Dopamine, epinephrine, or norepinephrine for refractory hypotension
- High-dose insulin (1 U/kg/hr to maximum of 10 U/kg/hr) and glucose (to maintain euglycemia) infusions
- Last-resort therapies: ECMO, cardiac pacing, intraaortic balloon
- Some evidence exists in support of intravenous (IV) lipid emulsion.
- Criteria for hospitalization: 24-hour observation, 24-hour monitoring if large ingestion or sustained release

CANNABIS

Most commonly used illicit substance in the United States; also used medically; derived from the cannabis plant

OXICOLOGY/PHARMACOLOGY

- Bind to and partially agonize cannabinoid receptors
- Principle psychoactive cannabinoid is tetrahydrocannabinol (THC)
- Rapid effects after smoking (minutes); delayed absorption after ingestion (1–2 hours)

CLINICAL MANIFESTATIONS

- Lethargy, alterations in perception, tachycardia, postural hypotension, slurred speech, panic reactions; severe toxicity is rare. Cannabinoid hyperemesis syndrome, consisting of abdominal pain, nausea, and hyperemesis, may occur in chronic heavy users.
- Abuse, dependence, and withdrawal can also occur in chronic users

DIAGNOSTICS

- Based on history and clinical presentation
- Urine toxicologic screen can identify THC for several days to weeks after exposure

MANAGEMENT

- Decontamination: not indicated
- Supportive care: Treat anxiety with reassurance and benzodiazepines as needed
- Cannabinoid hyperemesis syndrome: treat with anti-emetics and frequent hot water shower/bath; capsaicin cream and/or haloperidol may be effective for refractory emesis; ultimate treatment is cessation of marijuana use
- Criteria for hospitalization: Observe patients until asymptomatic. If persistent signs of toxicity, then require further work-up and admission. Patients with hyperemesis may require admission if unable to tolerate fluids.

CANNABINOIDS, SYNTHETIC

Common names: Spice, yucatan fire, aroma, incense, potpourri, K2. Attractive to users because they are not typically detected by drug screens and are advertised as "safe and legal."

TOXICOLOGY/PHARMACOLOGY

- Similar to THC in function by binding to cannabinoid receptors
- The limited data on human toxicity and high variability in preparations contribute to danger.

CLINICAL MANIFESTATIONS

- Common effects include nausea, vomiting, tachycardia, hypertension, agitation, and altered mental status; chest pain and ischemia occur in more severe cases, psychiatric effects include anxiety, depression, and psychosis; seizures reported.

DIAGNOSTICS

- Chemistry (synthetic cannabinoids have been reported to cause hypokalemia), ECG
- Drug screens may identify co-ingestions and high-performance liquid chromatography/tandem mass spectroscopy might identify more rare drugs but are rarely useful in the immediate setting.

MANAGEMENT

- Supportive care and close cardiorespiratory monitoring. Patients may benefit from benzodiazepines for agitation and/or psychiatric symptoms

CARBAMAZEPINE

Medication used for seizures (Tegretol, Carbatrol), neuropathic pain, some psychiatric disorders

TOXICOLOGY/PHARMACOLOGY

- Blocks sodium channels in the brain, preventing high-frequency firing; at high doses, also blocks cardiac sodium channels
- Mild anticholinergic activity
- Absorption can be erratic owing to anticholinergic-induced delayed gastric emptying.
- Peak level reached from 4 to 24 hours.
- Metabolized via cytochrome P450 to active compound, so drug level may not reflect magnitude of clinical toxicity

CLINICAL MANIFESTATIONS

- CNS: Ataxia, mydriasis, nystagmus, altered mental status, nausea, vomiting, dystonic posturing, coma, seizures; status epilepticus indicates poor prognosis
- Cardiac: Sinus tachycardia, hypotension from myocardial depression, AV block, bradycardia, QRS or QT prolongation, ventricular dysrhythmias
- Chronic toxicity: Syndrome of inappropriate antidiuretic hormone secretion, leukopenia, thrombocytopenia
- Symptom onset may be delayed due to delayed absorption.

DIAGNOSTICS

- Based on history and clinical signs
- Obtain immediate carbamazepine level; repeat levels every 4–6 hours; levels >40 mg/L associated with severe toxicity in adults; toxic level is even lower in children.
- Laboratory studies: CBC, electrolytes, glucose, arterial blood gases
- ECG

MANAGEMENT

- Treatment based on clinical status, not drug levels
- Supportive care
- Recognize that carbamazepine can significantly slow gastrointestinal (GI) motility and that neurologic status may warrant early airway management
- Activated charcoal
- Massive ingestion: Consider multidose activated charcoal (MDAC) or WBI
- Life-threatening toxicity: Hemodialysis
- Treat seizures with benzodiazepines and phenobarbital, not phenytoin (has same intracellular mechanism as carbamazepine).
- Criteria for hospitalization: Observe asymptomatic patients for 6 hours; admit symptomatic patients to monitored bed if levels or clinical picture are concerning.

CARBON MONOXIDE

Fire (indoor charcoal or house fire), automobile exhaust, gasoline engines operating in enclosed spaces (car or generator in garage), faulty furnaces or gas stoves, wood-burning stoves, inhaled spray paint; also, the main ingredient in paint remover is metabolized to carbon monoxide.

TOXICOLOGY/PHARMACOLOGY

- Children are at higher risk from CO poisoning because of their higher metabolic and respiratory rates.
- Toxicity results from CO binding hemoglobin with higher affinity than oxygen, which results in decreased oxygen saturation tissue delivery.
- CO also can bind myoglobin, resulting in cardiac toxicity by decreasing contractility.
- Mild symptoms of toxicity can be seen at carboxyhemoglobin levels of 5% and death at levels of 50%.

CLINICAL MANIFESTATIONS

- Most mild exposures present with flu-like symptoms, headache, visual changes, dizziness, nausea, and/or weakness.
- More severe exposure can present with syncope, seizures, coma, cardiac ischemia or infarction, dysrhythmias, pulmonary edema, or death.
- Physical exam findings can include tachycardia, hypotension or hypertension, tachypnea, and pallor; skin and soft tissue also more susceptible to trauma, with pressure points most affected.
- Classic description of cherry red skin is actually a late finding.
- Delayed neurologic sequelae may develop days to weeks after exposure; symptoms include headache, disorientation, dementia, apraxia, peripheral neuropathy, ataxia, chorea, and Parkinson-like signs.
  - ✓ 25% of patients with delayed neurologic sequelae may have permanent neurologic findings

DIAGNOSTICS

- CO hemoglobin (COHgb) levels: Remember, pulse oximetry may be normal.
- CBC, BUN, creatinine, cardiac enzymes, glucose, pregnancy test
- Chest x-ray
- ECG to look for ischemia or dysrhythmias
- Obtain history of risk factors for CO poisoning (e.g., fuel-burning space heaters, charcoal grills, portable generators)

MANAGEMENT

- Give 100% oxygen to reduce half-life of carboxyhemoglobin.
- Consider hyperbaric oxygen in several situations: COHgb >25%, pregnancy, or significant cardiac or neurologic symptoms.
  ✓ Hyperbaric oxygen may decrease the likelihood neurologic sequelae
- Continue therapy until COHgb <5–10%.
- Monitor for metabolic acidosis, which may require therapy with sodium bicarbonate in extreme cases.
- Criteria for hospitalization: (1) Adults with COHgb >25%; (2) children with COHgb >15%; (3) metabolic acidosis; (4) ECG changes; (5) neuropsychiatric symptoms; (6) abnormal thermoregulation; (7) partial pressure of oxygen <60 mm Hg

CAUSTICS

Acids or alkali; oven or drain cleaner; powdered laundry and dishwasher detergents; hair relaxers; industrial products

TOXICOLOGY/PHARMACOLOGY

- Causes burns when inhaled or ingested, but also with skin and eye contact
- Acids result in coagulation necrosis, and alkalis cause liquefaction necrosis.
  ✓ Although liquefaction necrosis is deeper, the clinical course is similar in both acid and alkali ingestions.

CLINICAL MANIFESTATIONS

- Stridor, hoarseness, dyspnea, aphonia, vomiting, or drooling
- May initially be asymptomatic
- Symptoms do not reliably predict presence or absence of esophageal injury.
- Usually present with burning of exposed areas
- Airway edema and obstruction can be delayed up to 48 hours in alkali exposures.
- Acids and alkali both can cause esophageal injury.
- Acid ingestions usually also cause damage to stomach with risk for gastric perforation and peritonitis.
- Alkali ingestions are more likely to damage esophagus with possibility of perforation and resulting mediastinitis.
- May present with acute GI bleed or acute gastric perforation
- Third-degree esophageal burns at risk for developing strictures.

DIAGNOSTICS

- Based on history of exposure and symptoms
- Determine whether the substance was only and irritant or whether it was actually a corrosive.

- Determined by pH, concentration, and viscosity
- Contact poison center for information
- Laboratory studies: CBC, type and screen, electrolytes, glucose, blood gas
- Chest x-ray and abdominal x-rays to look for free air

MANAGEMENT

- Stabilize airway: May need intubation under direct visualization (fiberoptic)
  ✓ Blind intubation can worsen damage or cause perforation.
- IV access; keep patient on a regimen of nothing-by-mouth (NPO), perform a chest x-ray.
- No GI decontamination, no ipecac, no lavage. Simple dilution may pose the risk of fluid leakage into surrounding tissues in the event of perforation, may worsen damage depending on the pH of administered fluids, and negates NPO status.
- Perform endoscopy in symptomatic patients and/or those with intentional ingestions as soon as possible to determine extent of burn.
- Surgery consult in all patients with significant burns
- Careful examination of the eyes, with irrigation if indicated
- Corticosteroids may be beneficial in some esophageal burns to prevent strictures (controversial).
- Pain control
- Antibiotics: If evidence of perforation or if steroids are used
- H_2 blocker to reduce gastric acid formation
- Criteria for hospitalization: All symptomatic patients with caustic ingestions

CLONIDINE

Imidazoline class, along with dexmedetomidine (Precedex®), tetrahydrozoline (Visine®), oxymetazoline (Afrin®), guanfacine (Tenex®, Intuniv®). Medication to treat hypertension and attention-deficit/hyperactivity disorder; has been used to treat withdrawal symptoms from opioids and nicotine.

TOXICOLOGY/PHARMACOLOGY

- Agonist at central alpha-2-receptors, resulting in decreased sympathetic outflow
- Binds to peripheral alpha-1-receptors, resulting in vasoconstriction and hypertension early in the course
- Can cause significant toxicity in small doses
- Rapidly absorbed and distributed, so symptoms appear soon after ingestion

CLINICAL MANIFESTATIONS

- Neurologic: Altered mental status with irritability, lethargy, or coma
- Respiratory depression, occasionally necessitating endotracheal intubation, apnea
- Cardiac: Most commonly see hypotension and bradycardia, but can also see tachycardia, transient hypertension, or AV nodal blockade
- Other: Miosis, pallor, hypothermia
- Clinical effects typically last 8–24 hours

DIAGNOSTICS

- Based on history and physical finding
- Drug levels not available

- Laboratory studies: Electrolytes, glucose, blood gas
- ECG

MANAGEMENT

- Activated charcoal
- Treatment primarily supportive
- Hypotension: Give fluids; if refractory can also use dopamine or epinephrine
- Bradycardia: Atropine
- Hypertension, when present, rarely needs treatment.
- Naloxone is sometimes effective in reversing respiratory, cardiac, and neurologic effects. Initial dose is usually 1–2 mg, though larger amounts may be necessary.
- Criteria for hospitalization: Observe asymptomatic patients for 6 hours; admit all symptomatic patients.

COCAINE

Used medically as local anesthetic; popular street drug

TOXICOLOGY/PHARMACOLOGY

- Toxic effects are via CNS stimulation and inhibited catecholamine uptake
- Toxicity develops though multiple routes (ingestion, inhalation, injection)
- Toxic dose is highly variable; however, toxicity is usually decreased with ingestion given time for absorption.
- "Body packers" swallow many tightly wrapped packets or condoms of cocaine in attempt to hide or smuggle drugs.
  - ✓ Toxicity results when packets break open, releasing drugs into GI tract, with potentially fatal effect.
- "Body stuffers" hastily ingest smaller packets sold on the street to avoid detection by law enforcement.
  - ✓ Body stuffing associated with a higher risk of rupture because drugs are not securely enclosed.
  - ✓ Risk of mortality, however, is lower than with body packing because relatively small quantities are typically ingested.

CLINICAL MANIFESTATIONS

- CNS: Euphoria, agitation, psychosis, seizures, stroke
- Cardiac: Hypertension, tachycardia, arrhythmias including ventricular fibrillation, myocardial ischemia, and infarction
- Respiratory: Bronchospasm, pneumothorax, pneumomediastinum, hemoptysis
- Other: Dilated pupils, hyperthermia, rhabdomyolysis, renal failure, nasal septum perforation
- Cocaine adulterants may cause otherwise unexpected toxicity.
  - ✓ For example, levamisole, a veterinary antihelminthic, has caused outbreaks of fever and agranulocytosis in cocaine users.

DIAGNOSTICS

- Based on history of use and clinical presentation
- Urine toxicologic screen: Metabolites may be found up to 3 days after exposure.

- Laboratory studies: Electrolytes, glucose, BUN, creatinine, creatine phosphokinase, urinalysis
- ECG
- Chest x-ray if respiratory symptoms present
- Head CT if stroke is suspected
- Abdominal x-rays and CT of abdomen/pelvis if suspect body packing; body stuffer packets not well visualized on radiographs

MANAGEMENT

- Decontamination: Give activated charcoal if cocaine taken orally; if suspect body packer give MDAC and consider WBI or surgical removal, given high mortality associated with cocaine packet rupture
- Supportive care: Benzodiazepines are used to decrease agitation, tachycardia, and hypertension and to treat seizures.
- Severe hypertension: Do not use beta-blocker, which can cause unopposed alpha-adrenergic effect, leading to increase in blood pressure and increased coronary vasospasm.
- Treat hyperthermia with active cooling (i.e., ice water immersion) and benzodiazepines for sedation
- Consider co-ingestions.
- Treat arrhythmias and rhabdomyolysis.
- Criteria for hospitalization: Admit patient with ECG changes, seizures, or neurologic deficits; "body packers"

CYANIDE

Naturally occurring in some plants but also present in car exhaust and cigarette smoke in small amounts; toxic exposure usually from the burning of cyanide-containing natural or synthetic products and industrial exposure.

TOXICOLOGY/PHARMACOLOGY

- Cyanide inhibits electron transport in mitochondria, impairing aerobic metabolism and causing metabolic acidosis.
- Small amounts are metabolized under normal circumstances, symptoms occur when the systems are overwhelmed.

CLINICAL MANIFESTATIONS

- Cardiac: Tachycardia, hypertension, myocardial toxicity, bradycardia, arrhythmias, and cardiovascular collapse
- Respiratory: Tachypnea, dyspnea, no cyanosis (cherry-red skin is classically described but not reliably seen)
- Neurologic: Headaches, light-headedness, ataxia, posturing, seizures
- Patients may have a "bitter almond" odor.

DIAGNOSTICS

- Blood gas with lactate: Often reveals high mixed venous saturation and severe lactic acidosis
- Electrolytes
- CBC
- ECG

MANAGEMENT

- Decontamination by removal of wet clothes in the appropriate context (environmental exposure)
- Supportive care: 100% oxygen, support of circulation with fluids and pressors if needed, correction of acidosis with sodium bicarbonate, and treatment of seizures with benzodiazepines
- Antidotes:
  - ✓ Older therapy: Nitrites (amyl and sodium nitrite) and sodium thiosulfate. Nitrites can cause hypotension and affect oxygen-carrying capacity by inducing methemoglobinemia, so are contraindicated if there is concern for concomitant carbon monoxide poisoning.
    - In pediatric patients, thiosulfate alone may be used; thiosulfate dose is 400 mg/kg for children <25 kg, with a maximum of 12.5 g.
  - ✓ Newer therapy: Involves use of hydroxocobalamin without attendant side effects of nitrites
    - Dose is 70 mg/kg IV given over 15 minutes; dose may need to be repeated.
    - Side effects include hypertension and reddish discoloration of skin, mucous membranes, and urine; also can interfere with colorimetric laboratory results, so blood for lab testing should be collected prior to treatment if possible.
    - May be given with or without thiosulfate.

DIGOXIN

Medication used to treat congestive heart failure and supraventricular tachycardias; digitoxin also found in plants (oleander, rhododendron, foxglove)

TOXICOLOGY/PHARMACOLOGY

- Inhibits sodium–potassium adenosine triphosphatase pump, increases vagal tone, slows AV conduction
- Toxicity can occur from chronic use or with overdose, symptoms may be more striking in patients with chronic toxicity.
- Doses as small as 250 mcg can be toxic in children.
- Absorption and redistribution occur rapidly; therefore, digoxin levels can decrease rapidly after ingestion.
- Elimination half-life is 30–50 hours, renal clearance is the major mode of elimination.

CLINICAL MANIFESTATIONS

- Symptoms include nausea, vomiting, lethargy, visual changes (halos or changes in color vision).
- Higher levels of intoxication can cause lethargy, mental status changes, electrolyte abnormalities (the most prognostic of which is hyperkalemia), bradycardia, ventricular dysrhythmias, and cardiac arrest.

DIAGNOSTICS

- Obtain digoxin level immediately; therapeutic level is 0.9–1.2 ng/mL.
- Laboratory findings include hyperkalemia, or with chronic toxicity, may see hypokalemia if concurrent diuretic use
- Other laboratory studies: Electrolytes, calcium, magnesium, BUN, creatinine

- ECG changes may vary; most common ECG abnormalities are sinus bradycardia and AV block.
  ✓ Ventricular dysrhythmias may occur precipitously, so early treatment advised in the patient with ECG abnormalities and elevated serum digoxin concentration

MANAGEMENT

- Decontamination; activated charcoal may be of benefit.
- Correction of hyperkalemia will not prevent dysrhythmias. Digoxin-specific Fab (Digibind) will correct hyperkalemia and rhythm disturbances: consider in any patient with ECG abnormalities, high serum digoxin concentration, and/or hyperkalemia (>5 mEq/L, depending on source).
- Calculating Digibind dosing
  ✓ If amount of digoxin ingested is known: 38 mg Digibind to bind 0.5 mg digoxin
  ✓ If amount unknown: Number of vials = [(serum digoxin level in ng/mL) × (body weight in kg)]/100
  ✓ Potential side effects include hypersensitivity reactions, decreased potassium, worsening of heart failure.
  ✓ Recognize that serum digoxin level may increase after administration, but this reflects inactive drug.
- Additional treatment of hyperkalemia
  ✓ Calcium salts are *contraindicated* and may cause cardioplegia ("stone heart").
  ✓ Adjunctive therapies such as insulin/glucose and sodium bicarbonate may be useful.
- Criteria for hospitalization: Admit patients with symptoms of digoxin toxicity, ECG abnormalities, hypokalemia, hyperkalemia, or elevated serum digoxin concentration or any patient getting Digibind.
  ✓ Patients with normal digoxin levels, no electrolyte abnormalities, and a normal ECG can be discharged after 6 hours of observation.

ETHANOL

Beer, wine, liquors; used as solvent, topical antiseptic; ingredient in perfume, cologne, mouthwash; used as antidote in treatment of methanol and ethylene glycol overdoses

TOXICOLOGY/PHARMACOLOGY

- Acts as a direct CNS depressant by binding to gamma aminobutyric acid receptors
- Ethanol can also have effects on cardiac muscle, thyroid, and liver.
- Ethanol is metabolized by the liver.
- Dose-independent fasting hypoglycemia in children results from ethanol-inhibiting gluconeogenesis.
- Levels at which symptoms appear are highly variable.

CLINICAL MANIFESTATIONS

- Mild acute toxicity: Nausea, vomiting, euphoria, incoordination, ataxia, nystagmus, impaired judgment; hypoglycemia and seizures seen in younger age group
- More severe acute toxicity: Coma, respiratory depression, metabolic acidosis; can have death from apnea
- Presentation in infants and children includes hypothermia, hypoglycemia, metabolic acidosis, and coma.
  ✓ These occur at levels of 50–100 mg/dL

DIAGNOSTICS

- Obtain blood glucose levels immediately.
- Laboratory studies: Electrolytes, BUN, creatinine, liver enzymes, prothrombin time, blood gas
- Ethanol level
- Chest x-ray if suspicious for aspiration

MANAGEMENT

- Supportive care: Assess airway and establish access; treat hypoglycemia, seizures, hypothermia
- Decontamination: Indicated only if concern for co-ingestion
- Hemodialysis effective, but rarely needed (consider in patients with hepatic impairment or very high blood alcohol levels)
- Criteria for hospitalization: In acute ingestions, observe until mental status is at baseline
  - ✓ Admit all young children with detectable ethanol levels and/or toxicity, all patients with hypoglycemia; for adolescents, determine admission based on clinical status.

ETHYLENE GLYCOL

Main ingredient in antifreeze; occasionally used by alcoholics in place of ethanol

TOXICOLOGY/PHARMACOLOGY

- Metabolized by alcohol dehydrogenase to toxic glycolaldehyde, glycolic, glyoxylic, and oxalic acids, causing metabolic acidosis and acute renal failure
- Oxalic acid chelates serum calcium, causing hypocalcemia and calcium oxalate precipitation in renal tubules.

CLINICAL MANIFESTATIONS

- Initially, patients will have CNS depression and coma from direct intoxicating effect.
- As compound is metabolized, anion-gap metabolic acidosis ensues, with tachycardia and hyperpnea, elevated WBC count, GI distress, and hypocalcemia.
  - ✓ Cardiovascular compromise may result from metabolic derangements and dysrhythmias from hypocalcemia.
- Acute kidney injury appears as calcium oxalate crystal precipitate in the kidney, causing direct tubular injury beginning approximately 24 hours after exposure

DIAGNOSTICS

- Anion-gap metabolic acidosis, elevated osmolar gap
- Hypocalcemia
- Ethylene glycol levels are available, but may be low if already converted to toxic metabolite
- Other laboratory studies: Electrolytes, glucose, BUN, creatinine, liver enzymes, urinalysis (which may demonstrate oxalate crystals), blood gas
- ECG
- Urine: Some antifreeze contains fluorescein, so urine may fluoresce under Wood's lamp; can see calcium oxalate crystals on microscopic urinalysis

MANAGEMENT

- Supportive: Cardiac monitoring; correct hypocalcemia with IV calcium salts; correct acidosis with sodium bicarbonate.
- Decontamination: *No* charcoal (ineffective); consider gastric lavage if presents within 1 hour
- Antidote: Fomepizole and ethanol bind ADH with higher affinity than ethylene glycol and thereby prevent formation of toxic metabolites
  - ✓ Treat with fomepizole (preferred) for ethylene glycol level >20 mg/dL or patients with presumed ingestion and metabolic acidosis
  - ✓ IV ethanol infusion is a second-line option that is effective but difficult to administer.
  - ✓ Other options include pyridoxine, folate, and thiamine to prevent toxic metabolite formation.
- Hemodialysis can be used to enhance elimination; indicated in renal failure or in cases of severe metabolic derangement.
- Criteria for hospitalization: Any known ingestion of ethylene glycol; clinical or laboratory abnormalities suggestive of ethylene glycol toxicity

HYDROCARBONS

Solvents, degreasers, fuels, pesticides, gasoline, kerosene, lighter fluid, torch fuels

TOXICOLOGY/PHARMACOLOGY

- Three categories of hydrocarbons
  - ✓ Aliphatic (petroleum distillates, furniture polish, lamp oils, lighter fluid)
  - ✓ Aromatic (benzene, toluene, xylene, camphor found in glues, solvents, and nail polish)
  - ✓ Otherwise "toxic" (halogenated, hydrocarbons that serve as a vehicle for other substances)
- Toxicity can be due to inhalation, skin absorption, or ingestion with systemic toxicity (in aromatic, halogenated hydrocarbons or those with toxic additives).
- Aspiration of as little as 1 mL of fluid can lead to severe pneumonitis.

CLINICAL MANIFESTATIONS

- Respiratory symptoms are the primary consequence of most aliphatic hydrocarbon ingestions, due to spillage into tracheobronchial tree: Tachypnea, dyspnea, cyanosis, grunting, cough
  - ✓ Severe pneumonitis and acute respiratory distress syndrome may develop.
- Lower viscosity associated with higher aspiration risk
- Neurologic symptoms usually result from systemic toxicity: Seizures, lethargy, coma (usually with aromatic hydrocarbons)
- Gastrointestinal symptoms usually result from ingestion: Nausea, vomiting, liver failure (carbon tetrachloride)
- Hematologic: Hemolysis, hemoglobinuria
- Cardiac: Dysrhythmias (with halogenated hydrocarbons)
- Fever
- Skin or eye contact can result in burns or corneal injury.

DIAGNOSTICS

- Based on history of exposure
  - ✓ If respiratory symptoms, check blood gas and obtain chest x-ray

- Repeat chest x-ray in 4–6 hours if initially negative.
- If concern over significant ingestion, check electrolytes, glucose, BUN, creatinine, liver enzymes, and an ECG

MANAGEMENT

- In general, no charcoal, no lavage, and no induction of emesis
  ✓ Aspiration poses the greatest risk, and prevention of aspiration is a mainstay of management.
  ✓ Exceptions to above "no" rules: (1) Consider charcoal if hydrocarbon contains a toxic substance (e.g., heavy metal, insecticide, camphor); (2) consider lavage (after intubating to protect airway) if massive amount is ingested
- Supportive respiratory care: Supplemental oxygen, continuous positive airway pressure, intubation as needed
- ECMO has been used successfully in some patients.
- Antibiotics and steroids are not routinely indicated.
- Avoid epinephrine if dysrhythmia is thought to be due to myocardial sensitization (i.e., sudden sniffing death syndrome).
- Criteria for hospitalization: All symptomatic patients and those with abnormal chest x-rays; monitor for at least 6 hours if asymptomatic
  ✓ Symptoms can begin up to 24 hours after exposure; therefore, appropriate discharge instructions are needed.

IRON

Ingredient in both pediatric and adult multivitamins; adult preparations have greater toxicity due to more elemental iron per tablet

TOXICOLOGY/PHARMACOLOGY

- In overdose, transferrin becomes saturated and unbound iron causes injury to cells.
- Toxicity can be due to direct corrosive injury or to impaired cellular metabolism.
- Toxic dose is 20–30 mg/kg of elemental iron.

CLINICAL MANIFESTATIONS

- Four stages
  ✓ Direct injury to GI mucosa results in vomiting and diarrhea, both of which can be bloody. Massive blood loss resulting in shock and death may result.
  ✓ GI symptoms are seen to resolve over the next 12–24 hours. In mild ingestions, this may indicate recovery. However, it may represent a brief quiescence prior to phase III, and patients should be monitored closely
  ✓ Up to 48 hours after ingestion, systemic symptoms may begin with GI bleeding, metabolic acidosis, coagulopathy, liver failure, seizures, shock, and possibly death.

DIAGNOSTICS

- Based on history of exposure and symptoms
- Laboratory studies: Obtain iron level immediately, if possible; should be done 4–6 hours after ingestion and then repeated 8–12 hours after ingestion to evaluate possibility of delayed absorption.
  ✓ Level >350 mcg/dL is likely to be toxic.
  ✓ Level >500 mcg/dL suggests more severe toxicity.

- Blood gas, lactate, CBC, electrolytes, glucose, BUN, creatinine, liver function tests, pro-thrombin time, partial thromboplastin time, type and cross-match
  - ✓ Elevated WBC (>15,000 mm³) and glucose (>150 mg/dL) levels are consistent with ingestion.
  - ✓ Acidosis is most concerning for toxicity.
- Abdominal radiograph at presentation and again after WBI, though a negative x-ray does not necessarily rule out a significant ingestion.

MANAGEMENT

- Decontamination: If <30 minutes since ingestion, consider gastric lavage; WBI if iron tablets seen on abdominal films (*do not* use phosphate-containing solutions); activated charcoal is *not effective*.
- Supportive care: Treat hypotension with fluids; may need to give blood products to treat GI blood loss
- Chelation with continuous IV deferoxamine for severe toxicity (iron level >500 mcg/dL, metabolic acidosis, persistent vomiting, lethargy, hypotension, and/or shock)
  - ✓ 10–15 mg/kg/hr; maximum dose, 6 g/day
  - ✓ Chelation treatment results in pink/orange appearance of urine (helpful to forewarn patient and family).
  - ✓ Discontinue when asymptomatic, with normal laboratory studies and normal appearance of urine
  - ✓ Adverse effects: Hypotension (infusion rate-related), acute respiratory distress syndrome if given >24 hours
- Criteria for hospitalization: Symptomatic patients; patients with iron level >500 or if iron tablets seen on abdominal radiographs; asymptomatic patients should have iron levels repeated at 8–12 hours—if levels normal and still asymptomatic, can be discharged

ISOPROPYL ALCOHOL

Solvent, antiseptic, disinfectant; main ingredient in rubbing alcohol; often ingested by alcoholics as a substitute for ethanol

TOXICOLOGY/PHARMACOLOGY

- Less toxic than other alcohols
- Toxicity can result from ingestion, inhalation, or via absorption through the skin.
- Causes CNS depression; large doses can also cause direct vasodilation, resulting in hypotension.
- Metabolized via alcohol dehydrogenase to acetone, which is also a CNS depressant

CLINICAL MANIFESTATIONS

- GI: Abdominal pain, vomiting, hemorrhagic gastritis
- CNS: Slurred speech, ataxia, stupor, coma, respiratory arrest
- Cardiac: Myocardial depression
- Respiratory: Tracheobronchitis

DIAGNOSTICS

- Based on history of ingestion, presence of osmolar gap without metabolic acidosis (unlike other toxic alcohols)
- Odor of acetone may be detected
- Ketones (acetone) present in blood and urine

MANAGEMENT

- Supportive care
- Activated charcoal adsorbs alcohols poorly.
- For large, recent ingestions, consider gastric lavage.
- Hemodialysis indicated for hemodynamic instability (very rare)
- Criteria for hospitalization: Any patient with symptomatic isopropanol ingestion; symptoms do not rely as heavily on toxic metabolites as for other alcohols, so symptoms emerge soon after ingestion.

LEAD

Most common source is chipping paint in homes built before the 1970s; also found in pipes, electric cable, munitions, batteries, glaze used for ceramics, imported toys, jewelry, cosmetics, and food

TOXICOLOGY/PHARMACOLOGY

- Majority of toxicity results from chronic exposure
- Toxicity from enzyme inhibition, resulting in blocked heme synthesis
- Can also affect neurotransmitter functioning

CLINICAL MANIFESTATIONS

- Most children are actually asymptomatic.
- Gastrointestinal: Can be nonspecific; abdominal pain, vomiting, constipation, anorexia
- Neurologic: Seen at higher lead levels (>70 mcg/dL); irritability, lethargy, ataxia, seizures, encephalopathy or death; may have increased intracranial pressure
- Renal: Clinical picture similar to Fanconi syndrome; aminoaciduria and glycosuria

DIAGNOSTICS

- Venous whole-blood lead level
- CBC will show microcytic anemia with basophilic stippling.
- Elevated free erythrocyte protoporphyrin
- Long bone radiograph: May see metaphyseal "lead lines"
- Abdominal radiographs: May see opacities
- Avoid lumbar puncture, if possible, owing to potential for increased ICP

MANAGEMENT

- Symptomatic patients and asymptomatic patients with elevated blood lead level are at increased risk of CNS involvement.
- Prevention: Screening should start at 9–12 months of age at well-child visit
- Decontamination: For acute ingestion, consider inducing vomiting or doing gastric lavage.
  ✓ Activated charcoal does not bind lead.
  ✓ Perform WBI if there are findings (paint chips) on abdominal radiographs.
- Identify and remove the source.
- Need for subsequent treatment based on blood lead levels: Should be <5 mcg/dL
  ✓ Level >45 mcg/dL: start oral chelation with succimer or with IV edetate calcium disodium (CaEDTA)
  ✓ Level >69 mcg/dL or signs of encephalopathy: Hospitalize for two-drug chelation therapy with British anti-Lewisite (BAL) and CaEDTA (give BAL first and then both together 4 hours later) or BAL and succimer

- Chelation dosing
  - ✓ Succimer (dimercaptosuccinic acid): Dose is 1050 mg/m^2/day (or 30 mg/kg/day) divided every 8 hours for 5 days, then 700 mg/m^2/day (or 20 mg/kg/day) divided every 12 hours for 14 days.
  - ✓ CaEDTA: 1000 mg/m^2/day IV divided every 12 hours for 3–5 days; for lead level greater than 69 mcg/dL or signs of encephalopathy, use 1500 mg/m^2/day as a continuous infusion for first 48 hours; maintain adequate hydration.
  - ✓ Dimercaprol or BAL: Used if lead level >69 mcg/dL or signs of encephalopathy; dose is 75 mg/m^2 per dose intramuscularly (IM) every 4 hours for 3–5 days; give first dose alone, then give BAL with CaEDTA; at 48 hours obtain lead level to decide whether to continue chelation.
    - *Do not* use BAL in patients with hepatic insufficiency, peanut allergy, or glucose-6-phosphate dehydrogenase deficiency.
    - Use cautiously in patients with hypertension or renal insufficiency.
- Criteria for hospitalization: Lead level >69 mcg/dL or signs of encephalopathy; if only option for removing child from source of lead exposure
- Supportive care (in lead encephalopathy): Anticonvulsants; manage increased intracranial pressure, adequate hydration to maintain urine output

METHANOL

Windshield washer fluid; Sterno fuel; solvents, paint remover, antifreeze; used by alcoholics as substitute for ethanol

TOXICOLOGY/PHARMACOLOGY

- Metabolized by alcohol dehydrogenase to formaldehyde and formic acid, which are responsible for the toxicity
- Metabolism is slow and symptoms may be delayed for hours, though in large ingestions, CNS depression and acidosis may manifest more acutely.
- In children, small ingestions (5 mL of 100% methanol) can result in death.

CLINICAL MANIFESTATIONS

- Ophthalmologic: Snowfield vision, retinal toxicity, papilledema, ophthalmoplegia, loss of pupillary light reflex, blindness
- CNS: Inebriation, CNS depression, seizures, coma, death
- Cardiovascular: Hypotension, reflex tachycardia
- These findings may not appear for up to 24–30 hours.

DIAGNOSTICS

- Based on history and symptoms
- Fundus exam may show optic disk hyperemia, venous engorgement, or papilledema
- Anion-gap metabolic acidosis may be preceded by an elevated osmolar gap
- Other laboratory studies: Electrolytes, glucose, BUN, creatinine, serum osmolality, blood gas, methanol level, lactate level

MANAGEMENT

- Decontamination: Do not induce emesis; activated charcoal is *not* effective.
  - ✓ May perform gastric lavage.
  - ✓ Treat metabolic acidosis with IV sodium bicarbonate.

- Antidote: Fomepizole and ethanol bind alcohol dehydrogenase with higher affinity than methanol and thereby prevent formation of toxic metabolites.
  ✓ Treat with fomepizole (preferred) for methanol level >25 mg/dL or patients with presumed ingestion and metabolic acidosis.
  ✓ If not available, IV ethanol infusion is also effective but difficult to administer.
- Folic acid helps conversion of formic acid to carbon dioxide and water.
- Hemodialysis is indicated in cases of severe metabolic acidosis or blood methanol concentrations >50 mg/dL
- Criteria for hospitalization: Any known methanol ingestion or clinical and lab findings suggestive of methanol ingestion

NICOTINE

Derived from the tobacco plant. Commonly found in tobacco cigarettes and electronic cigarettes (e-cigarettes), as well as other nicotine-containing products or pesticides

TOXICOLOGY/PHARMACOLOGY

- Well absorbed via inhalation, ingestion, or dermal exposure
- Binds to nicotinic receptors in the brain, sympathetic and parasympathetic ganglia, and neuromuscular junction, and stimulates acetylcholine release
- Lethal dose is 0.5–1 mg/kg in adults; severe toxicity in children can occur at lower doses.
- E-cigarettes contain varying but substantial concentrations of liquid nicotine; the products may be flavored and brightly colored, making them appealing to young children.

CLINICAL MANIFESTATIONS

- Early (first hour after ingestion): Diaphoresis, salivation, bronchorrhea, vomiting, diarrhea, hypertension, tachycardia, neurologic symptoms (headache, dizziness, tremor, fasciculations, ataxia, confusion, seizures)
- Late (1–4 hours after ingestion): Bradycardia, hypotension, dysrhythmias, coma, neuromuscular blockade with respiratory muscle paralysis and apnea

DIAGNOSTICS

- Based on history, vital signs, and neurologic status
- Laboratory studies: electrolytes, glucose, blood gas, ECG
- Serum concentrations are not useful in acute management.

MANAGEMENT

- Decontamination: Activated charcoal if normal mental status and no risk of aspiration
- Mild symptoms should resolve within 12 hours.
- Treatment of severe toxicity is primarily supportive: Atropine for excess secretions, wheezing, or bradycardia; treat hypotension with IV fluids and vasopressors if necessary; treat seizures with benzodiazepines.
- Criteria for hospitalization: Asymptomatic patients or those with only mild symptoms (vomiting) can be observed for several hours and then discharged home; patients with signs or symptoms of severe toxicity require admission to an intensive care unit for continuous monitoring and management.

OPIOIDS

Can be natural or synthetic; most commonly used to treat severe pain, can also be used as antitussive; opioid abuse can result from use of prescription medication or illegal street drugs.

TOXICOLOGY/PHARMACOLOGY

- Opioid effects result by the drug binding directly to opioid receptors in the CNS.
- Tolerance develops with chronic use, though miosis and constipation will still occur
- Buprenorphine is an opioid partial agonist with low potential for abuse that can also block the effect of full opioid agonists at high doses; prescribed for opioid addiction.
- Rising exploratory pediatric ingestions; increased toxicity in children

CLINICAL MANIFESTATIONS

- Classic triad of pinpoint pupils, coma, and respiratory depression
- GI: Decreased motility and increased sphincter tone can result in constipation; effects on biliary sphincter may cause right upper quadrant pain that mimics other biliary conditions.
- Cardiac: Hypotension; propoxyphene may cause arrhythmias.
- CNS: Lethargy, respiratory depression, coma, seizures (primarily with meperidine)
- Pulmonary: Pulmonary edema
- Diphenoxylate results in delayed onset of symptoms secondary to formulation that includes atropine.

DIAGNOSTICS

- Can be based on clinical findings
- Can perform urine or blood toxicologic screen, though methadone, fentanyl, and oxycodone may not be detected on routine drug screens
- Laboratory studies: Electrolytes, glucose, BUN, creatinine, blood gas
- Chest x-ray

MANAGEMENT

- Decontamination: Activated charcoal for oral ingestion; consider MDAC or WBI for "body stuffers."
- Supportive care: Provide adequate ventilation with bag-valve-mask ventilation; may need to intubate to maintain airway; treat hypotension, seizures, pulmonary edema if they occur.
- Naloxone is an opioid antagonist; it is available in IV, IM, and intranasal formulations
    - ✓ Dosing is dependent on risk of precipitated withdrawal (if chronic opioid use)
        - For patients taking opioids long term or those with suspected opioid abuse (mostly adolescents), dose is 0.04 mg IV; may repeat if no response after 2–3 minutes
        - For opioid-naive patients (mostly young children), can treat with higher doses because no concern for withdrawal. Start with 2 mg IV; may repeat if no response after 2–3 minutes.
    - ✓ May need to use repeat doses or an infusion to maintain response
    - ✓ May precipitate withdrawal in addicted patients; therefore, detoxification of an addicted patient is usually done with methadone.
- Criteria for hospitalization: In general, patients should be admitted for observation; length of observation is based on half-life of specific drug.

ORGANOPHOSPHATES

Insecticides; ingredient in chemical warfare agents

TOXICOLOGY/PHARMACOLOGY

- Toxicity is a result of inhibition of acetylcholinesterase; clinical findings are result of accumulation of acetylcholine at muscarinic, nicotinic, and CNS receptors
  - ✓ Enzyme inhibition can become irreversible with increasing time of exposure, a process known as "aging."
- Can be from inhalation, ingestion, or absorption from skin
- Rapid onset of symptoms after exposure
- Children and pregnant women are at increased risk of toxicity owing to lower baseline cholinesterase levels.
- Note that carbamate insecticides act similarly on acetylcholinesterase but do not cause irreversible inhibition ("aging").

CLINICAL MANIFESTATIONS

- CNS: Headache, agitation, seizures, coma
- Nicotinic: Weakness, fasciculations, increased heart rate and blood pressure; can result in death from respiratory muscle paralysis
- Muscarinic: Abdominal pain, vomiting, diarrhea, urinary and fecal incontinence, bronchospasm, bronchorrhea, bradycardia, hypotension, salivation, diaphoresis, miosis
- Can occasionally see a delayed, permanent, peripheral neuropathy

DIAGNOSTICS

- Diagnosis based on history of exposure and classic clinical presentation
- Not detected on urine toxicologic screens
- Can measure plasma pseudocholinesterase levels or red blood cell cholinesterase activity, but this is not very helpful unless baseline levels have been obtained
- Laboratory studies: Electrolytes, glucose, BUN, creatinine, liver function tests, blood gas
- ECG

MANAGEMENT

- Avoid contact with contaminated clothing, skin, or gastric aspirates.
- Decontamination: Contaminated clothing must be removed and discarded as toxic waste, skin should be cleaned with soap and water.
  - ✓ No ipecac; consider gastric lavage for recent ingestions; give activated charcoal
- Antidote: Atropine in doses of 0.05–0.1 mg/kg should be repeated until asymptomatic and lungs are clear; administer either IV or IM.
  - ✓ Pralidoxime (used in conjunction with atropine) is used specifically to treat muscle weakness and prevent "aging"—dose is 20–40 mg/kg either IV or IM; doses can be repeated every hour as needed until muscle weakness and other cholinergic signs and symptoms resolve.
- Avoid any concurrent therapy with drugs that affect acetylcholine uptake (i.e., phenothiazines).
- Criteria for hospitalization: Any patient requiring treatment

PHENOTHIAZINES (ANTIPSYCHOTICS)

Used for depression, psychosis, aggression, emotional instability, sleep disturbance, and acute management of agitation and delirium

TOXICOLOGY/PHARMACOLOGY

- Typical antipsychotics: Phenothiazines/butyrophenones—chlorpromazine, thioridazine, haloperidol, droperidol
  - ✓ Toxicity is due to effects on CNS, anticholinergic effects, alpha-adrenergic blocking effects.
  - ✓ Have variable antagonism at the D2 dopamine receptor, but cause nonspecific blockade throughout the brain, leading to side effects
  - ✓ Toxicity can be seen with therapeutic doses.
- Atypical antipsychotics (risperidone, clozapine, olanzapine, quetiapine)
  - ✓ Serotonin receptor antagonists or partial agonists in addition to dopamine receptor blockade
  - ✓ Lower risk of extrapyramidal side effects
  - ✓ Can bind with high affinity leading to long lasting adverse effects

CLINICAL MANIFESTATIONS

Typical antipsychotics

- Toxicity
  - ✓ Mild toxicity
    - CNS: Sedation, ataxia, slurred speech
    - Anticholinergic symptoms: constipation, urinary retention, dry mouth; orthostatic hypotension, tachycardia
  - ✓ Severe toxicity
  - ✓ CNS: Hypothermia or hyperthermia, coma, seizures, respiratory arrest
  - ✓ Cardiac: QRS or QT prolongation, dysrhythmias, hypotension
  - ✓ Extrapyramidal effects: Torticollis, rigidity, tremor, cogwheel rigidity
- Dystonic reactions: Can be seen regardless of amount ingested
- Neuroleptic malignant syndrome: Rigidity, hyperthermia, rhabdomyolysis, lactic acidosis

Atypical antipsychotics

- Mild toxicity: Sialorrhea (clozapine), orthostasis, sedation, metabolic and endocrinologic abnormalities, nausea and vomiting, urinary retention, sleep abnormalities, blurred vision
- Severe toxicity: Coma, respiratory depression, seizures, movement disorders, hypotension, myocardial depression, myocarditis, QT prolongation, hepatic toxicity, severe allergic reactions, delirium, agranulocytosis, neuroleptic malignant syndrome

DIAGNOSTICS

- Based on history of ingestion and symptoms
- Drug levels not generally available: Some cause a false positive tricyclic screen
- Laboratory studies: Electrolytes, BUN, creatinine, glucose, creatine phosphokinase, blood gas, liver function tests
- Abdominal x-ray: Pills can be radiopaque
- ECG to look for conduction delays

MANAGEMENT

- Decontamination: Activated charcoal, WBI for some sustained-release formulations. In specific cases, a lipid emulsion may be helpful in consultation with local poison control center.
- Supportive care: Treat dystonic reactions with either diphenhydramine (0.5–1.0 mg/kg IV or IM) or benztropine (0.02 mg/kg IV or IM for children >3 years of age)
  ✓ Be alert for other sequelae, such as arrhythmias (requires cardiac monitoring), seizures, and hypotension
- Neuroleptic malignant syndrome
  ✓ Ice-water immersion for severe hyperthermia
  ✓ Benzodiazepines for muscular rigidity
  ✓ Intubation and paralysis, if needed
  ✓ Dantrolene or bromocriptine for severe cases
- Criteria for hospitalization: Admit patients with signs of toxicity; observe asymptomatic ingestions for 6 hours.

PHENYTOIN (ANTICONVULSANT)

TOXICOLOGY/PHARMACOLOGY

- Phenytoin increases brain concentrations of gamma aminobutyric acid, reduces high-frequency neuronal firing, and affects cardiac conduction through class Ib antidysrhythmic effect (sodium channel blockade).
- Toxicity can be seen at doses of 20 mg/kg.
- Erratic oral absorption
- Drug is highly protein-bound, and toxicity can develop from decreased protein binding or displacement of drug by other drugs.
- With IV preparations, toxicity may be due to the diluent propylene glycol.

CLINICAL MANIFESTATIONS

- Cardiac: Can see tachycardia or bradycardia; hypotension (ventricular fibrillation and asystole can be seen with IV overdose)
- Neurologic: Ataxia, encephalopathy, tremor, agitation, nystagmus, confusion, hallucinations; seizures are rare (must rule out co-ingestion)
- GI: Nausea, vomiting, hepatitis
- Can also see hypersensitivity reactions
- Rapid IV administration can result in hypotension (due to propylene glycol) and arrhythmias

DIAGNOSTICS

- Diagnosis based on history of ingestion
- Obtain phenytoin concentration immediately (10–20 mg/L considered therapeutic); need to recheck due to possibility of delayed absorption
- Laboratory studies: Electrolytes, BUN, creatinine, glucose, albumin
- ECG if drug was given IV

MANAGEMENT

- Decontamination: Activated charcoal, may consider MDAC
- Supportive care: Treat hypotension, manage dysrhythmias (ACLS/PALS guidelines)
- Criteria for hospitalization: Cardiac or neurologic symptoms; unable to tolerate fluids due to severity of nausea and vomiting, fall risk due to ataxia

SALICYLATES (ASPIRIN)

OTC analgesics and cold medications; Pepto-Bismol (bismuth subsalicylate); liniments, oil of wintergreen (methyl salicylate)

TOXICOLOGY/PHARMACOLOGY

- Direct CNS stimulation of respiration resulting in respiratory alkalosis
- Uncouples oxidative phosphorylation and inhibits Krebs cycle, causing elevated anion-gap metabolic acidosis
- A unique mixed acid–base disorder ensues: Concomitant respiratory alkalosis and metabolic acidosis
  ✓ Young children are more likely to present with acidosis.
- 60% of cases of salicylism are from acute ingestion.
- Start to see toxicity at doses of 150 mg/kg.
- Elimination half-life can be as high as 36 hours in cases of overdose because of loss of first-order kinetics as drug concentrations increase.

CLINICAL MANIFESTATIONS

- Acute toxicity
  ✓ Mild symptoms: Vomiting, tinnitus, lethargy, tachypnea.
  ✓ Moderate symptoms: Agitation, diaphoresis, fever
  ✓ Severe symptoms: Seizures, coma, pulmonary edema; death results from CNS toxicity and inhibition of cardiorespiratory centers in the brain.
- Chronic toxicity: Symptoms can appear at much lower serum concentrations
- Can be nonspecific with only confusion or dehydration
- Can see metabolic acidosis and pulmonary and cerebral edema

DIAGNOSTICS

- Salicylate level: Therapeutic level is 15–30 mg/dL
  ✓ Mild toxicity (tinnitus) at levels of 30–40 mg/dL
  ✓ CNS depression at levels >80 mg/dL
  ✓ Severe toxicity at levels >100 mg/dL
- Chronic toxicity may manifest at lower levels.
- Obtain serial salicylate levels (every 2–4 hours) and blood gases until levels are falling into the nontoxic range.
- Other
  ✓ Electrolytes (repeat every 2 hours during alkalinization and then every 12 hours until acid–base disturbances resolve; early hyperglycemia followed by hypoglycemia and hypokalemia)
  ✓ Arterial or venous blood gas (combined respiratory alkalosis and anion gap metabolic acidosis)
  ✓ Liver function tests
  ✓ CBC, prothrombin time, and partial thromboplastin time (coagulopathy may occur)
  ✓ Urinalysis (every 2 hours; for pH and specific gravity; maintain urine pH of 7.5–8)
  ✓ ECG

MANAGEMENT

- Decontamination: Activated charcoal, may consider MDAC
- Treat fluid deficits (often profound) and electrolyte abnormalities

- Alkalinize to enhance salicylate excretion: Give 100–150 mEq sodium bicarbonate/L of 5% dextrose in water at 2× maintenance; goal serum pH 7.45–7.55; goal urine pH 7.5–8.0
- Maintain normal serum potassium (>4.0 mEq/L)
- Avoid intubation, if possible, to prevent worsening acidemia. If intubation needed, attempt to mimic the patient's own respiratory rate and tidal volume, as a decrease in minute ventilation can lead to worse neurologic outcomes and death.
- Hemodialysis should be considered for metabolic acidosis not easily reversed with alkalinization, CNS dysfunction impairing patient's ability to maintain hyperpnea, salicylate levels >100 mg/dL, renal failure, pulmonary edema, or deterioration despite therapy.
- Criteria for hospitalization: Admit all symptomatic patients; observe asymptomatic patients for at least 6 hours.

SELECTIVE SEROTONIN REUPTAKE INHIBITORS (SSRIS) AND SELECTIVE SEROTONIN–NOREPINEPHRINE REUPTAKE INHIBITORS (SNRIS)

Used to treat depression and obsessive–compulsive disorder and other behavioral disorders; examples include fluoxetine, paroxetine, and sertraline (SSRIs) and venlafaxine, duloxetine (SNRIs)

TOXICOLOGY/PHARMACOLOGY

- CNS depression
- Safer than tricyclic or monoamine oxidase inhibitor antidepressants; death from overdose uncommon
- Trazadone is a serotonin antagonist/reuptake inhibitor and can cause syndrome of inappropriate antidiuretic hormone and priapism

CLINICAL MANIFESTATIONS

- Neurologic: Confusion, sedation, coma
- Respiratory depression can occur, more likely after co-ingestion of other sedatives
- Cardiac: Usually mild, can get tachycardic and hypotensive or hypertensive; arrhythmias due to QT prolongation
- GI: Nausea, vomiting, and anorexia
- Serotonin syndrome: Can be seen after starting drug, switching drugs, increasing dose, or overdose; presents with rigidity, clonus, hyperreflexia, autonomic instability, alteration in mental status, restlessness, hyperthermia; may resemble neuroleptic malignant syndrome

DIAGNOSTICS

- Drug levels are not useful
- Laboratory studies: Electrolytes, glucose, creatine phosphokinase, urinalysis, blood gas, ECG

MANAGEMENT

- Decontamination: Activated charcoal
- Supportive care: Hydration; alkalinize urine if signs of rhabdomyolysis; manage seizures and rigidity with benzodiazepines; manage severe hyperthermia with ice-water immersion; may require neuromuscular paralysis and intubation if no improvement in rigidity with benzodiazepines
- In some reports, serotonin syndrome has been successfully treated with cyproheptadine, a serotonin receptor antagonist.

TRICYCLIC ANTIDEPRESSANTS

Used to treat depression, enuresis, neuropathic pain

TOXICOLOGY/PHARMACOLOGY

- Due to anticholinergic effects, peripheral alpha-blocking effects, and sodium-channel blockade causing ventricular conduction delay and myocardial depression, and inhibition of nor-epinephrine and serotonin reuptake
- Large volumes of distribution

CLINICAL MANIFESTATIONS

- Anticholinergic syndrome: Urinary retention, delayed gastric emptying, flushed and dry skin, delirium, dilated pupils, hyperthermia
- Extreme hyperthermia can result in rhabdomyolysis.
- Cardiac: Hypotension from peripheral vasodilation; sinus tachycardia; conduction abnormalities (prolongation of PR, QRS, or QT intervals); QRS interval >100 milliseconds is predictive of significant morbidity; various arrhythmias, including premature ventricular contractions, ventricular tachycardia, ventricular fibrillation
- Neurologic: Can range from lethargy to seizures to coma

DIAGNOSTICS

- Drug levels usually not helpful
- Most can be detected on urine screening
- Laboratory studies: Electrolytes, BUN, creatinine, glucose, blood gas, creatine phosphokinase, urinalysis
- ECG: Width of QRS interval >100 milliseconds is predictive of ventricular dysrhythmias and seizures.

MANAGEMENT

- Decontamination: Consider lavage, activated charcoal
- Sodium bicarbonate reverses cardiac sodium-channel blockade and narrows QRS complex by alkalinizing the blood (thereby trapping the drug in the circulation and not the myocardium) and overcoming channel blockade with sodium loading; 1–2 mEq/kg bolus dosing to narrow QRS, repeat as needed for wide complex. Consider infusion if repeated doses needed.
- Supportive care: Treat seizures with benzodiazepines. Norepinephrine can be used for persistent hypotension. Lidocaine can be used for persistent arrhythmias. Prevent hyperthermia. Consider ECMO for refractory poisoning.
- Physostigmine *should not* be given and will worsen cardiac toxicity.
- Criteria for hospitalization: Observe all patients for at least 6 hours. If any signs of toxicity, admit for 24 hours of observation.

DESIGNER DRUGS

Can refer to any synthetic form of a controlled substance

TOXICOLOGY/PHARMACOLOGY

Synthetic cannabinoids (see "Cannabis" section)

Synthetic stimulants

- Can be marketed as "bath salts" or "plant food."
- Derivatives of a stimulant called cathinone, a controlled substance
- Can be taken orally, intranasally, or intravenously
- Inhibit dopamine and norepinephrine reuptake
- Common effects include tachycardia and hypertension, agitation, diaphoresis, hyperthermia, psychosis, and hallucinations. Dysphoric reactions causing panic and anxiety have also been described.

DIAGNOSTICS

- Chemistry (synthetic cannabinoids have been reported to cause hypokalemia), ECG
- Drug screens may identify co-ingestions, and high-performance liquid chromatography/tandem mass spectrometry might identify more rare drugs but is rarely useful in the immediate setting,

MANAGEMENT

- Recognize that even designer drugs of the same name can have unreliable chemical compositions and can cause variable reactions,
- Management consists largely of supportive care and close cardiorespiratory monitoring. Patients may benefit from benzodiazepines for agitation and psychiatric symptoms,

FOREIGN BODY INGESTIONS

Button batteries, detergent pods, magnet toys, and expanding toys

- See page on foreign body ingestion at http://www.chop.edu/pathways.

TOXICOLOGY/PHARMACOLOGY

- Button batteries
  - ✓ Increased number of objects powered by button batteries (toys, remote controls, children's books with musical push buttons), with a resultant increase in ingestions
  - ✓ Injury occurs primarily from direct electrical current and caustic alkaline injury with liquefactive necrosis; heavy metal leaching and direct pressure can also be factors.
  - ✓ Increasing number of fatal cases in recent years, most of which are associated with 20 mm 3V lithium disk batteries
- Detergent pods
  - ✓ Agents thought to contribute to symptoms include propylene glycol, ethoxylated alcohols, and highly concentrated detergents.
- Magnet toys
  - ✓ Increasing incidence, as magnets are becoming more common in toys and household objects
- Expanding toys
  - ✓ Commonly balls made of superabsorbent polymers that expand when exposed to water
  - ✓ Generally attractive to toddlers because of their size and color; easy to swallow
  - ✓ Superabsorbent polymer technology more common now in household products and gardening supplies in addition to toys

CLINICAL MANIFESTATIONS

- Button battery ingestions
  - ✓ May be asymptomatic or may cause respiratory symptoms, pain, drooling, or dysphagia
- Detergent pods:
  - ✓ May cause drooling, coughing or gagging, respiratory distress, vomiting, and mental status changes, which may be profound
- Magnet toys
  - ✓ Number of magnets is important, as more than one may attract and cause intestinal obstruction, necrosis, and perforation
  - ✓ Magnet ingestions are often asymptomatic but may cause abdominal obstruction or fistulas.
- Expanding toys
  - ✓ Ingestion of expanding toys may also be initially asymptomatic but can rapidly cause symptoms of GI obstruction, including nausea and vomiting, abdominal distention, and pain.

DIAGNOSTICS

- Plain film of the chest and abdomen (does not rule out foreign body, as many are radiolucent)
- For detergent pods, a blood gas, electrolytes, BUN, creatinine, glucose, ECG, and CBC may be useful for further evaluation if there are mental status changes or concern for severe toxicity.

MANAGEMENT

- Supportive care, including close airway monitoring; in patients with worsening respiratory distress or mental status changes, securing the airway early might be indicated.
- Call for gastrointestinal and ear, nose, and throat consults for emergency removal of all button batteries located in the esophagus (serious injury can occur within 2 hours after ingestion).
  - ✓ For other proximal foreign bodies (esophageal and prepyloric) involve gastrointestinal and ear, nose, and throat to discuss removal. *Emergency* removal is necessary for multiple magnets or symptomatic patients and is highly recommended for expanding toys.
  - ✓ Admission criteria: Admit all patients requiring an acute intervention for proximal foreign bodies (as described above); also admit any other symptomatic patients for serial exams and monitoring to determine the need for possible intervention.

TABLE 1A	Suggested HR Cut Points Based on Average Predicated Value Within Each Age Group and Percentile						
Age group	1st	5th	10th	50th	90th	95th	99th
0–<3 mo	103	113	119	140	164	171	186
3–<6 mo	98	108	114	135	159	167	182
6–<9 mo	94	104	110	131	156	163	178
9–<12 mo	91	101	107	128	153	160	176
12–<18 mo	87	97	103	124	149	157	173
18–<24 mo	82	92	98	120	146	154	170
2–<3 years	77	87	93	115	142	150	167
3–<4 years	71	82	88	111	138	146	164
4–<6 years	66	77	83	106	134	142	161
6–<8 years	61	71	77	100	128	137	155
8–<12 years	56	66	72	94	120	129	147
12–<15 years	51	61	66	87	112	121	138
15–<18 years	48	57	62	82	107	115	132

Reproduced with permission from Bonafide CP, Brady PW, Keren R, et al. Development of heart and respiratory rate percentile curves for hospitalized children. *Pediatrics*. 2013;131(4):e1150-e1157.

TABLE 1B	Suggested RR Cut Points Based on Average Predicated Value Within Each Age Group and Percentile						
Age group	1st	5th	10th	50th	90th	95th	99th
0–<3 mo	22	27	30	41	56	62	76
3–<6 mo	21	25	28	38	52	58	71
6–<9 mo	20	23	26	35	49	54	67
9–<12 mo	19	22	24	33	46	51	63
12–<18 mo	18	21	23	31	43	48	60
18–<24 mo	16	20	21	29	40	45	57
2–<3 years	16	18	20	27	37	42	54
3–<4 years	15	18	19	25	35	40	52
4–<6 years	14	17	18	24	33	37	50
6–<8 years	13	16	17	23	31	35	46
8–<12 years	13	15	16	21	28	31	41
12–<15 years	11	13	15	19	25	28	35
15–<18 years	11	13	14	18	23	26	32

Reproduced with permission from Bonafide CP, Brady PW, Keren R, et al. Development of heart and respiratory rate percentile curves for hospitalized children. *Pediatrics*. 2013;131(4):e1150-e1157.

TABLE 1C		Range of Blood Pressure Values for Children of Average Height*	
Age		Blood Pressure Percentile[†]	Value or Range[‡]
Neonate (term)	Systolic	5th	63
		50th	78
		95th	92
	Diastolic	5th	30
		50th	45
		95th	60
1–5 years	Systolic	50th	85–95
		95th	103–112
	Diastolic	50th	37–53
		95th	56–72
6–10 years	Systolic	50th	96–102
		95th	114–119
	Diastolic	50th	55–61
		95th	74–80
11–18 years	Systolic	50th	104–118
		95th	121–136
	Diastolic	50th	61–67
		95th	80–87

*Please consult alternative sources such as the AAP 2017 Clinical Practice Guidelines for Screening and Management of High Blood Pressure in Children and Adolescents (https://pediatrics.aappublications.org/content/140/3/e20171904) for more precise classification of normal blood pressure, since the values vary slightly by sex, age, and height.

[†]Hypotension for children 1–10 years of age can be crudely estimated as a systolic blood pressure less than $70 + 2 \times$ Age in years.

[‡]By convention, the inflatable bladder width of an appropriately sized cuff covers at least 40% of the arm circumference at a point midway between the olecranon and the acromion (for more information, consult the American Heart Association or search their website at www.americanheart.org).

Data from National High Blood Pressure Education Program Working Group on High Blood Pressure in Children and Adolescents. The fourth report on the diagnosis, evaluation, and treatment of high blood pressure in children and adolescents. *Pediatrics.* 2004;114(2 Suppl 4th Report):555-576; Zubrow AB, Hulman S, Kushner H, et al. Determinants of blood pressure in infants admitted to neonatal intensive care units: a prospective multicenter study. Philadelphia Neonatal Blood Pressure Study Group. *J Perinatol.* 1995;15(6):470-479; Rusconi F, Castagneto M, Gagliardi L, et al. Reference values for respiratory rate in the first 3 years of life. *Pediatrics.* 1994;94(3):350-355.

Index

Note: Page numbers with an f and/or t indicate a figure or table on the designated page.

Index

Index